A Concise Dictionary of Novel Medical and General Hebrew Terminology from the Middle Ages

A Concise Dictionary of Novel Medical and General Hebrew Terminology from the Middle Ages

By

Gerrit Bos

BRILL

LEIDEN | BOSTON

Cover illustration: *A Cross Section of the Eye, identifying the membranes with the four humors*. Manuscript from Provence, c. 1400. Ms. Paris, BN, héb. 1181, fol. 265.

The Library of Congress Cataloging-in-Publication Data is available online at http://catalog.loc.gov
LC record available at http://lccn.loc.gov/2019942330

Typeface for the Latin, Greek, and Cyrillic scripts: "Brill". See and download: brill.com/brill-typeface.

ISBN 978-90-04-39865-8 (hardback)
ISBN 978-90-04-39866-5 (e-book)

This book is printed on acid-free paper and produced in a sustainable manner.

Contents

Abbreviations

NM 1 Gerrit Bos, *Novel Medical and General Hebrew Terminology from the 13th Century: Translations by Hillel Ben Samuel of Verona, Moses Ben Samuel Ibn Tibbon, Shem Tov Ben Isaac of Tortosa, Zeraḥyah Ben Isaac Ben She'altiel Ḥen*, Oxford 2011 (*Journal of Semitic Studies*, Suppl. 27).

NM 2 Gerrit Bos, *Novel Medical and General Hebrew Terminology from the 13th Century*, vol. 2, Oxford 2013 (*Journal of Semitic Studies*, Suppl. 30).

NM 3 Gerrit Bos, *Novel Medical and General Hebrew Terminology*, vol. 3: *Hippocrates'* Aphorisms *in the Hebrew Tradition*, Oxford 2016 (*Journal of Semitic Studies*, Suppl. 37).

NM 4 Gerrit Bos, *Novel Medical and General Hebrew Terminology from the 13th Century*, vol. 4, Leiden 2019.

Introduction

This dictionary has two major objectives:

1) to map the medical terminology featuring in medieval Hebrew medical works, especially those terms that do not appear in the current dictionaries at all or are inadequately[1] represented and thus to facilitate study of these medical works, and
2) to identify the medical terminology used by specific authors/translators and thus to enable the identification of anonymous medical material.

Unfortunately, the terminology in medieval Hebrew medical literature, both original works and translations, has been sorely neglected by modern research.[2] Moreover, medical terminology is virtually lacking in the standard dictionaries for the Hebrew language, such as *Ha-Millon he-ḥadash* composed by Abraham Even-Shoshan.[3] The only medieval medical work to which Even-Shoshan refers is the Hebrew translation of Ibn Sīnā's *K. al-Qānūn fī al-ṭibb* by Nathan ha-Me'ati;[4] and even those references are indirect, having been borrowed from the dictionary composed by Eliezer Ben-Yehuda. Ben-Yehuda's dictionary is indeed the only one containing a significant number of medical terms.[5] Unfortunately, Ben-Yehuda's use of the medieval medical texts listed in the dictionary's introduction is inconsistent at best. The only dictionary exclusively devoted to medical terms, both medieval and modern, is that by A.M. Masie, entitled *Dictionary of Medicine and Allied Sciences*.[6] However, like the dictionary by Ben-Yehuda, it only makes occasional use of the sources registered in the introduction and only rarely differentiates between the various medieval translators. Further, since Masie's work is alphabetized according to

1 By "inadequately," I mean that the dictionary in question quotes the term without a proper translation and/or definition of its (novel) meaning, or that the dictionary contains no witness for the usage in the period in question. The introduction to this volume is a revised version of the introduction to G. Bos, "Medical Terminology in the Hebrew Tradition: Shem Tov Ben Isaac, Sefer ha-Shimmush, book 30," *Journal of Semitic Studies* 55.1 (2010): 53–101, and of the introduction to NM 1: 1–8.

2 The following survey does not take into consideration the field of the medieval plant names and remedies, with the exception of some characteristic examples.

3 The edition I consulted is the renewed and updated edition in 5 vols., Jerusalem 2000.

4 Ibid., 1:16.

5 E. Ben-Yehuda, *Millon ha-Lashon ha-Ivrit: Thesaurus Totius Hebraitatis et Veteris et Recentioris*, 17 vols., 1910–59; repr., Tel Aviv 1948–59.

6 A.M. Masie, *Dictionary of Medicine and Allied Sciences: Latin-English-Hebrew*, ed. by S. Tchernichovsky, Jerusalem 1934.

 | DOI:10.1163/9789004398665_002

the Latin or English term, it cannot be consulted for Hebrew terms. The *Historical Dictionary of the Hebrew Language*, which is currently being created by the Academy of the Hebrew Language, has not been taken into account consistently as it is not a dictionary in the proper sense of the word;[7] moreover, consultation of this resource suggests that it is generally deficient in medieval medical terminology.[8] The Bar Ilan Responsa Project has also been excluded as a source despite the fact that it contains a larger number of medieval medical terms than the *Historical Dictionary*.

Apart from the comprehensive dictionaries, the secondary literature dealing with the subject of the medieval Hebrew medical terminology is extremely limited and generally addresses only a small number of medical terms.[9] An early study is Joseph Hyrtl's "Das Arabische und Hebräische in der Anatomie," which was published in 1879.[10] Although it was a pioneering work, it is of little use for scholars today for the following reasons: 1) it deals with very few terms; 2) most of these terms are derived from a single source, namely a printed edition of the Hebrew translation of Ibn Sīnā's *K. al-Qānūn fī al-ṭibb*, which was published in Naples in 1491–2;[11] 3) it does not identify particular translators. Thus, Hyrtl remarks that the term *almagabani* (fauces), i.e., larynx, was translated in the Hebrew Avicenna as לוֹעַ from לוּע (to devour). He fails to specify to which of the different translations of Avicenna he refers. Shortly after Hyrtl, David Kaufmann's monograph on the five senses, entitled *Die Sinne: Beiträge zur Geschichte der Physiologie und Psychologie im Mittelalter aus hebräischen und arabischen Quellen*, was published in Budapest 1884.[12] The work is admittedly very useful even today; however, the medical terminology he discusses is limited to that of the physiology of the five senses.

7 Cf. the definition of the term 'dictionary' in *The New Oxford Dictionary of English* (Oxford 1998), 512: "A book that lists the words of a language in alphabetical order and gives their meaning, or that gives the equivalent words in a different language."

8 Cf. Bos, "Medical Terminology in the Hebrew Tradition," 53–101.

9 The following survey does not pretend to be complete or exhaustive.

10 J. Hyrtl, *Das Arabische und Hebräische in der Anatomie*, Vienna 1879.

11 For the Hebrew translations of the *K. al-Qānūn fī al-ṭibb* by Nathan ha-Me'ati, Zeraḥyah ben Isaac ben She'altiel Ḥen, Joseph Lorki, and an anonymous translator, as well as the manuscripts of these translations, see C. Rabin, "Toledot Targum Sefer ha-Qanun le-Ivrit," *Melilah* 3–4 (1950): 132–46; B. Richler, "Manuscripts of Avicenna's *Kanon* in Hebrew Translation: A Revised and Up-to-Date List," *Koroth* 30.8 (1982): 145–68; L. Ferre, "Avicena Hebraico: La traducción del Canon de Medicina (The Hebrew Translation of Avicenna's Canon)," *Miscelánea de Estudios Árabes y Hebraicos* 52 (2003): 163–82.

12 It was published as part of the *Jahresbericht der Landes-Rabbinerschule in Budapest für das Schuljahr 1883–84*; repr. in: D. Kaufmann, *Die Spuren al-Baṭaljûsi's (Budapest 1880), and Studien über Salomon Ibn Gabirol (Budapest 1899), and Die Sinne (Budapest 1884)*, intr. by L. Jacobs, Farnborough 1972.

A more general study dealing with medieval medical terminology was undertaken by Hermann Kroner, a Rabbi practicing in Bopfingen, southern Germany, and published in 1921 under the title *Zur Terminologie der arabischen Medizin und zu ihrem zeitgenössischen hebräischen Ausdrucke*.[13] However, it discusses a relatively small number of terms since it is based primarily on the Hebrew translations of some of Maimonides' minor works, and only distinguishes between two translators, Zeraḥyah ben Isaac ben She'altiel Ḥen and Moses ben Samuel ibn Tibbon. It also suffers from a variety of errors, some resulting from the fact that Kroner only had access to corrupt manuscripts. Thus the term منهرم is translated as "Apathischer (Lässiger)"[14] and should be corrected into منهزم, meaning "defeated, vanquished." And ibid., تَسجيع ("Rhythmus (des Herzens) geben") should be read as تَشجيع, meaning "strengthening," which was translated by Ibn Tibbon as לתת גבורה.

In 1945, Asher Goldstein published an article entitled "Ha-Refu'ah we-ha-Lashon ha-Ivrit (Medicine and the Hebrew Language)," in which he discusses different ways in which novel medieval Hebrew medical terminology was created. However, he only considers a few terms. Moreover, he seems to have had a certain bias against the Arabic medical terminology as he denies the important role it played in the formation of the medieval medical terminology in general, as he states explicitly:

> I allow myself to remind [the reader] of my warning published in "Ha-Rofe ha-Ivri," I (1927), p. 18, about the danger of using the Arabic [for the innovation of Hebrew medical terms], for it does not have any scientific value in our days. And also in the Golden Age of the Arabic medical science, in the Middle Ages, when it left its mark on medicine worldwide, [Hebrew] authors, doctors and translators of Arabic medical works were careful not to use Arabic medical terms. Only a few medical terms in Arabic infiltrated the Hebrew language.[15]

Accordingly, when discussing the term חולי הפיל (elephantiasis) as it features in the *Sefer Ṣori ha-Guf* by Nathan ben Jo'el Falaquera,[16] Goldstein simply

13 H. Kroner, *Zur Terminologie der arabischen Medizin und zu ihrem zeitgenössischen hebräischen Ausdrucke: An der Hand dreier medizinischer Abhandlungen des Maimonides*, Berlin 1921.

14 Ibid., 55.

15 A. Goldstein, "Ha-Refu'ah we-ha-Lashon ha-Ivrit," *Harofé haivri: The Hebrew Medical Journal* 2 (1945): 95 (trans. from the Hebrew by G. Bos).

16 See G. Bos and R. Fontaine, "Medico-Philosophical Controversies in Nathan b. Jo'el Falaquera's *Sefer Ṣori ha-Guf*," *Jewish Quarterly Review* 90 (1999): 27–60.

states that it is a translation of Latin *elephantiasis*.[17] However, since the work is based on Arabic sources, it would have been more appropriate to suggest that it is a loan translation from the Arabic داء الفيل. Again, in an article entitled "Munaḥim refu'iyyim be-Ivrit mi-beḥinah historit (Medical Nomenclature in Hebrew from a Historical Point of View)," which was published in 1967, Goldstein's discussion of some medical terms, like hernia, duodenum, cirrhosis, and their Hebrew counterparts, is primarily based on the Hebrew translation of Ibn Sīnā's *K. al-Qānūn fī al-ṭibb* and some of Maimonides' medical writings, such as the *Sefer ha-Peraqim* (*Medical Aphorisms*).[18] However, he does not specify which of the Hebrew translations he used. For instance, when discussing the disease called "hemorrhagia" (i.e., bleeding), he mentions as Hebrew equivalents from Maimonides' writings and Ibn Sīnā's *K. al-Qānūn fī al-ṭibb*: שטף דם, תשפוכת דם, רעף דם, without providing sources.[19]

Following Goldstein, the research into medieval Hebrew medical terminology was generally limited to a study of the anatomical terms featuring in Vesalius' *Tabulae Anatomicae Sex*, which was published in 1538, and his *De Humani Corporis Fabrica Libri Septem*, commonly known as *Fabrica*, which was published in 1543. As Vesalius himself knew no Hebrew, the Hebrew (and Arabic) equivalents and their transliterations for the *Tabulae* hail from an anonymous friend; for the *Fabrica*, bk. 1: *On Osteology*, he consulted his friend Lazarus de Frigeis of Venice, who relied, in turn, on the Naples edition of Ibn Sīnā's *K. al-Qānūn fī al-ṭibb* mentioned above. However, the Hebrew terminology in the *Fabrica* edition of 1543 is very corrupt. De Frigeis' knowledge of Hebrew and Arabic may have been rudimentary; further, the transcriber and the typesetter, who were evidently unfamiliar with Hebrew, introduced many typographical errors.[20]

Mordecai Etziony studied the Hebrew material in two articles, published in 1945 and 1946. The first article deals with the Hebrew anatomical terminology featuring in Vesalius' *Tabulae*,[21] while the second article covers the Hebrew

17 Goldstein, "Ha-Refu'ah," 91, actually reads: אלשופנאטטיאזיס.

18 Id., "Munaḥim refu'iyyim be-Ivrit mi-beḥinah historit," *Koroth* 4.5–7 (1967): 452–62; 4.8–10 (1968): 625–36, and 4.11–2 (1968): 773–86.

19 Ibid., 459.

20 See A. Vesalius, *On the Fabric of the Human Body: An Annotated Translation of the 1543 and 1555 Editions of Andreas Vesalius' "De Humani Corporis Fabrica Libri Septem,"* ed. by D.H. Garrison and M.H. Hast, bk. 1, ch. 40, 166, esp. n. 5 (vesalius.northwestern.edu); see also: B.L. Gordon, "C. Singer and C. Rabin, *Prelude to Modern Science: Being a Discussion of the History Sources and Circumstances of the 'Tabulae Anatomicae Sex' of Vesalius*, Cambridge 1946" (Review), *Jewish Quarterly Review* 38.2 (1947), 201.

21 M. Etziony, "The Hebrew-Aramaic Element in Vesalius' *Tabulae Anatomicae Sex*: A Critical Analysis," *Bulletin of the History of Medicine* 18 (1945): 413–24.

terms featuring in the *Fabrica*.[22] The value of both articles lies primarily in their elucidation of the Hebrew terminology; the author does not analyse the medieval source(s), but refers to Rabbinic parallels on the basis of Marcus Jastrow's dictionary,[23] as in the case of the term שלבים (see below). In addition to Etziony, Charles Singer and C. Rabin studied the Hebrew material in Vesalius' *Tabulae* in their monograph entitled: *Prelude to Modern Science: Being a Discussion of the History Sources and Circumstances of the "Tabulae Anatomicae Sex" of Vesalius*, which was published in 1946 as well.[24] The authors trace the Semitic terminology in the *Tabulae* to contemporary oral usage in Arabic, Hebrew and Romance.[25] They state explicitly that this work was not influenced by the printed Hebrew Avicenna.[26] The study is valuable insofar, as the authors extensively discuss these Hebrew terms, compare them with the terminology in the *Fabrica* and that of the different medieval Hebrew translations of Ibn Sīnā's *K. al-Qānūn fī al-ṭibb*. Take for example, their discussion regarding the term זרוע:

> ZĔROAʿ is biblical, being mostly applied to the forearm. It is thus employed by Meathi and Lorci. The printed Hebrew edition of the Canon of Avicenna (1491), however, following Graciano (= Zeraḥyah Ḥen), used it for the upper arm. Doubtless on account of this confusion, Vesalius or Lazarus in the Fabrica give the phrase of the printed Hebrew Avicenna QĔNEH HA-ZEROAʿ = shaft of the upper arm.[27]

One more study was devoted to the Hebrew elements in Vesalius' *Fabrica* by Juan Jose Barcia Goyanes and published under the title "Los terminos osteologicos de la Fabrica y la evolucion del lenguaje anatomico Hebreo en la edad media" in 1982.[28] As the title indicates, the author, contrary to Etziony, dealt

22 Id., "The Hebrew-Aramaic Element in Vesalius: A Critical Analysis," *Bulletin of the History of Medicine* 20.1 (1946): 36–57.

23 M. Jastrow, *A Dictionary of the Targumim, the Talmud Bavli and Yerushalmi, and the Midrashic Literature*, 2 vols., 1903; repr. New York 1950. Cf. Etziony's statement in "The Hebrew-Aramaic Element," 38: "References are given only in the case of some Hebrew terms. The occurrence of those equivalents which are common use in old and modern Hebrew has not been traced to any particular place in literature. Practically all references quoted are those found in Jastrow."

24 C. Singer and C. Rabin, *Prelude to Modern Science: Being a Discussion of the History Sources and Circumstances of the "Tabulae Anatomicae Sex" of Vesalius*, Cambridge 1946, esp. lxxv–lxxxvi.

25 Ibid., lxxvii.

26 Ibid.

27 Ibid., 24, n. 131.

28 J.J. Barcia Goyanes, "Los terminos osteologicos de la Fabrica y la evolucion del lenguaje anatomico Hebreo en la edad media," *Sefarad* 42.2 (1982): 299–326.

with the origin of medieval Hebrew terminology featuring in the *Fabrica*, bk. 1. Thus he consulted the Hebrew translations of Ibn Sīnā's *K. al-Qānūn fī al-ṭibb* by Nathan ha-Me'ati, Zeraḥyah ben Isaac ben She'altiel Ḥen, and Joseph Lorki. The following comparative table illustrates the differences in approach by both scholars:

Goyanes	**Etziony** ***Fabrica* (ed. 1543), 166, l. 20**
Suturae ... שלבים scelauim: The proper transliteration is shlabim meaning mortised boards, steps of a ladder, plural of שלב shalv or shalav, of the root שלב, joint.[a] N (= Nathan): שלב and שלבים šalab̲, šělab̲îm. L (= Joseph Lorki): idem, Az.:[b] idem; Z (= Zeraḥyah): חוליה ḥulyâ, member, joint, vertebra. Av (= Avicenna) uses the terms درز and دروز, which are transliterated by Alpago[c] as adorem and feature in Vesalius as direzan, adorem. AH[d] has: šěleb̲, pl. šělab̲îm, pl. c. šilb̲ê. The term darz used by Avicenna is a translation of the Greek ῥοφή as used by Galen ...	Suturae ... שלבים scelauim: The proper transliteration is shlabim meaning mortised boards, steps of a ladder, plural of שלב shalv or shalav, the derivative of the root שלב join, fit in with mortise and tenon. Compare the synonym with מחוברים mechubarim, Tabula VI, 1. For שלב see Jastrow, Taanith Yerushalmi, IV 68.

a For this term, see the extensive discussion in Rabin, "Toledot Targum," 146.

b Az. is the abbreviation used by Goyanes to refer to Azriel ben Joseph of Gunzenhausen, who, with his father Joseph ben Jacob, printed the Hebrew edition of the *K. al-Qānūn fī al-ṭibb* (Naples 1491–2). However, this edition is, according to Richler, "Manuscripts of Avicenna's *Kanon*," 148, based on the translation of Nathan for bks. 2–5, while the edition of bk. 1 is based mainly on Lorki's translation, which is a revision of that by Nathan. Thus, Az. is nothing else but N. In an earlier comparative study, Rabin, "Toledot Targum," 137, came to the conclusion that this edition is mainly based on Nathan's translation, but that the editor sometimes prefers the version of Joseph Lorki or Zeraḥyah.

c I.e., Andrea Alpago (sixteenth century), who revised the Latin translation by Gerard of Cremona.

d AH: I.e., The Academy of the Hebrew Language.

In a second article entitled "Medieval Hebrew Anatomical Names: A Contribution to Their History," published in 1985,[29] Goyanes studied nineteen (mainly

29 J.J. Barcia Goyanes, "Medieval Hebrew Anatomical Names: A Contribution to Their History," *Koroth* 8.11–2 (1985): 192–202.

anatomical) terms in the previously mentioned translations of Ibn Sīnā's *K. al-Qānūn fī al-ṭibb*, and in Shem Tov ben Isaac's Hebrew translation of al-Rāzī's *K. al-Manṣūrī*.

The usefulness of the published studies is unfortunately limited because they discuss so few terms. Thus, they do not contribute significantly to our knowledge of medieval medical terminology and do not make it easier to read the pertinent texts. Moreover, none of them is devoted to the technical vocabulary or translation technique of a particular translator. These eclectic studies do not help the reader of medieval Hebrew medical literature solve the most common problem, namely, that many of the extant medical texts do not name their translator. To deal with this unsatisfactory situation and to facilitate the study of these texts I published several volumes with a considerable number of novel Hebrew medical terms based on a wide variety of medical texts and translations. The dictionary following below is based on these volumes.[30] Since research into this field is ongoing and constantly yielding more material, it is my intention to publish the dictionary not only as a printed volume, but also in the form of an online database to which new terms can be added.

30 I thank Felix Hedderich and Jessica Kley for helping me compile and arrange the terms from the following volumes: NM 1 = G. Bos, *Novel Medical and General Hebrew Terminology from the 13th Century: Translations by Hillel Ben Samuel of Verona, Moses Ben Samuel Ibn Tibbon, Shem Tov Ben Isaac of Tortosa, Zeraḥya Ben Isaac Ben She'altiel Ḥen*, Oxford 2011 (*Journal of Semitic Studies*, Suppl. 27); NM 2 = id., *Novel Medical and General Hebrew Terminology from the 13th Century*, vol. 2, Oxford 2013 (*Journal of Semitic Studies*, Suppl. 30); NM 3 = id., *Novel Medical and General Hebrew Terminology*, vol. 3: *Hippocrates'* Aphorisms *in the Hebrew Tradition*, Oxford 2016 (*Journal of Semitic Studies*, Suppl. 37); NM 4 = id., *Novel Medical and General Hebrew Terminology from the 13th Century*, vol. 4, Leiden 2019.

Sources and Structure of the Dictionary

The terms discussed in this dictionary hail from both dated and undated texts and translations.

The dated texts are the following:

(1) *Sefer Agur*: Do'eg ha-Edomi's translation (between 1197 and 1199) of a Latin version of Hippocrates' *Aphorisms*.[1]

(2) *Sefer Issur ha-Qevurah le-Galienus*: Judah ben Solomon al-Ḥarizi's translation (around 1200) of Pseudo-Galen's *Prohibition of Burial*.[2]

(3) *Sefer Keritut*: Hillel ben Samuel of Verona's translation (in the year 1254) of the *Cyrurgia Magna*, composed by Bruno Longobucco.[3]

(4) *Sefer ha-Shimmush*: Shem Tov ben Isaac of Tortosa's translation of the *K. al-taṣrīf li-man ʿağiza ʿan at-taʾlīf* (*The Arrangement of Medical Knowledge for One Who is Not Able to Compile a Book for Himself*), written by Abū l-Qāsim Khalaf ibn ʿAbbās al-Zahrāwī. Shem Tov started his translation in 1254 and completed it at an unknown date.[4]

(5) Hippocrates' *Aphorisms*, translated by Hillel ben Samuel (around 1260) and incorporated in the commentary by Moses Rieti.[5]

(6) *Sefer Almansur*: Translation of al-Rāzī's *K. al-Manṣūrī* by Shem Tov ben Isaac, which he completed in 1264.[6]

(7) *Pirqei Abuqraṭ*: Moses ben Samuel ben Judah ibn Tibbon's translation of Maimonides' *Commentary on Hippocrates' Aphorisms* (*Šarḥ fuṣūl Abūqrāṭ*), dated 1257 or 1267.[7]

(8) *Sefer Ṣedat ha-Derakhim*: Moses ibn Tibbon's translation (probably hailing from the year 1259) of Ibn al-Jazzār's *Zād al-musāfir wa-qūt al-ḥādir* (*Provisions for the Traveller and the Nourishment for the Sedentary*).[8]

(9) *Sefer ha-Peraqim*: Zeraḥyah ben Isaac ben She'altiel Ḥen's translation (dated 1277) of Maimonides' *K. al-fuṣūl fī al-ṭibb* (*Medical Aphorisms*).[9]

---

1 Cf. NM 3:3–6, 21–248.
2 Cf. NM 4:4–5, 11–224.
3 Cf. NM 1:9–46.
4 Cf. NM 1:73–120; 4:2–3, 11–224.
5 Cf. NM 3:6–7, 21–248.
6 Cf. NM 2:1–20.
7 Cf. NM 3:11–2, 21–248.
8 Cf. NM 1:47–72; 4:1–2, 11–224.
9 Cf. NM 1:121–95.

 | DOI:10.1163/9789004398665_003

(10) *Sefer ha-Qanun*: Nathan ha-Me'ati's translation (completed in 1279) of Ibn Sīnā's *K. al-Qānūn fī al-ṭibb*.[10]

(11) *Sefer ha-Peraqim*: Nathan ha-Me'ati's translation (ca. 1280) of Maimonides' *K. al-fuṣūl fī al-ṭibb* (*Medical Aphorisms*).[11]

(12) Hippocrates' *Aphorisms*: Nathan ha-Me'ati's translation (dated 1283) from the Arabic version (*Fuṣūl Abūqrāṭ*) incorporated in his translation of Galen's commentary.[12]

(13) *Pirqei Abuqraṭ*: Zeraḥyah Ḥen's translation of Hippocrates' *Aphorisms*, incorporated in his translation (ca. 1277–90) of Maimonides' commentary (*Šarḥ fuṣūl Abūqrāṭ*).[13]

(14) *Sefer ha-Qanun*: Zeraḥyah Ḥen's translation (ca. 1280) of Ibn Sīnā's *K. al-Qānūn fī al-ṭibb*.[14]

(15) *Hanhagat ha-Beri'ut le-Abu 'Ali ben Zuhr*: Jacob ben Machir ibn Tibbon's translation (end thirteenth century) of a *Regimen of Health* by Abū 'l-Alā' ibn Zuhr.[15]

(16) *Sefer Ro'a Mezeg Mitḥallef*: David ben Abraham Caslari's translation (ca. 1300) of Galen's *De inaequali intemperie* from a Latin vorlage.[16]

(17) *Shemot ha-Mashqim*: Estori ha-Parḥi's translation (completed at some time before 1306) of the *Tabula Antidotarii*, composed by Armengaud Blaise.[17]

(18) *Qibbuṣei Ma'amarei Galenus bi-Yemei ha-Buḥran*: Shimshon ben Shlomo's translation (in the year 1322) of an abridgement (in Arabic, Ḥunayn ibn Isḥāq's *K. ayyām al-buḥrān*) of Galen's *De diebus decretoriis* (*On Critical Days*).[18]

(19) *Pirqei Arnauṭ de Vilanova*: Arnau de Vilanova's *Medicationis Parabole*, translated into Hebrew (probably in 1388) by Abraham Avigdor of Arles.[19]

(20) *Sefer ha-Qanun*: Joseph ben Joshua Lorki's translation (ca. 1400) of Ibn Sīnā's *K. al-Qānūn fī al-ṭibb*.[20]

10 Cf. NM 4:3, 11–224.

11 Cf. NM 2:21–94.

12 Cf. NM 3:10, 21–248.

13 Cf. NM 3:12–3, 21–248.

14 Cf. NM 4:4, 11–224.

15 Cf. NM 4:5, 11–224.

16 Cf. NM 2:165–70.

17 Cf. NM 4:5, 11–224.

18 Cf. NM 2:171–3.

19 Cf. NM 4:6, 11–224.

20 Cf. NM 4:4, 11–224.

(21) Hippocrates' *Aphorisms*: Hebrew translation by Judah (Astruc) ben Samuel Shalom, included in his commentary (ca. 1450).[21]

Undated texts consulted:

(1) *On the Treatment of Small Children*, attributed to al-Rāzī: Translation (from a Latin vorlage, *De curis puerorum*) by Azariah ben Yosef ibn Abba Mari (also known as Bonfos (Bonafus) Bonfil Astruc).[22]

(2) *On the Treatment of Small Children*, attributed to al-Rāzī: Translation (from a Latin vorlage) by an anonymous author.[23]

(3) *Sammim Libbiyim*: Anonymous translation (from the Arabic) of Ibn Sīnā, *K. al-adwiya al-qalbiya* (*On Cardiacs*).[24]

(4) *Sefer ha-Refu'ot ha-Libbiyot*: Anonymous translation (from the Latin) of Ibn Sīnā, *K. al-adwiya al-qalbiya* (*On Cardiacs*).[25]

(5) *Pirqei Abuqraṭ*: Anonymous Hebrew translation incorporated in the translation of Maimonides' commentary (*Šarḥ fuṣūl Abūqrāṭ*).[26]

(6) *Sefer Hanhagat ha-Beri'ut* by Judah ben Jacob.[27]

(7) Hippocrates' *Aphorisms*: Hebrew translation by Joseph ben Solomon Delmedigo.[28]

Some of the terms featuring in the dictionary hail from anonymous medical glossaries, extant in the following manuscripts:

(1) Ms. Vatican, Biblioteca Apostolica, ebr. 361, fols. 176–81.[29]

(2) Ms. Oxford, Bodleian Library, Mich. Add. 22 (cat. Neubauer 2129), fols. (5^b)–(16^a).[30]

(3) Ms. Leiden, Universiteitsbibliotheek, Cod. Or. 4732/1 (SCAL 15), fols. 1^a–17^b.[31]

---

21 Cf. NM 3:7–9, 21–248.

22 Cf. NM 2:175–81.

23 Cf. ibid.

24 Cf. NM 4:6, 11–224.

25 Cf. ibid.

26 Cf. NM 3:13, 21–248.

27 Cf. NM 4:6, 11–224.

28 Cf. NM 3:14, 21–248.

29 Cf. NM 4:7, 11–224.

30 Cf. ibid.

31 Cf. ibid.

Each entry is generally structured as follows:

> ① אָבָה · ② **to pay attention:** ③ Arab. أَبِهَ · ④ Maimonides, *K. al-fuṣūl fī al-ṭibb* · ⑤ trans. Zeraḥyah Ḥen (*Sefer ha-Peraqim*), ⑥ 25.64: גליאנוס לא יאבה בשום דבר מזה ולא ידענו אבל הוא מכה לבד. → ⑦ NM 1:128.

① Hebrew term;
② English translation;
③ Arabic, Latin, and/or Greek equivalent;
④ title of original source;
⑤ Hebrew translator;
⑥ a quotation of the term in its Hebrew context;[32]
⑦ bibliographical reference.[33]

Entries of nouns featuring without a definite article may feature with a definite article in the quotations and vice versa, and entries of nouns featuring in singular can refer to nouns quoted in plural. Entries of verbs featuring in an active conjugation (Qal, Piʿel, Hifʿil) may appear in the corresponding passive conjugation (Nifʿal, Puʿal, Hofʿal) in the quotations, and entries of verbs featuring in a perfect conjugation can refer to verbs quoted as participles and infinitives. In a few entries, especially those derived from anonymous glossaries and original Hebrew texts, a reference to an Arabic, Latin, or Greek equivalent is missing. Regarding the translation into English: It should be noted that sometimes a singular Hebrew term has been translated as a plural one and vice versa in accord with the grammatical number of the term it has been translated from. The terms and quotations featuring in the dictionary are not always completely identical to those featuring in the different volumes of NM, as quotations have been harmonized and errors have been corrected; some of the errors found in NM 1–3 have been corrected and listed separately in NM 4.

32 Some terms are quoted for more than one source. In that case, the earliest occurrence is quoted first. In this way I hope to show the wider distribution of the term.

33 I.e., one of the NM 1–4 vols., in which the term in question is discussed extensively.

Dictionary

א

אָבָה · **to pay attention:** Arab. أبه · Maimonides, *K. al-fuṣūl fī al-ṭibb* · trans. Zeraḥyah Ḥen (*Sefer ha-Peraqim*), 25.64: גליאנוס לא יאבה בשום דבר מזה ולא ידענו אבל הוא מכה לבד. → NM 1:128.

אֶבֶן · **mineral:** *Anonymous Glossary*, Ms. Vatican, Biblioteca Apostolica, ebr. 361, fol. 181[b]: תותיאה היא טוטיאה והיא אבן דומה למרתק אבל היא יותר אדומה. → NM 4:11.

• **אבן הדם** · **hematite:** Arab. شاذنة · Maimonides, *K. al-fuṣūl fī al-ṭibb* · trans. Nathan ha-Me'ati (*Sefer ha-Peraqim*), 21.73: שאדנה הוא אבן הדם. → NM 2:27.

אַבְנֵט · **truss:** Lat. braccale · Bruno Longobucco, *Cyrurgia Magna* · trans. Hillel ben Samuel (*Sefer Keritut*), fol. 93[b]: ומונעין אותו שלא ירחב בתקון האבנט. → NM 1:16–7.

אבניי • עצם אבניי → עֶצֶם.

אבעבועה → אֲבַעְבֻּעָה.

אֲבַעְבֻּעָה • *Plur.* **אבעבועות** · **watery vesicles:** Arab. نفّاخات · Maimonides, *Šarḥ fuṣūl Abūqrāṭ* · trans. Zeraḥyah Ḥen (*Pirqei Abuqraṭ*), 7.55 (407): יתחדשו אלו האבעבועות מאד בכבד ומאמרו שמי שנתמלא בטנו מים ימות ברוב. → NM 3:21.

אָבָק · **powder:** Arab. سفوف / Lat. pulvis · Ibn al-Jazzār, *Zād al-musāfir wa-qūt al-ḥādir* · trans. Moses ibn Tibbon (*Sefer Ṣedat ha-Derakhim*), bk. 1, ch. 23: תאר אבק חברו יצחק לפלג והרפיון וכאיבי הפרקים והרעש ומותר העב. → NM 4:11.

• **אבק מקרר** · **cooling remedy:** Arab. برود · Ibn al-Jazzār, *Zād al-musāfir wa-qūt al-ḥādir* · trans. Moses ibn Tibbon (*Sefer Ṣedat ha-Derakhim*), bk. 2, ch. 2: תאר אבק מקרר חברו בן מאסויה יסיר הלובן וירפאהו. → NM 4:11.

אֵבֶר • **האבר המושל** · **the major organ:** Arab. العضو الرئيس · Al-Zahrāwī, *K. al-taṣrīf li-man ʿağiza ʿan at-taʾlīf* · trans. Shem Tov ben Isaac (*Sefer ha-Shimmush*), bk. 30, 2.40 (fol. 215[a]): ויהיה הצמח לפעמים קרוב מאבר מושל שהמאחר לדקרו וממתין עד שיתבשל יזיק לאותו האבר המושל. → NM 1:76.

• **אבר שיש לו מתרים רבים** · **a limb with many muscles:** Arab. عضو عضلي · Ibn al-Jazzār, *Zād al-musāfir wa-qūt al-ḥādir* · trans. Moses ibn Tibbon (*Sefer Ṣedat ha-Derakhim*), bk. 7, 25.10: ואם היה הרצוץ באבר שיש לו מתרים רבים או עצבים שים עם מה שספרתי מעט שמן איריאוש או שמן נרקיט ומעט יין ריחני. → NM 1:60.

• **האבר הקטן** · **(lit., small member); penis:** Judah ben Jacob, *Sefer Hanhagat ha-Beri'ut*, 8.1: והכליות מושכות המים הרעים אשר בדם ומתפרנסות ממעט האדמימות הנשאר בו ושולחות המותר אל כיס המים והוא מזומן לקבלו ולהוציאו לחוץ על פי האבר הקטן והוא השתן. → NM 4:12.

• *Plur.* **אברים** · **joints:** Lat. articulus, *Plur.* articuli · Hippocrates, *Aphorisms* · trans. Hillel ben Samuel, 4.45 (182) (fol. 25[b]): א"א: מי שיבא לו מורסא או כאב באברים אחר סור הקדחת מורה שאוכל מזון יותר ממה שהוא סובל. → NM 3:21.

• **האברים הישרים** · 1. **the noble members (organs):** Lat. membra nobilia · Armengaud Blaise, *Tabula Antidotarii* · trans. Estori ha-Parḥi (*Shemot ha-Mashqim*), 7 (35): משקה רושאד ורדים הפרח נודע קר בא' יבש בב' מטהר האדומה בהיות לחה. מטהר האדומה והדם מחזק הלב והאברים הישרים. → NM 4:11.

› II. **the spiritual members (organs):** Lat. membra spiritualia · Armengaud Blaise, *Tabula Antidotarii* · trans. Estori ha-Parḥi (*Shemot ha-Mashqim*), 2 (25): משקה אסיטוס מעט החמוץ ... משקיט הצמא מלחלח פותח מבשל האברים הישרים כמו שהוא בשלישית מהנהגות החדות. → NM 4:11.

• **האברים המגדלים** › **the nutritive members (organs):** Lat. membra nutritiva · Armengaud Blaise, *Tabula Antidotarii* · trans. Estori ha-Parḥi (*Shemot ha-Mashqim*), 33 (87): גיראופילאטום ... מועיל לרוע העכול וחולשתו ולסתום האברים המגדלים והרוחניים. → NM 4:12.

• **האיברים המיוחסים** › **the principal or noble organs:** Lat. membra principalia vel nobilia · Bruno Longobucco, *Cyrurgia Magna* · trans. Hillel ben Samuel (*Sefer Keritut*), fol. 40[b]: ובאמת הנגע הבא אל המעים או אל השלפוחית או אל האיברים המיוחסים לא יבריא לגמרי. → NM 1:17.

• **האיברים המעולים** › **the noble organs:** Arab. الأعضاء الشريفة · Maimonides, *K. al-fuṣūl fī al-ṭibb* · trans. Zeraḥyah Ḥen (*Sefer ha-Peraqim*), 3.79: מורסות האברים המעולים ממיתים. → NM 1:128.

• **האיברים הנפשיים** › **the spiritual members (organs):** Lat. membra spiritualia · Armengaud Blaise, *Tabula Antidotarii* · trans. Estori ha-Parḥi (*Shemot ha-Mashqim*), 62 (145): פאולינום: אם ינתן לעצור הגרת השעול אל האיברים הנפשיים יותכו ששה או ארבעה בבשול סוס נקי ופפאברי לבן (זנב). → NM 4:12.

• **האברים הפנימיים** › **viscera:** Lat. viscera / Arab. الأحشاء · Galen, *De inaequali intemperie* · trans. David Caslari (*Sefer Roʿa Mezeg Mitḥallef*), 3.3: והקבוצים המתחדשים באברים הפנימיים בקיעתם בגידים הדופקים והבלתי דופקים אשר בהם, או אצל הקרום אשר יקיפם אשר הוא להם במקום העור. → NM 2:165–6.

• **איברי הרוח** › **the spiritual members (organs):** Lat. membra spiritualia · Armengaud Blaise, *Tabula Antidotarii* · trans. Estori ha-Parḥi (*Shemot ha-Mashqim*), 20 (61): דיאה פינדיאון פניד ברקוח עשוי עם סוכר חם לח מועיל ליובש הריאה ולכל איברי הרוח. → NM 4:13.

• **האיברים הרוחיים** › **the spiritual members (organs):** Lat. membra spiritualia · Armengaud Blaise, *Tabula Antidotarii* · trans. Estori ha-Parḥi (*Shemot ha-Mashqim*), 6 (33): משקה ויאולד ויאוליש הפרח נודע קר בסוף הא׳ לח בראש הג׳ מלחלח [המעים] ומניע האדומה ישקיט ההתלהבות ובפרט מהכבד ואיברים הרוחיים. → NM 4:12–3.

• **האברים הרוחניים** › **the spiritual members (organs):** Lat. membra spiritualia · Armengaud Blaise, *Tabula Antidotarii* · trans. Estori ha-Parḥi (*Shemot ha-Mashqim*), 33 (87): גיראופילאטום ... מועיל לרוע העכול וחולשתו ולסתום האברים המגדלים והרוחניים. → NM 4:13.

• **רפיון האברים** → רִפְיוֹן.

• **תרדמת האברים** → תַּרְדֵּמָה.

אָבָשׁ › **apricot** [***Prunus armeniaca*** **L.**]: Arab. برقوق · Al-Zahrāwī, *K. al-taṣrīf li-man ʿağiza ʿan at-taʾlīf* · trans. Shem Tov ben Isaac (*Sefer ha-Shimmush*), bk. 27, fol. 138[a], col. b: האבש יש ממנו פג בלתי מבושל כל צרכו ויש ממנו מבושל כל צרכו קוסס. → NM 4:13.

אֲגֻדָּה • *Plur.* **אגודות** ‣ I. **buboes**: Arab. غدد · Al-Zahrāwī, *K. al-taṣrīf li-man ʿağiza ʿan at-taʾlīf* · trans. Shem Tov ben Isaac (*Sefer ha-Shimmush*), bk. 30, 2.36 (fol. 214[a]): לפעמים תקרנה בגרון אגודות דומות אל האגודות אשר תקרנה מחוץ. → NM 1:76; corr. 2:198.

‣ II. **callus**: Arab. تعقّد · Al-Zahrāwī, *K. al-taṣrīf li-man ʿağiza ʿan at-taʾlīf* · trans. Shem Tov ben Isaac (*Sefer ha-Shimmush*), bk. 30, 3.20 (fol. 236[b]): ברפואת האגודות המתהוות בעקבות קצת השברים. → NM 1:76.

‣ III. **cysts**: Arab. سلع · Al-Zahrāwī, *K. al-taṣrīf li-man ʿağiza ʿan at-taʾlīf* · trans. Shem Tov ben Isaac (*Sefer ha-Shimmush*), bk. 30, 2.41 (fol. 215[a]): יקרו בעור הראש צמחים קטנים והם ממיני האגודות יקיפום קרומות הם להם נאדות דומים לזפק התרנגולת. → NM 1:76.

‣ IV. **hoarseness**: Lat. branchus, *Plur.* branchi · Hippocrates, *Aphorisms* · trans. Hillel ben Samuel, 2.40 (92) (fol. 14[a]): האגודות והנזל בזקנים לא התבשלו. → NM 3:21.

‣ V. **nodules**: Arab. عقد · Al-Zahrāwī, *K. al-taṣrīf li-man ʿağiza ʿan at-taʾlīf* · trans. Shem Tov ben Isaac (*Sefer ha-Shimmush*), bk. 30, 2.27 (fol. 202[b]): בהוצאת האגודות אשר תקרנה בשפתים. → NM 1:76.

• **אגודות חבשר** ‣ **cysts**: Arab. سلع · Al-Zahrāwī, *K. al-taṣrīf li-man ʿağiza ʿan at-taʾlīf* · trans. Shem Tov ben Isaac (*Sefer ha-Shimmush*), bk. 30, 2.45 (fol. 216[a]): שער מ״ה בבקיעה על מיני אגודות הבשר. → NM 1:77.

אגודה → אֲגֻדָּה.

אֵד ‣ **bad breath**: Arab. بَخَر · Al-Rāzī, *K. al-Manṣūrī* · trans. Shem Tov ben Isaac (*Sefer Almansur*), Samekh 18 (60): יועיל מדפיקת הלב והאד סאדג ובלעז מלאבטרום. → NM 2:8–9.

אדום → אָדֹם.

אֲדִיּוּת ‣ **transudation**: Arab. رشح · Maimonides, *Šarḥ fuṣūl Abūqrāṭ* · trans. Anonymous (*Pirqei Abuqraṭ*), 7.54 (406): אמר המפרש: כבר נאמר כי זה הפרק אינו דברי אבוקרט ואמר ג׳אלינו׳ כי לא ימנע עבור אלו הליחות לעורקים באידיות כי הטבע מתעסק לדקק הליחות ולהוציאם בכל דרך שיוכל ואפילו מאחרי הקרומים כמו שידחה המוגלא המתקבצת במה שבין החזה והריאה. → NM 3:21

• **אידיות הדבש** ‣ **honeycomb**: Lat. favositas mellis · Al-Rāzī, attr., *On the Treatment of Small Children* · trans. Bonfos, ch. 1: ועשניות או אידיות הדבש הוא מין ממיני החולי הזה וימתיח על הנגע ותראה כמו קשקשים כי הוא מקשקש העור עם חכוך רב ומעט ממנו הוא כמו הדבש. → NM 2:176.

[אדם] • *Part. Piʿel* מְאַדֵּם • **הסם המאדם** → סַם.

אָדָם • **זיו האדם** → זִיו.

אָדֹם ‣ I. **erysipelas**: Arab. حمرة · Maimonides, *Šarḥ fuṣūl Abūqrāṭ* · trans. Anonymous (*Pirqei Abuqraṭ*), 5.43 (263): אמר אבוקרט: כשתתחדש באשה הרה המורסא הנקראת האדום ברחמה ודאי זה הוא מאותות מות. → NM 3:22.

‣ II. **livid**: Arab. كمد / Gr. πελιδνός · Maimonides, *Šarḥ fuṣūl Abūqrāṭ* · trans. Zeraḥyah Ḥen (*Pirqei Abuqraṭ*), 4.47 (184): אמר בקראט: בקדחת אשר לא תבדיל הרוק האדום והדומה לדם והמוסרח ואשר הוא מסוג המרירות כלם רעות. → NM 3:21–2.

• **אדומה** ‣ **choler (yellow bile)**: Lat. colera / Arab. صفراء · Galen, *De inaequali intem-*

perie · trans. David Caslari (*Sefer Ro'a Mezeg Mitḥallef*), 4.3: והאבר גם כן אשר בו המורסא או הוא קרוב לאברים אשר הם רבי הדם או רחוק מהם. ועוד, כי הדם שתגבר האדומ׳ או השחורה או הליחה או הרוח. → NM 2:166.

• צמח אדום → צֶמַח.

אֹדֶם · **blood-spot in the eye:** Arab. طرفة / Gr. ὑπόσφαγμα · Ibn al-Jazzār, *Zād al-musāfir wa-qūt al-ḥādir* · trans. Moses ibn Tibbon (*Sefer Ṣedat ha-Derakhim*), bk. 2, ch. 3 (fol. 43[b]): השער הג׳ באודם באשר באחת קצוות העין הנקרא בער׳ טרפא. → NM 4:13–4.

• **אודם הביצה** · **egg yolk:** Arab. صفرة البيض · Maimonides, *Šarḥ fuṣūl Abūqrāṭ* · trans. Zeraḥyah Ḥen (*Pirqei Abuqraṭ*), 2.3: המרה האדומה צבועה הרבה או בלתי צבועה הרבה וכן כשתתרבה בה החמימות עד שתשוב כאודם הביצה תתילד בעורקים ובגידים הדופקים. → NM 1:128.

אֲדַמְדֶּמֶת · **erysipelas:** Arab. حمرة · Maimonides, *Šarḥ fuṣūl Abūqrāṭ* · trans. Anonymous (*Pirqei Abuqraṭ*), 2.6 (58): אמר המפרש: ירצה בכאב בכאן סבת הכאב כמו אם יהיה בחולה מורסא חמה או אדמדמת או מכה או פצע או חבורה והדומה לזה ולא ירגישנו ודאי שכלו מעורבב. → NM 3:22.

אֲדַמְימוּת · **blood-spot in the eye:** Arab. طرفة / Gr. ὑπόσφαγμα · Ibn al-Jazzār, *Zād al-musāfir wa-qūt al-ḥādir* · trans. Moses ibn Tibbon (*Sefer Ṣedat ha-Derakhim*), bk. 2, ch. 3 (fol. 44[a]): ואם לא יקבל תועלת ברפואות האלו יקח מרישארמה וישים אותה בקדרה וישפוך עליה מים וירתיחם ואחר כן יקח חתיכה מבגד פשתן ויטבול אותה במים ההם וישימה על העין כי זה יסיר האדמימות ההוא. → NM 4:14.

אדרופיקי · **dropsy patients:** Lat. ydropici · Bruno Longobucco, *Cyrurgia Magna* · trans. Hillel ben Samuel (*Sefer Keritut*), fol. 32[b]: לכן כבדה רפואת האדרופיקי אשר לחותם עודפת והיא לחות זרה. → NM 1:43.

אודם → אֹדֶם.

אוזן → אֹזֶן.

אוטם → אֹטֶם.

אוֹיֵב · **harmful:** Lat. inimicus / Gr. πολέμιος · Hippocrates, *Aphorisms* · trans. Hillel ben Samuel, 5.18 (238) (fol. 32[a]): א״א: הקור אויב לעצמות ולעצבים ולשינים ולמוח ולחוט השדרה אבל החום מועיל ואוהב. → NM 3:22.

אומץ → אֹמֶץ.

אומר → אֹמֶר.

אופל → אֹפֶל.

אופן → אֹפֶן.

אוֹצֵר · **firm:** Arab. مكتنز / Gr. στερεός · Maimonides, *Šarḥ fuṣūl Abūqrāṭ* · trans. Moses ibn Tibbon (*Pirqei Abuqraṭ*), 5.52 (272): אמר אבקראט: כשיצא החלב משדי המעוברת יורה זה על חולשת העובר וכאשר יהיו אוצרים יורה זה על שהעובר יותר בריא. → NM 3:23.

אורובי • קמח אורובי → קֶמַח.

אוריטי · **aorta:** Arab. أوريطى · Ibn al-Jazzār, *Zād al-musāfir wa-qūt al-ḥādir* · trans. Moses ibn Tibbon (*Sefer Ṣedat ha-Derakhim*), bk. 1 (fol. 61[a]): אמנם החלק העולה משני חלקי האוריטי הנה הוא מתחלק לשני חלקים. → NM 4:14.

אורך → אֹרֶךְ.

אַזְהָרָה · I. **care:** a) Arab. توقّ · Maimonides, *K. al-fuṣūl fī al-ṭibb* · trans. Nathan ha-Me'ati (*Sefer ha-Peraqim*), 13.38: ראוי שתעשה האזהרה והכונה כפי האפשר בשאר מיני ההרקה ממי שיהיה ענין גופו שיהיה בשרו רך ורפה ואספוגי מהיר ההתכה. → NM 2:27.

b) Arab. وثيقة · Maimonides, *K. al-fuṣūl fī al-ṭibb* · trans. Nathan ha-Me'ati (*Sefer ha-Peraqim*), 15.12: כשתחתך אבר שכבר נתעפש או שכבר מת התחזק באזהרה ושמירה ועשה הרפואות אשר זכרתים אחר שתעיין בטבע מי שתרפאהו וטבע האבר. → NM 2:27–8.

· II. **caution:** Arab. حذر · Maimonides, *K. al-fuṣūl fī al-ṭibb* · trans. Nathan ha-Me'ati (*Sefer ha-Peraqim*), 12.14: וכשיתראו סמנים מרבוי הדם עם חוזק שלשת הכחות ר״ל הנפשיי והחיוני והטבעי אז תקרב להקיז מִבלי אזהרה. → NM 2:27.

אִזּוּן · **rhythm:** Arab. وزن · Maimonides, *K. al-fuṣūl fī al-ṭibb* · trans. Nathan ha-Me'ati (*Sefer ha-Peraqim*), 4.2: כוונת האזון הנזכר במיני הדפק הוא ההקש בין זמן ההתפשטות עם זמן המנוחה אשר אחריה. → NM 2:28.

אֹזֶן • **נקב האזן** → נֶקֶב.

• **פתיחת האזן** → פְּתִיחָה.

• **קצה העין מצד האזן** → קָצֶה.

• *Plur.* **אזנים** • **שרש האזנים** → שֹׁרֶשׁ.

אָח[1] • *Plur.* **אחים** • **דם שני האחים** → דָּם.

אָח[2] · **brazier:** Arab. كانون · Al-Zahrāwī, *K. al-taṣrīf li-man ʿağiza ʿan at-taʾlīf* · trans. Shem Tov ben Isaac (*Sefer ha-Shimmush*), bk. 27, fol. 125ᵃ, col. 1: הלחם האפוי באח הטמון בדשן רע מפני שנוי חלקיו כי חצונו נשרף כמו אש ותוכו בלתי מצטמק. → NM 4:14.

אֶחָד · **odd:** Arab. فرد / Gr. περισσός · Maimonides, *Šarḥ fuṣūl Abūqrāṭ* · trans. Zeraḥyah Ḥen (*Pirqei Abuqraṭ*), 4.61 (198): אמר בקראט: אם לא תהיה סר הקדחת מהמוקדח ביום מימי האחדים מטבעה לשוב. → NM 3:23.

אָחוֹר • **העצל המחזיר לאחור** → עָצָל.

• **הרתיע לאחור** → [רתע].

אֲחוֹרֵי • **העומק אשר בעליון אחורי הצואר** → עֹמֶק.

[אחז] • *Hitpaʿel* הִתְאַחֵז · **to settle:** Arab. تمكّن / Gr. στηρίζω · Maimonides, *Šarḥ fuṣūl Abūqrāṭ* · trans. Zeraḥyah Ḥen (*Pirqei Abuqraṭ*), 4.33 (170): אמר בקראט: ואם כמו כן הקדים והטריח אבר מן האיברים קודם שיחלה בעליו באותו האבר יתאחז החולי. → NM 3:23.

אַחֲרוֹן • **המעי האחרון** → מְעִי.

אַחֲרֵי • **אחרי צאת המאכל מן האצטומכא** · **on an empty stomach:** Arab. على الريق · Ibn al-Jazzār, *Zād al-musāfir wa-qūt al-ḥādir* · trans. Moses ibn Tibbon (*Sefer Ṣedat ha-Derakhim*), bk. 1, ch. 23 (fol. 36ᵃ): הלקיחה ממנו ד׳ שקלים במים חמים אחרי צאת המאכל מן האצטומכא. → NM 4:169.

אַחֲרִית · **after:** Arab. بعقب · Maimonides, *K. al-fuṣūl fī al-ṭibb* · trans. Nathan ha-Me'ati (*Sefer ha-Peraqim*), 13.6: ולכן בחרו אבקראט וגאלינוס כשך השעורים ומי השעורים ולהרגילם מאד נאה אצלם שיוקח ממנו דבר מועט שירחוץ אחרית הרפואה. → NM 2:28.

אֹטֶם · **blockage; obstruction:** Arab. انسداد / Lat. opilatio · Ibn al-Jazzār, *Zād al-musāfir* *wa-qūt al-ḥādir* · trans. Moses ibn Tibbon (*Sefer Ṣedat ha-Derakhim*), bk. 1, ch. 23 (fol. 33b): יסור תנועת הלשון ויתבטל הדבור אם מנפילת הכח המניע אותה אשר יבא מן המח ואם מפני סבה מאוטם או מורסא יקרה בעצב אשר ילך בו מן המח אל הלשון כח התנועה. → NM 4:14–5.

• *Plur.* **אטמים** · **obstructions**: Arab. سدد · Al-Rāzī, *K. al-Manṣūrī* · trans. Shem Tov ben Isaac (*Sefer Almansur*), Ṭet 2 (40): טין מכתום ובלע׳ בול שגלאטום וב״ח טיט חתום הארמי: טוב לרקיקת הדם ולשלשולו והנאכל ממנו יוליד אטמים בכבד וגורם הפסד מזג אלא שהוא מחזק פי האצטומכה ויסיר ממנה זוהמת המטעם המזוהם וישקיט אסטניסות וייטיב הנפש. → NM 2:9.

אַטְמָא (*Aram.*) • **בוקא דאטמא** → **בּוּקָא**.

איבר → **אֵבֶר**.

אידיות → **אֲדִיּוֹת**.

איכול → **אִכּוּל**.

אִילָן • **אילן מרים** · **cyclamen** [*Cyclamen europaeum* L.]: Arab. شجرة مريم · Maimonides, *K. al-fuṣūl fī al-ṭibb* · trans. Nathan ha-Me'ati (*Sefer ha-Peraqim*), 23.99: ואמנם הסם העב העצם נקרא פותח כי הוא פותח פיות העורקים מלמטה כגון השום והבצל ואילן מרים ומררת הפר. → NM 2:28.

• **אילן השועל** · **black nightshade** [*Solanum nigrum* L.]: Arab. عنب الثعلب / Lat. solatrum · Ibn al-Jazzār, *Zād al-musāfir wa-qūt al-ḥādir* · trans. Moses ibn Tibbon (*Sefer Ṣedat ha-Derakhim*), bk. 1, ch. 5 (fol. 11b): או יקח ממי אילן השועל הוא שולטרי שתים עשרה אוקיות ומירבולנש סיטרינש עשר אוקיות ויערבם עם מי אילן השועל. → NM 4:15.

אישרוב · **syrup**: Arab. شراب · Al-Zahrāwī, *K. al-taṣrīf li-man ʿağiza ʿan at-taʾlīf* · trans. Shem Tov ben Isaac (*Sefer ha-Shimmush*), bk. 27, fol. 142b, col. a: ויש שעושין מהם אישרוב להועיל מהשלשול. → NM 4:15.

• **אישרוב אסיטוש** · **oxymel**: Arab. سكنجبين · Al-Zahrāwī, *K. al-taṣrīf li-man ʿağiza ʿan at-taʾlīf* · trans. Shem Tov ben Isaac (*Sefer ha-Shimmush*), bk. 27, fol. 141a, col. b: והמתילדים בארצות חזקות הקרירות הם בהפך ממה שזכרתי שהם לא יוכלו להתבשל ותתגבר עליהם הקביצות ותקונם ודחיית נזקם לבעלי החמימות למהר תכף אכילתם למצוץ מן הרמונים הקוססים ולשתות מן האישרוב אסיטוש. → NM 4:15.

• **אישרוב ג׳לאבי** · **julep (rose water syrup)**: Arab. جلّاب · Al-Zahrāwī, *K. al-taṣrīf li-man ʿağiza ʿan at-taʾlīf* · trans. Shem Tov ben Isaac (*Sefer ha-Shimmush*), bk. 27, fol. 145a, col. b: ואם תתעורר אחריו חמימות וצמא חזק צריך לשתות עליו אישרוב ג׳לאבי או אישרוב אסיטוס במים קרים. → NM 4:15.

אִכּוּל · I. **canker**: Arab. أكلة · Maimonides, *K. al-fuṣūl fī al-ṭibb* · trans. Nathan ha-Me'ati (*Sefer ha-Peraqim*), 23.35: כל שחין שאינו עובר העור והם יתרחבו נקראם נמלה וכל שחין יעבר העור ויתרחב בבשר ובעור נקרא אכול. → NM 2:28–9.

· II. **corrosion**: a) Arab. أكل · Maimonides, *K. al-fuṣūl fī al-ṭibb* · trans. Zeraḥyah Ḥen (*Sefer ha-Peraqim*), 7.60: האיכול יתחדש מליחות נושכות והליחות הנושכות הם החריפות והחמוצות והמלוחות. → NM 1:128.

b) Arab. تأكّل · Maimonides, *K. al-fuṣūl fī al-ṭibb* · trans. Nathan ha-Me'ati (*Sefer

הליחות המחדשות הכאב באחד משׁשׁה פנים אם ברבוים אם בעבים *ha-Peraqim*), 7.19: אם בדבקותם אם בחומם אם בקורם אם בעקיצתם ואיכולם לאבר. → NM 2:28.

› III. **gangrene:** Arab. آكلة · Al-Zahrāwī, *K. al-taṣrīf li-man ʿağiza ʿan at-taʾlīf* · trans. Shem Tov ben Isaac (*Sefer ha-Shimmush*), bk. 30, 1.52 (fol. 208[a]): האיכול אמנם הוא הפסד מתפשט באבר ויאכלנו כאכילת האש העצים היבשים. → NM 1:77; corr. 2:198.

› IV. **irritation:** Arab. أكال · Al-Zahrāwī, *K. al-taṣrīf li-man ʿağiza ʿan at-taʾlīf* · trans. Shem Tov ben Isaac (*Sefer ha-Shimmush*), bk. 30, 2.96 (fol. 231[a]): ומהם מי שימצא חכוך בפניו ובמצחו וחשיכות ואיכול בעיניו. → NM 1:77; corr. 2:198.

• **אכול השנים** › **corrosion of the teeth (caries):** Arab. تأكّل الأسنان · Ibn al-Jazzār, *Zād al-musāfir wa-qūt al-ḥāḍir* · trans. Moses ibn Tibbon (*Sefer Ṣedat ha-Derakhim*), bk. 2, ch. 18 (fol. 59[a]): וכאשר יכאבו ויפסדו יחסר פעולתם ויראו בהם חליים מתחלפים ומהם חליים נראה אותם לעין כמו אכול השנים ונקובם ועפושם ותנועתם ולכלוכם אשר יהיה עליהם ומה שדומה לזה. → NM 4:15–6.

אכחל • **האכחל** › **the median vein:** Arab. الأكحل · Ibn Sīnā, *K. al-Qānūn fī al-ṭibb* · trans. Nathan ha-Me'ati (*Sefer ha-Qanun*), bk. 1 (fol. 66[a]): והרביעי והוא הגדול שבהם והוא אותו אשר יראה ויעלה וישתלח ענף מאסף עמו שריג מן הקיפאל ויתהוה ממנו האכחל ושאריתו הוא הבאסליק. → NM 4:16.

• **גיד הראש הנקרא אכחל** → **גִּיד**.

אֲכִילָה › **corrosion:** Arab. تأكّل · Maimonides, *K. al-fuṣūl fī al-ṭibb* · trans. Zeraḥyah Ḥen (*Sefer ha-Peraqim*), 16.7: יקרה לנשים החולי הנקרא הגרת דם בהנקות בזה הגוף כולו. וברוב יהיה זה לנשים אשר גופן יהיה לח ושמן. והדבר אשר יהיה מורק בהגרת הדם בקצת העתים הוא טרי אדום ולפעמים טרי מימיי או שיהיה נוטה אל הכרכומות. אבל אם ראית אותו כדם ההקזה תרגיש אם יוכל להיות מאכילה שתהיה בצואר הרחם. → NM 1:129.

• **המתון מן האכילה** → **מִתּוּן**.

[אכל] • *Part. Nifʿal* **נֶאֱכָל** › **being affected by caries:** Arab. متآكل · Ibn al-Jazzār, *Zād al-musāfir wa-qūt al-ḥāḍir* · trans. Moses ibn Tibbon (*Sefer Ṣedat ha-Derakhim*), bk. 2, ch. 19 (fol. 61[b]): ואם היה האיכול בשרשי השנים נקח עפץ בלתי נקוב וישחוק אותו ויולש בליציאום או בטרבנטינה או בקטרן ואחר כן יחבש בה השן הנאכלת. → NM 4:16.

• **הטיט הנאכל** → **טִיט**.

• *Part. Piʿel* **מְאַכֵּל** • **הסם המאכל** → **סַם**.

• *Part. Hitpaʿel* **מִתְאַכֵּל** › **corrosive:** Lat. corrosivus · Arnau de Vilanova, *Medicationis Parabole* · trans. Abraham Avigdor (*Pirqei Arnauṭ de Vilanova*), 5.96 (110): הנגעים המתאכלים אשר יתרחבו ויתפשטו אל העומק מעצמם ראוי לרפאם עם דברים קובצים ומיבשים בלתי עוקצים ואם יהיו ארסיים כמו חולי הזאב יצטרך שיהיו בזהריים. → NM 4:16.

אַלְיָה › **buttock:** Arab. ألية · Al-Zahrāwī, *K. al-taṣrīf li-man ʿağiza ʿan at-taʾlīf* · trans. Shem Tov ben Isaac (*Sefer ha-Shimmush*), bk. 30, 4.14 (fol. 235[b]): אך הדוקו ראוי להיותו על זה התאר והוא לכרוך על השבר במצנפת גסה שלש כריכות או ארבע ולהעדיף ממנה מותר ואחר כך לקפול השוק עד שוב העקב אצל שרש האליה. → NM 1:77.

אליל › **cartilage:** Arab. غضروف / Gr. χόνδρος · Maimonides, *Šarḥ fuṣūl Abūqrāṭ* · trans.

Moses ibn Tibbon (*Pirqei Abuqraṭ*), 6.19 (311): אמר אבקראט: כאשר נחתך עצם או אליל או עצב או המקום הדק מן הלחי או קצה הגיד לא יצמח ולא יתחבר. → NM 3:24.

אֲלַכְסוֹנִי · **diagonal; oblique**: Arab. مورّب · Ibn Sīnā, *K. al-Qānūn fī al-ṭibb* · trans. Nathan ha-Me'ati (*Sefer ha-Qanun*), bk. 1 (fol. 46[a]): ואיזה שנים מצד אחד שיכוונו יטה הראש אליהם נטיה בלתי אלכסונית. → NM 4:17.

אֲלַכְסוֹנִינַּה · **going in a diagonal, oblique line (diagonality; obliqueness)**: Arab. توريب · Ibn Sīnā, *K. al-Qānūn fī al-ṭibb* · trans. Nathan ha-Me'ati (*Sefer ha-Qanun*), bk. 1 (fol. 46[a]): וסגולתו שהוא מקיים נטיית הראש בעת התהפכו אל הענין הטבעי לאלכסוניותו. → NM 4:17.

[אלם] • *Inf. Nif'al* **הֵאָלֵם** • **האלם לשון החולה** · **stroke**: Hippocrates, *Aphorisms* · trans. Do'eg ha-Edomi (*Sefer Agur*), 2.42 (94) (fol. 45[a]): אמר אפוקרט: קשה הוא בחולי חזק בהאלם לשון החולה כי לא ישוב עוד לדבר אך בחולי קל. → NM 3:24–5.

אֶלֶף • **אלף עלים** · **poss., yarrow; milfoil** [*Achillea millefolium* L.]; **water milfoil** [*Myriophyllum spicatum* L.]: Gr. στρατιώτης ὁ χιλιόφυλλος; μυριόφυλλον · *Anonymous Glossary*, Ms. Oxford, Bodleian Library, Mich. Add. 22, fol. 6[b]. → NM 4:17.

אִלְפָּס • **הלחם האפוי באלפס** → לֶחֶם.

אֵם • **אם הדם** · **aneurism**: Arab. أمّ الدم · Maimonides, *K. al-fuṣūl fī al-ṭibb* · trans. Nathan ha-Me'ati (*Sefer ha-Peraqim*), 12.38: אך הקזת העורקים הדופקים סכנה גדולה כי לפעמים לא יפסק הדם או שיתחדש אֵם הדם. → NM 2:29.

• **חניקת האם** → חֲנִיקָה.

• **אם הילדים** · **mother of children** (a collective notion for a variety of female demons who in the Indian medico-magical tradition were believed to take possession of small children): Lat. mater puerorum · Al-Rāzī, attr., *On the Treatment of Small Children* · trans. Bonfos, ch. 7: מתעורה ופחד יקרה לילדים וימשך מזה החולי אשר נקרא אם הילדים וזה החולי אשר יקרה לילד בזמן היניקה ואותותיו שיבכה הנער ופחד גדול בשינה והיקיצה ויתוסף החום בם ויצא מפיהם ריח מוסרח. → NM 2:176; cf. BM 262.

• **אם הנערים** · **mother of children** (a collective notion for a variety of female demons who in the Indian medico-magical tradition were believed to take possession of small children): Lat. mater puerorum · Al-Rāzī, attr., *On the Treatment of Small Children* · trans. Anonymous, ch. 8: מחולי אשר יקרא אם הנערים יתחייב מחולי אחד הנקרא אם הנערים זה החולי יקרה לנערים בפרק הראשון מהשנים תמיד והאות שלו בכיית הנער תמיד פחד גדול בשינה וביקיצה ירבה החום ויצא מפיו ריח מסריח. → NM 2:176; cf. BM 262.

אַמָּה · I. **foreskin**: Lat. praeputium · Hippocrates, *Aphorisms* · trans. Hillel ben Samuel, 6.19 (311) (fol. 40[a]): א"א: אם יכרת העצם או התנוך או הדק מהלחיים או האמה לא ידבקו ולא יצמחו. → NM 3:25.

· II. **urethra**: a) Arab. إحليل / Gr. οὐρήθρα · Maimonides, *Šarḥ fuṣūl Abūqrāṭ* · trans. Moses ibn Tibbon (*Pirqei Abuqraṭ*), 4.82 (219): אמר אבקראט: מי שיצא באמתו מורסא הנה כאשר תתבשל ותפתח יתך חליו. → NM 3:25.

b) Galen, attr., *Prohibition of Burial* · trans. Judah al-Ḥarizi (*Sefer Issur ha-Qevurah le-Galienus*), par. 31: והמקום השלישי העורק בין צדי האמה והאמה כשיהודקו הדוק חזק ירגיש האדם כמו התלהבות האש ואם תראה זה הנה הוא חי. → NM 4:17.

• זקיפת האמה → זְקִיפָה.
• העצם שעל האמה → עֶצֶם.
• צדי האמה → צַד.
• קצה האמה → קָצֶה.
• ראש האמה → רֹאשׁ.
• *Plur.* **אמות** ‣ I. **elbows**: Gr. ἀγκών, *Plur.* ἀγκῶνες · Hippocrates, *Aphorisms* · trans. Joseph Delmedigo, 6.22 (314): הנזילות היורדות מהגב לאמות תתיר ההקזה. → NM 3:25.
‣ II. **forearms**: Gr. πῆχυς, *Plur.* πήχεις · Hippocrates, *Aphorisms* · trans. Joseph Delmedigo, 5.69 (289): הסימורים מתחילים בנשים על הרוב מהכסלים ובאים דרך הגב אל הראש ובגברים כמו כן על הרוב באחורי הגוף יותר מבפנים רצוני מהאמות ומהירכים ואמתות זה הוא ספוגיות שמראה השער. → NM 3:25.

אִמּוּן ‣ **administration; application**: Lat. administratio · Bruno Longobucco, *Cyrurgia Magna* · trans. Hillel ben Samuel (*Sefer Keritut*), fol. 38b: אימון הרפואות המצמיחות בשר שכתבנו בשער שעבר. → NM 1:17.

אֲמִיצָה ‣ **strengthening**: Arab. تقوية · Ibn Sīnā, *K. al-Qānūn fī al-ṭibb* · trans. Nathan ha-Me'ati (*Sefer ha-Qanun*), bk. 1 (fol. 55b): ואותה שהיא במקרה הוא חוזק הבשר ואמיצת הגוף. → NM 4:17.

אֲמִיצוּת • **אמיצות המעים** ‣ **constipation**: Arab. حبس البطن · Al-Zahrāwī, *K. al-taṣrīf li-man ʿağiza ʿan at-taʾlīf* · trans. Shem Tov ben Isaac (*Sefer ha-Shimmush*), bk. 27, fol. 124a, col. 1: ומי שנזרקו עליו מים מלוחים עד שתסור ממנו רוב לחותו הנותרת בו הבלתי מבושלת יהיה מזונו פחות ממזון המהובהב ויהיה דקותו יותר וימעטו רוחותיו ויסור ממנו העפוש ויתחזק על אמיצות המעים ועכולו יהיה קשה. → NM 4:18.

[אמן] • *Part. Nifʿal* **נֶאֱמָן** ‣ **chronic**: Judah ben Jacob, *Sefer Hanhagat ha-Beriʾut*, 10.1: ומוליד עליו חלאים רבים רעים ונאמנים. → NM 4:110.
• *Piʿel* **אִמֵּן** ‣ **to administer; to apply**: Lat. administratio · Bruno Longobucco, *Cyrurgia Magna* · trans. Hillel ben Samuel (*Sefer Keritut*), fol. 22b: אם כן הוא כמו שאמרנו שאם חזז הארר יהיה יבש צריך שתאמן בו הרפואה המיבשת. → NM 1:17.

[אמץ] • *Piʿel* **אִמֵּץ** • **אימץ המעים** ‣ **to cause constipation**: Arab. عقل البطن · Al-Rāzī, *K. al-Manṣūrī* · trans. Shem Tov ben Isaac (*Sefer Almansur*), Alef 13 (16): אקאקיא: קר יבש מפסיק הדם ישיב בליטת פי הטבעת ויאמץ המעים. → NM 2:9.

אֹמֶץ • **אומץ המעים** ‣ **constipation**: Arab. اعتقال الطبع · Al-Zahrāwī, *K. al-taṣrīf li-man ʿağiza ʿan at-taʾlīf* · trans. Shem Tov ben Isaac (*Sefer ha-Shimmush*), bk. 30, 2.81 (fol. 223b): והפלחים יקרו הרבה מצד נגוב הצואה ואומץ המעים. → NM 1:77.

אֶמְצַע • **אמצע החזה** ‣ I. **jugular fossa**: Arab. لبّة / Gr. σφαγή / Lat. fossa iugularis · Ibn Sīnā, *K. al-Qānūn fī al-ṭibb* · trans. Joseph Lorki (*Sefer ha-Qanun*), bk. 1 (fol. 18a): אמנם החלק העולה מחלקי אוריטי יחלק לשני חלקים היותר גדול שבהם אוחז למעלה כנגד אמצע החזה. → NM 4:18.
‣ II. **sternum**: Arab. قصّ · Ibn Sīnā, *K. al-Qānūn fī al-ṭibb* · trans. Nathan ha-Me'ati (*Sefer ha-Qanun*), bk. 1 (fol. 36b): אמצע החזה מחובר מעצמות שבעה ולא נבראו עצם אחד כמו שנודע בשאר המקומות מן התועלת. → NM 4:18.

• צלעות אמצע החזה → צֵלָע.

אֶמְצָעִי · **moderate:** Lat. mediocris / Gr. μέτριος · Hippocrates, *Aphorisms* · trans. Judah Shalom, 5.25 (245) (fol. 81[a]): אותם המורסות אשר בפרקים והכאבים אשר הם בלי נגע וכאבי הנקראס ובעלי הקווץ רבים מאלו משקיט וממעט שפיכת מים רבים קרים ומתיך הכאבים כי ההרדמה האמצעית משקטת הכאב. → NM 3:26.

• הגיד האמצעי → גִּיד.

אָמַר • **אמר ב-** · **to profess:** Arab. قال ب · Maimonides, *K. al-fuṣūl fī al-ṭibb* · trans. Nathan ha-Me'ati (*Sefer ha-Peraqim*), 25.64: ואמנם כפי סברת מי שיאמר בקדמות העולם הנה כל אלו האפשריים לפי דעתנו הם לפי דעתו מהנמנעות. → NM 2:29.

אֹמֶר • **גוזר אומר** → גָּזַר.

[אנש] • *Hif'il* **הֶאֱנִישׁ** · I. **to cause pain:** Arab. آلم · Maimonides, *K. al-fuṣūl fī al-ṭibb* · trans. Nathan ha-Me'ati (*Sefer ha-Peraqim*), 15.16: מה שיהיה מן האברים מרגיש ראוי לך שתרפאהו רפואה רחוקה בתכלית מהכאיב ומהאניש. → NM 2:29.

· II. **to cause severe pain:** Arab. برّح · Maimonides, *K. al-fuṣūl fī al-ṭibb* · trans. Nathan ha-Me'ati (*Sefer ha-Peraqim*), 8.38: הרפואות המשקיטות הכאבים והם אותם אשר יעורב בהם המרדימים החוש והמישנים אין ראוי שיוקחו אלא במקום שהכאבים הם חזקים וקשים המאנישים. → NM 2:29.

אִסְטוֹמְכָא (*Aram.*) → אִצְטוֹמְכָא.

אִסְטְנִיסוּת (also: אִצְטְנִיסוּת; אִסְתְּנִיסוּת) · I. **nausea; sickness in the stomach; urge to vomit:** a) Arab. غثيان · i. Al-Zahrāwī, *K. al-taṣrīf li-man 'ağiza 'an at-ta'līf* · trans. Shem Tov ben Isaac (*Sefer ha-Shimmush*), bk. 27, fol. 142[a], col. b: ופעולתם על דרך הסם שהם מפסיקים האסתניסות והקיא ומועילים אל המעי הצם ומוציאים התולעים הגדולים והקטנים מבטן המרבה באכילתם. → NM 4:19.

· ii. Maimonides, *K. al-fuṣūl fī al-ṭibb* · trans. Nathan ha-Me'ati (*Sefer ha-Peraqim*), 13.54: זכר אלתמימי בספר מרשד שהבצל אם יפולח ויורח בעת שתות הרפואה המשלשלת יבטל האסטניסות וימנע קיא הרפואה בסגולה שיש בה. → NM 2:30.

b) Arab. قيء · Al-Rāzī, *K. al-Manṣūrī* · trans. Shem Tov ben Isaac (*Sefer Almansur*), Qof 5 (70): קאקלא ובלעז קרדמומי: חמה מחממת האצטומכא ומשקטת האצטניסות. → NM 2:10.

· II. **want of appetite:** Lat. fastidium / Gr. ἀποσιτία · Hippocrates, *Aphorisms* · trans. Hillel ben Samuel, 4.17 (154) (fol. 20[b]): מי שיש לו קדחת ויש לו אסטניסות ועקיצה בלב ואופל העינים ומרירות בפה מורה שצריך אליו שינקהו מלמעלה. → NM 3:26.

• גרם אסטניסות → גֶּרֶם.

• עורר אסטנסות → [עור].

אסטנסות → אִסְטְנִיסוּת.

אסיטוש • **אישרוב אסיטוש** → אישרוב.

אסילם • **האסילם** · **the vena salvatella:** Arab. الأسيلم · Ibn Sīnā, *K. al-Qānūn fī al-ṭibb* · trans. Nathan ha-Me'ati (*Sefer ha-Qanun*), bk. 1 (fol. 66[a]): והולך ענף שני ממנו והוא האסילם ומתפרד במה שבין האמה והקמיצה. → NM 4:18.

אספוגות · looseness; porousness; rarefaction: Arab. تخلخل · Maimonides, *K. al-fuṣūl fī al-ṭibb* · trans. Zeraḥyah Ḥen (*Sefer ha-Peraqim*), 3.99: בהתקבץ דקות הליחה ואספוגות האבר וחמימות האויר הסובב וכח הרפואה הנעשית וחוזק כח החולה אז תתיר המורסה במהרה ואפשר שתתיר פתאם. → NM 1:129–30; corr. 4:229.

אספידבאג׳ה · white stew: Arab. إسفيدباجة · Al-Zahrāwī, *K. al-taṣrīf li-man ʿağiza ʿan at-taʾlīf* · trans. Shem Tov ben Isaac (*Sefer ha-Shimmush*), bk. 27, fol. 148ᵃ, col. a: ותקונם לבשלם אספידבאג׳ה פשוטה וכל שכן השחורים מהם. → NM 4:18–9.

אִסְפְּלָנִית · plaster; salve: Arab. مرهم · Ibn al-Jazzār, *Zād al-musāfir wa-qūt al-ḥāḍir* · trans. Moses ibn Tibbon (*Sefer Ṣedat ha-Derakhim*), bk. 1 (Ms. Oxford, Bodleian Library, Poc. 353, Uri Heb. 314, fol. 10ᵇ): יתקן מהם אספלנית בדונג ויעשה בו. → NM 4:19.

אספרגוס • **תבשיל האספרגוס** → **תַּבְשִׁיל**.

אֱסָר (also: **אִסָּר**) · ligament: Arab. رباط · Al-Zahrāwī, *K. al-taṣrīf li-man ʿağiza ʿan at-taʾlīf* · trans. Shem Tov ben Isaac (*Sefer ha-Shimmush*), bk. 30, 2.88 (fol. 226ᵇ): כשנתחדש צמח במקצת האיברין הבשריים וארך זמנו עד שקבץ מוגלא ואחר נתבקע או שדקרוהו ויצא כל מה שהיה בו מן המוגלא ונשאר המקום ריקן ככיס והעור אשר עליו כבגד שכבר נתדקדק ולא הגיע אל ההפסד לגמרי לעשות רושם בעצם ולא בעצב ולא באסר. → NM 1:77–8; corr. 4:229.

אסתניסות → **אִסְטְנִיסוּת**.

אַף • **הגרת הדם מהאף** → **הַגָּרָה**.

• **הקטיר האף בדבר** → [קטר].

• **מסננת האף** → **מְסַנֶּנֶת**.

• **נזלת האף** → **נַזֶּלֶת**.

אָפָה • *Pass. Part.* **אָפוּי** • **הלחם האפוי באלפס** → **לֶחֶם**.

אָפוּי (*Pass. Part.*) → **אָפָה**.

אֲפִיסָה • **אפיסת הדעת** · madness: Hippocrates, *Aphorisms* · trans. Do'eg ha-Edomi (*Sefer Agur*), 3.20 (126) (fol. 54ᵇ): ספור המדוים אשר יחולו בזמן האביב והם תחלואי הקדחת והדם והאדומה והשחורה גם אפיסת הדעת סתימת הגידים והחולי הנופל וזיבת הדם ונזלת האף שעול ואפיסת הקול. → NM 3:27.

• **אפיסת הלב** · cardialgia: Hippocrates, *Aphorisms* · trans. Do'eg ha-Edomi (*Sefer Agur*), 4.65 (202) (fol. 75ᵃ): דמה לעלות שלהבת בקרב העליון ואפיסת הלב עם קדחת אות רע הוא. → NM 3:27.

• **אפיסת המים הרעים** · dropsy: Hippocrates, *Aphorisms* · trans. Do'eg ha-Edomi (*Sefer Agur*), 3.22 (128) (fol. 55ᵇ): אמר אפוקרט: פגרי החורף להביא על הגופים קצת המדוים אשר באו עליו בימי הקייץ פרצת קדחת רביעית נפח טחול אפיסת המים הרעים החולי היבש יציאת השתן במכאוב הזלת הבטן והדם וכאב הירכים פוקות מיני השעול וכאב המעי הגדול והחולי המפיל רעת הליחה השחורה וכאב הגרון. → NM 3:28.

• **אפיסת המראה** · dimsightedness: Hippocrates, *Aphorisms* · trans. Do'eg ha-Edomi (*Sefer Agur*), 3.31 (137) (fol. 58ᵇ): קול נמוך אפיסת המראה וכובד השמע. → NM 3:28.

• **אפיסת הקול** · hoarseness: Hippocrates, *Aphorisms* · trans. Do'eg ha-Edomi (*Sefer Agur*), 3.20 (126) (fol. 54ᵇ): ספור המדוים אשר יחולו בזמן האביב והם תחלואי הקדחת והדם והאדומה והשחורה גם אפיסת הדעת סתימת הגידים והחולי הנופל וזיבת הדם ונזלת האף שעול ואפיסת הקול. → NM 3:28–9.

אֹפֶל › I. **dullness [of sight]**: Arab. ظلمة / Gr. ἀμαύρωσις / Lat. continua tenebrositas oculorum · Ibn al-Jazzār, *Zād al-musāfir wa-qūt al-ḥāḍir* · trans. Moses ibn Tibbon (*Sefer Ṣedat ha-Derakhim*), bk. 2, ch. 6 (fol. 45[b]): השער הו׳ באופל אשר יתחדש בעין. פעמים יחלש הראות מפני שנוי מזג העין או מפני עשן יעלה אליה מן האצטומכא. → NM 4:20.

› II. **eclipse**: Arab. كسوف · Maimonides, *K. al-fuṣūl fī al-ṭibb* · trans. Zeraḥyah Ḥen (*Sefer ha-Peraqim*), 24.1: ספר כאבי הנשים לאבקראט הוציאו חונין וביארו גליאנוס ונמצא תוספת באותו הספר הוציאו זולתי חונין וביארו זולתי גליאנוס ונמצא באותו התוספת עניינים זרים מהם שאמר שפוריפירויס אמר שהיה לשמש בסקליאה אופל גדול ובאותה השנה קרה שהנשים ילדו בנים משונים בצורתם בעלי שני ראשים ושקצת הנשים קרה להם שרואות דם וסתן מפיהן בקיא. → NM 1:130.

• **אופל העינים** › **dizziness**: Lat. tenebrositas oculorum / Gr. σκοτόδινος · Hippocrates, *Aphorisms* · trans. Hillel ben Samuel, 4.17 (154) (fol. 21[b]): א״א: מי שיש לו קדחת ויש לו אסטניסות ועקיצה בלב ואופל העינים ומרירות בפה מורה שצריך אליו שינקהו מלמעלה. → NM 3:29.

אֹפֶן • **אופן העצירה** › **the mode of binding (tightly)**: Lat. modus stringendi · Bruno Longobucco, *Cyrurgia Magna* · trans. Hillel ben Samuel (*Sefer Keritut*), fol. 57[a]: אחר כן כשתקל המורסא עצור השבר כמו שאמרנו ואופן העצירה הוא כמו שאמרנו. → NM 1:35.

אפר › **ophthalmia**: Arab. رمد · Al-Rāzī, *K. al-Manṣūrī* · trans. Shem Tov ben Isaac (*Sefer Almansur*), Alef 17: אנזרות: טוב לצואת העין והאפר והחבורות הטריות. → NM 2:10.

• **אפר העינים** › **ophthalmia**: Arab. رمد · Al-Zahrāwī, *K. al-taṣrīf li-man ʿaǧiza ʿan at-taʾlīf* · trans. Shem Tov ben Isaac (*Sefer ha-Shimmush*), bk. 30, 2.95 (fol. 228[b]): והשני ורידין אשר בשתי הרקות תועלת הקזתם לכאב הצלחתא הישנה והכאב הקשה ואל אפר העינים המתמיד והגרת המותרות הנשפכות החדות אל העינים. → NM 1:78.

אֵפֶר • **מי האפר** → מַיִם.

אֶפְרוֹחַ • *Plur.* **אפרוחים** • **אפרוחי הדבורים** › **young bees**: Arab. فراخ النحل · Al-Zahrāwī, *K. al-taṣrīf li-man ʿaǧiza ʿan at-taʾlīf* · trans. Shem Tov ben Isaac (*Sefer ha-Shimmush*), bk. 27, fol. 133[a], col. a: והדבש החדש אשר יהיה מאפרוחי הדבורים הוא יותר רטוב וחומו יותר מועט. → NM 4:20.

אֶפְשָׁר › **almost; to be near to; to tend to**: Arab. كاد · Maimonides, *Šarḥ fuṣūl Abūqrāṭ* · trans. Moses ibn Tibbon (*Pirqei Abuqraṭ*), 1.17 (44): ואולם אמצע האביב וכאשר קרב מן הקיץ הנה ראוי שיזונו במזון מעט במה שבין עתים ארוכים כי הזמן הזה אפשר שיהיו הגופות מלאים. → NM 3:29.

• **אי אפשר** › **hardly; scarcely**: Arab. لا يكاد / Gr. οὐδὲ εἴωθα · Maimonides, *Šarḥ fuṣūl Abūqrāṭ* · trans. Moses ibn Tibbon (*Pirqei Abuqraṭ*), 2.27 (79): אמר אבקראט: אין ראוי שתבטח בקלות החולי שימצא החולה שלא בדרך ההקש ולא שיפחידוך ענינים קשים יתחדשו שלא בדרך ההקש כי רוב מה שיקרה מזה אינו קיים ואי אפשר שיעמוד ולא תאריך עמידתו. → NM 3:29–30.

אֶצְבַּע › **index finger**: Arab. سبابة · Ibn Sīnā, *K. al-Qānūn fī al-ṭibb* · trans. Nathan ha-Me'ati (*Sefer ha-Qanun*), bk. 1 (fol. 50[a]): ואם יתנועע הראשון לבדו ירחיק בין הגודל והאצבע. → NM 4:20.

• **אצבע קטנה** ‹ I. **little finger**: Arab. خنصر · Al-Zahrāwī, *K. al-taṣrīf li-man ʿağiza ʿan at-taʾlīf* · trans. Shem Tov ben Isaac (*Sefer ha-Shimmush*), bk. 30, 3.12 (fol. 235[a]): ולהיות האצבע הקטנה למטה מכל האצבעות. → NM 1:78.

‹ II. **little toe**: Arab. خنصر · Al-Zahrāwī, *K. al-taṣrīf li-man ʿağiza ʿan at-taʾlīf* · trans. Shem Tov ben Isaac (*Sefer ha-Shimmush*), bk. 30, 2.95 (fol. 230[b]): ואם לא ימצא ולא יראה לחוש כלל ראוי להקיז קצת סעיפיו והם הנראים בגב הרגל בין אצבע קטנה והשני לו. → NM 1:78.

• *Plur.* **אצבעות** • **המעי הנקרא י״ב אצבעות** → מְעִי.

• **פרקי האצבעות** → פֶּרֶק.

• **קרב בעל השתים עשרה אצבעות** → קֶרֶב.

• **קשרי האצבעות** → קֶשֶׁר.

אִצְטוֹמְכָא (*Aram.*) (also: אִסְטוֹמְכָא; אִצְטוֹמְכָה) • **אחרי צאת המאכל מן האצטומכא** → אַחֲרֵי.

• **נשיכה בפי האצטומכה** → נְשִׁיכָה.

• **עיבד האצטומכה** → [עבד].

• **עקיצה בפי האצטומ׳** → עֲקִיצָה.

• **צער באסטומכא** → צַעַר.

• **קמטי האסטוכמה** → קֶמֶט.

• **קערורית האצטומכא** → קַעֲרוּרִית.

• **רוע בשול האצטומכא** → רֹעַ.

אִצְטוֹמְכָה → אִצְטוֹמְכָא.

אִצְטְנִיסוּת → אִסְטְנִיסוּת.

אַצִּיל ‹ **axilla**: Arab. إبط · Al-Zahrāwī, *K. al-taṣrīf li-man ʿağiza ʿan at-taʾlīf* · trans. Shem Tov ben Isaac (*Sefer ha-Shimmush*), bk. 30, 1.25 (fol. 205[b]): שער כה׳ בכוית האצילה. → NM 1:78.

אַצִּילִי ‹ **the axillary vein**: Arab. إبطي · a) Al-Zahrāwī, *K. al-taṣrīf li-man ʿağiza ʿan at-taʾlīf* · trans. Shem Tov ben Isaac (*Sefer ha-Shimmush*), bk. 30, 2.95 (fol. 228[b]): והבאסליק הוא בזרוע למטה מן הגיד האמצעי לעמת הלב ויקרא גם כן האצילי ויקראוהו עם הארץ גיד הבטן. → NM 1:79.

b) Ibn Sīnā, *K. al-Qānūn fī al-ṭibb* · trans. Nathan ha-Me'ati (*Sefer ha-Qanun*), bk. 1 (fols. 65[b]–66[a]): והשני פונה אל מקום כפיפת המרפק בחיצוני הקנה ומתערב בעומק בשריג גם כן מן האצילי. → NM 4:20.

אֲרוּכִי • **השלב הארוכיי** → שָׁלָב.

אָרוֹן • **ארון החזה** ‹ **thorax**: Arab. صندوق الصدر · Al-Zahrāwī, *K. al-taṣrīf li-man ʿağiza ʿan at-taʾlīf* · trans. Shem Tov ben Isaac (*Sefer ha-Shimmush*), bk. 27, fol. 145[a], col. a: מקומות הבשר החשובים מגוף בעלי חיים: החשוב שבאיברי בעלי חיים הוא האבר שהוא תדיר התנועה כבשר הצואר והזרוע והכתף ודומיהם ומה שנמשך אל פני הבטן ואל ארון החזה הוא יותר חשוב מן הנמשך בירך לקרבתו מן הלב. → NM 4:20–1.

אֲרִיגָה • **אריגת העכביש** ‹ **a spider's web**: Lat. aranee tela · Bruno Longobucco, *Cyrurgia Magna* · trans. Hillel ben Samuel (*Sefer Keritut*), fol. 27[b]. → NM 1:17.

אַרְיֵה • חולי האריה → חָלִי.

אֹרֶךְ • החוליא ההולכת באורך → חֻלְיָה.

אַרְכֻּבָּה • חולית הארכובה → חֻלְיָה.

• כפיפת הארכובה → כְּפִיפָה.

• כפל הארכובה → כֶּפֶל.

• מגן הארכובה → מָגֵן.

• עגול הארכובה → עִגּוּל.

• עין הארכובה → עַיִן.

• פלך הארכובה → פֶּלֶךְ.

• תחת הארכובה → תַּחַת.

ארכובה → אַרְכֻּבָּה.

אַרְנֶבֶת · **wing of the nostrils**: Arab. أرنبة / Lat. ala nasi · Ibn Sīnā, *K. al-Qānūn fī al-ṭibb* · trans. Nathan ha-Me'ati (*Sefer ha-Qanun*), bk. 1 (fol. 43^{a}): מה שידוע שעצלי הפנים הם כמספר האיברים המתנועעים בפנים והאיברים המתנועעים בפנים הם המצח ושתי העפעפים התחתונים ושתי העפעפים העליונים והרקה בשתוף עם השפתים ⟨והשפתים⟩ לבדם ושתי קצוות הארנבת והלחי התחתון. → NM 4:21.

• **הארנבת הימית** · **sea-hare; shelled sea-slug [*Aplysia leporina*]**: Arab. الأرنب البحري / Gr. ὁ θαλάττιος λαγωός · Al-Zahrāwī, *K. al-taṣrīf li-man ʿağiza ʿan at-taʾlīf* · trans. Shem Tov ben Isaac (*Sefer ha-Shimmush*), bk. 27, fol. 146^{b}, col. a: חלב הנשים יותר שוה מכל החלבים ... ולפיכך הוא מועיל מן העקיצה אשר תקרה באסטומ׳ ומשחין הריאה והמעים ומשתיית הארנבת הימית ומשתית הסם הנודע בהורג הזאב. → NM 4:21.

אֶרֶס · **anything, esp., liquid substance that powerfully affects or changes the condition of the body**: Lat. venenum · Al-Rāzī, attr., *On the Treatment of Small Children* · trans. Anonymous, ch. 10: מהארס. זה החולי יקרה לנערים גם כן מאבעבוע או מכה שהכה באזן. → NM 2:177.

אֵשׁ • **אש זרה** · **artificial fire (i.e., saltpeter)**: *Anonymous Glossary*, Ms. Leiden, Universiteitsbibliotheek, Cod. Or. 4732/1, fol. 8^{a}: שלניטרי הוא מלח אחר יתקנו ממנו אש זרה. → NM 4:21–2.

• הכרמל המהובהב באש → כַּרְמֶל.

• מכות אש → מִכְוָה.

• **האש הפרסי** · **erysipelas**: Lat. ignis sacer · Arnau de Vilanova, *Medicationis Parabole* · trans. Abraham Avigdor (*Pirqei Arnauṭ de Vilanova*), 5.102: כמו שהקושי הנקרא אשקלירושיש כאשר יתישן שרשו יעתק אל החולי המכונה אירפיטים, כן בנגעים אשר יקרו באיברים החמים הבשר המת אם לא יעקר משרש, יוליד שם האש הפרסי בפתע. → NM 4:22.

• צלי אש → צָלִי.

אִשָּׁה • נקב אותו מקום של אשה → נֶקֶב.

• קיבת האשה → קֵבָה.

אֶשֶׁךְ · **ovary**: Arab. خصية · Ibn Sīnā, *K. al-Qānūn fī al-ṭibb* · trans. Nathan ha-Me'ati (*Sefer ha-Qanun*), bk. 1, fol. 52^{b}: ואמנם הנשים יספיק להם אחד לכל אשך נפרד. → NM 4:22.

• **האשך הבשרי** · **a fleshy hernia**: Arab. الأدرة اللحمية · Al-Zahrāwī, *K. al-taṣrīf li-man*

ʿağiza ʿan at-taʾlīf · trans. Shem Tov ben Isaac (*Sefer ha-Shimmush*), bk. 30, 2.63 (fol. 219[b]): שער ס״ג בבקוע על האשך הבשרי ורפואתו. → NM 1:79.

• **האשך הזמורי** · **hernia with varix:** Arab. الأدرة التي مع دالية · Al-Zahrāwī, *K. al-taṣrīf li-man ʿağiza ʿan at-taʾlīf* · trans. Shem Tov ben Isaac (*Sefer ha-Shimmush*), bk. 30, 2.64 (fol. 220[a]): שער ס״ד ברפואת האשך הזמורי ר״ל אשר יהיה עם זמורה. → NM 1:79.

• **האשך המימי** · **a watery hernia:** Arab. الأدرة المائية · Al-Zahrāwī, *K. al-taṣrīf li-man ʿağiza ʿan at-taʾlīf* · trans. Shem Tov ben Isaac (*Sefer ha-Shimmush*), bk. 30, 2.62 (fol. 219[a]). → NM 1:79.

• **האשך המעיי** · **intestinal hernia:** Arab. الأدرة المعائيّة · Al-Zahrāwī, *K. al-taṣrīf li-man ʿağiza ʿan at-taʾlīf* · trans. Shem Tov ben Isaac (*Sefer ha-Shimmush*), bk. 30, 2.65 (fol. 220[a]). → NM 1:79.

• **האשך הרוחיי** · **flatulent hernia:** Arab. الأدرة الريحيّة · Al-Zahrāwī, *K. al-taṣrīf li-man ʿağiza ʿan at-taʾlīf* · trans. Shem Tov ben Isaac (*Sefer ha-Shimmush*), bk. 30, 2.66 (fol. 220[a]). → NM 1:79.

• *Plur.* **אשכים** · **אשכי השועל** · **(lit., testicles of the fox); salep:** *Anonymous Glossary*, Ms. Oxford, Bodleian Library, Mich. Add. 22, fol. 5[b]: אשכי השועל שטריאון. → NM 4:22.

אַשְׁכְּנַז · **the Skyths; the Slavs:** Arab. الصقالبة · Al-Zahrāwī, *K. al-taṣrīf li-man ʿağiza ʿan at-taʾlīf* · trans. Shem Tov ben Isaac (*Sefer ha-Shimmush*), bk. 27, fol. 145[b], col. a: הבשר השלוק וקוראים אותו אנשי המזרח אספגדבאג׳ה ואנחנו קוראים אותו גם כן שלוק האשכנז והוא חם בשוי ונאות ברוב העתים והענינים לכל בני אדם לבד מי שיגבר על מזגו החמימות. → NM 4:23.

אֶתְמוֹלִי · **pertaining to (from) yesterday:** Judah ben Jacob, *Sefer Hanhagat ha-Beriʾut*, 6: ומן הראוי לבלתי התעצל מהתיגע ומהתנועע יום יום קודם האכילה ואחר תום טחינת המאכל האתמולי באחת ממיני התנועות הראויות לו. → NM 4:23.

אֶתְרוֹג • **חמיצות האתרוג** → חֲמִיצוּת.

• *Plur.* **אתרוגים** • **חימוץ האתרוגים** → חִמּוּץ.

ב

בֵּאוּר · **distinction**: Arab. تبيين · Maimonides, *K. al-fuṣūl fī al-ṭibb* · trans. Zeraḥyah Ḥen (*Sefer ha-Peraqim*), 6.8: אמר משה הסתכל איך שם הפרש בין החיכוך והפלצות והריגור מדרגות חידוד הליחה לבד ובזה תוספת ביאור ממה שאמרו במאמרו ברעדה וברפפות ובריגור ובכיווץ. → NM 1:130.

באסאליק → **באסליק**.

באסליק • **הבאסליק** · **the basilic vein**: Arab. الباسليق · Ibn Sīnā, *K. al-Qānūn fī al-ṭibb* · trans. Nathan ha-Me'ati (*Sefer ha-Qanun*), bk. 1 (fol. 66[a]): והרביעי והוא הגדול שבהם והוא אותו אשר יראה ויעלה וישתלח ענף מאסף עמו שריג מן הקיפאל ויתהוה ממנו האכחל ושאריתו הוא הבאסליק. → NM 4:23.

[**באר**] • *Part. Pu'al* **מְבֹאָר** · **different**: Arab. مباين · Maimonides, *K. al-fuṣūl fī al-ṭibb* · trans. Zeraḥyah Ḥen (*Sefer ha-Peraqim*), 3.40: וישובו אלו הגידים המשותפים התחלתם מבוארת להתחלת שאר העורקים. → NM 1:160.

• *Hitpa'el* **הִתְבָּאֵר** · **to exfoliate**: Arab. تبيّن · Hippocrates, *Aphorisms* · trans. Nathan ha-Me'ati, 6.45 (337) (fol. 121[a]): אמר אבוקרט: כשיעבור בשחין שנה או זמן יותר ארוך מזה ראוי בהכרח שיתבאר ממנו עצם ושיהיה מקום הרושם אחר שיבריא שוקע. → NM 3:30.

בֶּגֶד · I. **pannus**: Lat. pannus · Bruno Longobucco, *Cyrurgia Magna* · trans. Hillel ben Samuel (*Sefer Keritut*), fol. 66[b]: הבגד המתילד בעינים מחמת המכות או מחמת פישטולי הוא מכת נמנעי הרפואה. → NM 1:18.

· II. **papyrus**: Arab. قرطاس / Lat. carta · Ibn al-Jazzār, *Zād al-musāfir wa-qūt al-ḥāḍir* · trans. Moses ibn Tibbon (*Sefer Ṣedat ha-Derakhim*), bk. 1, ch. 7 (fol. 12[a]): או יקח בגד שרופה וישחקהו בחומץ חזק ויטוח אותו על הנגעים. → NM 4:24.

• **לט בבגד חם** → [לוט].

• *Plur.* **בגדים** · **membranes**: Lat. velamina; panniculi · Bruno Longobucco, *Cyrurgia Magna* · trans. Hillel ben Samuel (*Sefer Keritut*), fol. 46[a]: המוח יש לה ב׳ בגדים אחת נקרא דורא מטרי ואחרת נקרא פיאה מטרי. → NM 1:17–8.

[**בדל**] • *Part. Hif'il* **מַבְדִּיל** · **spine of the scapula**: Arab. حاجز · Ibn Sīnā, *K. al-Qānūn fī al-ṭibb* · trans. Zeraḥyah Ḥen (*Sefer ha-Qanun*), bk. 1 (fol. 26[b]): וחמשה מושקולים צומחים מעצם הכתף ויעסוק מה שבין המבדיל והצלע העליון מן הכתף. → NM 4:94.

• **המכסה המבדיל** → [כסה].

בדלי · **cartiliginous**: Arab. غضروفي · Ibn Sīnā, *K. al-Qānūn fī al-ṭibb* · trans. Joseph Lorki (*Sefer ha-Qanun*), bk. 1 (fol. 12[a]): העצה מחובר מחוליות ג׳ בדליים אין תוספת להם. → NM 4:24.

בָּדַק • **בדק עצמו** · **to open one's bowel (i.e., to defecate)**: Arab. تبرّز · Al-Zahrāwī, *K. al-taṣrīf li-man 'ağiza 'an at-ta'līf* · trans. Shem Tov ben Isaac (*Sefer ha-Shimmush*), bk. 30, 2.81 (fol. 223[a]): ורפואת הטחורים אשר יהיו מבפנים לצוות אל החולה לבדוק עצמו ולהרגיל העיצום עד שיבלוט פי הטבעת ויראו היבלות. → NM 1:79.

בֶּהָלָה · I. **confusion**: Arab. حيرة / Gr. ἔκστασις · Maimonides, *Šarḥ fuṣūl Abūqrāṭ* · trans. Moses ibn Tibbon (*Pirqei Abuqraṭ*), 7.5 (357): אמר אבקראט: כשיתחדש אחר השטות שלשול דם או שקוי או בהלה הנה הוא אות טוב. → NM 3:30–1.

‣ II. **forgetfulness; heedlessness; inadvertence; neglectfulness; unmindfulness:** Arab. غفلة · Ibn al-Jazzār, *Zād al-musāfir wa-qūt al-ḥāḍir* · trans. Moses ibn Tibbon (*Sefer Ṣedat ha-Derakhim*), bk. 1, ch. 14 (fol. 21[a]): ונצוהו גם כן להתמיד לקיחת הרפואה הזאת כי כבר ניסינו אותה ושבחנוה והוא גרגרים חברם אצחק בן עמרם יועילו בע"ה מן הבהלה והשכחה וכאב הראש המתילד מן הליחה הלבנה. → NM 4:24.

‣ III. **stupor:** Arab. بهتة / Gr. ἔκπληξις · Maimonides, *Šarḥ fuṣūl Abūqrāṭ* · trans. Zeraḥyah Ḥen (*Pirqei Abuqraṭ*), 7.14 (366): אמר בקראט: ובעבור ההכאה על הראש הבהלה ובלבול הדעת רע. → NM 3:30.

בֹּהַק • **בחק שחור** ‣ **black *bahaq* (i.e., a kind of melanoderma):** Arab. بهق أسود · Al-Zahrāwī, *K. al-taṣrīf li-man ʿağiza ʿan at-taʾlīf* · trans. Shem Tov ben Isaac (*Sefer ha-Shimmush*), bk. 27, fol. 134[b], col. b: והתמדת אכילתו גורמת השטות והסרטן ומדוה השועל והדליות והטחורים והבהק השחור ודומיהם מן החליים השחוריים. → NM 4:24–5.

[בוא] • **בא לו חולי הרגלים** ‣ **to suffer from gout:** Gr. ποδαγριάω · Hippocrates, *Aphorisms* · trans. Joseph Delmedigo, 6.28 (320): לסריסים אינו בא לא חולי הרגלים ולא קרחה. → NM 3:86–7.

• **קדחת חבאה בכל יום** → **קַדַּחַת**.

• *Hifʿil* **הֵבִיא** • **הביא שתי שערות** ‣ **to reach puberty:** Hippocrates, *Aphorisms* · trans. Do'eg ha-Edomi (*Sefer Agur*), 5.7 (227) (fol. 80[b]): אמר אפוקרט: גזור על סובל חולי הנפילה אם לא הביאה שתי שערות תאחר רפואתו. → NM 3:233.

• *Part. Hifʿil* **מֵבִיא** • **הסם המביא חדם** → **סַם**.

בּוּקָא (*Aram.*) • **בוקא דאטמא** ‣ **hip joint:** Lat. vertebrum · Hippocrates, *Aphorisms* · trans. Hillel ben Samuel, 6.59 (351) (fol. 44[a]): א"א: בעלי השיאטיקה אם הבוקא דאטמא יצא לחוץ ותשוב למקומה נעשו שם להם רירים. → NM 3:31.

בורקי ‣ I. **alkaline:** Arab. بورقي · Maimonides, *K. al-fuṣūl fī al-ṭibb* · trans. Nathan ha-Me'ati (*Sefer ha-Peraqim*), 21.59: ויש בדברים המרים גם כן כח מדקדק איננו למטה מן הכח אשר יש בדברים הבורקיים והמלוחים. → NM 2:30.

‣ II. **nitrous:** Lat. nitrosus · Arnau de Vilanova, *Medicationis Parabole* · trans. Abraham Avigdor (*Pirqei Arnauṭ de Vilanova*), 4.13 (50): הדם הנוטה לצדדי העור בורקי או חלודי הנה יורק באופן נאות עם הנחת קרני המציצה וביחוד אם יהיה הדם עב או עמוק אמנם אם יהיה דק או שטחי הנה העלוקות יריקוהו. → NM 4:25.

• **המים הגפריתיים והבורקיים** → **מַיִם**.

בורקיות ‣ **alkalinity:** Arab. بورقية · Maimonides, *K. al-fuṣūl fī al-ṭibb* · trans. Nathan ha-Me'ati (*Sefer ha-Peraqim*), 21.59: וכל מה שיהיה בטעמו בורקיות או מליחות הנה ברב מה שזהו ענינו יש בו כח מדקדק והוא מרכך הבטן. → NM 2:30–1.

בושמיות → **בְּשָׂמִיּוּת**.

בזהרי ‣ **antidotal:** Lat. theriacalis · Arnau de Vilanova, *Medicationis Parabole* · trans. Abraham Avigdor (*Pirqei Arnauṭ de Vilanova*), 5.96 (110): הנגעים המתאכלים אשר יתרחבו ויתפשטו אל העומק מעצמם ראוי לרפאם עם דברים קובצים ומיבשים בלתי עוקצים, ואם יהיו ארסיים כמו חולי הזאב יצטרך שיהיו בזהריים. → NM 4:25.

בְּחִינָה ‣ I. **experience:** Lat. experimentum · Bruno Longobucco, *Cyrurgia Magna* · trans.

Hillel ben Samuel (*Sefer Keritut*), fol. 24[a]: הרפואות המחברות שסמכתי מטובם ומרוב הבחינה ומעדות הקדמונים הם אלו. → NM 1:18.

‣ II. **expression**: Arab. عبارة · Maimonides, *K. al-fuṣūl fī al-ṭibb* · trans. Nathan ha-Me'ati (*Sefer ha-Peraqim*), introduction: ואם יפקפק אחד בלשון גאלינוס באותו הפרק או בכונתו ישוב אל המאמר ההוא בנקלה בספר גליאנוס עצמו וימצא אותו הפרק וימצא לשון גליאנוס או רובו או ימצא אותו הענין בלי חסרון ובלי תוספת בדברי גאלינוס באותו המאמר ואם תתחלף הבחינה אז יסולק הספק. → NM 2:31.

בָּטוּחַ · **healthy**: Arab. سالم · Maimonides, *Šarḥ fuṣūl Abūqrāṭ* · trans. Moses ibn Tibbon (*Pirqei Abuqraṭ*), 7.45 (397): אמר המפרש: כשתהיה המוגלא במכסה וגרם הכבד הוא בטוח ואפשר לו הבריאות. → NM 3:31.

בִּטּוּל · **numbness**: Arab. خدر · Maimonides, *K. al-fuṣūl fī al-ṭibb* · trans. Zeraḥyah Ḥen (*Sefer ha-Peraqim*), 22.38: אכילת ראשי הארנבת כל מה שאפשר יועיל מן הרעש ונמצא בנסיון שיועיל כמו כן מבטול והפלג ואכילת בשר הארנבת ישבר החול. → NM 1:130.

• **ביטול הגוף** · **paralysis**: Judah ben Jacob, *Sefer Hanhagat ha-Beri'ut*, 8.5: אז ינקה הגוף ממנה בסמים המנקים אותה נפרדים או מורכבים פן תוליד בו בטול כל הגוף או חציו ועקימת הפה. → NM 4:25.

• **בטול החוש** · **numbness**: Lat. stupor / Arab. خدر · Hippocrates, *Aphorisms* · trans. Hillel ben Samuel, 5.25 (245) (fol. 32[b]): א"א: נפח הפרקים ומכאובם אשר הוא בלא נגע ופודגרא וקווץ נחלאים רבים מזה המין הטבילה במים קרים רבים מקררת ומזירה ומסירה הכאב מפני שבטול החוש מסיר הכאב. → NM 3:31.

• **ביטול חצי הגוף** · **hemiplegia**: Judah ben Jacob, *Sefer Hanhagat ha-Beri'ut*, 8.5: אז ינקה הגוף ממנה בסמים המנקים אותה נפרדים או מורכבים פן תוליד בו בטול כל הגוף או חציו ועקימת הפה. → NM 4:25.

[בטח] • *Hif'il* **הִבְטִיחַ** · **to hope**: Arab. رجا · Maimonides, *K. al-fuṣūl fī al-ṭibb* · trans. Zeraḥyah Ḥen (*Sefer ha-Peraqim*), 8.22: ובאלהים כי כל מי ששתה המים הקרים מאותם שאני הבטחתי שיהיו ניצלים ניצלו ונתרפאו. → NM 1:131.

[בטל] • *Pi'el* **בִּטֵּל** · **to benumb**: Arab. خدّر · Maimonides, *K. al-fuṣūl fī al-ṭibb* · trans. Zeraḥyah Ḥen (*Sefer ha-Peraqim*), 8.39: זאת הרפואה המחוברת לשכך הכאב אשר יכנסו בה הדברים המבטלים החוש ראוי לאדם שיכוין בחיבורה אל ג׳ סגולות: האחת שיבטל החוש. → NM 1:131.

• *Hitpa'el* **הִתְבַּטֵּל** · **to turn numb**: Arab. خدر · Maimonides, *K. al-fuṣūl fī al-ṭibb* · trans. Zeraḥyah Ḥen (*Sefer ha-Peraqim*), 23.23: הביטול הנקרא בערבי כדר בכף רפה הוא דבר מורכב מעוצר החוש ועוצר התנועה ויהיה מקרירות האויר ומלחיצת הגופות העצביות וממישוש הבעל חיים הימיי. והאברים יקרה להם תחלה שיתבטלו ואחרי כן ישובו אין להם חוש ולא תנועה ויאמר לזה המין מההזק רפיון בערבי איסתירכא ברפה הכף. → NM 1:131.

[בטן] • *Part. Hof'al* **מֻבְטָן** · **abdominal patient**: Arab. مبطون · a) Maimonides, *K. al-fuṣūl fī al-ṭibb* · trans. Zeraḥyah Ḥen (*Sefer ha-Peraqim*), 23.93: בהתחדש במעים הדקים מורסא קשה או סתימה גדולה ממותר עד שיקיא האדם צואתו אותו החולי נקרא איליאוס ומעט הם שיהיו נצלים ממנו. ובהתבטל המעים כולם והאסטומכא ולא יוכל להחזיק מה שבהם ואפילו שעה מועטת ולא תהיה החולי עוקץ אותו החולי נקרא המעדת המיעים וחוליי הבטן. ונקרא בעל זה החולי כמו כן מובטן. → NM 1:132.

b) Maimonides, *K. al-fuṣūl fī al-ṭibb* · trans. Nathan ha-Me'ati (*Sefer ha-Peraqim*), 23.93: וכשהמעים יהיו עלולים והאסטו׳ ולא יוכלו לאחוז מה שיש בגרמם ואפילו זמן מועט ולא תהיה העלה עוקצת הנה אותה העלה נקראת המעדת המעים ותקרא גם כן עלות הבטן ויקרא בעליו מובטן. → NM 2:56.

בֶּטֶן · I. **bowels:** Hippocrates, *Aphorisms* · trans. Do'eg ha-Edomi (*Sefer Agur*), 3.31 (137) (fol. 58[b]): רוך הבטן ורוך העינים וזוב הנחירים. → NM 3:32.

· II. **cavity:** Lat. venter · Hippocrates, *Aphorisms* · trans. Judah Shalom, 7.38 (390) (fol. 120[b]): נזילה בעליונות הבטן יושב אל מוגלא בעשרים יום. → NM 3:32.

· III. **hollowness:** Arab. بطن · Maimonides, *K. al-fuṣūl fī al-ṭibb* · trans. Zeraḥyah Ḥen (*Sefer ha-Peraqim*), 15.3: אין ראוי שיהיה אבר שיהיה לו עומק או בטן ואין בגוף אבר אלא ולו בטן עם עומק מלבד הידים והרגלים והחלצים. → NM 1:131.

• **גרישת הבטן** → גְּרִישָׁה.
• **הגרת הבטן** → הֲגָרָה.
• **הותר בטנו** → [נתר].
• **הזלת הבטן** → הֲזָלָה.
• **הזלת דם הבטן** → הֲזָלָה.
• **החליק הבטן** → [חלק].
• **התרת הבטן** → הַתָּרָה.
• **זחילת הבטן** → זְחִילָה.
• **חדרי הבטן** → חֶדֶר.
• **חולי מכרס הבטן** → חֳלִי.
• **חלקות הבטן** → חֲלָקוּת.
• **מכסה הבטן** → מִכְסֶה.
• **מקום הבטן** → מָקוֹם.
• **נשמט הבטן** → [שמט].
• **עוצר הבטן** → עֹצֶר.
• **עיוות הבטן** → עֲוּוּת.
• **עיצור הבטן** → עִצּוּר.
• **עצור הבטן** → עָצַר.
• **עצירת הבטן** → עֲצִירָה.
• **העצל הישר מעצלי הבטן** → עָצָל.
• **צירים בבטן** → צִיר.
• **צמח השער בשפל הבטן** → צָמַח.
• **קלוח הבטן** → קִלּוּחַ.
• **שלשול הבטן** → שִׁלְשׁוּל.
• **שפולי הבטן** → שִׁפּוּל.
• **שפל הבטן** → שֵׁפֶל.

בָּטְנָה • *Plur.* בטנים · **pine cone(s):** Arab. صنوبر · Ibn al-Jazzār, *Zād al-musāfir wa-qūt al-ḥāḍir* · trans. Moses ibn Tibbon (*Sefer Ṣedat ha-Derakhim*), bk. 2, ch. 8 (fol. 48[b]): או יקח סחיטת כרתי עם חלב אשה ויעורב עם שמן ורדים ויטיף ממנו באזן או יתיך מרישארמה הוא אישוף בשמן בטנים ויטיף ממנו בהם. → NM 4:25–6.

ביטול → בִּטּוּל.

בֵּיצָה · ovary; testicle: Arab. خصية · Ibn Sīnā, *K. al-Qānūn fī al-ṭibb* · trans. Zeraḥyah Ḥen (*Sefer ha-Qanun*), bk. 1 (fol. 28ᵃ): אבל הנשים יספיק להן זוג לכל ביצה אחת. → NM 4:26.

• **אודם הביצה** → אֹדֶם.

• **מוח הביצה** → מֹחַ.

• *Plur.* **בצים** • **חוטי הבצים** → חוט.

בישול → בִּשּׁוּל.

בַּיִת · ventricle [of the brain]: Arab. بطن · Ibn Sīnā, *K. al-Qānūn fī al-ṭibb* · trans. Zeraḥyah Ḥen (*Sefer ha-Qanun*), bk. 1 (fol. 17ᵇ): ואמר גאלינוס ואי איפשר שיהיה לראש צורה רביעית בלתי טבעית עד שיהיה האורך יותר מחוסר מן הרוחב אלא אם יהיה חסור ממנו מבתי המוח או חלק אחד ממנו וזה הפך לכל חיי האדם נמנע מבריאות ההרכבה. → NM 4:26.

• **בית הבליעה** · anterior part of the throat; gorge; pharynx: Arab. حلق · Ibn Sīnā, *K. al-Qānūn fī al-ṭibb* · trans. Zeraḥyah Ḥen (*Sefer ha-Qanun*), bk. 1 (fol. 25ᵃ): האחד הוא הקלפיי אשר יבואנו החוש לפני בית הבליעה ותחת הזקן. → NM 4:26.

• **בית יד** · handle: Arab. مقبض · Galen, attr., *Prohibition of Burial* · trans. Judah al-Ḥarizi (*Sefer Issur ha-Qevurah le-Galienus*), par. 37: הרפואה הראשונה היא לזקנים ושוכני הארצות הקרות ומקבלי המקרה בסתיו. תרופתו שתצוה לקחת שתי לוחות ברזל כל לוח אר⟨ו⟩כה כמו אמה ויהיה לה בית יד וימשחנה בשמן אגוזים ותניחנה על האש ונפח במפוח. → NM 4:26–7.

• **בית הערוה** · genitals: Arab. فرج · Maimonides, *Šarḥ fuṣūl Abūqrāṭ* · trans. Anonymous (*Pirqei Abuqraṭ*), 2.35 (87): אמר המפרש: שפל הבטן הוא מה שבין בית הערוה והטבור כי חלקי הבטן שלושה: המקום אשר מתחת לצלעות ומה שאצל הטיבור ושפל הבטן. → NM 3:32.

• **בית הפרשות** · perineum: Arab. فضاء · Al-Zahrāwī, *K. al-taṣrīf li-man ʿağiza ʿan at-taʾlīf* · trans. Shem Tov ben Isaac (*Sefer ha-Shimmush*), bk. 30, 2.80 (fol. 220ᵃ): ולפעמים יהיה מהם טחורים כשיהיו בבית הפרשות מפולשים אל כיס מקוה המים ואל מעבר השתן. → NM 1:79–80.

• **צמוח השיער בבית הערוה** → צָמַח.

בִּלְבּוּל • **בלבול הדעת** · I. delirium: Arab. اختلاط العقل · Maimonides, *K. al-fuṣūl fī al-ṭibb* · trans. Zeraḥyah Ḥen (*Sefer ha-Peraqim*), 6.37: סימני קראניטס י״ו עלאמה והם התעורה או השינה המצטערת ובלבול הדעת. → NM 1:132.

· II. madness: Gr. μανία · Hippocrates, *Aphorisms* · trans. Joseph Delmedigo, 5.40 (260): האשה שמתקבץ דם בדדיה מורה על בלבול הדעת שיבא. → NM 3:33.

· III. phrenitis: Gr. φρενῖτις · Hippocrates, *Aphorisms* · trans. Joseph Delmedigo, 7.12 (364): ממורסת הריאה בלבול הדעת רע. → NM 3:33.

• **הבלבול הקורה מן השחורה** · melancholic delusion: Arab. الوسواس السوداوي · Hippocrates, *Aphorisms* · trans. Nathan ha-Me'ati 3.14 (120) (fol. 47ᵃ): אמר אבוקרט: כשיהיה החורף צפוני ויבש יהיה נאות למי שיהיה טבעו רטוב ולנשים ואמנם שאר האנשים יקרה להם רמד יבש וקדחות חדות וזכאם נושן ויש מהם שיקרה להם הבלבול הקורה מן השחורה. → NM 3:33.

• **בלבול בראש** · dizziness: Arab. دوار / Gr. σκότωμα · Maimonides, *K. al-fuṣūl fī al-ṭibb* · trans. Nathan ha-Me'ati (*Sefer ha-Peraqim*), 6.34: מי שימצאהו סבוב בראש ובלבול בראש יחשכו עיניהם ויפלו ויקיף בהם מסבות מועטות. → NM 2:31.

• **בלבול הראש השחור** › **melancholic delusion**: Arab. الوسواس السوداوي / Gr. τὰ μελαγχολικά · Maimonides, *Šarḥ fuṣūl Abūqrāṭ* · trans. Moses ibn Tibbon (*Pirqei Abuqraṭ*), 3.20 (126): אמר אבקראט: פעמים יקרה באביב בלבול הראש השחור והשטות וחולי הנופל והגרת הדם והאסכרא והרבמאס והרבקיי והשעול והחולי אשר יתקלף בו העור והקואבי והבהק והשחין הרב אשר יפתח ויתנגע והמורסות וכאבי הפרקים. → NM 3:33–4.

• **הבלבול השחורי** › **melancholic delusion**: Arab. الوسواس السوداوي · Maimonides, *K. al-fuṣūl fī al-ṭibb* · trans. Nathan ha-Me'ati (*Sefer ha-Peraqim*), 9.16: הבלבול השחורי לפעמים יהיה מפני שכל מה שיש בעורקים מן הדם השחורי נשפך אליו או שנתחדש בו מפני חום שיש שם שחורך ושורף המרה האדומה או הדם העב. → NM 2:31–2.

• **בלבול השכל** › I. **madness**: Arab. جنون / Gr. μανία · Maimonides, *Šarḥ fuṣūl Abūqrāṭ* · trans. Moses ibn Tibbon (*Pirqei Abuqraṭ*), 5.40 (260): אמר אבקראט: כשיקפא לאשה בשדיה דם מורה מעניינה על בלבול השכל. → NM 3:34; corr. 4:229.

› II. **melancholy; melancholic delusion**: Arab. الوسواس السوداوي / Gr. μελαγχολιά · Maimonides, *Šarḥ fuṣūl Abūqrāṭ* · trans. Moses ibn Tibbon (*Pirqei Abuqraṭ*), 3.14 (120): אמר אבקראט: ואם היו רוחותיו צפוניות יבשות הנה יהיה נאות למי שהיה טבעו לח ולנשים ואולם שאר האנשים הנה יקרה להם קצידה יבשה וקדחות חדות ורבמאס מתמיד ומהם מי שיקרה להם בלבול השכל מן המרה השחורה. → NM 3:34.

• **בלבול השכל השחורי** › **melancholic delusion**: Arab. الوسواس السوداوي · Hippocrates, *Aphorisms* · trans. Nathan ha-Me'ati, 3.20 (126) (fol. 51[a]): אמר אבוקרט: לפעמים יקרה באביב בלבול השכל השחורי והשטות והכפיון והזביחה וזכאם הוא קוריזא וצרידות קול והזלת הדם והשעול והעלה אשר יקולף ממנה העור והספחת והבהק והבתור הרבים המשתחנים ומורסות הנקראות יציאות וכאיבי הפרקים. → NM 3:34–5.

[בלבל] • *Pu'al* **בֻּלְבַּל** • **בולבל בטנו** › **to suffer from diarrhea**: Lat. venter turbatur / Arab. استطلق بطنه · Hippocrates, *Aphorisms* · trans. Hillel ben Samuel, 4.60 (197): א"א: אותם שבקדחות תחרשנה אזניהם אם יצא דם מחוטמם או יבולבל בטנם יעדר החלי. → NM 3:35.

• *Part. Pu'al* **מְבֻלְבָּל** › I. **heterogeneous**: Arab. متشتّت · Hippocrates, *Aphorisms* · trans. Nathan ha-Me'ati, 7.33 (385) (fol. 133[b]): אמר אבוקרט: מי שיהיה שתנו מבולבל הנה זה יורה שיש בגופו התגעשות חזקה. → NM 3:124.

› II. **turbid**: Arab. متثوّر / Gr. ἀνατεταραγμένος · Hippocrates, *Aphorisms* · trans. Nathan ha-Me'ati, 4.70 (207) (fol. 79[b]): אמר אבוקרט: מי שישתין בקדחות שתן מבולבל דומה לשתן החמורים יש בו כאב ראש עתה או שיתחדש בו עדין. → NM 3:123–4.

• *Hitpa'el* **הִתְבַּלְבֵּל** › **to become turbid**: Arab. تثوّر · Maimonides, *Šarḥ fuṣūl Abūqrāṭ* · trans. Anonymous (*Pirqei Abuqraṭ*), 4.70 (207): אמר המפרש: אמנם יהיה השתן כן כשיעשה החום בחומר עבה ורב. ומה שהיה מן החמרים על זה התואר ובפרט כשתעשה בו החום הנכרי יתילד ממנו הרוחות עד שיתבלבל כמי השעוה או הזפת והראתינג. → NM 3:35.

בָּלָה › **to develop pus**: Arab. تقيّح · Maimonides, *Šarḥ fuṣūl Abūqrāṭ* · trans. Anonymous (*Pirqei Abuqraṭ*), 6.27 (319): וכבר יראה גם כן בשאר האיברים כשנתחדש באחד מהם מורסא גדולה ובלתה והורק הבלוי ממנה בפתע מסתכן כי יקרה לבעליו ממנו העלוף לאלתר ונפילת הכח ואחר כן כשישאר בחלישותו קשה להשיבו. → NM 3:35.

• *Pass. Part.* **בָּלוּי** • **המוגלא הבלויה** → **מֻגְלָא**.

• *Plur.* בלויים ‣ **patients with empyema:** Arab. المتقيّحون · Maimonides, *Šarḥ fuṣūl Abūqrāṭ* · trans. Anonymous (*Pirqei Abuqraṭ*), 6.27 (319): אמר אבוקרט: מי שנכוה או נכרת מן הבלויים או מן המשוקים ונגר ממנו מוגלא או מים הרבה מאד בפתע הוא יאבד בלי ספק. → NM 3:37.

בָּלוּי (*Pass. Part.*) → **בָּלָה**.

בְּלוּי ‣ I. **irritation:** Arab. تقيّح · Hippocrates, *Aphorisms* · trans. Do'eg ha-Edomi (*Sefer Agur*), 3.25 (131) (fol. 56[b]): רעות רבות תקרינה לנערים בעת יצמחו שניהם: קדחת קיבוץ הגידים הזלת בטנם בלוי בשר שניהם אף כי בעת צאת הטוחנת. → NM 3:36.

‣ II. **suppuration:** Arab. تقيّح · Maimonides, *Šarḥ fuṣūl Abūqrāṭ* · trans. Anonymous (*Pirqei Abuqraṭ*), 7.20 (372): אמר אבוקרט: ומן המורסא הנקרא חומרה העפוש והבלוי. → NM 3:35–6.

• בלוי הטיט ‣ **pus:** Hippocrates, *Aphorisms* · trans. Do'eg ha-Edomi (*Sefer Agur*), 2.47 (99) (fol. 46[b]): ראשית ירידת בלוי הטיט בצמחים יחול הכאב לבוא והקדחת לעלות. → NM 3:36.

• בלוי עב טיט ‣ I. **empyema:** Hippocrates, *Aphorisms* · trans. Do'eg ha-Edomi (*Sefer Agur*), 6.27 (319) (fol. 101[b]): טנף הסובל בלוי עב טיט או המים הרעים ועשה מכות אש להוציא מן המים לרוב בפעם אחת בלי ספק ימות. → NM 3:36–7.

‣ II. **suppuration:** Hippocrates, *Aphorisms* · trans. Do'eg ha-Edomi (*Sefer Agur*), 7.20 (372) (fol. 113[b]): אמר אפוקרט: חולי הצמח הנקרא חמרה אם יקרה עמו בלוי עב טיט ועפוש אות טוב הוא. → NM 3:36.

בָּלַט ‣ **to become convex:** Arab. احدودب · Maimonides, *K. al-fuṣūl fī al-ṭibb* · trans. Nathan ha-Me'ati (*Sefer ha-Peraqim*), 1.70: העצלים אשר בידים וברגלים והפנים כשימתחו יבלטו. → NM 2:32.

בְּלִיטָה ‣ I. **convex part of a vertebra; epiphysis:** Arab. لقمة · Ibn Sīnā, *K. al-Qānūn fī al-ṭibb* · trans. Nathan ha-Me'ati (*Sefer ha-Qanun*), bk. 1, ch. 13 (fol. 36[a]): ובהיות שתי קצוות השדרה נוטים אל השכיבה לא נוצר להם בליטות אבל נקרות. → NM 4:27.

‣ II. **prominence [of the head]:** Arab. نتوء · Ibn Sīnā, *K. al-Qānūn fī al-ṭibb* · trans. Nathan ha-Me'ati (*Sefer ha-Qanun*), bk. 1, ch. 2 (fol. 29[a]): ואמנם תבניתי הראש הבלתי טבעיים הם ג' אחד מהם כשיחסר הבליטה הקודמת. → NM 4:27.

‣ III. **protuberance:** Arab. نتوء · Al-Zahrāwī, *K. al-taṣrīf li-man ʿağiza ʿan at-taʾlīf* · trans. Shem Tov ben Isaac (*Sefer ha-Shimmush*), bk. 30, 2.16 (fol. 211[b]): אמנם בליטת בשר ראש העין אם תהיה הבליטה מזקת העין נזק מכוער ראוי לתלות הבליטה ההיא בחכה ולחתוך ממנה קצתה מבלי רבוי חתוך פן תתחדש הגרת הדמעות. → NM 1:80.

• בליטת הרחם ‣ **prolapse of the uterus:** Arab. نتوء الرحم · Ibn al-Jazzār, *Zād al-musāfir wa-qūt al-ḥāḍir* · trans. Moses ibn Tibbon (*Sefer Ṣedat ha-Derakhim*), introduction (fol. 4[a]): השער הי"ד בבליטת הרחם. → NM 4:27.

• בליטת הרקה ‣ **cheekbone; upper part of the cheek:** Arab. وجنة · Ibn Sīnā, *K. al-Qānūn fī al-ṭibb* · trans. Nathan ha-Me'ati (*Sefer ha-Qanun*), bk. 1 (fol. 44[b]): ואמנם יורדים מצד בליטת הרקה כי תנועתם אליהם. → NM 4:27.

בְּלִיעָה • בית הבליעה → **בַּיִת**.

בָּלַל · **to moisten**: Arab. بلّ · Ibn al-Jazzār, *Zād al-musāfir wa-qūt al-ḥādir* · trans. Moses ibn Tibbon (*Sefer Ṣedat ha-Derakhim*), bk. 7, 26.5: תאר אבק לסוקרא או למי שהוכה בסיף או סכין או במקל: יקח אלובי ומירא ואמוניאק וסרקא קולא מ״א אוקיא וירדיט וסוכר קשה מ״א שני שקלים יודק היטב וימלא בו הנגע או הסוקרא ואחר כן יבלול חתיכת בגד דק ברוק ויושם עליו. → NM 1:53–4.

• *Hofʿal* **הֻבְלַל** · **to become moist**: Arab. ابتلّ · Maimonides, *Šarḥ fuṣūl Abūqrāṭ* · trans. Moses ibn Tibbon (*Pirqei Abuqraṭ*), 6.59 (351): אמר המפרש: בעבור הליחה ההיא המדובקת יובללו המיתרים ויקל להוקע כף הירך. → NM 3:37.

בֵּן • *Plur.* **בנים** • **חלקות חבני מעים** → **חֲלָקוֹת**.

בסליק → **באסליק**.

בֹּסֶר • **תבשיל בסר הכרם** → **תַּבְשִׁיל**.

[בעבע] • *Nitpaʿel* **נִתְבַּעְבֵּעַ** • **נתבעבע הצמח** · **to break out in open ulceration**: Arab. تقرّح · Al-Zahrāwī, *K. al-taṣrīf li-man ʿağiza ʿan al-taʾlīf* · trans. Shem Tov ben Isaac (*Sefer ha-Shimmush*), bk. 30, introduction (fol. 201b): וראיתי רופא אחר דקר צמח סרטני ונתבעבע הצמח אחר ימים. → NM 1:80.

בַּעַל • **בעל הטחול** · **a splenetic patient**: Arab. المطحول / Gr. σπληνώδης · Maimonides, *Šarḥ fuṣūl Abūqrāṭ* · trans. Moses ibn Tibbon (*Pirqei Abuqraṭ*), 6.43 (335): אמר אבקראט: כשימצא בעל הטחול שלשול דם וארך בו יתחדש בו שקוי או קלוח המעים וימות. → NM 3:37.

• *Plur.* **בעלים** • **בעלי מוגלא** · **those suffering from an empyema**: Arab. المتقيّحون · Hippocrates, *Aphorisms* · trans. Nathan ha-Me'ati, 6.27 (319) (fol. 113b): אמר אבקראט: כשיכוה או יכרת דבר מבעלי המוגלא ובעלי השקוי ויזול מהם מוגלא או מן המים דבר רב בבת אחת הנה הוא ימות בלי ספק. → NM 3:37–8.

• **בעלי העמל** · **those who do physical exercise**: Arab. أصحاب رياضة · Maimonides, *Šarḥ fuṣūl Abūqrāṭ* · trans. Moses ibn Tibbon (*Pirqei Abuqraṭ*), 1.3 (30): אמר אבקראט: שומן הגוף המופלג לבעלי העמל סכנה כאשר הגיעו ממנה בתכלית האחרון. → NM 3:176–7.

• **בעלי שקוי** · **dropsy patients**: Lat. hydropici · Hippocrates, *Aphorisms* · trans. Hillel ben Samuel, 6.27 (319) (fol. 40b): א״א: כל אימפיסי וכל בעלי שקוי יעשו רויה או יררחו ותצא בחוץ מוגלא או מים רבים ימותו פתאום. → NM 3:38.

בַּעֲלָה • **בעלת הצד** · **pleuritis**: Arab. ذات الجنب · Maimonides, *K. al-fuṣūl fī al-ṭibb* · trans. Nathan ha-Me'ati (*Sefer ha-Peraqim*), 6.40: לפעמים יזלו בקצת החליים החדים ליחות רעות אל הריאה ויהיה שעורם מועט ולא יחדשו מורסא ויצאו ברקיקה ויחשב מי שאין לו הרגל שיש בעלול בעלת הצד ובעלת הריאה ואינם בו. → NM 2:32.

• **בעלת הריאה** · **pneumonia**: Arab. ذات الرئة · Maimonides, *K. al-fuṣūl fī al-ṭibb* · trans. Nathan ha-Me'ati (*Sefer ha-Peraqim*), 6.40: לפעמים יזלו בקצת החליים החדים ליחות רעות אל הריאה ויהיה שעורם מועט ולא יחדשו מורסא ויצאו ברקיקה ויחשב מי שאין לו הרגל שיש בעלול בעלת הצד ובעלת הריאה ואינם בו. → NM 2:32.

בְּעֵרָה · **heat**: Lat. cauma · Arab. التهاب · Hippocrates, *Aphorisms* · trans. Hillel ben Samuel, 4.65 (202) (fol. 27b): א״א: בקדחת בערה רבה קרוב לבטן נשיכה בלב רע. → NM 3:38.

בצלי • **המכסה הבצלי** → **מִכְסֶה**.

בָּצֵק • **הגבנה הטפלה בבצק** → **גְּבִנָּה**.

בְּקִיעָה · **hernia:** a) Arab. فتق · i. Ibn al-Jazzār, *Zād al-musāfir wa-qūt al-ḥādir* · trans. Moses ibn Tibbon (*Sefer Ṣedat ha-Derakhim*), introduction (fol. 4[a]): השער הח' בבקיעה המתילד בביצים. → NM 4:28.

· ii. Maimonides, *K. al-fuṣūl fī al-ṭibb* · trans. Zeraḥyah Ḥen (*Sefer ha-Peraqim*), 9. 123: זכר התמימי בספר הנקרא אלמרשד זה העניין מרפואת הבקיעה קודם שיאריך. → NM 1:132.

· iii. Maimonides, *K. al-fuṣūl fī al-ṭibb* · trans. Nathan ha-Me'ati (*Sefer ha-Peraqim*), 9.123: זכר החכם אלתמימי בספר נקרא אלמרשד כלומר המיישר זה הענין מרפואת הבקיעה קודם שתתישן. → NM 2:32.

b) Lat. crepatura · Al-Rāzī, attr., *On the Treatment of Small Children* · trans. Bonfos, ch. 21: בבקיעת הילדים. כבר אמרנו מכמה סבות יקרה הבקיעה ולא נצטרך כי אם ברפואות פשוטות מצטרכות. → NM 2:177.

• **בקיעת דם** · **hemorrhage:** Arab. انفجار الدم / Gr. αἱμορραγεῖν · Hippocrates, *Aphorisms* · trans. Nathan ha-Me'ati, 5.19 (239) (fol. 89[b]): אמר אבוקרט: כל מקום שנתקרר ראוי שיחומם אם לא שיפוחד עליו בקיעת דם ממנו. → NM 3:38–9.

• **בקיעת השפתים** · **lip fissures:** Arab. تشقيق الشفتين · Ibn al-Jazzār, *Zād al-musāfir wa-qūt al-ḥādir* · trans. Moses ibn Tibbon (*Sefer Ṣedat ha-Derakhim*), introduction (fol. 2[b]): השער הי"ו בבקיעת השפתים. → NM 4:28.

[בקע] • *Nif'al* **נִבְקַע** · **to be incised:** Arab. بُطّ / Gr. τέμνω, Pass. τέμνομαι · Maimonides, *Šarḥ fuṣūl Abūqrāṭ* · trans. Moses ibn Tibbon (*Pirqei Abuqraṭ*), 6.27 (319): אמר אבקראט: מי שנכוה או נבקע מן הנפוחים או המשוקים ויגר ממנו מן החומר או מן המים שעור רב פתאום הנה הוא ימות בלא ספק. → NM 3:39.

בָּקָר • **שפות הבקר** → שְׂפוֹת.

בַּר • **שור הבר** → שׁוֹר.

בַּרְזֶל · I. **scalpel:** a) Arab. مبضع · Ibn al-Jazzār, *Zād al-musāfir wa-qūt al-ḥādir* · trans. Moses ibn Tibbon (*Sefer Ṣedat ha-Derakhim*), bk. 7, 13.3: ואם היה צר הנה ראוי שנפתח שפתיו בברזל ונרחיב ראשו ונשרוט סביב הנגע שריטות גדולות כדי שיצא הדם יציאה רבה או יכוה המקום באש כי היא תעצור ותעכב הארס ממרוצת הגרתו וימנענו מהכנס תוך הגוף. → NM 1:54.

b) Arab. حديدة · Ibn al-Jazzār, *Zād al-musāfir wa-qūt al-ḥādir* · trans. Moses ibn Tibbon (*Sefer Ṣedat ha-Derakhim*), bk. 7, 16.3: ואם סרו במה שזכרנו טוב ואם לא יעקרם בברזל או בכויה ויכוה בקני הדס כמו שאמר אפלטון. → NM 1:54.

· II. **surgery:** Arab. حديد · Maimonides, *K. al-fuṣūl fī al-ṭibb* · trans. Nathan ha-Me'ati (*Sefer ha-Peraqim*), 15.18: אם אתה רשאי לרפאת הסרטאן בברזל אז שים התחלתך הרקת הליחה השחורית בשלשול. → NM 2:33.

• **כלי ברזל** → כְּלִי.

• **הכריתה בברזל** → כְּרִיתָה.

• **רפואות הברזל** → רְפוּאָה.

בְּרִיאוּת · I. **correctness:** Arab. صحّة · Maimonides, *Šarḥ fuṣūl Abūqrāṭ* · trans. Zeraḥyah Ḥen (*Pirqei Abuqraṭ*), 4.76 (213): ורפואת זה החולי יורה על בריאות ההקש בסבתו כי אותם שקרה להם זה החולי אמנם נתרפאו ברפואה המחתכת. → NM 3:39.

· II. recovery: Lat. sanitas / Arab. برؤ / Gr. ὑγίεια · Hippocrates, *Aphorisms* · trans. Hillel ben Samuel, 2.19 (71) (fol. 10[a]): א״א: הקדמת ההכרה בחלאים החדים בכלם אינה אמיתית הן לא מהבריאות ולא מהמות. → NM 3:39.

[ברק] • *Hif'il* **הִבְרִיק** · **to become pale; to turn yellow**: Arab. اصفرّ · Galen, attr., *Prohibition of Burial* · trans. Judah al-Ḥarizi (*Sefer Issur ha-Qevurah le-Galienus*), par. 142: ואות מי שיקרהו זה כי שיניו יהיו דופקות ועצביו יתקבצו וידיו ורגליו יזיעו ויבריק חוטמם. → NM 4:28.

בִּשּׁוּל · **digestion**: Arab. هضم · Maimonides, *Šarḥ fuṣūl Abūqrāṭ* · trans. Moses ibn Tibbon (*Pirqei Abuqraṭ*), 2.7 (59): ואולם הגופות אשר רזו וכחשו בזמן ארוך הנה כבר נתך מהם הבשר והודק וחלשו מהם שאר האיברים אשר בהם יהיה הבשול והתפזר המזון בגוף והולדת הדם ולא יוכלו שיבשלו מן המזון השעור אשר יצטרך אליו הגוף. → NM 3:39–40.

• **בשול המחלה** · **crisis**: Hippocrates, *Aphorisms* · trans. Do'eg ha-Edomi (*Sefer Agur*), 2.12 (64) (fol. 36[a]): דעתך שים להכיר בישול המחלה ואז כפי הכח תתיר המאכל. → NM 3:40.

• **רוע בשול** → **רֹעַ**.

• **רוע בשול האצטומכא** → **רֹעַ**.

• **תירוש ענבים קרוש בבשול** → **תִּירוֹשׁ**.

בָּשׂוֹם · **aroma**: Arab. عطرية · Al-Zahrāwī, *K. al-taṣrīf li-man ʿağiza ʿan at-taʾlīf* · trans. Shem Tov ben Isaac (*Sefer ha-Shimmush*), bk. 27, fol. 131[a], col. b: ויש לו סגולה מופלאה איננה לשאר היינות כי כשישתה נודף ריחו ובשומו מבגדי שותהו. → NM 4:28.

בשורה → **בְּשֹׂרָה**.

[בשל] • *Part. Pi'el* **מְבַשֵּׁל** • **הסם המבשל** → **סַם**.

• *Part. Pu'al* **מְבֻשָּׁל** • **יין מבושל עד שׁשב כדבש** → **יַיִן**.

• **(ה)תירוש (ה)מבושל** → **תִּירוֹשׁ**.

• *Hitpa'el* **הִתְבַּשֵּׁל** · **to suppurate**: Arab. تقيّح / Gr. διαπυέω · Hippocrates, *Aphorisms* · trans. Do'eg ha-Edomi (*Sefer Agur*), 4.82 (219) (fol. 36[a]): אמר אבקראט: מי שיצא באמתו מורסא הנה כאשר תתבשל ותפתח יתך חליו. → NM 3:40.

בְּשָׂמוּת · **fragrance**: Arab. عطرية · Maimonides, *K. al-fuṣūl fī al-ṭibb* · trans. Zeraḥyah Ḥen (*Sefer ha-Peraqim*), 20.75: הפירה יחזק האסטומכא ויש להם סגולה שהם מכבים הצמא כשהם נאכלים אחר המזון ומיצם כשיונח ישוב חומץ שיחזק האסטומכא חיזוק מופלא ולא יזיק בעצבים מפני שיש בו מן הקיבוץ והבשמות. → NM 1:132–3.

בָּשְׂמִיּוּת · **aroma**: Arab. عطرية · Ibn Sīnā, *K. al-adwiya al-qalbiya* · trans. Anonymous (*Sammim Libbiyim*), fol. 126[a]: ויש לו עם זה דקות והוא בסבת הבושמיות אשר בו נאות לעצם הרוח [ו]למה שיש בו מן הקביצות עם הדקות מקשר אותו מנקה לעצמיותו מפשיט אותו. → NM 4:28–9.

[בשר] • *Pi'el* **בִּשֵּׂר** · **to indicate**: Arab. أنذر · Hippocrates, *Aphorisms* · trans. Nathan ha-Me'ati, 2.28 (80) (fol. 31[b]): אמר אבוקרט: מי שיהיה בו קדחת איננה קשה מאד אם ישאר גופו על ענינו ולא יחסר דבר ממנו או שימס ביותר ממה שראוי יהיה זה רע כי הראשון מבשר באורך מן החולי והשני מורה על חולשה מן הכח. → NM 3:41.

• *Part. Pi'el* **מְבַשֵּׂר** · **[day of] announcement (warning) (i.e., indicatory [day])**: a) Arab. إنذار · Maimonides, *K. al-fuṣūl fī al-ṭibb* · trans. Nathan ha-Me'ati (*Sefer ha-*

Peraqim), 11.13: האותות המורים על טוב הבחראן ההוה עתה הם חמשה: הראשון שבהם והיותר גדול שבהם הוא הקדמת הבשול ולא ראיתי אחד שמת מאותם שבאהו הבחראן אחר הבשול. והשני שיהיה ביום מימי הבחראן. השלישי שיקדימהו מבשר ביום מחובר אליו. והרביעי שיהיה הבחראן קל ונקל. והחמישי שתהיה ההרקה דומה לטבע החולי ופונה לצדו. → NM 2:56.

b) Galen, *De diebus decretoriis* · trans. Shimshon ben Shlomo (*Qibbușei Ma'amarei Galenus bi-Yemei ha-Buḥran*), 18: הבחראן השלם והבחראן החסר: וכבר ראוי שיתקבץ בבחראן שיהיה שלם ושיהיה שמור ושיהיה ביום הבחראן בטוח ושיהיה מבואר ואשר לו מבשר. → NM 2:172–3.

• **יום מבשר** → **יוֹם**.

בָּשָׂר · **pulp (of fruit)**: Arab. شحم · Ibn al-Jazzār, *Zād al-musāfir wa-qūt al-ḥādir* · trans. Moses ibn Tibbon (*Sefer Ṣedat ha-Derakhim*), bk. 2, ch. 18 (fol. 60[b]): ואם היה כאב השנים מפני קור ... או יבשל בשר קולוקונטידא או עורקיו בחומץ ויגמא אותו. → NM 4:29.

• **אגודות הבשר** → **אֲגֻדָּה**.

• **הגרת הבשר בכיס** → **הַגָּרָה**.

• **כיס הבשר** → **כִּיס**.

• **מורסת הבשר חרך** → **מֻרְסָא**.

• **מורסת הבשר הרפה** → **מֻרְסָא**.

• **הבשר המליח המתובל** · **(lit., salted, spiced meat); jerked meat**: Arab. اللحم المقدد · Al-Zahrāwī, *K. al-taṣrīf li-man 'ağiza 'an at-ta'līf* · trans. Shem Tov ben Isaac (*Sefer ha-Shimmush*), bk. 27, fol. 145[a], col. a: הבשר המליח המתובל הנקרא בלשונם אלקדיד מיוחס אל הבשר החי אשר הומלח ממנו כי המלח יקנהו מותר יבשות וחמימות ואחור עכול. → NM 4:29.

• **בשר נוסף** · **nasal polyps**: Arab. بواسير / Gr. πολύπους · Ibn al-Jazzār, *Zād al-musāfir wa-qūt al-ḥādir* · trans. Moses ibn Tibbon (*Sefer Ṣedat ha-Derakhim*), bk. 2, ch. 13 (fol. 53[b]): ואם יקרה בחוטם בשר נוסף. → NM 4:29.

• **נקביות הבשר** → **נְקֵבִיּוּת**.

• **הבשר הסחוסי** · **cartilage**: Gr. χονδρός · Hippocrates, *Aphorisms* · trans. Joseph Delmedigo, 6.19 (311): העצם שנחתך או הבשר הסחוסי או העצב או החלק הדק שבלחי או הערלה לא יגדל ולא ידבק. → NM 3:40–1.

• **העגול השחור שבבשר** → **עִגּוּל**.

• **צמח בבשר דומה לדמיון הבשר** → **צֶמַח**.

• **בשר השינים** · **gums**: Lat. gingiva, *Plur.* gingivae · Hippocrates, *Aphorisms* · trans. Hillel ben Samuel, 3.25 (131) (fol. 19[a]): א"א: כשצומחים שיניהם יקרה להם חכוך בשר השינים וקדחות וקווץ ודיאריאה וביחוד כשיצמחו השינים הכלביים ובשמן מן הנערים ואשר בטנם עצור. → NM 3:41.

• **הבשר השלוק** · **dish with boiled meat**: Arab. اللحم المسلوق · Al-Zahrāwī, *K. al-taṣrīf li-man 'ağiza 'an at-ta'līf* · trans. Shem Tov ben Isaac (*Sefer ha-Shimmush*), bk. 27, fol. 145[b], col. a: הבשר השלוק וקוראים אותו אנשי המזרח אספגדבאג'ה ואנחנו קוראים אותו גם כן שלוק האשכנז והוא חם בשוי ונאות ברוב העתים והענינים לכל בני אדם לבד מי שיגבר על מזגו החמימות ובעתים החמים מאד ולמי שיש לו אסתניסות והפוך נפש. → NM 4:29–30.

• תלוליות של בשר → תְּלוּלִית.

• תשית הבשר → תשיה.

בְּשׂוֹרָה • ימי הבשורה → יוֹם.

בְּשָׂרִי • האשך הבשרי → אֶשֶׁךְ.

• השקוי הבשריי → שִׁקּוּי.

בַּת • **בת עין** · **eyeball**: Arab. مقلة · Ibn Sīnā, *K. al-Qānūn fī al-ṭibb* · trans. Zeraḥyah Ḥen (*Sefer ha-Qanun*), bk. 1 (fol. 23b): הפרק הרביעי בנתוח המושקולו שלבת עין. → NM 4:30.

בֶּתֶק · **opening; rupture**: Arab. فتق · Al-Zahrāwī, *K. al-taṣrīf li-man ʿağiza ʿan at-taʾlīf* · trans. Shem Tov ben Isaac (*Sefer ha-Shimmush*), bk. 30, 2.65 (220a): שער ס"ה ברפואת האשך המעיי. התחדש זה האשך יהיה מבקוע יקרה בקרום הנמתח על הבטן לעמת עיקרי הירכים וישפך המעי מן הבתק ההוא אל אחד מן הבצים. → NM 1:80.

ג

גַּב • **גב הערוה** · I. **hip bone; pubic bone:** Arab. عظم العانة · Ibn Sīnā, *K. al-Qānūn fī al-ṭibb* · trans. Nathan ha-Me'ati (*Sefer ha-Qanun*), bk. 1 (fol. 60[a]): ובעבור כי אין לעצלים הצומחים מצד עצבי גב הערוה דרך ⟨אל⟩ הרגלים מאחורי הגוף ומפנימי הפחדים לרוב מה שיש שם מן העצלים והעורקים. → NM 4:30.

· II. **lower abdomen:** Arab. ثنة · Hippocrates, *Aphorisms* · trans. Nathan ha-Me'ati, 2.35 (87) (fol. 35[a]): אמר אבוקרט: הנה היותר טוב בכל חולי שיהיה מה שנטה לטבור ולגב הערוה ויש לו עובי. → NM 3:42.

· III. **pubes:** Arab. عانة · a) Maimonides, *K. al-fuṣūl fī al-ṭibb* · trans. Nathan ha-Me'ati (*Sefer ha-Peraqim*), 1.67: צמיחת האמה היא מעצם גב הערוה היא אלעאנה. → NM 2:33.

b) Hippocrates, *Aphorisms* · trans. Nathan ha-Me'ati, 4.80 (217) (fol. 84[b]): אמר אבוקרט: מי שישתין דם עב ויהיה בו טפטוף שתן וימצאהו כאב בשפל בטנו וגב ערותו הנה מה שהוא אצל מקותו כואב. → NM 3:42.

• **עצמות גב הערוה** → **עֶצֶם**.

• **צמיחת השער בגב הערוה** → **צְמִיחָה**.

גְּבוּל · **crisis:** Arab. بحران · Maimonides, *K. al-fuṣūl fī al-ṭibb* · trans. Nathan ha-Me'ati (*Sefer ha-Peraqim*), introduction: המאמר האחד עשר פרקים כוללים בעתות החלאים וגבוליהם הנקראים בחראנים. → NM 2:33.

[גבל] • *Nif'al* **נִגְבַּל** · **to come to a crisis:** Gr. κρίνομαι · a) Hippocrates, *Aphorisms* · trans. Joseph Delmedigo, 2.23 (75): החולאים החדים נגבלים בארבעה עשר יום → NM 3:42.

b) Hippocrates, *Aphorisms* · trans. Joseph Delmedigo, 4.59 (196): הקדחת השלישית האמתית היותר ארוכה שתהיה נגבלת בשבע הקפות. → NM 3:42.

• *Hif'il* **הִגְבִּיל** · **to bring to a crisis:** Hippocrates, *Aphorisms* · trans. Judah Shalom, 4.36 (173) (fol. 62[a]): הזיעות במוקדחים טובות אם מתחילות בשלישי ובחמישי ובשביעי ובתשיעי ובאחד עשר ובארבעה עשר ובשבעה עשר ובעשרים ובארבעה ועשרים ובשלושים וארבעה כי אלו הזיעות מגבילות החליים ואשר בלתי נעשות כך מורות יגיעה ואורך החולי וחזרה. → NM 3:42–3.

• *Hof'al* **הֻגְבַּל** · **to come to a crisis:** Hippocrates, *Aphorisms* · trans. Judah Shalom, 4.59 (196) (fol. 67[a]): השלישית היותר ארוכה תוגבל בשבעה הקפים. → NM 3:43.

[גבן] • *Part. Pu'al* **מְגֻבָּן** · **convex:** Arab. محدّب · Maimonides, *K. al-fuṣūl fī al-ṭibb* · trans. Nathan ha-Me'ati (*Sefer ha-Peraqim*), 1.16: אותו שימהר אליו סתימה בכבדו הוא שיהיו צרים קצוות העורקים אשר יעלה בהם המזון מהצד המקוער מן הכבד אל הצד המגובן. → NM 2:57.

• *Hitpa'el* **הִתְגַּבֵּן** · **to become convex:** Arab. احدودب · Maimonides, *K. al-fuṣūl fī al-ṭibb* · trans. Nathan ha-Me'ati (*Sefer ha-Peraqim*), 1.70: ויסתר אז הגבנינות במקומות הנטמנים והנשפלים וכשיתרפו יתגבנו. → NM 2:33–4.

גְּבִנָּה • **הגבננה הטפלה בבצק** · **cheese pie** (some are filled with cheese and fried and others baked in the oven); **a pastry made from meal and cheese:** Arab. الجبّنة · Al-Zahrāwī, *K. al-taṣrīf li-man ʿağiza ʿan at-taʾlīf* · trans. Shem Tov ben Isaac (*Sefer ha-Shimmush*), bk. 27, fol. 147b, col. a: הגבנה הטפלה בבצק וקלויה בשמן ראוי להיות בצקה שוה השאור. → NM 4:30.

• מי הגבנה → מַיִם.

גַּבְנוּת · **hunchback:** a) Arab. حدب · Ibn al-Jazzār, *Zād al-musāfir wa-qūt al-ḥādir* · trans. Moses ibn Tibbon (*Sefer Ṣedat ha-Derakhim*), bk. 1, ch. 23 (fol. 35b): תאר גרגרי אבפורבי למה שתקנו יצחק מועיל מן הפלג שסבתו הקור והרעש ורוח הגבנות ולכל חולי יתילד בפרקים ממותר עב וניסיתיהו. → NM 4:30–1.

b) Arab. حدبة · Maimonides, *Šarḥ fuṣūl Abūqrāṭ* · trans. Zeraḥyah Ḥen (*Pirqei Abuqraṭ*), 6.46 (338): אמר בקראט: מי שמצאו גבנות מפני שעול הנק׳ רבו או שעול אחר קודם שיגדל זה ימות. → NM 3:43.

גַּבְנִינוּת · **hunchback:** Arab. حدبة / Gr. ὗβος · Hippocrates, *Aphorisms* · trans. Nathan ha-Me'ati, 6.46 (338) (fol. 121b): אמר אבוקרט: מי שימצאהו גבנינות מן גניחה ושעול קודם שיצמח השער הנה הוא ימות. → NM 3:43.

[גבר] • *Hitpa'el* **הִתְגַּבֵּר** · **to boil (over); to bubble; to simmer:** Arab. فار · Ibn al-Jazzār, *Zād al-musāfir wa-qūt al-ḥādir* · trans. Moses ibn Tibbon (*Sefer Ṣedat ha-Derakhim*), bk. 1, ch. 18 (fol. 26a): ותתילד משתי סבות אחת מהן התלהבות מרה כרכומית והתלקח בחלקי המוח והאחרת מרתיחת דם הלב והתגברו כי דם הלב כשירתח ויתלהב בחום מרה אדומה יתגבר ויעלה חזקתו אל הראש. → NM 4:31.

גָּדוֹל • **הקנה הגדול** → קָנֶה.

• **קצה העין הגדול** → קָצֶה.

• **התולעים הגדולים** → תּוֹלַעַת.

[גדל] • *Part. Pi'el* **מְגַדֵּל** • **האברים המגדלים** → אֵבֶר.

גדמי • **הצרעת הגדמיית** → צָרַעַת.

גומות → גֻּמְמוּת.

גומי → גֻּמְמִי.

[גוס] • *Hif'il* **הֵגִיס** · **to stir:** Arab. ضرب · Ibn al-Jazzār, *Zād al-musāfir wa-qūt al-ḥādir* · trans. Moses ibn Tibbon (*Sefer Ṣedat ha-Derakhim*), bk. 2, ch. 13 (fol. 53a): ויגיס אותו עד שישוב אספלנית. → NM 4:31.

גּוּף · **cavity:** Lat. venter / Arab. جوف · Hippocrates, *Aphorisms* · trans. Hillel ben Samuel, 7.38 (390) (fol. 46b): הנזילות היורדות אל עליוני הגוף באות לידי מוגלה בעשרים יום. → NM 3:43–4.

• **ביטול הגוף** → בִּטּוּל.

• **ביטול חצי הגוף** → בִּטּוּל.

• **מורך הגוף** → מֹרֶךְ.

• **תרדמת הגוף** → תַּרְדֵּמָה.

גָּזַר • **הקדים הגזר דין** → קָדַם.

גָּזַר • **גזר אומר** · **to make a definite statement:** Arab. أطلق القضيّة · Maimonides, *Šarḥ fuṣūl Abūqrāṭ* · trans. Anonymous (*Pirqei Abuqraṭ*), 5.40 (260): אמר המפרש: הקרוב אצלי שראה זה פעם או פעמים וגזר אומר כמו שנהג מנהגו בספר אפידימיא. → NM 3:44.

• *Inf.* **גְּזוֹר** • **החקדמה לגזור** → הַקְדָּמָה.

גְּזָרָה • **incision**: Arab. قَطْع • Al-Zahrāwī, *K. al-taṣrīf li-man ʿağiza ʿan at-taʾlīf* • trans. Shem Tov ben Isaac (*Sefer ha-Shimmush*), bk. 30, 2.95 (fol. 228ᵇ): ואחר להרים היד בגיד ובעור כלפי מעלה ולגזור הגיד עם העור לשנים ולהיות הגזרה שתי אצבעות מצומצמות. → NM 1:81.

גַּחֶלֶת • **carbuncle**: Arab. جمر • a) Maimonides, *K. al-fuṣūl fī al-ṭibb* • trans. Zeraḥyah Ḥen (*Sefer ha-Peraqim*), 23.38: הגחלת הוא מן המורסות החמות אלא שתולדת הגחלת תהיה בקרות לדם כמו הרתיחה עד שהעור יהיה נשרף ויחדש עם זה קרושטא. → NM 1:133.

b) Maimonides, *K. al-fuṣūl fī al-ṭibb* • trans. Nathan ha-Meʾati (*Sefer ha-Peraqim*), 23.38: הגחלת הוא מן המורסות החדות אלא שהולד הגחלת יהיה כשיקרה לדם דומה לרתיחה עד ששורף העור ויחדש עם זה כשכרישה. → NM 2:34.

גִּיד • I. **artery**: Arab. شريان • Al-Zahrāwī, *K. al-taṣrīf li-man ʿağiza ʿan at-taʾlīf* • trans. Shem Tov ben Isaac (*Sefer ha-Shimmush*), bk. 30, 2.42 (fol. 215ᵇ). → NM 1:81.

• II. **penis**: a) Lat. virga • Bruno Longobucco, *Cyrurgia Magna* • trans. Hillel ben Samuel (*Sefer Keritut*), fol. 97ᵃ: שער ארבע עשר. מן הוורוג׳׳ והפורי הבאים בגיד. → NM 1:18.

b) Arab. قضيب • i. Al-Zahrāwī, *K. al-taṣrīf li-man ʿağiza ʿan at-taʾlīf* • trans. Shem Tov ben Isaac (*Sefer ha-Shimmush*), bk. 30, 2.70 (fol. 220ᵇ): אמנם בנשים הוא מין אחד ויהיו למעלה מן הקיבה על הזקן התחתון כבצי אדם קטנים בולטים לחוץ האחד מהם כגיד האדם והבצים כבציו. → NM 1:81.

• ii. Maimonides, *K. al-fuṣūl fī al-ṭibb* • trans. Zeraḥyah Ḥen (*Sefer ha-Peraqim*), 16.10: כל הגידים הדופקים ושאינם דופקים בכל הגוף מהזכרים והנקיבות הם על דמיון אחד לא במספר לבדו אלא ביצירתם ותכונתם ומקומם אבל ישתנו בכלי ההריון ויתבאר בניתוח כי כלי ההריון בזכרים ובנקבות זה נוכח זה בדמיון כי בזכרים יוצאים ובנקבות הם בפנים עד שהרחם אילו נתהפך שטחו הפנימי לחוץ היה דומה לכיס הביצים והביצים אשר בצדי הרחם יהיו בתוך כיס ויהיה צואר הרחם דומה לגיד. → NM 1:133.

• III. **vein; vessel**: Arab. عرق • a) Al-Zahrāwī, *K. al-taṣrīf li-man ʿağiza ʿan at-taʾlīf* • trans. Shem Tov ben Isaac (*Sefer ha-Shimmush*), bk. 30, 1.35 (206ᵇ): הגיד אשר יגר ממנו הדם. → NM 1:81

b) Al-Zahrāwī, *K. al-taṣrīf li-man ʿağiza ʿan at-taʾlīf* • trans. Shem Tov ben Isaac (*Sefer ha-Shimmush*), bk. 30, 2.95 (228ᵇ): הקזת הגידים. → NM 1:81.

• **הגיד האמצעי** • **the median cubital vein**: Arab. الأكحل • Ibn al-Jazzār, *Zād al-musāfir wa-qūt al-ḥādir* • trans. Moses ibn Tibbon (*Sefer Ṣedat ha-Derakhim*), bk. 7, 17.3: ואם ראינו שהדם הוא הגובר נצוה להקיז הגיד האמצעי אם לא ימנע ממנו מונע ויצא הדם כל זמן שהתמיד לצאת נפסד והכח סובל אותו. → NM 1:54.

• **גיד הדופק** • **artery**: Arab. العرق • Maimonides, *K. al-fuṣūl fī al-ṭibb* • trans. Zeraḥyah Ḥen (*Sefer ha-Peraqim*), 4.21: בהיות בגיד הדופק רוע המזג משתנה כי החלק ממנו שהוא יותר לחות וחמימות יהיה דפקו יותר גדול ויותר מהיר. → NM 1:134.

• **הגיד הדופק הורידי** • **pulmonary vein; venous artery**: Arab. الشريان الوريدي • Ibn Sīnā, *K. al-Qānūn fī al-ṭibb* • trans. Joseph Lorki (*Sefer ha-Qanun*), bk. 1 (fol. 18ᵃ): ולכן נקרא הגיד הדופק הורידי. → NM 4:31.

• **הגיד הורידי** • **pulmonary vein; venous artery**: Arab. الشريان الوريدي • Ibn Sīnā, *K. al-*

Qānūn fī al-ṭibb · trans. Zeraḥyah Ḥen (*Sefer ha-Qanun*), bk. 1 (fol. 32[a]): ועל כן נקרא הגיד הורידי. → NM 4:31.

• **הגיד המדני** ‧ **the Medina vein**: Arab. العرق المدني / Lat. dracunculus medinensis · Al-Zahrāwī, *K. al-taṣrīf li-man ʿağiza ʿan at-taʾlīf* · trans. Shem Tov ben Isaac (*Sefer ha-Shimmush*), bk. 30, 2.91 (fol. 227[b]): בהוצאת הגיד המדני. → NM 1:82.

• **הגיד העליון** ‧ **cephalic vein**: Arab. القيفال · Ibn al-Jazzār, *Zād al-musāfir wa-qūt al-ḥādir* · trans. Moses ibn Tibbon (*Sefer Ṣedat ha-Derakhim*), bk. 1, ch. 3 (fol. 8[b]): ויקיז הגיד העליון אם יעזור הזמן והשנים והמנהג והכח ויוציא מן הדם בשיעור כדי שיצא עמו מה שיהיה ממותר חד. → NM 4:31.

• **גיד הערוה** ‧ **urethra**: Hippocrates, *Aphorisms* · trans. Doʾeg ha-Edomi (*Sefer Agur*), 4.82 (219) (fol. 79[a]): אמר אפוקרט: למי שצמח לו שחין בתוך גיד הערוה כאשר יעלה נפח ויצא עם השתן עב טיט קרבה רפואתו. → NM 3:44.

• **קצה הגיד** → קָצֶה.

• **קצה גיד הערוה** → קָצֶה.

• **גיד הראש** ‧ **cephalic vein**: Arab. القيفال · a) Al-Zahrāwī, *K. al-taṣrīf li-man ʿağiza ʿan at-taʾlīf* · trans. Shem Tov ben Isaac (*Sefer ha-Shimmush*), bk. 30, 2.95 (fol. 229[a]): ושני הגידים אשר תחת הלשון תועלת הקזתם אחר הקזת גיד הראש אל החניקה אשר תהיה בגרון וחלי ערלתו ותחלאי הפה. → NM 1:82.

b) Ibn al-Jazzār, *Zād al-musāfir wa-qūt al-ḥādir* · trans. Moses ibn Tibbon (*Sefer Ṣedat ha-Derakhim*), bk. 1, ch. 1 (fol. 5[a]): ואם היה מראה המקום אדום נדע שהוא ממותר דם נפסד ואם עזר הזמן והשנים והמנהג והכח נקיז לו גיד הראש ונוציא מן הדם בשיעור הצורך והכח. → NM 4:31–2.

• **גיד הראש הנקרא אכחל** ‧ **median vein**: Arab. الأكحل · Ibn Sīnā, *K. al-Qānūn fī al-ṭibb* · trans. Zeraḥyah Ḥen (*Sefer ha-Qanun*), bk. 1 (fol. 34[b]): והרביעי הוא היותר גדול והוא אשר הוא נראה ויעלה וישתלח לשעיפים יתחבר שעיף מן הקיפל ויבא מהם גיד הראש הנקרא אכחל והנשאר הוא הנקר׳ באסאליק. → NM 4:32.

• *Plur.* **גידים** ‧ I. **nerves**: Lat. nervus · Bruno Longobucco, *Cyrurgia Magna* · trans. Hillel ben Samuel (*Sefer Keritut*), fol. 5[a]: כגון בבשר ובגידים ובורדים. → NM 1:18.

‧ II. **vessels**: Arab. عروق · Maimonides, *K. al-fuṣūl fī al-ṭibb* · trans. Zeraḥyah Ḥen (*Sefer ha-Peraqim*), 6.6: הגידים הנראים יהיו מליאים מתמשכים ולא יהיו הפנימיים כן. → NM 1:133–4.

• **דפק הגידים** → דֹּפֶק.

• **גידי ההרגש** ‧ **nerves**: Hippocrates, *Aphorisms* · trans. Doʾeg ha-Edomi (*Sefer Agur*), 5.18 (238) (fol. 83[a]): זכור כי המים הקרים יזיקו לעצמות ולגידי ההרגש ולמוח הראש והשזרה והחמים יועילו לכל אלה. → NM 3:44.

• **הגידים הנחים** ‧ **veins**: Judah ben Jacob, *Sefer Hanhagat ha-Beriʾut*, 2.1: ועבדי הכבד הם הגידים הנחים היוצאים ממנו השולחים להם הדם הטהור והנקי להתפרנס בו. → NM 4:32.

• **נפח הגידים השפלים** → נֶפַח.

• **צנורות הגידים** → צִנּוֹר.

• **קבוץ הגידים** → קִבּוּץ.

גיעוש → גְעוּשׁ.

גירגור → גִּרְגּוּר.

ג׳לאבי • **אישרוב ג׳לאבי** → אִישְׁרוֹב.

גָּלָב • *Plur.* **גלבים** • **תער הגלבים** → תַּעַר.

גִּלְגּוּל · **dizziness:** Arab. سدر / Lat. vertigo vel scotomia · a) Ibn al-Jazzār, *Zād al-musāfir wa-qūt al-ḥādir* · trans. Moses ibn Tibbon (*Sefer Ṣedat ha-Derakhim*), bk. 1, ch. 13 (fol. 20ª): הגלגול הוא שיתדמה לאדם שמה שיראה יתגלגל סביבו ויאבד הרגש הראות פתאום עד שיחשוב שכסה כל מה שהיה רואה חשך. → NM 4:32.

b) Maimonides, *Šarḥ fuṣūl Abūqrāṭ* · trans. Zeraḥyah Ḥen (*Pirqei Abuqraṭ*), 4.17 (154): אמר המפרש: הגלגול הוא שידמה לאדם שכל מה שהוא רואה יקיף סביבו ויעדר ממנו חוש הראות פתאום עד שיחשוב שהכל יתכסה מאפילה. → NM 3:44–5.

• **גלגול הראש** · **dizziness:** Arab. دوار · a) Ibn al-Jazzār, *Zād al-musāfir wa-qūt al-ḥādir* · trans. Moses ibn Tibbon (*Sefer Ṣedat ha-Derakhim*), bk. 1, ch. 23 (fol. 35ᵇ): תאר גירא בן מאסויה לניקוי הראש מליחה לבנה ומה שיתלד ממנה מן השתוק והפלג ותרדמת האיברים וגלגול הראש. → NM 4:32–3.

b) Maimonides, *Šarḥ fuṣūl Abūqrāṭ* · trans. Zeraḥyah Ḥen (*Pirqei Abuqraṭ*), 2.37 (89): אמר המפרש: הבריאים כשעושים הקיא או השלשול יקרה להם גלגול הראש ועקיצה ויקשה עליהם מה שיצא מגופם. → NM 3:45.

גַּלְגַּל · **speculum; a surgical instrument:** Arab. لولب · Al-Zahrāwī, *K. al-taṣrīf li-man ʿağiza ʿan at-taʾlīf* · trans. Shem Tov ben Isaac (*Sefer ha-Shimmush*), bk. 30, 2.77 (fol. 222ª): זאת צורת גלגל לפתוח בו הרחם. → NM 1:82.

גֻּלְגֹּלֶת • **מדוה הגלגלת** → מַדְוֶה.

גֶּלֶד • **הגלד הענבי** · **uveal membrane:** Arab. الطبقة العنبية · Al-Zahrāwī, *K. al-taṣrīf li-man ʿağiza ʿan at-taʾlīf* · trans. Shem Tov ben Isaac (*Sefer ha-Shimmush*), bk. 30, 2.21 (fol. 212ª): כשתקרה בליטה (= בקיעה) בגלד הענבי. → NM 1:82.

גלדי · **crystalline:** Arab. جليدي · Maimonides, *K. al-fuṣūl fī al-ṭibb* · trans. Nathan ha-Meʾati (*Sefer ha-Peraqim*), 3.52: הלחות הגלדיית והבציית והזכוכיית וכן הכתונת הקרניית אין עורקים בהם כלל בשום פנים. → NM 2:34.

[גלה] • *Part. Nifʿal* **נִגְלֶה** • **הודאג הנגלה** → וּדְאג.

גְּלִידָה · **adhesion:** Arab. التحام · Al-Zahrāwī, *K. al-taṣrīf li-man ʿağiza ʿan at-taʾlīf* · trans. Shem Tov ben Isaac (*Sefer ha-Shimmush*), bk. 30, 2.63 (fols. 219ᵇ–220ª): ואם תהיה הגלידה בין כלום מן הקרומות או במה שיש בין הכיסים ראוי להפריד כל הגלידה ההיא ולחתכה חתיכות חתיכות עגולות. → NM 1:82–3.

[גלל] · *Part. Puʿal* **מְגֻלָּל** · I. **damped:** Arab. مبلول · Al-Zahrāwī, *K. al-taṣrīf li-man ʿağiza ʿan at-taʾlīf* · trans. Shem Tov ben Isaac (*Sefer ha-Shimmush*), bk. 30, 1.17 (fol. 205ª): ואחרי כן לשית צמר גפן מגולל בחלבון ביצה או בריר שיליות (= שיליום) על העין. → NM 1:99.

· II. **soaked:** a) Arab. مشرّب · Al-Zahrāwī, *K. al-taṣrīf li-man ʿağiza ʿan at-taʾlīf* · trans. Shem Tov ben Isaac (*Sefer ha-Shimmush*), bk. 30, 1.16 (fol. 204ᵇ): ולתת תחת העין צמר גפן מגולל בחלבון ביצה וראש החולה בחיק הרופא. → NM 1:99.

b) Arab. مغموس · Al-Zahrāwī, *K. al-taṣrīf li-man ʿağiza ʿan at-taʾlīf* · trans. Shem Tov ben Isaac (*Sefer ha-Shimmush*), bk. 30, 1.22 (fol. 205[b]): ולתת עליו צמר גפן מגולל בחמאה. → NM 1:99.

גָּמָא · **to rinse the mouth:** Arab. تمضمض / Gr. διακλύζω · Ibn al-Jazzār, *Zād al-musāfir wa-qūt al-ḥādir* · trans. Moses ibn Tibbon (*Sefer Ṣedat ha-Derakhim*), bk. 2, ch. 18 (fol. 60[b]): ואם היה כאב השנים מפני קור ... או יבשל בשר קולוקונטידא או עורקיו בחומץ ויגמא אותו. → NM 4:33.

גָּמוּר (*Pass. Part.*) → **גָּמַר**.

גֻּמְמוּת · **concavity:** Lat. concavitas · Bruno Longobucco, *Cyrurgia Magna* · trans. Hillel ben Samuel (*Sefer Keritut*), fol. 11[a]: ואם בחבלה יתחדש שום גוממות ועומק אז לא תהיה כוונתך על הדרך שזכרנו. → NM 1:18–9.

גֻּמְמִי • **החבלות הגממיות** → **חַבָּלָה**.

גָּמַר • **גמר מוגלא** · **to suppurate:** Lat. sanie fieri · Hippocrates, *Aphorisms* · trans. Hillel ben Samuel, 4.82 (219) (fol. 30[a]): מי שנולדו לו באמה צמחים כשתגמר המוגלא ויפתחו יותרו. → NM 3:46.

• *Pass. Part.* **גָּמוּר** · I. **indefinite:** Arab. مهمل · Maimonides, *Šarḥ fuṣūl Abūqrāṭ* · trans. Zeraḥyah Ḥen (*Pirqei Abuqraṭ*), 2.20 (72): אמר המפרש: כשתבקש על האמת תדע שזה העניין בלתי מקויים אם כן הוא פסק דינו שקר בלא ספק. והאמת אצלי כי אבקראט ראה שני אנשים או שלשה שעניינם כן ושמו כפסק דין גמור כמו שהיה מנהגו ברוב ספר פידימיאי. → NM 3:45–6.

· II. **unmixed:** Arab. صرف / Gr. ἀκρατής · Hippocrates, *Aphorisms* · trans. Nathan ha-Me'ati, 7.23 (375) (fol. 131[a]): אמר אבוקרט: ומהיציאה הגמורה שלשול הדם. → NM 3:45.

• *Nifʿal* **נִגְמַר** · **to become chronic (of an illness):** Arab. استحكم / Lat. morbi dominium · Ibn al-Jazzār, *Zād al-musāfir wa-qūt al-ḥādir* · trans. Moses ibn Tibbon (*Sefer Ṣedat ha-Derakhim*), bk. 1, ch. 18 (fol. 27[b]): ונזכיר רפואת זה לפי דרך הרפואה ונאמר כי ראוי שנקיז בעל מורסת הראש קודם שיגמר חליו. → NM 4:33.

גְּנוּחַ · **asthma:** Arab. ربو · Al-Zahrāwī, *K. al-taṣrīf li-man ʿağiza ʿan at-taʾlīf* · trans. Shem Tov ben Isaac (*Sefer ha-Shimmush*), bk. 30, 2.96 (fol. 231[a]): אמנם נתינת הרבידות על המקום הנקרא אל כאהל והוא אמצע הצואר הוא תמורת הקזת הגיד הנקרא אל אכחל ... והקזת הבאסליק ולפיכך יועילו מן הגנוח וצרות הנשימה וקריעת כלי הנשימה והשעול והמלוי. → NM 1:83.

גְּנִיחָה · **asthma:** Arab. ربو · Maimonides, *K. al-fuṣūl fī al-ṭibb* · trans. Nathan ha-Me'ati (*Sefer ha-Peraqim*), 8.19: החליים הנושנים יצטרכו אל הנהגה דקה עד שרבים מהם יספיק להם בארוכתם בהנהגה הזאת לבדה. וכבר ראיתי אנשים רבים מאותם שהיה בהם כאב פרקים והגניחה ומי שיהיה בו כפיה מעוטה יהיה בהנהגה הזאת הדקה תועלת איננו מועט. → NM 2:34–5.

גָּסוּס · **snoring (h.l., breathing stertorously):** Arab. غطيط / Gr. ῥέγκω · Maimonides, *Šarḥ fuṣūl Abūqrāṭ* · trans. Moses ibn Tibbon (*Pirqei Abuqraṭ*), 6.51 (343): אמר אבקראט: מי שהתחדש בו והוא בריא כאב פתאום בראשו ונשתתק מיד וקרה לו כמו גסוס הנה הוא ימות בשבעה ימים אם לא התחדש בו קדחת. → NM 3:46.

גָּסַס · **to snore (h.l., to breath stertorously):** Lat. sterto · Hippocrates, *Aphorisms* · trans.

Judah Shalom, 6.51 (343) (fol. 110[a]): כל מי שהוא בריא ופתאום יהיה לו כאב ראש ופתאום יהיה בבלתי קול ויגסוס הנה ימות תוך ז׳ ימים אם לא תתחדש בו קדחת. → NM 3:46.

גְּעוּשׁ • **גיעוש הנקרא רוט** › **eructation**: Arab. جشاء · Maimonides, *K. al-fuṣūl fī al-ṭibb* · trans. Nathan ha-Me'ati (*Sefer ha-Peraqim*), 7.55: כשתאכל מאכל ולא יקרה לך ממנו קרקור ולא נפח ולא רפרוף ולא פוקות אך שימצאך באסטומכה מצוק אין הרגלך בו בכיוצא בו ויכבד עליך אותו המאכל ותשתוקק שירד או שיתחדש לך גיעוש הנקרא רוט ותמצא עם זה בקצת העתים צרות הנשימה אין ספק אז שהאסטומכה כבר נתקבצה על המאכל על צד ההתגעשות. → NM 2:35; corr. 4:229.

גַּעַשׁ › **belching; eructation**: Arab. جشاء · Al-Zahrāwī, *K. al-taṣrīf li-man ʿağiza ʿan at-ta'līf* · trans. Shem Tov ben Isaac (*Sefer ha-Shimmush*), bk. 27, fol. 135[a], col. b: וכבר נאמר שהוא מעפש המזון באסטו׳ והראיה על זה געשו. → NM 4:33–4.

גֶּפֶן • *Plur.* **גפנים** › **varicose veins**: Arab. دوالي · Maimonides, *K. al-fuṣūl fī al-ṭibb* · trans. Zeraḥyah Ḥen (*Sefer ha-Peraqim*), 23.47: כל המורסות הסרטניות אמנם תהיה תולדתם ממותר מלינקוניקו. ואם יטה אותו המותר אל שפל הגוף וידחהו הכח הדוחה אשר בגידים מפיותיהם אשר בפי הטבעת או ברחם נקרא זו ההרקה טחורים שיצא מהם הדם. ולפעמים תדחה אל הרגלים ותעשה חולי הנקרא גפנים. → NM 1:134.

• **דשן גפנים** → דֶּשֶׁן.

גָּפְרִית • **גפרית חי** › **natural sulphur**: Lat. sulphur vivum · Bruno Longobucco, *Cyrurgia Magna* · trans. Hillel ben Samuel (*Sefer Keritut*), fol. 41[b]. → NM 1:19.

גָּפְרִיתִי • **המים הגפריתיים והבורקיים** → מַיִם.

גֶּפֶת › **kernels; stones**: Arab. نوى · Al-Zahrāwī, *K. al-taṣrīf li-man ʿağiza ʿan at-ta'līf* · trans. Shem Tov ben Isaac (*Sefer ha-Shimmush*), bk. 27, fol. 138[b], col. a: וכשיבוקע יתפרד מן הגפת שלו. → NM 4:34.

גָּרָב › I. **granular conjunctiva (i.e., trachoma)**: Arab. جرب · Al-Zahrāwī, *K. al-taṣrīf li-man ʿağiza ʿan at-ta'līf* · trans. Shem Tov ben Isaac (*Sefer ha-Shimmush*), bk. 30, 2.95 (fol. 229[a]): ושני הגידים אשר בראשי העינים תועלת הקזתם לתחלאי העינים מן הגרב והאדימות והגידים המסתבכים האדומים הנקראים בלשונם סבל. → NM 1:83.

› II. **itch**: Lat. scabies / Arab. جرب / Gr. ψωροφθαλμία · Al-Rāzī, attr., *On the Treatment of Small Children* · trans. Anonymous, ch. 11: ואמנם אם יקרה להם שום חולי מן החולאים האחרים כמו הגרב והלובן והדומין לאילו יונהגו עם רפואות אשר הם נאמרות בפרקי הנערות והבחרות ובאחרים אבל מהקלות בלבד. → NM 2:177.

› III. **psoriasis**: Hippocrates, *Aphorisms* · trans. Do'eg ha-Edomi (*Sefer Agur*), 4.77 (214) (fol. 78[b]): תראה השתן עב ובתוכו כמראה קליפת חטים תדין כי בתוך המקוה גרב. → NM 3:47.

› IV. **pustules**: Arab. بثور / Gr. ἐξανθήματα · Maimonides, *Šarḥ fuṣūl Abūqrāṭ* · trans. Moses ibn Tibbon (*Pirqei Abuqraṭ*), 6.9 (301): אמר אבקראט: הגרב הרחב אי אפשר שיהיה עמו חכוך. → NM 3:47.

גִּרְגּוּר • *Plur.* **גירגורים** › **gargles**: Arab. غراغر · a) Al-Zahrāwī, *K. al-taṣrīf li-man ʿağiza ʿan at-ta'līf* · trans. Shem Tov ben Isaac (*Sefer ha-Shimmush*), bk. 30, 1.6 (fol. 204[a]): כשירפא הרופא זה המין מן הנטייה במיני הג׳ירא פיקרא והעיטושים והגרגורים. → NM 1:83–4.

b) Ibn al-Jazzār, *Zād al-musāfir wa-qūt al-ḥādir* · trans. Moses ibn Tibbon (*Sefer Ṣedat ha-Derakhim*), bk. 2, ch. 7 (fol. 48[a]): ויצוק המימות המבושל בהם הסמים החמים אשר יפתחו הסתומים ויעוטש בסמים הדקים המפתחים ויגרגר בגירא פיגרא עם דבש ובגירגורים אשר ימשכו הליחה וינקו הראש. → NM 4:34.

גַּרְגַּר • *Plur.* **גרגרים • גרגרי הדלעת** · **tapeworms:** Arab. حبّ القرع · Maimonides, *K. al-fuṣūl fī al-ṭibb* · trans. Nathan ha-Me'ati (*Sefer ha-Peraqim*), 7.31: התולעים הנקראים גרגרי הדלעת והם נקראים דלועיים אוכלים כל מה שיזון בו האדם לכן מרזים הגוף. → NM 2:35.

• **גרגרי הדלועים** · **tapeworms:** Arab. حبّ القرع · a) Al-Zahrāwī, *K. al-taṣrīf li-man ʿağiza ʿan at-taʾlīf* · trans. Shem Tov ben Isaac (*Sefer ha-Shimmush*), bk. 27, fol. 141[b], col. a: ורבוי אכילתם יוציא התולעים מהבטן הנקראים גרגרי הדלועים. → NM 4:34.

b) Al-Rāzī, *K. al-Manṣūrī* · trans. Shem Tov ben Isaac (*Sefer Almansur*), Kaf 7 (44): כילדארוא: חם רך יוציא התולעים הנקראים גרגרי הדלועים. → NM 2:11.

• **הגרגרים המוסרחים** · **malodorous pills:** Arab. حبّ المنتن / Lat. fetidi pilluli · Ibn al-Jazzār, *Zād al-musāfir wa-qūt al-ḥādir* · trans. Moses ibn Tibbon (*Sefer Ṣedat ha-Derakhim*), bk. 1, ch. 23: וזה תאר הגרגרים המוסרחים לפי נסחת סאבור והוא מועיל בע"ה מן הפלג ועקום הפה וכאב הפרקים והנקרס והרוחות העבות והקולון והנאות וכאב העצבים והרפיון ויגיר הנדות והוא מנוסה עירובו יקח אלואי סיקוטרי ודיליום וקולוקונטידא וסרפי ואפופנק ואמוניאק וזרע סיקודא מ"א דרהם יקובצו אלה הסמים שחוקים ומנופים וישרה מהם מה שראוי לשרותו במי כרתי ויעשה ממנו גרגרים קטנים ויוצנעו והלקיחה מהם ב' דרהם וחצי במים חמים. → NM 4:35.

גַּרְגֶּרֶת · **throat; trachea:** Arab. حلقوم / Gr. βρόγχος · Maimonides, *Šarḥ fuṣūl Abūqrāṭ* · trans. Moses ibn Tibbon (*Pirqei Abuqraṭ*), 6.37 (329): אמר אבקראט: כשתראה המורסא בגרגרת מחוץ במי שקרה לו האסכרא יהיה אות טוב. → NM 3:47.

גַּרְגַּתְנִי · **fistula:** Arab. ناصور · Al-Zahrāwī, *K. al-taṣrīf li-man ʿağiza ʿan at-taʾlīf* · trans. Shem Tov ben Isaac (*Sefer ha-Shimmush*), bk. 30, 1.17 (fol. 205[a]): שער י"ז בכוית הגרגתני אשר יקרה בראש העין. → NM 1:84.

גָּרַד · I. **to abrade:** Arab. سحج · Maimonides, *Šarḥ fuṣūl Abūqrāṭ* · trans. Anonymous (*Pirqei Abuqraṭ*), 4.24 (161): אמ' המפר': כאשר התחיל לצאת המרה הכרכומית וגרדה את המעים או נגעה אותם ובא הדם אחר זה יתכן שיבריא זו הגרידה או זה הנגע. → NM 3:47–8.

· II. **to rub:** Arab. حكّ · Maimonides, *K. al-fuṣūl fī al-ṭibb* · trans. Zeraḥyah Ḥen (*Sefer ha-Peraqim*), 22.53: ואבן עקיק כשתשחקנו ותגרד בו השנים ילבנם וימנע איכולם. → NM 1:134.

· III. **to strip:** Arab. جرد · Al-Zahrāwī, *K. al-taṣrīf li-man ʿağiza ʿan at-taʾlīf* · trans. Shem Tov ben Isaac (*Sefer ha-Shimmush*), bk. 30, 1.17 (fol. 205[a]): ואם עברו עליו ארבעים יום ולא נרפא ראוי לתת עליו הסם החד האוכל עד שיתגלה העצם ולגרדו על מה שיבא זכרו מן המלאכה במקומו. → NM 1:84.

גֵּרָה · I. **collarbone:** Arab. ترقوة · Al-Zahrāwī, *K. al-taṣrīf li-man ʿağiza ʿan at-taʾlīf* · trans. Shem Tov ben Isaac (*Sefer ha-Shimmush*), bk. 30, 3.5 (fol. 235[a]): בחבוש הגרה כשתשתבר. → NM 1:84.

‣ II. **the weight of one barley corn (i.e., 0.05 grams):** Arab. حبّة · Ibn al-Jazzār, *Zād al-musāfir wa-qūt al-ḥādir* · trans. Moses ibn Tibbon (*Sefer Ṣedat ha-Derakhim*), bk. 2, ch. 10 (fol. 50[a]): אם יגר מן האזן מוגלא והיה עם זה כאב חזק הנה ראוי שנתחיל במה שישקיט הכאב כמו שיקח משקל קיראט אופי ומשקל שתי גרות שעוה ויתיכהו במעט שמן ורדים ויטוח ממנו בפתילה וישים אותה באזן. → NM 4:35–6.

גָּרוֹן • **חולי הגרון** → **חֳלִי**.

• **נחרת הגרון** → **נַחֲרָה**.

• **ניחור הגרון** → **נִחוּר**.

גְּרִידָה ‣ I. **abrasion:** Arab. سَحْج · Maimonides, *Šarḥ fuṣūl Abūqrāṭ* · trans. Anonymous (*Pirqei Abuqraṭ*), 4.24 (161): אמ׳ המפר׳: כאשר התחיל לצאת המרה הכרכומית וגרדה את המעים או נגעה אותם ובא הדם אחר זה יתכן שיבריא זו הגרידה או זה הנגע. → NM 3:48.

‣ II. **scarification:** Lat. scarificatio · Bruno Longobucco, *Cyrurgia Magna* · trans. Hillel ben Samuel (*Sefer Keritut*), fol. 5[a]: אבל אותה הנעשית באיברים הרכים היא נחלקת לשלשה פנים: א׳ הנעשית בבשר לבד ונקרא׳ גרידה. → NM 1:19.

‣ III. **shred:** Arab. خراطة · Maimonides, *K. al-fuṣūl fī al-ṭibb* · trans. Nathan ha-Me'ati (*Sefer ha-Peraqim*), 6.82: שלשול הדם מעלת הכבד לפעמים יתחדש פתאם. ואמנם אותו שהוא מן המעים לא יתחדש פתאם אבל יתחדש תחלה שלשול מררי עוקץ תכלית העקיצה ואחר ימשך לזה גרידת המעים ואחר יצא אחר זה עם הגרידה דם מעט. → NM 2:35–6.

• **גרידת המעים** ‣ I. **abrasion of the intestines:** Arab. سحج الأمعاء / Gr. δυσεντερία · Maimonides, *Šarḥ fuṣūl Abūqrāṭ* · trans. Anonymous (*Pirqei Abuqraṭ*), 3.30 (136): אמר אבוקרט: מי שעבר אלו השנים יקרה לו נזילה על הריאה וחולי הצד וחולי הריאה ושכחה והקדחת אשר תהיה עמה התעורה והקדחת אשר יהיה עמה ערבוב השכל וקדחת השורפת ושלשול היוצא הקיא ושלשול הארוך וגרידת המעים וחליקות המעים והתפתח פיות העורקים ממטה. → NM 3:48–9.

‣ II. **shreds of intestinal tissue:** Arab. خراطة الأمعاء · Maimonides, *K. al-fuṣūl fī al-ṭibb* · trans. Zeraḥyah Ḥen (*Sefer ha-Peraqim*), 6.82: שלשול הדם הבא מחולי הכבד יתחדש פתאום אבל אותו שיבוא מהמעים לא יתחדש פתאום אבל יתחדש שלשול מרות ינשוך בתכלית הנשיכה ואחר כן יהיה נמשך אחר זה גרידת המעים. → NM 1:134–5.

גְּרִיס • *Plur.* **גריסים** ‣ I. **the meal of the different kinds of grain (mostly barley) that was parched:** Arab. سويق / Gr. ἄλφιτον · Al-Zahrāwī, *K. al-taṣrīf li-man ʿağiza ʿan at-taʾlīf* · trans. Shem Tov ben Isaac (*Sefer ha-Shimmush*), bk. 27, fol. 124[a], col. 2: גריסי החטה חמים במעלה הראשונה יבשים באמצעה זנין מעט מזער אלא שהם יותר זנין מגריסי השעורים. → NM 4:36.

‣ II. **the meal of parched or dried mealy fruits:** Arab. سويق / Gr. ἄλφιτον · Al-Zahrāwī, *K. al-taṣrīf li-man ʿağiza ʿan at-taʾlīf* · trans. Shem Tov ben Isaac (*Sefer ha-Shimmush*), bk. 27, fol. 139[a], col. a: וגריסי המנוגבים מהם עצירתם לבטן יותר חזקה. → NM 4:36.

• **שחיקת הגריסים** → **שְׁחִיקָה**.

גריקא • **זפת גריקא** → **זֶפֶת**.

גְּרִירָה · saw cut: Arab. نَشْر · Al-Zahrāwī, *K. al-taṣrīf li-man ʿağiza ʿan at-taʾlīf* · trans. Shem Tov ben Isaac (*Sefer ha-Shimmush*), bk. 30, 2.86 (fol. 225[b]): וראוי להיות הגרירה במגרה למעלה ממקום ההפסד מעט פן יהיה בתוך העצם הפסד ולא יראה מחוץ לחוש ויביא הצורך לגררו במגרה פעם שנית. → NM 1:84–5.

גְּרִישׁ • **גריש החטה** · pounded wheat; wheat groats: Ibn Zuhr, *Regimen of Health* · trans. Jacob ibn Tibbon (*Hanhagat ha-Beri'ut le-Abu ʿAli ben Zuhr*), ch. 17: ועשית הקיא על המלוא מועיל מחולי המקוה מאד ואכילת המתיקה הידועה באכילתה והוא גריש החטה בלולה בחמאה טובה ולושה בדבש יש לה סגולה לחזק המקוה. → NM 4:36.

גְּרִישָׁה • **גרישת הבטן** · diarrhea: Arab. اسطلاق البطن / Gr. ταραχή τῆς κοιλίης · Maimonides, *Šarḥ fuṣūl Abūqrāṭ* · trans. Anonymous (*Pirqei Abuqraṭ*), 1.2 (29): אמר אבוקרט: אם היה מה שיורק מן הגוף עם גרישת הבטן והקיא אשר תהיינה נאותות מן המין אשר צריך שינוקה הגוף ממנו יועיל זה ויקל סובלו ואם לא היה כן הנה הענין להפך. → NM 3:49.

גָּרַם • **גרם אסטניסות** · to cause nausea: Arab. أغثى · Al-Rāzī, *K. al-Manṣūrī* · trans. Shem Tov ben Isaac (*Sefer Almansur*), Ḥet 3 (36): חב אלניל ובלע' גראנא דאינדי וב״ח גרגרי האיסטיס: ישלשל הליחה הלבנה ויועיל מן הצרעת והבהק הלבן אלא שהוא יצער וגורם אסטניסות. → NM 2:9–10.

• **גרם חוג** · to cause dizziness (stupefaction): Arab. أسدر · Al-Rāzī, *K. al-Manṣūrī* · trans. Shem Tov ben Isaac (*Sefer Almansur*), Ḥet 1 (36): חמאמא ובלעז אממו: חם יבש טוב לסתומי הכבד כשיהיו עם קור ומועיל למכאובי הרחמים ויכביד הראש ויגרום חוג. → NM 2:12.

• **גרם קבסא** · to cause indigestion: Arab. أتخم · Al-Zahrāwī, *K. al-taṣrīf li-man ʿağiza ʿan at-taʾlīf* · trans. Shem Tov ben Isaac (*Sefer ha-Shimmush*), bk. 27, fol. 139[a], col. a: ובעל מזג חם אין ראוי לתקנם על הרוב אם לא יגרמו לו קבסא. → NM 4:177–8.

גֶּרֶם · flesh; pulp: Arab. جسم / Gr. σάρξ · Al-Zahrāwī, *K. al-taṣrīf li-man ʿağiza ʿan at-taʾlīf* · trans. Shem Tov ben Isaac (*Sefer ha-Shimmush*), bk. 27, fol. 137[a], col. a: וגרם הצמוקים על הכלל חם ולח וחרצניהם קרים ויבשים. → NM 4:36–7.

גָּרָע · one who carries out venesection: Arab. فاصد · Al-Zahrāwī, *K. al-taṣrīf li-man ʿağiza ʿan at-taʾlīf* · trans. Shem Tov ben Isaac (*Sefer ha-Shimmush*), bk. 30, 2.95 (fol. 229[b]): וצריך הגרע להיותו נזהר בעת הקזתו כי יש תחתיו וריד ואם פשע ויוסיף בתחיבת המסמר ויחתוך הוריד ההוא תתחדש ממנו רעיפת דם. → NM 1:85.

• **מסמר הגרע** → **מַסְמֵר**.

גַּרְעִין • *Plur.* **גרעינים** · pills: Arab. حبّ · Maimonides, *K. al-fuṣūl fī al-ṭibb* · trans. Zeraḥyah Ḥen (*Sefer ha-Peraqim*), 13.13: כשתרצה להריק הגוף ממה שיש בו מן הליחות ותנקה הראש עמו עד שלא ירד ממנו קטרא ראוי לך שתהיה הרפואה מחוברת מרפואה משונה בכחותיה כמו הגרעינים אשר חברנו אנחנו. → NM 1:135.

גָּרַר • **גרר במגרה** · to saw: Arab. نشر · Al-Zahrāwī, *K. al-taṣrīf li-man ʿağiza ʿan at-taʾlīf* · trans. Shem Tov ben Isaac (*Sefer ha-Shimmush*), bk. 30, 2.86 (fol. 225[b]): ואחר כך שבתי וגליתי העצם שנית למעלה מן הגלוי הראשון ומצאתי ההפסד הגיע אל העצם וגררתי במגרה מה שנראה לו גם כן מן ההפסד ההוא. → NM 1:85.

[גרש] • *Piʿel* **גֵּרֵשׁ** · to push (upon): Lat. impellere · Bruno Longobucco, *Cyrurgia Magna*

· trans. Hillel ben Samuel (*Sefer Keritut*), fol. 63a–63b: עם כל זה יהיה הרופא משגיח שיגרש הפרק בידיו ורגליו עד שיושב למקומו הטבעי. → NM 1:19–20.

גֶּרֶשׂ • גרש כרמל · **coarse meal**: Arab. سويق الجريش / Gr. κρίμνον · Hippocrates, *Aphorisms* · trans. Nathan ha-Me'ati, 7.3 (383) (fol. 132b): מי שיהיה בו קדחת ויהיה שישקע בשתנו דומה לגרש כרמל הנה זה יורה שחליו יארך. → NM 3:49.

גֶּשֶׁם • *Plur.* **גשמים • ימות הגשמים** → **יום**.

גַּת · **confluence of sinuses; torcula**: Arab. معصرة / Lat. torcular herophili · Ibn Sīnā, *K. al-Qānūn fī al-ṭibb* · trans. Nathan ha-Me'ati (*Sefer ha-Qanun*), bk. 1 (fol. 65b): ואחר מתפרד ממנו במה שבין שתי המחיצות ונקרא מעצרה כלומר גת. → NM 4:37.

ד

דְּאָגָה • חולי הדאגה → חֳלִי.

• **הדאגה השחורי** › **melancholic delusion**: Arab. الوسواس السوداوي · Maimonides, *Šarḥ fuṣūl Abūqrāṭ* · trans. Anonymous (*Pirqei Abuqraṭ*), 3.22 (128): אמר אבוקרט: ואמנם בחורף יקרה הרבה מתחלואי הקיץ וקדחת רביעית ארוכה ומעורבת והטחול והשקוי והטפת השתן ושלשול הדם וחלקת המעים וכאב הירכים והאסכרה ונזילה על הריאה וחולי מעים החזק אשר יקראוהו היונים איליאוש והכפיה והדאגה השחורי והשטות. → NM 3:49–50.

דִּבּוּק • פרוד (ה)דבוק → פֵּרוּד.

• *Plur.* **דבוקים** • **דבוקי הזרוע** › **elbows**: Hippocrates, *Aphorisms* · trans. Judah Shalom, 6.22 (314) (fol. 100^b): כל הכאבים העוברים מן הגב לדבוקי הזרוע ההקזה תתיכם. → NM 3:50.

דְּבוֹרָה • *Plur.* **דבורים** • **אפרוחי הדבורים** → אֶפְרוֹחַ.

[דבק] • *Part. Nif'al* **נִדְבָּק** › **healed (of broken bones)**: Arab. المجبر · Maimonides, *K. al-fuṣūl fī al-ṭibb* · trans. Zeraḥyah Ḥen (*Sefer ha-Peraqim*), 15.63: העצמות במי שהוא בחור יהיו נדבקים קודם מהיותם נדבקים בילדים כי הילדים צריכים אל חומר יגדלו בו ויחליפו במקום מה שהותך מהם. זכר זה אסקליביוס במאמר הראשון מפירושו לספר הדבקות. → NM 1:135.

• *Pi'el* **דִּבֵּק** › I. **to seal**: Arab. لحم · Maimonides, *K. al-fuṣūl fī al-ṭibb* · trans. Nathan ha-Me'ati (*Sefer ha-Peraqim*), 3.13: ולכן ראוי שלא תדבק מקום השחין ושתניח עליו הדברים הרכים המחממים הרחוקים מהכאיב כדי שלא תתחדש מורסא. → NM 2:36.

› II. **to set (broken bones)**: Arab. جبر · Maimonides, *K. al-fuṣūl fī al-ṭibb* · trans. Zeraḥyah Ḥen (*Sefer ha-Peraqim*), 15.64: כל עצם שישבר שילך עליו ד׳ ימים ויותר לא תחשוב לדבקו כי היה גובר על החולה הזק גדול. → NM 1:135.

• *Part. Pu'al* **מְדֻבָּק** › **mucous**: Arab. مخاطي · Maimonides, *Šarḥ fuṣūl Abūqrāṭ* · trans. Moses ibn Tibbon (*Pirqei Abuqraṭ*), 6.60 (352): אמר המפרש: התנגב הליחה ההיא המדובקת בכויה וכאשר לא יתנגב הליחה ההיא בכויה יתחדש החגרות ולא ילך הרגל כמנהגו ויצמק. → NM 3:125.

• *Hitpa'el* **הִתְדַּבֵּק** › I. **to grow [together again]**: Arab. نمى · Maimonides, *Šarḥ fuṣūl Abūqrāṭ* · trans. Zeraḥyah Ḥen (*Pirqei Abuqraṭ*), 7.28 (380): אמר בקראט: כשיהיה שום דבר נחתך מן העצם או מן התנוך לא יתדבק. → NM 3:50.

› II. **to be regenerated**: Arab. تجبّر · Maimonides, *Šarḥ fuṣūl Abūqrāṭ* · trans. Zeraḥyah Ḥen (*Pirqei Abuqraṭ*), 4.26 (163): אמר המפרש: כי זה ראיה על התאחז חבלת המעיים עד שתחתוך עצמותם ואי אפשר שיתדבק אותו הבשר. → NM 3:50.

• *Hif'il* **הִדְבִּיק** › **to cause to heal up**: Arab. ألحم · Maimonides, *K. al-fuṣūl fī al-ṭibb* · trans. Nathan ha-Me'ati (*Sefer ha-Peraqim*), 15.17: אם ימצאהו עקיצה או דקירה לעצב מן העצבים עצמו אז אין ספק בהכרח ליתרון הרגש העצב מן הכאב החד אז הערים להשקיט הכאב ולמנוע חדוש המורסא. וזה שתשאיר האבר פתוח שלא תדביקהו. → NM 2:36.

• *Part. Hif'il* **מַדְבִּיק** › **a sticking plaster**: Arab. لصوق · Ibn al-Jazzār, *Zād al-musāfir wa-qūt al-ḥādir* · trans. Moses ibn Tibbon (*Sefer Ṣedat ha-Derakhim*), bk. 7, 26.6: אבק יולש ברוק יאכל הבשר המת ויצמיח הבשר החי וכשהיה הנגע מכה טריה בדמו ימלאהו בו בראש או בפנים או בגוף פעם אחת יבריאהו: יקח דם שני האחים וסרקא קולא מ״א אוקיא כאנפר דרהם יודק וינופה ויולש ברוק וימלא ממנו הנגע וישים עליו מדביק ויזרה זריה. → NM 1:59.

• מדביק הזהב · **chrysocolla**: Arab. لصاق الذهب · Maimonides, *K. al-fuṣūl fī al-ṭibb* · trans. Nathan ha-Me'ati (*Sefer ha-Peraqim*), 23.101. → NM 2:57.

• סם המדביק או המחליק → סַם.

• *Part. Hof'al* מֻדְבָּק • *Plur.* מודבקים · **joints**: Lat. iuncturae · Bruno Longobucco, *Cyrurgia Magna* · trans. Hillel ben Samuel (*Sefer Keritut*), fol. 59[a]: המודבקים ממקומם ההשמטה היא ההפרדה או יציאת. → NM 1:28.

דָּבֵק • הקדחת הדבקה → קַדַּחַת.

• ריח דבק → רֵיחַ.

דֶּבֶק • דבק היד · (lit., joint of the hand); **wrist**: Lat. iunctura manus · Bruno Longobucco, *Cyrurgia Magna* · trans. Hillel ben Samuel (*Sefer Keritut*), fol. 61[b]: וכאשר תבוא ההשמטה בדבק היד השבתו קלה. → NM 1:20.

• *Plur.* דבקים · **joints**: Lat. iuncturae · Bruno Longobucco, *Cyrurgia Magna* · trans. Hillel ben Samuel (*Sefer Keritut*), fol. 40[b]: וכאשר יגיע לאחד מן האשפונדלי חוליות בלשון הקודש או אל הצלעות או אל אחד מן הדבקים ביד או ברגל או בגיד או בווריד גדול או בווייתן בכל אלה לפי הרוב הם מכות נמנעות מרפואה. → NM 1:20.

• מחלת הדבקים וקשרי העצמות → מַחֲלָה.

• קשרי הדבקים → קֶשֶׁר.

דבקה • *Plur.* דבקות · **trusses**: Arab. جبائر · Maimonides, *K. al-fuṣūl fī al-ṭibb* · trans. Zeraḥyah Ḥen (*Sefer ha-Peraqim*), 15.69: ראוי שתקשור תחלה תחת הרפידות ותתחיל ממקום החולי ותכלה אל המקום העליון למען מנוע הרקת הלחויות ויהיה מונע המורסא. ואחרי כן תשים הרפידות ואחר כן תרפד ממעלה לרפידות כדי שלא יסתער ותתחיל ממקום המחלה ותכלה למטה לדחוק הדם המעופש מן האבר החולה עד הקצה. ואחר זאת הקשירה השנייה תשים והיא תקיים ותחזק כל מה שהוא מאחריה ויסמוך אותו. ויהיה כל אשר יקיף באבר ארבעה דברים. הקשירה הנעשית על האבר והרפידות והקשירה שעליהם והדבקות. → NM 1:135–6.

דְּבֵקוּת · **setting (of broken bones)**: Arab. جبر · Maimonides, *K. al-fuṣūl fī al-ṭibb* · trans. Zeraḥyah Ḥen (*Sefer ha-Peraqim*), 15.63: העצמות במי שהוא בחור יהיו נדבקים קודם מהיותם נדבקים בילדים כי הילדים צריכים אל חומר יגדלו בו ויחליפו במקום מה שהותך מהם. זכר זה אסקליביוס במאמר הראשון מפירושו לספר הדבקות. → NM 1:136.

• הפרדת הדבקות → הַפְרָדָה.

• התרת הדבקות → הַתָּרָה.

• דבקות הזהב · **chrysocolla**: Arab. لصاق الذهب · Maimonides, *K. al-fuṣūl fī al-ṭibb* · trans. Zeraḥyah Ḥen (*Sefer ha-Peraqim*), 23.101: הרפואה אשר תחמם ותלחלח עד שתפסיד מה שתמצא היא באמת הרפואה המעפשת. וכן נקראות כמו כן כל הרפואות החמות היבשות העבות בעצמותם בהיותם נושכים מעט או שורפות מעט מבלתי חדש כאב נקראות מעפשות כי הם יתיכו ויאכלו הבשר ויעשו בו מה שיעשה המעפשת באמת והם כמו הארסניץ ודבקות הזהב והפיניי וממית הזאב. → NM 1:136.

• *Plur.* דבקיות · **viscous matters**: Arab. لزوجة, *Plur.* لزوجات · Maimonides, *Šarḥ fuṣūl Abūqrāṭ* · trans. Moses ibn Tibbon (*Pirqei Abuqraṭ*), 3.53 (190): אלו הדבקיות אמנם יתחדשו מחום חזק פעלו בלחיות לבנות עד שנגבו אותם. → NM 3:50.

[דבר] • *Pi'el* דִּבֵּר • דיבר בלא עיון · **to make an error**: Arab. وهم · Maimonides, *Šarḥ fuṣūl*

Abūqrāṭ · trans. Moses ibn Tibbon (*Pirqei Abuqraṭ*), introduction (8): אמר כל זה כדי שלא יאמר כי אבוקראט טעה או דבר בלא עיון בזה המאמר. → NM 3:175.

דָּבָר • הקטיר האף בדבר → [קטר].

• **דבר מעטיש** · **sternutatory:** Hippocrates, *Aphorisms* · trans. Do'eg ha-Edomi (*Sefer Agur*), 5.49 (269) (fol. 90ª): צוה ברצונך לגרש השלייא להריח לאפי האשה דבר מעטיש ולסתום מיד את נחיריה ואת פיה. → NM 3:134–5.

• **דבר נאמר בלי עיון** · **error:** Arab. وَهْم · Maimonides, *Šarḥ fuṣūl Abūqrāṭ* · trans. Moses ibn Tibbon (*Pirqei Abuqraṭ*), introduction (7): אבל כי ג'אלינוס ימאן זה ואינו רואה בשום פנים שיהיה בדברי אבוקראט דבר נאמר בלי עיון. → NM 3:175.

• *Plur.* **דברים • דברים מחליקים** · **mollifacients:** Lat. lenificantia · Bruno Longobucco, *Cyrurgia Magna* · trans. Hillel ben Samuel (*Sefer Keritut*), fol. 96ª: וחובש המקום בדברים מתיכים מחליקים כמו כממילא קמח פולים ודומיהם. → NM 1:26.

דְּבַשׁ • אידיות הדבש → אֲדִיּוּת.

• **יין מבושל עד ששב כדבש** → יַיִן.

• **יין הדבש השרוי** → יַיִן.

• **יערת הדבש** → יַעֲרָה.

• **דבש מקוצף** · **skimmed honey:** Lat. mel dispumatum · Bruno Longobucco, *Cyrurgia Magna* · trans. Hillel ben Samuel (*Sefer Keritut*), fol. 41ᵇ. → NM 1:20.

• **משקה הדבש** → מַשְׁקֶה.

• **עשניות הדבש** → עֲשָׁנִיּוֹת.

• **צוף הדבש** → **צוּף**.

• **דבש רושד** · **roses confected with honey:** Arab. جلنجبين · Al-Zahrāwī, *K. al-taṣrīf li-man ʿağiza ʿan at-taʾlīf* · trans. Shem Tov ben Isaac (*Sefer ha-Shimmush*), bk. 27, fol. 132ª, col. b: ואחר להרגיל אחד מן העסיסים החמוצים אם הוא בעל מזג חם ומן הדבש רושד אם הוא בעל מזג קר. → NM 4:37.

דִּבְשִׁי • הדבשי · **honey dish:** Arab. معسّل · Al-Zahrāwī, *K. al-taṣrīf li-man ʿağiza ʿan at-taʾlīf* · trans. Shem Tov ben Isaac (*Sefer ha-Shimmush*), bk. 27, fol. 145ᵇ, col. a: הדבשי הנקרא בלשונם מעשל הוא תבשיל עשוי בדבש ובשר ותבלין ושקדים והוא חם וטוב לבעלי הקרירות ובזמן הקר. → NM 4:37.

דַּבֶּשֶׁת · **hunchback:** Arab. حدبة · Al-Zahrāwī, *K. al-taṣrīf li-man ʿağiza ʿan at-taʾlīf* · trans. Shem Tov ben Isaac (*Sefer ha-Shimmush*), bk. 30, 1.43 (fol. 202ᵇ): בכוית התחלת הדבשת. → NM 1:85.

דִּגְדּוּג · **pruritus:** Arab. دغدغة · Maimonides, *K. al-fuṣūl fī al-ṭibb* · trans. Nathan ha-Me'ati (*Sefer ha-Peraqim*), 7.21: הדגדוג יתחדש מפני ליחות חריפות עוקצות יעקצו האבר ויתחדש בו דמיון התנועה המתחדשת מן ההנעה באצבעות תחת האצילים וכיוצא בו. → NM 2:36.

דוחק → דֹּחַק.

[דון] • דן · **to bring to a crisis:** Lat. iudicare / Arab. كان به بحران · Hippocrates, *Aphorisms* · trans. Hillel ben Samuel, 4.36 (173) (fol. 24ᵇ): א"א: הזיעות הבאות למוקדחים הם טובות בשלישי ובחמישי ובשביעי ובתשיעי ובי"א וי"ד ובי"ז ובכ' ובכ"ד ובכ"ז ובל"א ובל"ד ובל"ז מפני שאלו הזיעות דנין החלי אך אותן שלא נעשו בימים אלו מורים מכאוב ואורך חולי והשבתו. → NM 3:51; corr. 4:229.

• *Nif'al* נָדוֹן • **to reach a crisis**: Lat. iudico, *Pass.* iudicor / Arab. انقضى • Hippocrates, *Aphorisms* • trans. Hillel ben Samuel, 4.59 (196) (fol. 27[a]): א״א: שלישית אמתית אם לא תדון בשבעה הקפים היא ארוכה. → NM 3:51.

דּוֹפֵק (*Part.*) → דָּפַק.

דּוֹפֶק → **דֹּפֶק**.

[דות] • *Part. Nitpa'el* **מדיית** • **destined; sweating; transuding**: Arab. مرشح • Ibn Sīnā, *K. al-Qānūn fī al-ṭibb* • trans. Nathan ha-Me'ati (*Sefer ha-Qanun*), bk. 1 (fol. 61[a]): אמנם נברא המדיית לירידה נוסף בשעורו על האחר כי הוא מנהיג אברים הם רבים יותר במספר והם יותר גדולים בשעורים והם האברים המונחים למטה מן הלב. → NM 4:37–8.

דְּחִיקָה • **bandage**: Lat. strictura • Bruno Longobucco, *Cyrurgia Magna* • trans. Hillel ben Samuel (*Sefer Keritut*), cf. fol. 57[b]: וכבר ידעת אופן דחיקת הקשר בכלל כלומר כשתהיה הדחיקה על מקום השבר יותר חזקה. → NM 1:20.

דְּחִיקוּת • **density**: Arab. كثافة • Maimonides, *Šarḥ fuṣūl Abūqrāṭ* • trans. Zeraḥyah Ḥen (*Pirqei Abuqraṭ*), 1.2 (15): החלק הראשון מה שצריך לרופא לדעת מקום המלאכה והם גוף האדם וזהו לדעת חכמת הניתוח ולדעת מזג כל אבר ואבר מן האברים בכלל ולדעת פעולתו ותועלתו ועניין עצמותו בקושי ובחלקות ובדחיקות ובספוגות. → NM 3:51.

דָּחַק • **to bind (tightly)**: Lat. stringere • Bruno Longobucco, *Cyrurgia Magna* • trans. Hillel ben Samuel (*Sefer Keritut*), fol. 56[a]: אחר כן יוחבש כראוי וידחוק השבר עם לוח אם יצטרך. → NM 1:21.

דֹּחַק • **בדוחק** • **forcefully; strongly**: Lat. fortiter • Bruno Longobucco, *Cyrurgia Magna* • trans. Hillel ben Samuel (*Sefer Keritut*), fol. 62[b]: ויניח פסותיו על האשפונדלי ויעצור בדוחק עד שובם. → NM 1:21.

דִּיּוּת • **transudation**: Arab. رشح • Maimonides, *Šarḥ fuṣūl Abūqrāṭ* • trans. Moses ibn Tibbon (*Pirqei Abuqraṭ*), 7.54 (406): אמר המפרש: הנה אמרו כי זה אינו לאבקראט ואמר ג׳אלינוס שהוא בלתי נמנע שתעבור הליחה הזאת לעורקים בדיות כי הטבע תעשה תחבולה לדקדק החמרים ולהוציאם בכל דרך שיוכל ואפילו בדרך רחוק כמו שיוציא המוגלא המתקבצת במה שבין הריאה והחזה ובכלל הוא מאמר שיקרה מעט ומעט התועלת מאד. → NM 3:52.

דִּין • **בדין** • **in the case**: Arab. في حقّ • Maimonides, *Šarḥ fuṣūl Abūqrāṭ* • trans. Moses ibn Tibbon (*Pirqei Abuqraṭ*), 0 (8): ואפילו יהיה זה בדין נכבד וידוע. → NM 3:52.

• **הקדים הגזר דין** → קָדַם.

• **התיר הפסק דין** → [נתר].

• **יום דין** → יוֹם.

דַּיְסָא (*Aram.*) • **coarsely pounded wheat or barley eaten alone or mixed with honey**: Arab. هريسة • Al-Zahrāwī, *K. al-taṣrīf li-man ʿağiza ʿan at-taʾlīf* • trans. Shem Tov ben Isaac (*Sefer ha-Shimmush*), bk. 27, fol. 124[b], cols. 1–2: הדיסא היא גם כן מזה המין והיא בטבעה עבה וחלוקה ומתאחרת להתעכל ומולידה סתומים כהולדת הגריסין אלא שהיא כשתתעכל בגופי הבריאים תוליד דם יש בו לחות וחלוקה ותזון מזון רב. → NM 4:38.

דיקוק → דִּקּוּק.

דָּלִית • *Plur.* **דליות** • **1. varices**: Arab. دالية, *Plur.* دوالٍ / Gr. κιρσός, *Plur.* κιρσόι • Al-Zahrāwī, *K. al-taṣrīf li-man ʿağiza ʿan at-taʾlīf* • trans. Shem Tov ben Isaac (*Sefer ha-Shimmush*), bk. 30, 2.90 (fol. 227[a]): הדליות הם גידים נפתלים עבים מלאים מהעדפות שחוריות מתחדשות ברוב איברי הגוף. → NM 1:85; corr. 4:229.

‣ II. **varicose veins**: Arab. دوال · Al-Zahrāwī, *K. al-taṣrīf li-man ʿaǧiza ʿan at-taʾlīf* · trans. Shem Tov ben Isaac (*Sefer ha-Shimmush*), bk. 27, fol. 134[b], col. b: והתמדת אכילתו גורמת השטות והסרטן ומדוה השועל והדליות והטחורים והבהק השחור ודומיהם מן החליים השחוריים. → NM 4:38–9.

דְּלַעַת • גרגרי הדלעת → **גַּרְגַּר**.

• *Plur.* **דלועים • גרגרי הדלועים** → **גַּרְגַּר**.

• **התולעים הדלועיים** → **תּוֹלַעַת**.

דָּם • אבן הדם → **אֶבֶן**.

• **דם שני האחים** ‣ **(lit., the blood of the two brothers); red resin derived from the dragontree** [*Dracaena Draco* L.]: Arab. دم الأخوين · Ibn al-Jazzār, *Zād al-musāfir wa-qūt al-ḥādir* · trans. Moses ibn Tibbon (*Sefer Ṣedat ha-Derakhim*), bk. 7, 26.3. → NM 1:71.

• **אם הדם** → **אֵם**.

• **בקיעת דם** → **בְּקִיעָה**.

• **הגרת הדם** → **הַגָּרָה**.

• **הגרת הדם מהאף** → **הַגָּרָה**.

• **הגרת דם מהנחירים** → **הַגָּרָה**.

• **הזלת הדם** → **הַזָּלָה**.

• **הזלת דם הבטן** → **הַזָּלָה**.

• **הזלת דם הנחירים** → **הַזָּלָה**.

• **הטפת דם מהנחירים** → **הַטָּפָה**.

• **הרעיף דם** → [**רעף**].

• **השתנת הדם** → **הַשְׁתָּנָה**.

• **זוב דם הנחירים** → **זוֹב**.

• **זלוף הדם מן החוטם** → **זִלּוּף**.

• **יציאת דם הנחירים** → **יְצִיאָה**.

• **מעבה דם** → [**עבה**].

• **נזלת דם** → **נַזֶּלֶת**.

• **הסם המביא הדם** → **סַם**.

• **הסם המגיר הדם** → **סַם**.

• **הסם העוצר הדם** → **סַם**.

• **עירוב הדם** → **עֵרוּב**.

• **עריפת דם החוטם** → **עֲרִיפָה**.

• **עריפת דם הנחירים** → **עֲרִיפָה**.

• **צאת דם הנחירים** → **יָצָא**.

• **דם קרוש** ‣ **blood clots**: Arab. عبيط / Gr. θρομβώδης · Hippocrates, *Aphorisms* · trans. Nathan ha-Me'ati, 4.69 (206) (fol. 79[a]): אמר אבוקרט: מי שיהיה שתנו עב דומה לדם קרוש מעט ואין גופו נקי מן הקדחת הנה הוא אם ישתין שתן רב רקיק יקבל תועלת בו. → NM 3:52–3.

• **רעיפת הדם** → **רְעִיפָה**.

• רְעִיפָה → רעיפת דם מן החוטם •.

• רְעִיפָה → רעיפת דם מן הנחירים •.

• רְקִיקָה → רקיקת הדם •.

• **דם שותת** · dysentery: Arab. اختلاف دم / Gr. δυσεντερία · Maimonides, *Šarḥ fuṣūl Abūqrāṭ* · trans. Zeraḥyah Ḥen (*Pirqei Abuqraṭ*), 3.11 (117): אמר בקראט: אמנם בזמני השנה אני אומר כי כשיהיה האוירנו במטר מועט ורוחו שמאלי והיה הויר בעל מטר והרוח רוח האלגנוב ראוי בהכרח שיתחדש בקייץ קדחות חדות וחולי העיניים הנק׳ רמד ודם שותת ורוב מה שיקרה שלשול הדם לנשים ולבעלי הטבעים הלחים. → NM 3:53.

• שִׁלּוּחַ → שילוח הדם •.

• שִׁנּוּי → שינוי דם •.

• שִׁלְשׁוּל → שלשול (ה)דם •.

• שִׁלְשׁוּל → שלשול עם דם •.

דִּמְיוֹן • צֶמַח → צמח בבשר דומה לדמיון הבשר.

דֶּמַע · **persistent flow of tears (epiphora)**: Arab. دمعة / Gr. ἐπιφορά · Ibn al-Jazzār, *Zād al-musāfir wa-qūt al-ḥādir* · trans. Moses ibn Tibbon (*Sefer Ṣedat ha-Derakhim*), bk. 2, ch. 4 (fol. 45[a]): כשיקרה לו הדמע ולא יהיה לו סבה מחוץ ידענו כי הגרת הלחות ההוא אל העינים מן הראש והגרתו תהיה אם בעורקים אשר למעלה מגולגולת הראש ואם בעורקים אשר תחת הגלגולת. → NM 4:39.

• נָצוּר → הנצור אשר יהיה בדמע העין •.

• קָצָה → הקצוות אשר הדמע יורד מהן •.

דִּמְעָה · **rhyas (i.e., a continuous weeping discharge caused by a wasting of flesh at the great canthus)**: Arab. دمعة / Gr. ρυάς · Al-Rāzī, *K. al-Manṣūrī* · trans. Shem Tov ben Isaac (*Sefer Almansur*), Bet 11 (20): בסד: קר יבש מועיל כשישחק היטב וישתה מרקיקת הדם ומחזק העין ומפסיק הדמעה. → NM 2:11.

דְּעִיכָה · **lividness**: Arab. كمودة · Maimonides, *K. al-fuṣūl fī al-ṭibb* · trans. Nathan ha-Me'ati (*Sefer ha-Peraqim*), 15.50: וכן המורסא הנקר׳ חמרה אם יטה ענינה אל הדעיכה או אל הירקות או אל השחרות אז תשרט. → NM 2:37.

דַּעַת • אֲפִיסָה → אפיסת הדעת.

• בִּלְבּוּל → בלבול הדעת •.

• רָאָה → ראה בדעת •.

דְּפוּס · **cast**: Arab. قالب · Maimonides, *K. al-fuṣūl fī al-ṭibb* · trans. Nathan ha-Me'ati (*Sefer ha-Peraqim*), 15.68: שבירת הרגל תצטרך לדפוס פן יתנועע ויתגעש האבר בעת התנועה וראוי שתטיב לעין בחולי המחייב הדפוס כי שאם יהיה ההיזק המתחדש מן הדפוס יותר רב מתועלתו אז לא תעשהו. → NM 2:37; corr. 4:229.

דְּפִיקָה · **throbbing pain**: Arab. ضربان · Ibn al-Jazzār, *Zād al-musāfir wa-qūt al-ḥādir* · trans. Moses ibn Tibbon (*Sefer Ṣedat ha-Derakhim*), bk. 2, ch. 1 (fol. 42[b]): ומזה תואר עגולים לבנים כוללים מועילים בע״ה לקצידה החמה והדפיקה. → NM 4:39.

• **דפיקת (ה)לב** · **cardialgia**: a) Arab. خفقان · Ibn al-Jazzār, *Zād al-musāfir wa-qūt al-ḥādir* · trans. Moses ibn Tibbon (*Sefer Ṣedat ha-Derakhim*), bk. 1, ch. 18 (fol. 26[a]): ויקרה לחולה עם עלות החולי וקרוב חזקתו מקרים מפחידים כמו צמא חזק ונגוב פה ושעירות לשון ושחרותה וסער ודפיקת לב. → NM 4:39.

b) Arab. خفقان في الفؤاد · Maimonides, *Šarḥ fuṣūl Abūqrāṭ* · trans. Anonymous (*Pirqei Abuqraṭ*), 4.65 (202): אמר אבוקרט: כשהיתה בעת הקדחת התלהבות חזקה בקיבה ודפיקת הלב כל זה הוא רע. → NM 3:53.

• **דפיקה במוראה** · **cardialgia:** Arab. خفقان في الفؤاد · Maimonides, *Šarḥ fuṣūl Abūqrāṭ* · trans. Moses ibn Tibbon (*Pirqei Abuqraṭ*), 4.65 (202): אמר אבקראט: כשתהיה בקדחת התלהבות גדול באצטו׳ ודפיקה במוראה הנה זה אות רע. → NM 3:53.

דָּפַק • *Part.* **דּוֹפֵק** • **הגיד הדופק הורידי** → **גִּיד**.

• **הוריד הדופק** → **וָרִיד**.

• **מקום שדופק** → **מָקוֹם**.

דֹּפֶק • **גיד הדופק** → **גִּיד**.

• **דפק הגידים** · **tetanus:** a) Hippocrates, *Aphorisms* · trans. Do'eg ha-Edomi (*Sefer Agur*), 4.57 (194) (fol. 73[a]): פוקת קבוץ הגידים או דפקם ובא אחרי כן קדחת יגיד על הסרת מדוה מעליו. → NM 3:54.

b) Hippocrates, *Aphorisms* · trans. Do'eg ha-Edomi (*Sefer Agur*), 5.20 (240) (fol. 84[b]): חרדת המים הקרים תכאיב חבורות הגוף ותקשה עורה ותעורר בהם כאב כאשר לא נקבץ שם עב טיט ותשחירם ותעורר עליהם קור וקדחת וקיבוץ הגידים ודפקם. → NM 3:53–4.

• **התפשטות הדפק** → **הִתְפַּשְּׁטוּת**.

• **דפק משורי** · **serrated pulse:** Arab. النبض المنشاري · Maimonides, *K. al-fuṣūl fī al-ṭibb* · trans. Nathan ha-Me'ati (*Sefer ha-Peraqim*), 6.54: המקרים הדבקים לבעלת הצד שלא יפרדו ממנה הם אלו: קדחת חדה כאב עוקץ בצד ונשימה קטנה תכופה דפק משורי ושעול. → NM 2:63.

דַּק • **הסם הדק** → **סַם**.

• **קדחת דקה** → **קַדַּחַת**.

• **שחין דק** → **שְׁחִין**.

• **התולעים הדקים** → **תּוֹלַעַת**.

דִּקְדּוּק · I. **intuition:** Arab. حدس · Maimonides, *Šarḥ fuṣūl Abūqrāṭ* · trans. Anonymous (*Pirqoi Abuqraṭ*), 1.7 (21): ולזה צריך אל הרגל ארוך בשמושי הראיות הפרטיות ואז תוכל לגזור מה שיתחדש בדקדוק טוב קרוב אל האמת. → NM 3:54.

· II. **thinness:** Arab. لُطْف · Maimonides, *Šarḥ fuṣūl Abūqrāṭ* · trans. Zeraḥyah Ḥen (*Pirqei Abuqraṭ*), 5.5 (225): אמר המפרש: זה הקווץ יקרה מפני מילוי העצבים ומטבע היין שימלא העצבים מהרה כי הוא שוקע מפני דקדוקו וחומו. → NM 3:54.

· III. **thinning:** Arab. تلطيف · Maimonides, *K. al-fuṣūl fī al-ṭibb* · trans. Nathan ha-Me'ati (*Sefer ha-Peraqim*), 9.113: רפרוף הלב ראינו מי שמצאו פתאם מרבים מהבריאים מאותם שלא היה חסר מבריאותם דבר בחורים וזקנים וכלם קבלו תועלת בהקזת העורק ודקדוק המזון. → NM 2:37.

[דקדק] • *Pi'el* **דִּקְדֵּק** · **to act with grace; to act with kindness:** Arab. تلطّف · Ibn Sīnā, *K. al-Qānūn fī al-ṭibb* · trans. Nathan ha-Me'ati (*Sefer ha-Qanun*), bk. 1 (fol. 42[b]): ודקדק הבורא והצמיח מן העצמות דבר דומה בעצבים נקרא עקבים וקשורים להתחבר עם העצבים ומסתבכים בו כדבר אחד. → NM 4:39–40.

• *Part. Pi'el* **מְדַקְדֵּק** • **הסם המדקדק** → **סַם**.

דִּקּוּק · **refining**: Arab. تلطيف · Maimonides, *Šarḥ fuṣūl Abūqrāṭ* · trans. Anonymous (*Pirqei Abuqraṭ*), 2.53 (104): וזהו הצד בעצמו יצדד במזונות ובמיני מה שינוקה בם הליחה ההיא המחליאה או בהתכה או בדיקוק או לבשל או לעבות החומר או להקפיא. → NM 3:54–5.

דְּקִירָה · **bursting**: Arab. انبثاق · Maimonides, *K. al-fuṣūl fī al-ṭibb* · trans. Zeraḥyah Ḥen (*Sefer ha-Peraqim*), 15.39: החבלות אשר יתרבה יציאת הדם מהם מפני דקירת העורקים יפסיק אותו הדם בכויה או ברפואה שיהיה כחה כח הכויה או בדבר שיקבץ וימעט או כשיעתיק החומר אל מקום אחר קרוב או במשכו אל הפך הצד או בקררו לכל הגוף וכל שכן לקרר האבר שבו החבלה. → NM 1:136–7.

דֶּקֶל • לוּלָב הדקל → לוּלָב.

דָּקַר · I. **to cut**: Arab. بتر · Maimonides, *K. al-fuṣūl fī al-ṭibb* · trans. Zeraḥyah Ḥen (*Sefer ha-Peraqim*), 12.38: וכשידוקר הגיד הדופק על רחבו בשני חצאיו אין בו פחד כי הוא יתקווץ כל אחד משני קצותיו אל הצד אשר הוא בו → NM 2:37.

· II. **to lance**: Arab. بطّ · Maimonides, *K. al-fuṣūl fī al-ṭibb* · trans. Zeraḥyah Ḥen (*Sefer ha-Peraqim*), 15.8: כשתדקור שום מקום והריקות מה שיש בו מן המים הטרי תהיה נזהר באותה שעה ובמה שאחריה מעשותך השמן עם. → NM 2:37.

דרדני · **gums**: Arab. لثة · a) Al-Zahrāwī, *K. al-taṣrīf li-man ʿağiza ʿan at-taʾlīf* · trans. Shem Tov ben Isaac (*Sefer ha-Shimmush*), bk. 27, fol. 141[a], col. a: ומזיקים אל הדרדני ומחדדים שחין דק בפה ומולידים האפר בעינים. → NM 4:40.

b) Al-Zahrāwī, *K. al-taṣrīf li-man ʿağiza ʿan at-taʾlīf* · trans. Shem Tov ben Isaac (*Sefer ha-Shimmush*), bk. 30, 2.95 (fol. 229[a]): וגידי השפה והפסד הדרדני והשחין הרע. → NM 1:85–6; corr. 4:229.

דֶּרֶךְ • **דרך השתן** · **urethra**: Lat. via urinalis · Hippocrates, *Aphorisms* · trans. Judah Shalom, 4.82 (219) (fol. 74[a–b]): כל מי שבדרך השתן הנה יולדו צמחים הנה בעשותו בהעשות באלו בשול ותפתחם תהיה ההתכה. → NM 3:55; corr. 4:230.

• *Plur.* **דרכים** · I. **passages (in the body)**: Arab. مجار · Maimonides, *Šarḥ fuṣūl Abūqrāṭ* · trans. Zeraḥyah Ḥen (*Pirqei Abuqraṭ*), 2.9 (61): אמר המפרש: יהיה זה בשתפתח ותרחיב כל דרכיו ותחתוך ותדקדק ותתיך הלחויית אשר בהם אם היה להם שום דבר מן העובי והדבקות. → NM 3:55.

· II. **rules**: Arab. قوانين · Maimonides, *Šarḥ fuṣūl Abūqrāṭ* · trans. Moses ibn Tibbon (*Pirqei Abuqraṭ*), 0 (16): והחלק הרביעי ידיעת דרכי הראיה והוא איך ילקח מן המקרים ההם המשיגים הנושא ראיות על מין ומין ממיני הבריאות ועל מין ומין ממיני החולי היה זה בגוף כלו או באיזה אבר שיהיה מאיבריו ואיך יבדיל בין חולי וחולי כי הנה יתדמו רוב הראיות. → NM 3:55.

דֶּשֶׁן · **ophthalmia**: Arab. رمد · Al-Rāzī, *K. al-Manṣūrī* · trans. Shem Tov ben Isaac (*Sefer Almansur*), Ḥet 4 (36): חי אלעאלם ובלעז כובא קורבינא ובי״ח חיי עולם: קר טוב למורסות החמות כשיטחו בו ומכבה שרפת האש והדשן כשיוטח בו. → NM 2:11.

• **דשן גפנים** · **ash of the grapevine**: Lat. cinis vitium · Al-Rāzī, attr., *On the Treatment of Small Children* · trans. Anonymous, ch. 1. → NM 2:177.

ה

הַאֲצָלָה • *Plur.* **ההאצלות הנפשיות • האצלות** · **the psychical faculties**: Arab. القوة النفسانية · Galen, attr., *Prohibition of Burial* · trans. Judah al-Ḥarizi (*Sefer Issur ha-Qevurah le-Galienus*), par. 15: ויקרה מזה לאדם עד ו׳ או ז׳ שעות שלא ישכיל ולא יאכל ולא ישתה אבן עורקיו דופקים ונשומו מתנועע וזה הסוג מן השעמום יסתום מעברי ההאצלות הנפשיות אשר לחושים. → NM 4:40.

[הבהב] • *Part. Pu'al* **מְהֻבְהָב** • **הכרמל המהובהב באש** → **כַּרְמֶל**.

הַבָּטָה • **יום החבטה** → **יוֹם**.

• **עוות החבטה** → **עִוּוּת**.

הַבְטָחָה · **confidence**: Arab. ثقة · Maimonides, *K. al-fuṣūl fī al-ṭibb* · trans. Zeraḥyah Ḥen (*Sefer ha-Peraqim*), 8.22: הייתי מקדים על הרבה בני אדם וקצתם השקיתים המים הקרים בהבטחה ונאמנות בבכל זמן שהם חולים ומהם בזמן בלתי זמן עם שזולתי מן הרופאים היו מניחים מהשקותם אילו. → NM 1:137–8.

הֲבָרָה · **[intestinal] rumblings (borborygmus)**: a) Arab. قراقر / Gr. διαβορυγμός · Al-Zahrāwī, *K. al-taṣrīf li-man 'ağiza 'an at-ta'līf* · trans. Shem Tov ben Isaac (*Sefer ha-Shimmush*), bk. 27, fol. 124[a], col. 1: החטה השלוקה כבדה מאד רבת הנפח וההברה ומתעכבת לרדת מן האצטומכא ומולידה חלט עב בתכלית העובי והחלוקה וכל שכן אם תהיה מן החטה הכבדה האדומה. → NM 4:40.

b) Arab. قرقرة · Al-Zahrāwī, *K. al-taṣrīf li-man 'ağiza 'an at-ta'līf* · trans. Shem Tov ben Isaac (*Sefer ha-Shimmush*), bk. 30, 2.90 (fol. 220[a]): ולפעמים הלך במעי הצואה ותתעכב שמה ויהיה ממנה אבדת החולה שהיא תחדש כאב קשה והברה וכל שכן בעת הסחיטה עליו. → NM 1:86.

הִגָּבְנוּת · **turning into cheese**: Arab. تجبّن · Maimonides, *K. al-fuṣūl fī al-ṭibb* · trans. Nathan ha-Me'ati (*Sefer ha-Peraqim*), 20.41: והיותר משובח בטוב כימוס מה שיהיה מבעלי חיים בריא ושמן כשישתה מיד שיחלב ומן הראוי שיושם בו דבש ומעט מלח להיות בטוח מההגבנות. → NM 2:38.

הַגְלָדָה · I. **healing (i.e., of a wound)**: Arab. اندمال · Al-Zahrāwī, *K. al-taṣrīf li-man 'ağiza 'an at-ta'līf* · trans. Shem Tov ben Isaac (*Sefer ha-Shimmush*), bk. 30, 2.89 (fol. 227[a]): והדבקות אשר יקרה אל האצבעות קצתם בקצתם יתכן היותו מזמן היצירה או מהגלדת חבורה או משרפת אש וזולתם. → NM 1:86.

· II. **mending**: Arab. التحم · Al-Zahrāwī, *K. al-taṣrīf li-man 'ağiza 'an at-ta'līf* · trans. Shem Tov ben Isaac (*Sefer ha-Shimmush*), bk. 30, 3.1 (fol. 232[a]): וידוע שהעצמות הנשברות כשתהיינה באנשים כחושים וזקנים לא יתכן חבורם והגלדתם על טבעם הראשון לעולם לנגוב עצמותם וקשים. → NM 1:86.

הַגָּרָה · **hernia**: Arab. قيلة · Maimonides, *K. al-fuṣūl fī al-ṭibb* · trans. Nathan ha-Me'ati (*Sefer ha-Peraqim*), 9.102: לא יפחידך ואל יבהילוך במלאכת היד גודל החליים אבל העיון בסכנתם וחזקם וחולשתם. ומזה שאין ראוי שיבהילך גודל ההגרה הנקראת בקיעה ועצמה כי אז תחשוב אותה חולי חזק אבל תעיין ותדע שההגרה אשר ירד בה הקרום המכסה המעים והאסטומכה והחלב הוא חולי חזק ועצום ואע״פ ששעורו אינו גדול. וההגרה שאינה חולי מועט ואע״פ שתהיה גדולת השיעור היא אותה שהיא מן המים. → NM 2:38.

• **הגרת הבטן** › **diarrhea**: Arab. استطلاق البطن · Maimonides, *Šarḥ fuṣūl Abūqrāṭ* · trans. Moses ibn Tibbon (*Pirqei Abuqraṭ*), 1.2 (29): אמר אבקראט: אם היה מה שיורק מן הגוף בעת הגרת הבטן והקיא אשר יהיו ברצון מן המין אשר ראוי שינקה ממנו הגוף יועיל זה ויהיה נקל לסבלו ואם לא יהיה כן יהיה הדבר בהפך. → NM 3:55–6.

• **הגרת הבשר בכיס** › **sarcocele**: Arab. قيلة اللحم · Maimonides, *K. al-fuṣūl fī al-ṭibb* · trans. Nathan ha-Me'ati (*Sefer ha-Peraqim*), 23.57: קשי האשכים נקרא קילה אללחם כלומר הגרת הבשר בכיס כמו שנקרא הלחות המתקבצת בכיס אשר סביב האשכים קילה אלמא כלומר הגרת המים. → NM 2:38.

• **הגרת הדם** › I. **bloody diarrhea; dysentery**: Arab. اختلاف الدم · Maimonides, *K. al-fuṣūl fī al-ṭibb* · trans. Zeraḥyah Ḥen (*Sefer ha-Peraqim*), 6.90: בתחלת הגרת הדם יקרה בטול תאות המזון. → NM 1:138.

› II. **hemophtysis**: Arab. نفث الدم · Maimonides, *K. al-fuṣūl fī al-ṭibb* · trans. Zeraḥyah Ḥen (*Sefer ha-Peraqim*), 9.61: בעל האיקטריזיאה יועילנו המראים הירוקים שהם יתירו הקולורא. והרחיקו בעלי הגרת הדם מראות המראה האדום כי הם ישלחו הדם. → NM 1:138.

• **הגרת הדם מהאף** › **nosebleed**: Arab. رعاف · a) Maimonides, *K. al-fuṣūl fī al-ṭibb* · trans. Zeraḥyah Ḥen (*Sefer ha-Peraqim*), 9.2: לא תמתין בהגרת הדם מהאף עד שיפול כח החולה. → NM 1:138.

b) Maimonides, *Šarḥ fuṣūl Abūqrāṭ* · trans. Zeraḥyah Ḥen (*Pirqei Abuqraṭ*), 5.33 (253): אמר בקראט: כשיפסק הווסת בהגרת הדם מהאף זה טוב. → NM 3:56.

• **הגרת דם מהנחירים** › **nosebleed**: Arab. رعاف · Maimonides, *Šarḥ fuṣūl Abūqrāṭ* · trans. Zeraḥyah Ḥen (*Pirqei Abuqraṭ*), 3.27 (133): אמר בקראט: אמנם מי שיעבור אלו השנים ויתקרב שיצמח בו השיער בעצם הערוה יקרה לו הרבה מאלו החליים וקדחות יותר ארוכים והגרת דם מהנחירים. → NM 3:56.

• **הגרת הזרע מבלי רצון** › **an involuntary flow of sperm (spermatorrhea)**: Arab. سيلان المني من غير إرادة · Ibn al-Jazzār, *Zād al-musāfir wa-qūt al-ḥādir* · trans. Moses ibn Tibbon (*Sefer Ṣedat ha-Derakhim*), introduction (fol. 4^a): השער הג׳ בהגרת הזרע מבלי רצון. → NM 4:41.

• **הגרת טיפות השתן** › **strangury**: Arab. تقطير البول · Maimonides, *Šarḥ fuṣūl Abūqrāṭ* · trans. Zeraḥyah Ḥen (*Pirqei Abuqraṭ*), 3.16 (122): אבל החוליים המתחדשים במעט מטר הם טיציש ורמד וכאב הפרקים והגרת טיפות השתן. → NM 3:56.

• **הגרת המים** › **hydrocele**: Arab. قيلة الماء · Maimonides, *K. al-fuṣūl fī al-ṭibb* · trans. Nathan ha-Me'ati (*Sefer ha-Peraqim*), 23.57: קשי האשכים נקרא קילה אללחם כלומר הגרת הבשר בכיס כמו שנקרא הלחות המתקבצת בכיס אשר סביב האשכים קילה אלמא כלומר הגרת המים. → NM 2:38.

• **הגרת השתן** › **micturiction**: Arab. إدرار البول · Maimonides, *Šarḥ fuṣūl Abūqrāṭ* · trans. Moses ibn Tibbon (*Pirqei Abuqraṭ*), 1.2 (29): אמר המפרש: אמרו וכן הרקת העורקים רוצה לומר הגרת השתן והזיעה ודם הנחירים ופתיחת פיות העורקים ויהיה זה הפרק כלו במה שיבא ברצון. → NM 3:56.

הַדְבָּקָה › **agglutination**: Lat. agglutinatio · Bruno Longobucco, *Cyrurgia Magna* · trans.

Hillel ben Samuel (*Sefer Keritut*), fol. 92[b]: ואימון רפואתו שיחבוש השבר במה שמגרש הרוחות ושיהיה בהן קבצות חזקה עם הדבקה קונגלוטינציאוני. → NM 1:21.

הִדּוּק · I. **ligature:** Arab. شدّ · Al-Zahrāwī, *K. al-taṣrīf li-man ʿağiza ʿan at-taʾlīf* · trans. Shem Tov ben Isaac (*Sefer ha-Shimmush*), bk. 30, 1.56 (fol. 208[a–b]): והמתעסק בהפסקתו בקשירה או בהדוק בבגדים או בתת הדברים השורפים וכיוצא בהם לשוא יטרח כי לא יועילנו כלל אלא במקרה. → NM 1:86.

· II. **solidity; strength:** Arab. وثاقة · Ibn Sīnā, *K. al-Qānūn fī al-ṭibb* · trans. Nathan ha-Me'ati (*Sefer ha-Qanun*), bk. 1 (fol. 39[a]): וכן לא נבראו מפחות משלשה כמו שאם היה נברא משתי עצמות היה ההדוק נוסף והתנועות כחסרות מן המספיק. → NM 4:41.

הַדְחָקָה · **coercion:** Arab. استكراه · Maimonides, *Šarḥ fuṣūl Abūqrāṭ* · trans. Zeraḥyah Ḥen (*Pirqei Abuqraṭ*), 2.42 (94): ואם השתוק נעדרה ממנו תנועת החזה זה יותר גדול ממה שאפשר וכשיתנפש ביותר חזק ממה שיהיה מן ההדחקה שיתוקו חזק כמו כן. → NM 3:56–7.

הַדְלָקָה • *Plur.* **הדלקות** · **burns:** Gr. καῦμα, *Plur.* καύματα · Hippocrates, *Aphorisms* · trans. Joseph Delmedigo, 7.13 (365): מהדלקות חזקות קיווץ או מתיחות רע. → NM 3:57.

[הדק] • *Puʿal* **הֻדַּק** · **to be palpated:** Arab. غمز · Galen, attr., *Prohibition of Burial* · trans. Judah al-Ḥarizi (*Sefer Issur ha-Qevurah le-Galienus*), par. 31: והמקום השלישי העורק בין צדי האמה והאמה כשיהודקו הדוק חזק ירגיש האדם כמו התלהבות האש ואם תראה זה הנה הוא חי. → NM 4:41.

הַדְרָאָה • **פת הדראה** → **פַּת**.

הדרוקן → **הִידְרוֹקָן**.

הדרקון → **הִידְרוֹקָן**.

הַוָּה · **affliction; disaster; harm:** Arab. آفة · Al-Zahrāwī, *K. al-taṣrīf li-man ʿağiza ʿan at-taʾlīf* · trans. Shem Tov ben Isaac (*Sefer ha-Shimmush*), bk. 27, fol. 137[a], col. a: אמנם מי שיקרה לו מאכילתו נפח ומשיכה בבטן או שיש בו הווה מההדרקון מתילד מן הרוח ראוי להזהר מאכילתו בזגו וחרצנו או עם לחם או לשתות עליו מים קרים. → NM 4:42.

הווה › **הַוָּה**.

הוזות · **mental confusion (delirium):** a) Lat. alienatio / Arab. اختلاط ذهنه · Hippocrates, *Aphorisms* · trans. Hillel ben Samuel, 6.26 (318): כל אותם שיבוא להם הפלצות בקואסון יבואם ההוזות ויוסר הקואסון. → NM 3:58–9.

b) Lat. desipientia / Arab. اختلاط في العقل · Hippocrates, *Aphorisms* · trans. Hillel ben Samuel, 4.50 (187) (fol. 26[a]): א"א: אם בקדחות שאין להם הפסקה תבוא להם דיסניאה היא רוע הנשימה וההוזות הוא אות מות. → NM 3:58.

הוֹמֶה (*Part.*) → **הָמָה**.

הוֹצָאָה • **הוצאת מוגלא** · **empyema:** Arab. تقييح · Maimonides, *Šarḥ fuṣūl Abūqrāṭ* · trans. Anonymous (*Pirqei Abuqraṭ*), 5.10 (230): אמר אבוקרט: מי שקרתהו שחיטה הנקרא אסכרה וימלט ממנו ונטה החומר אל ריאתו הוא ימות בשבעה ימים. ואם יעברם יחזור להוצאת מוגלא. → NM 3:59.

הוֹרָאָה · **indication; symptom:** Lat. significo (Honofredi) · Ibn Zuhr, *Regimen of Health* · trans. Jacob ibn Tibbon (*Hanhagat ha-Beri'ut le-Abu ʿAli ben Zuhr*), ch. 28: וכאשר

יהיה האדם רואה כאלו זבובים יפרחו נגד עיניו או שערות או יראה סביבו ענן או עשן פעמים יהיה הוראה לירידת המים בעין וישתדל ברפואתו. → NM 4:42.

• **יוֹם הוראה** → **יוֹם**.

• *Plur.* **הוראות** ‣ **prognostic signs**: Arab. استدلالات · Maimonides, *K. al-fuṣūl fī al-ṭibb* · trans. Nathan ha-Me'ati (*Sefer ha-Peraqim*), introduction: השׁשׁי בשׁאר ההוראות. → NM 2:39.

הוֹרֵג • **הורג הזאב** ‣ **aconite** [***Aconitum napellus***]: Arab. قاتل الذئب · a) Al-Zahrāwī, *K. al-taṣrīf li-man ʿağiza ʿan at-taʾlīf* · trans. Shem Tov ben Isaac (*Sefer ha-Shimmush*), bk. 27, fol. 146[b], col. a: חלב הנשים יותר שוה מכל החלבים ... ולפיכך הוא מועיל מן העקיצה אשר תקרה באסטומ׳ ומשחין הריאה והמעים ומשתיית הארנבת הימית ומשתית הסם הנודע בהורג הזאב ומשתית המאירות ועוד יועיל מאדמימות זנב העין. → NM 4:43.

b) Maimonides, *K. al-fuṣūl fī al-ṭibb* · trans. Nathan ha-Me'ati (*Sefer ha-Peraqim*), 23.101: הסמים המחממים והמרטיבים עד שמפסידים מה שיפגשו הם הנקראים באמת סמים מעפשים. וכן נקראים כל הסמים החמים היבשים עבי העצם כשיעקצו מעט או שישרפו מעט מבלי שיחדשו כאב נקראים מעפשים באמת והם שני זרניכים ומדביק הזהב ותולעת הצינובר והורג הזאב. → NM 2:39.

הוֹרָדָה ‣ **relaxation**: Arab. إنحطاط · Maimonides, *Šarḥ fuṣūl Abūqrāṭ* · trans. Anonymous (*Pirqei Abuqraṭ*), 1.7 (34): אמר אבוקראט: וכשיהיה החולי חד מאד והיו הכאבים אשר בקצה התכלית מן הדקות. וכשלא יהיה כן אמנם יסבול מן ההנהגה מה שהוא יותר עב מזה ויצטרך שיהיה ההורדה כפי רכות החולי וחסרונו מקצה התכלית. → NM 3:59.

הִזְדַּכְּכוּת ‣ **cleansing; purification**: Ibn Zuhr, *Regimen of Health* · trans. Jacob ibn Tibbon (*Hanhagat ha-Beri'ut le-Abu ʿAli ben Zuhr*), ch. 2: ואמר אחד מן החכמים: התמדת הטיולים וההזדככות עבדי השכל. → NM 4:43.

הֲזָיָה ‣ **raving**: Arab. هذيان · Maimonides, *Šarḥ fuṣūl Abūqrāṭ* · trans. Zeraḥyah Ḥen (*Pirqei Abuqraṭ*), 7.9 (361): אמר המפרש: בלבול הדעת אחר ההרקה יהיה בעבור הצטער המוח בתנועותיו ויהיה לעולם חלוש ובקראט יקרא לבלבול הדעת החלוש הזיה. → NM 3:60.

הֲזָלָה ‣ I. **diarrhea**: Hippocrates, *Aphorisms* · trans. Do'eg ha-Edomi (*Sefer Agur*), 3.30 (136) (fol. 58[a]): תגיע אליהם בהגיעם לארבעים צרת כאב הצדדים ולמטה מן הצלעות גם כאב הריאה וקדחות עם תעורה ואפיסת הדעת ההזלה הארוכה וקיא ונפח הגידים השפלים. → NM 3:60.

‣ II. **flux**: Arab. سيلان / Gr. ῥύσις · Hippocrates, *Aphorisms* · trans. Nathan ha-Me'ati, 7.16 (368) (fol. 130[a]): אמר אבוקרט: ומרקיקת המוגלא אלסל ואלסילאן הנקרא הזלה וכשיעצר הרוק ימות בעל החולי. → NM 3:60–1.

• **הזלת הבטן** ‣ I. **diarrhea**: Hippocrates, *Aphorisms* · trans. Do'eg ha-Edomi (*Sefer Agur*), 1.2 (29) (fol. 21[b]): אמר אפוקרט: בבא הזלת הבטן והקיא מן הנוסף הוא אות מרפא וחיים ומזולתו יהיה ההפך. → NM 3:61.

‣ II. **lientery**: Hippocrates, *Aphorisms* · trans. Do'eg ha-Edomi (*Sefer Agur*), 6.1 (293) (fol. 96[a]): אמר אפוקרט: אדם כי יקרהו להוציא דרך גרונו כיח חמוץ בחולי הזלת הבטן ארוך ואינו נהוג כן אות טוב הוא. → NM 3:61.

• **הזלת הדם** ‣ **dysentery**: Hippocrates, *Aphorisms* · trans. Do'eg ha-Edomi (*Sefer Agur*), 3.11 (117) (fols. 52[a–b]): אמר אפוקרט: העדרת הגשם בימי הקור עם חזקת רוח צפונית הירידה

ממנו החום עם מרוצת רוח דרומית הם סבות מולידים תחלואים חדים. אמר אפוקר׳: ומדוה עינים והזלת הדם. → NM 3:62.

• **הזלת דם הבטן** ‣ **dysentery**: Hippocrates, *Aphorisms* · trans. Do'eg ha-Edomi (*Sefer Agur*), cf. 4.26 (163) (fol. 64[b]): חתיכות קטנות דומות בשר מעורבות בהזלת דם הבטן הוא אות מות. → NM 3:62.

• **הזלת דם הנחירים** ‣ **nosebleed**: Hippocrates, *Aphorisms* · trans. Judah Shalom, 5.33 (253) (fols. 82[b]–83[a]): לנשים שיחסר הנדות הזלת דם הנחירים טובה. → NM 3:62.

• **כובד הזלת השתן** → **כֹּבֶד**.

• **הזלת מקור** ‣ **venesection**: Hippocrates, *Aphorisms* · trans. Do'eg ha-Edomi (*Sefer Agur*), 6.22 (314) (fol. 101[a]): זחלת המכאוב היוצא מאחרי הכתף והולך עד הזרוע יעבירנו הזלת מקור הזרוע. → NM 3:63.

• **הזלת השתן** ‣ **micturiction**: Arab. إدرار البول · Maimonides, *Šarḥ fuṣūl Abūqrāṭ* · trans. Anonymous (*Pirqei Abuqraṭ*), 1.2 (29): אמר המפרש: אמרו וכן הרקת העורקים ר״ל הזלת השתן או הזיעה או דם הנידות או פיתוח פיות העורקים ויהיה הפרק הזה כלו במה שהביא בו מצורך. → NM 3:63.

• *Plur.* **הזלות** • **הזלות הראש** ‣ **catarrhs**: Arab. نظلات · Al-Zahrāwī, *K. al-taṣrīf li-man ʿağiza ʿan at-taʾlīf* · trans. Shem Tov ben Isaac (*Sefer ha-Shimmush*), bk. 30, 2.95 (fol. 228[b]): אמנם שני הגידים אשר אחורי האזנים תועלת הקזתם מהזלות הראש הישנות ומכאב הצילחתא ומן השחין הנקרא בלשונם אל סעפה ומן השחין הרחב הישן אשר יהיה בראש. → NM 1:86–7.

הַזְמָנָה ‣ **disposition**: Arab. استعداد · Ibn Sīnā, *K. al-Qānūn fī al-ṭibb* · trans. Joseph Lorki (*Sefer ha-Qanun*), bk. 1 (fol. 12[b]): והעמוד העליון מעוקל כאלו לוקח מן הצד הפנימי ונוטה מעט אל החיצוני בעקום וקפול והתועלת בזה טוב ההזמנה לתנועת הקפול. → NM 4:43.

הֲזָעָה ‣ **inducing perspiration**: Arab. تعريق · Maimonides, *Šarḥ fuṣūl Abūqrāṭ* · trans. Moses ibn Tibbon (*Pirqei Abuqraṭ*), 1.20 (47): אמר המפרש: אמרו יבא אליהם ר״ל שהוכנו סיבותיו ונראו אותואיו והוא מזומן שיהיה ואמרו ולא בזולתה מן התנועות כמו הרחיצה וההזעה והורת השתן או דם הנדות והחפיפה. → NM 3:63.

הֶזֵּק ‣ **pain**: Gr. πόνος · Hippocrates, *Aphorisms* · trans. Joseph Delmedigo, 2.1 (53): החולאים שהשינה גורמת בהם היזק יש בהם סכנת מות ואם תועלת אין בהם סכנת מות. → NM 3:63–4.

הֲזָרָה ‣ I. **powder**: Arab. ذرور · Al-Zahrāwī, *K. al-taṣrīf li-man ʿağiza ʿan at-taʾlīf* · trans. Shem Tov ben Isaac (*Sefer ha-Shimmush*), bk. 30, 2.17 (fol. 211[b]): וכשישלם החתוך ויכלה כל הבשר ראוי למלא העין במלח שחוק או להטיף בו מן ההזרה האדומה. → NM 1:87.

‣ II. **rebounding; repelling**: Lat. repercussio · Bruno Longobucco, *Cyrurgia Magna* · trans. Hillel ben Samuel (*Sefer Keritut*), fol. 96[b]: ורפואת המורסא הקרה היא ההתכה לבד בלא הזרה. → NM 1:21.

‣ III. **repulsion; restraining; restraint**: a) Lat. refrenatio · Bruno Longobucco, *Cyrurgia Magna* · trans. Hillel ben Samuel (*Sefer Keritut*), fol. 78[a]: אלא שאין צריך בתחלה הזרה גדולה. → NM 1:21.

b) Arab. رَدْع · Maimonides, *K. al-fuṣūl fī al-ṭibb* · trans. Zeraḥyah Ḥen (*Sefer ha-*

Peraqim), 3.85: ולא ארמוז בהזרתו לעולם אלא לעתים רחוקות שנזיר במעט הזרה כשלא יהיה שם כאב ויהיה הגוף נקי. → NM 1:138, 143; corr. 4:229.

הֲטָחָה · **befouling; dirtying; soiling**: Arab. تلطيخ · Al-Zahrāwī, *K. al-taṣrīf li-man ʿağiza ʿan at-taʾlīf* · trans. Shem Tov ben Isaac (*Sefer ha-Shimmush*), bk. 27, fol. 144[a], col. b: והמוח הצלוי מתעכב לרדת מן האסטומכא יותר מן המבושל אלא שהטחתו אל האסטומ׳ יותר מעוטה. → NM 4:43.

הַטָּפָה • **הטפת דם מהנחירים** · **nosebleed**: Arab. رعاف · Maimonides, *K. al-fuṣūl fī al-ṭibb* · trans. Zeraḥyah Ḥen (*Sefer ha-Peraqim*), 12.42: הנשים אשר יתחיל להם ההדרוקן בסבת העצר הווסת וכן מי שקרה לו זה מהעצר דם שהיה נגר מפיות העורקים או בהטפת דם מהנחירים ראוי שתתחיל בהקזתם קודם שהכח יחלש ויפול. → NM 1:138–9.

• **הטפת השתן** · **strangury**: a) Hippocrates, *Aphorisms* · trans. Do'eg ha-Edomi (*Sefer Agur*), 5.58 (278) (fol. 92[a]): שמור בעלות צמח בקצה גיד הערוה או בפי הרחם כי יחול מזה הטפת השתן במכאוב ופוקות. → NM 3:64.

b) Arab. تقطير البول · Al-Zahrāwī, *K. al-taṣrīf li-man ʿağiza ʿan at-taʾlīf* · trans. Shem Tov ben Isaac (*Sefer ha-Shimmush*), bk. 27, fol. 141[b], col. a: האגוזים ההודיים ... קשי להתעכל ומקלקלין האסטו׳ אלא שהם מועילים מהטפת השתן ומכאב הגב הישן. → NM 4:44.

• *Plur.* **הטפות** · **embrocations**: Arab. تنطيلات · Al-Zahrāwī, *K. al-taṣrīf li-man ʿağiza ʿan at-taʾlīf* · trans. Shem Tov ben Isaac (*Sefer ha-Shimmush*), bk. 30, 2.37 (214[b]): ואחר כך לגמע במים קרים ולרפא מחוץ בהטפות ומבית בגרגורים עד שיבריא. → NM 1:87.

הַטְפָּחָה · **fomentation**: Arab. نطول · Al-Zahrāwī, *K. al-taṣrīf li-man ʿağiza ʿan at-taʾlīf* · trans. Shem Tov ben Isaac (*Sefer ha-Shimmush*), bk. 30, 3.26 (fol. 237[a]): ואם לא ישוב במה שזכרתי ותהיה לשמיטה מעת שנתחדשה ימים רבים ראוי להשיב החולה במים חמין במרחץ ולהרגיל ההטפחה המרפה והמרככה. → NM 1:87–8.

הִידְרוֹקָן (also: **הדרקון**) · I. **colic**: Arab. قولنج · a) Al-Zahrāwī, *K. al-taṣrīf li-man ʿağiza ʿan at-taʾlīf* · trans. Shem Tov ben Isaac (*Sefer ha-Shimmush*), bk. 27, fol. 129[b], col. b: המים ההולכים על מחצבי העופרת מולידים ההדרקון. → NM 4:42.

b) Al-Rāzī, *K. al-Manṣūrī* · trans. Shem Tov ben Isaac (*Sefer Almansur*), Bet 6 (18): בסבאיג ובלעז פוליפודיאו: חם משלשל המרה השחורה ומתיך ההדרוקן כשילקח עם המרק. → NM 2:11.

· II. **dropsy**: Arab. استسقاء · a) Maimonides, *K. al-fuṣūl fī al-ṭibb* · trans. Zeraḥyah Ḥen (*Sefer ha-Peraqim*), 6.45: מי שהוא בטבעו דומה לבעל ההידרוקן ההידרוקן ימהר אליו. → NM 1:139.

b) Maimonides, *Šarḥ fuṣūl Abūqrāṭ* · trans. Zeraḥyah Ḥen (*Pirqei Abuqraṭ*), 4.11 (148): אמר בקראט: מי שיהיה בו עקיצה וכאב סביב הטבור וכאב בבטן תמיד לא יסור לא ברפואה משלשלת ולא בזולתה עניינו ילך אל ההדרוקן היבש. → NM 3:57.

• **ההדרוקן אשר בו המים כמי הנאד** · **ascites**: Arab. الاستسقاء الزقّي · Maimonides, *Šarḥ fuṣūl Abūqrāṭ* · trans. Zeraḥyah Ḥen (*Pirqei Abuqraṭ*), 4.11 (148): אמר המפרש: כשלא יהיה סר זה בשום רפואה הוא ראיה על רוע מזג שגבר על אותם האיברים ונתאחז בהם ויתחדש ההדרקון התופיי הוא אשר קראו ההדרוקן היבש שהוא נוכח ההדרוקן אשר בו המים כמי הנאד ויתיילד מקרירות נוסף. → NM 3:57–8.

• **החדרקון התופיי** ‹ **tympanites**: Arab. الاستسقاء الطبلي · Maimonides, *Šarḥ fuṣūl Abūqrāṭ* · trans. Zeraḥyah Ḥen (*Pirqei Abuqraṭ*), 4.11 (148): אמר המפרש: כשלא יהיה סר זה בשום רפואה הוא ראיה על רוע מזג שגבר על אותם האיברים ונתאחז בהם ויתחדש ההדרקון התופיי הוא אשר קראו ההדרוקן היבש שהוא נוכח ההדרוקן אשר בו המים כמי הנאד ויתיילד מקרירות נוסף. → NM 3:58.

היזק → חֵזֶק.

הַכָּאָה ‹ I. **beat [of the pulse]**: Arab. ضربان / Lat. percussio · Ibn al-Jazzār, *Zād al-musāfir wa-qūt al-ḥādir* · trans. Moses ibn Tibbon (*Sefer Ṣedat ha-Derakhim*), bk. 1, ch. 20 (fol. 30[a]): ויהיו עיני בעליו בעבור זה עמוקים ממהרי התנועה בעבור סער הנפש במחשבה ותשוקתה להשיג מי שישתוקק אליו ויהיו עפעפיו כבדות ומראהו כרכומי לתנועת המרה האדומה בנדוד השינה ויהיה דפק עורקיו חזק ולא ימצא בו התפשטות הדפק הטבעי ולא ישפל הכאתו. → NM 4:44.

‹ II. **throbbing**: Arab. ضربان / Gr. σφυγμός · Maimonides, *Šarḥ fuṣūl Abūqrāṭ* · trans. Anonymous (*Pirqei Abuqraṭ*), 7.21 (373): אמר אבוקרט: ומן ההכאה החזקה בנגע השפך הדם. → NM 3:64.

הַכָּרָה • **הקדמת החכרה** → הַקְדָּמָה.

הָלַךְ • **החוליא ההולכת באורך** → חֻלְיָה.

• **החוליא ההולכת ברוחב** → חֻלְיָה.

• **העצב אשר בו ילך השמע** → עָצָב.

• *Inf.* **לֶכֶת** • **התנערות ללכת** → הִתְנַעֲרוּת.

הָמָה • *Part.* **הוֹמֶה** ‹ **suffering from [intestinal] rumbling**: Lat. subrugiens · Hippocrates, *Aphorisms* · trans. Hillel ben Samuel, 4.73 (210) (fol. 28[b]): א"א: אותם שנראים להם האפוקונדריאי נפוחים והומים אם יבא להם כאב למטה מהחלצים יותר להם הבטן אלא אם יצאו להם רוחות הרבה או ישתין שתן רב. → NM 3:59.

הֶמְיָה ‹ I. **colic**: Arab. مغص · Maimonides, *Šarḥ fuṣūl Abūqrāṭ* · trans. Anonymous (*Pirqei Abuqraṭ*), 5.41 (261): אמר אבוקרט: כשתרצה לדעת האם האשה הרה אם לא תשקנה כשרוצה לישן מי הדבש. ואם מצא אותה המיה בחטיה היא הרה ואם לא ימצאנה המיה אינה הרה. → NM 3:64.

‹ II. **rumblings**: Lat. rugire / Arab. قرقرة, *Plur.* قراقر · Hippocrates, *Aphorisms* · trans. Hillel ben Samuel, 5.64 (284) (fol. 37[a]): א"א: החלב רע למי שיש לו כאב הראש ורע למוקדחים ולאותם שיש להם המיה באיפוקונדריאה ורם. → NM 3:65.

הַמְעָדָה ‹ **lubrication**: Arab. إزلاق · Al-Zahrāwī, *K. al-taṣrīf li-man ʿağiza ʿan at-taʾlīf* · trans. Shem Tov ben Isaac (*Sefer ha-Shimmush*), bk. 30, 3.27 (fol. 237[b]): המעדת הפרק. → NM 1:88; corr. 2:198.

• **המעדת המעים** ‹ **lientery**: Arab. زلق الأمعاء · a) Maimonides, *K. al-fuṣūl fī al-ṭibb* · trans. Zeraḥyah Ḥen (*Sefer ha-Peraqim*), 23.80: אנמם שינוי המזונות באסטומכא אל איכות אחרת לא אל אותם אשר בטבע ויאמר לו רוע העיכול והוא האמפונימינטו בערבי תכמה וביטול הכח העוצר מן האסטומכא הוא שלא תתקבץ האסטומכא כלל ולא תרחף על המזון ולא תאסוף עליו בדבקות ואסיפה וזה יקרה לה בחולי הנקרא חלקות או המעדת המיעים. → NM 1:139; corr. 2:198.

b) Maimonides, *K. al-fuṣūl fī al-ṭibb* · trans. Nathan ha-Me'ati (*Sefer ha-Peraqim*), 23.93: וכשהמעים יהיו עלולים והאסטו' ולא יוכלו לאחוז מה שיש בגרמם ואפילו זמן מועט ולא תהיה העלה עוקצת הנה אותה העלה נקראת המעדת המעים ותקרא גם כן עלות הבטן ויקרא בעליו מובטן. → NM 2:39.

הַמְרָצָה · **accuracy; perfection; precision**: Arab. إحكام · Ibn Sīnā, *K. al-Qānūn fī al-ṭibb* · trans. Nathan ha-Me'ati (*Sefer ha-Qanun*), bk. 1 (fol. 61[a]): ואמנם נסתפק בשנים שאין שם מן הצורך אל הַמרצת התבנית מה שיש הנה. → NM 4:44–5.

הַמְשָׁכָה · **tetanus**: Arab. تمدد · Maimonides, *Šarḥ fuṣūl Abūqrāṭ* · trans. Zeraḥyah Ḥen (*Pirqei Abuqraṭ*), 4.57 (194): אמר אבקראט: מי שקרה לו קיוץ או המשכה בלע' טומור ואחרי כן אחזתו קדחת חליו יהיה נתך ויסור. → NM 3:65.

הַמְתָּחָה · **extension**: Lat. extensio · Ibn Sīnā, *K. al-adwiya al-qalbiya* · trans. Anonymous (*Sefer ha-Refu'ot ha-Libbiyot*), fol. 243[b]: והדבק הוא אותו אשר יסבול ההמתחה מבלי שיחתך. → NM 4:45.

הַמְתָּנָה • **ההמתנה מן המאכל** · **abstention from food (i.e., fasting)**: Arab. الصبر عن الطعام · Maimonides, *Šarḥ fuṣūl Abūqrāṭ* · trans. Anonymous (*Pirqei Abuqraṭ*), 1.13 (40): אמנם הישישים שהם בתכלית הזקנה לא יסבלו ההמתנה מן המאכל אבל צריכים שינתן להם מעט מעט פעם אחר פעם לקרוב חומם היסודי להכבות וצריך אל הנהגתם מי שיגיעם מעט אחר מעט. → NM 3:65.

הַנְהָגָה · **preparation**: Arab. تدبير · Al-Zahrāwī, *K. al-taṣrīf li-man 'ağiza 'an at-ta'līf* · trans. Shem Tov ben Isaac (*Sefer ha-Shimmush*), bk. 27, fol. 140[a], col. a: הזתים ישתנו פעולותיהם כפי השתנות מיניהם ושנוי הנהגתם. → NM 4:45.

• **הנהגת השמירה** · **diet**: Lat. dieta · Bruno Longobucco, *Cyrurgia Magna* · trans. Hillel ben Samuel (*Sefer Keritut*), fol. 4[a]: כי חלקי הרפואה הם שלשה שבאמצעותם יוכל הרופא מסיבות החולי לעזור: הראשון הנהגת השמירה הב' הנהגת המשקיות הג' הכריתות. השמירה הוא הראשון והמובחר כמאמר גלינו בספר הנהגת החדות. → NM 1:40.

• **שמירה והנהגה** → **שְׁמִירָה**.

הַנָּחָה · **subject**: Arab. موضوع · Maimonides, *K. al-fuṣūl fī al-ṭibb* · trans. Zeraḥyah Ḥen (*Sefer ha-Peraqim*), introduction: המאמר הראשון ישלם על פרקים יהיו נתלים בהנחת המלאכה. → NM 1:139.

• **הנחה חמה** · **hot compress**: Arab. تكميد · Maimonides, *K. al-fuṣūl fī al-ṭibb* · trans. Nathan ha-Me'ati (*Sefer ha-Peraqim*), 23.33: ההנחה החמה הנקרא בערבי תכמיד נופל על כל מה שמחמם הגוף מחוץ ומיני החנחה ארבעה: הרטוב והיבש והעוקץ וממוצע ושוה. → NM 2:39–40; corr. 4:229.

הִסְתַּבְּכוּת · **cramps; spasms**: Arab. تشبّك · Al-Zahrāwī, *K. al-taṣrīf li-man 'ağiza 'an at-ta'līf* · trans. Shem Tov ben Isaac (*Sefer ha-Shimmush*), bk. 27, fol. 127[b], col. b: ומין אחר רע מזיק לעצבים נזק גדול ויגרום למי שיישן עליו או יפרשהו תחתיו הסתבכות בשוקים עד שלא יכול בעליו ללכת. → NM 4:45.

הִסְתַּלְּקוּת · **abatement**: Arab. إقلاع · Maimonides, *K. al-fuṣūl fī al-ṭibb* · trans. Nathan ha-Me'ati (*Sefer ha-Peraqim*), 25.24: ומובן דברו השני הוא שלא יהיה הסתלקות מורגשת אלא כשתהיה הליחה המעופשת חוץ מן העורקים במקום אחר. → NM 2:40.

הִסְתַּעֲרוּת · **disturbance:** Arab. اضطراب · Maimonides, *Šarḥ fuṣūl Abūqrāṭ* · trans. Moses ibn Tibbon (*Pirqei Abuqraṭ*), 2.13 (65): אמר המפרש: בהבדל הטבע הדבר הרע מן הדבר הטוב ויכין לו הדחיה והיציאה יתחדש הסתערות. וראוי בהכרח בעת ההסתערות ההוא שיסתער החולה ויכבד עליו חליו. → NM 3:65–6.

הַעֲדָפָה • *Plur.* **העדפות** · **superfluities:** a) Lat. superfluitates · Bruno Longobucco, *Cyrurgia Magna* · trans. Hillel ben Samuel (*Sefer Keritut*), fol. 85ª: שער השביעי מן האישקורופולו ומשאר ההעדפות הדומות להם. → NM 1:22.

b) Arab. فضول · Al-Zahrāwī, *K. al-taṣrīf li-man ʿağiza ʿan at-taʾlīf* · trans. Shem Tov ben Isaac (*Sefer ha-Shimmush*), bk. 30, introduction (fol. 202ª): ומה שיזדמן בגופו מהתקבץ ההעדפות בו. → NM 1:88.

הַעֲמָדָה · I. **culmination:** Arab. منتهى · Maimonides, *K. al-fuṣūl fī al-ṭibb* · trans. Nathan ha-Me'ati (*Sefer ha-Peraqim*), 8.6: החלאים כלם בהתחלתם ובאחריתם הם יותר חלושים ובהעמדה יותר חזקים ובמה שהוא בין שני העתים האלו ענינם ממוצע בין החולשה והחוזק. → NM 2:40.

· II. **maturity:** Arab. وقوف · Ibn Sīnā, *K. al-Qānūn fī al-ṭibb* · trans. Nathan ha-Me'ati (*Sefer ha-Qanun*), bk. 1 (fol. 31ᵇ): והקצויות יצמחו ברוב באמצע זמן הגדול והוא אחר ההמרצה אל ההעמדה וזה כי ההעמדה קרובה מל׳ שנה ולכן נקראים שני אלחלם כלומ׳ החלימה. → NM 4:45.

• **העמדת התכלית** · **climax:** Arab. منتهى · Maimonides, *K. al-fuṣūl fī al-ṭibb* · trans. Nathan ha-Me'ati (*Sefer ha-Peraqim*), 25.11: כבר באר ג׳אלינוס במקומות רבים מהליחות בהשפכם ובעת הוספת המורסות החמות גם כן ובעת העמדת תכליתם תמשוך הליחה להפך הצד. → NM 2:40.

• **תכלית החעמדה** → **תַּכְלִית**.

הֶעְתֵּק · **change [of a disease] (i.e., cure):** Arab. انتقال / Gr. μεταστάσις · Maimonides, *Šarḥ fuṣūl Abūqrāṭ* · trans. Moses ibn Tibbon (*Pirqei Abuqraṭ*), 5.7 (227): אמר אבקראט: מי שמצאו חולי הנופל קודם צמיחת השער סביב הערוה הנה יתחדש לו העתק ואולם מי שקרה לו וכבר עָברו עָליו מן השנים חמישה ועֶשרים שנה הנה הוא ימות והוא בו. → NM 3:66.

הַעְתָּקָה · **removal [of a disease] (i.e., cure):** Arab. انتقال · Maimonides, *Šarḥ fuṣūl Abūqrāṭ* · trans. Anonymous (*Pirqei Abuqraṭ*), 5.7 (227): אמר אבוקרט: מי שמצאתהו הכפייה קודם שיצמח לו השיער של בית הערוה הוא יתחדש לו ההעתקה. ואמנם מי שקרה לו זה וכבר חלפו עליו מן השנים חמשה ועשרים הוא ימות והוא בו. → NM 3:66.

הִפּוּךְ • **הפוך נפש** · **(lit., upsetting the soul); nausea; sickness in the stomach:** Arab. تقلّب النفس / Gr. ἀσώδης · Al-Zahrāwī, *K. al-taṣrīf li-man ʿağiza ʿan at-taʾlīf* · trans. Shem Tov ben Isaac (*Sefer ha-Shimmush*), bk. 27, fol. 145ᵇ, col. a: הבשר השלוק וקוראים אותו אנשי המזרח אספגדבאג׳ה ואנחנו קוראים אותו גם כן שלוק האשכנז והוא חם בשוי ונאות ברוב העתים והענינים לכל בני אדם לבד מי שיגבר על מזגו החמימות ובעתים החמים מאד ולמי שיש לו אסתניסות והפוך נפש. → NM 4:45–6.

הָפַךְ • **הפך ל-** · **to have a contrary effect on:** Arab. ضادّ · Maimonides, *K. al-fuṣūl fī al-ṭibb* · trans. Zeraḥyah Ḥen (*Sefer ha-Peraqim*), 21.42: הקנמון הוא רפואה דקה מאד פותחת שבילי האסטומכא ויטהר הליחות וידקדקם ויהפך לטרי המוסרח כולו כשישנהו ויתירהו. → NM 1:139–40.

• *Pi'el* הִפֵּךְ · **to bend (the head):** Arab. نكس · Ibn Sīnā, *K. al-Qānūn fī al-ṭibb* · trans. Nathan ha-Me'ati (*Sefer ha-Qanun*), bk. 1 (fol. 45[b]): ואמנם העצלים המהפכים הראש ביחוד והם שני עצלים יורדים משני צדדים. → NM 4:46.

• **היפך על פניו** · **to supinate:** Arab. بطح · Ibn Sīnā, *K. al-Qānūn fī al-ṭibb* · trans. Zeraḥyah Ḥen (*Sefer ha-Qanun*), bk. 1 (fol. 27[a]): ואמנם המהפכת על פניו לזרוע הוא זוג אחד ממנו מונח מבחוץ. → NM 4:46.

• *Hitpa'el* הִתְהַפֵּךְ · **to be different; to vary:** Lat. diversificari · Bruno Longobucco, *Cyrurgia Magna* · trans. Hillel ben Samuel (*Sefer Keritut*), fol. 37[b]: אמנם הנגעים יתהפכו לפי התהפך הזמן כי מהן יש שהן חדשים ומהן ישנים. → NM 1:22.

• *Inf. Hitpa'el* הִתְהַפֵּךְ · **difference; diversity:** Lat. diversitas · Bruno Longobucco, *Cyrurgia Magna* · trans. Hillel ben Samuel (*Sefer Keritut*), fol. 7[a]: השער השני מן התכונה הכללית מהתרת הדבקות לפי התהפך האברים. → NM 1:23.

• *Part. Hitpa'el* מִתְהַפֵּךְ · **opposite:** Arab. متضادّ / Lat. oppositus · a) Ibn al-Jazzār, *Zād al-musāfir wa-qūt al-ḥāḍir* · trans. Moses ibn Tibbon (*Sefer Ṣedat ha-Derakhim*), bk. 1, ch. 15 (fols. 22[a–b]): ולכן אמר גאלינוס כי הכונה ברפואת החולי הזה הנקרא המוקץ נקוי המוח משתי אלו הליחות המתהפכות בעצמיהם ר"ל ליחה לבנה ומרה אדומה. → NM 4:46–7.
b) Maimonides, *Šarḥ fuṣūl Abūqrāṭ* · trans. Moses ibn Tibbon (*Pirqei Abuqraṭ*), 0 (4): והסבה השלישית אופני המאמר וזה כי רוב המאמרים בכל לשון יסבול הסברות ואפשר יהיה שיובן מן המאמר ההוא ענינים מתחלפים גם קצתם מתהפכים גם סותרים. → NM 3:66.

הַפְכִּיּוֹת · **alteration:** Lat. diversitas / Arab. استحالة · Galen, *De inaequali intemperie* · trans. David Caslari (*Sefer Ro'a Mezeg Mitḥallef*), 5.3: והנה ניסכמו על זה הפילוסופים הטבעיים בעיונם בחושים ואמרו, שאין הרגש אם לא בהפכיות. → NM 2:166.

הַפָּלָה · **miscarriage:** Arab. سقط / Gr. διαφθείρειν τὰ ἔμβρυα · Maimonides, *Šarḥ fuṣūl Abūqrāṭ* · trans. Moses ibn Tibbon (*Pirqei Abuqraṭ*), 5.53 (273): אמר אבקראט: כשיהיה ענין האשה הולך אל ההפלה הנה שדיה יצמקו. → NM 3:67.

הֶפְסֵד • **הפסד וחולשה** · **senility:** Arab. هرم · Maimonides, *Šarḥ fuṣūl Abūqrāṭ* · trans. Moses ibn Tibbon (*Pirqei Abuqraṭ*), 1.13 (40): וזה אשר זכר מסבול הזקנים הצום זכר ג'אלינוס שהוא הישיש שלא הגיע לגבול ההפסד והחולשה. → NM 3:67.

• **הפסד המזג** · **bad temperament:** Arab. سوء المزاج · Maimonides, *Šarḥ fuṣūl Abūqrāṭ* · trans. Moses ibn Tibbon (*Pirqei Abuqraṭ*), 4.35 (172): אמר המפרש: עוות הצואר ועוצר הבליעה יהיה מסור אחת מן החליות וסורה פעמים יהיה בעבור מורסא ופעמים יהיה לתגבורת היובש ואשר ירצה בו הנה הוא המתהווה מתגבורת היובש כי הוא ראיה על שקיעת הפסד המזג באיברים ותגבורת היובש. → NM 3:67–8.

• **הפסד הקול** · **hoarseness:** Arab. بحوحة · Maimonides, *Šarḥ fuṣūl Abūqrāṭ* · trans. Zeraḥyah Ḥen (*Pirqei Abuqraṭ*), 2.40 (92): אמר בקראט: מה שיקרה מן הנזל והפסד הקול לזקן הכלה לא יבואו לידי בישול. → NM 3:68.

הַפְעָמוּת · **disturbance:** Arab. اضطراب · Maimonides, *Šarḥ fuṣūl Abūqrāṭ* · trans. Anonymous (*Pirqei Abuqraṭ*), 2.13 (65): אמר המפרש: עם הבדלת הטבע לדבר הרע מן הדבר הטוב והכין אותו אל הדחיה והיציאה יחדש הפעמות שיצטער החולה ויכבד עליו חליו. וממנהג האנשים

שישנו בלילה וכאשר מנע ההצטערות ההוא מן השינה יתבאר סערת החולה וקושי חוליו מבואר נגלה. → NM 3:68.

הַפְרָדָה • הפרדת הדבקות • **dissolution of continuity:** Arab. تفرّق اتّصال · Maimonides, *K. al-fuṣūl fī al-ṭibb* · trans. Zeraḥyah Ḥen (*Sefer ha-Peraqim*), 7.6: סבות הכאבים הוא או הפרדת הדבקות או שינוי מה שיהיה פתאום. → NM 1:140.

הֶפְרֵשׁ • **distance:** Arab. مسافة · Ibn Sīnā, *K. al-Qānūn fī al-ṭibb* · trans. Nathan ha-Me'ati (*Sefer ha-Qanun*), bk. 1 (fol. 36ª): ואינם מתחברות מקדם אבל בהדרגה מעט ההפסק שיהיו העליונות בהם יותר קרובות ההפרש מה שבין שתי קצותיהן היוצאות. → NM 4:47.

הֶפְשֵׁט • **abrasion (of the intestines):** Arab. سَحْج · Maimonides, *K. al-fuṣūl fī al-ṭibb* · trans. Nathan ha-Me'ati (*Sefer ha-Peraqim*), 21.27: הסכנג'בין אם יפליג בעשייתו יחדש במעיים הפשט ומעורר שעול ומזיק לאברים העצביים. → NM 2:40–1.

הַפְשָׁטָה • **ulceration:** Lat. ulceratio · Bruno Longobucco, *Cyrurgia Magna* · trans. Hillel ben Samuel (*Sefer Keritut*), fol. 42ᵇ: וממנו שיתילד משחורה שהיא משרפה מאדומה טבעית וכאבו חזק מרוב הפשטה. → NM 1:22.

• **העיצום וההפשטה** → **עִצּוּם**.

הִצְטַעֲרוּת • **agitation; disturbance; unrest:** a) Arab. قلق / Gr. ταραχή · Ibn al-Jazzār, *Zād al-musāfir wa-qūt al-ḥādir* · trans. Moses ibn Tibbon (*Sefer Ṣedat ha-Derakhim*), bk. 1, ch. 17 (fol. 24ª): ואם היה עם היובש חום יקרה עם התעורה הצטערות וערבוב שכל ומחשב. → NM 4:47.

b) Arab. اضطراب · Maimonides, *Šarḥ fuṣūl Abūqrāṭ* · trans. Anonymous (*Pirqei Abuqraṭ*), 2.13 (65): אמר המפרש: עם הבדלת הטבע לדבר הרע מן הדבר הטוב והכין אותו אל הדחיה והיציאה יחדש הפעמות שיצטער החולה ויכבד עליו חליו. וממנהג האנשים שישנו בלילה וכאשר מנע ההצטערות ההוא מן השינה יתבאר סערת החולה וקושי חוליו מבואר נגלה. → NM 3:68.

הַקְדָּמָה • החקדמה לגזור • **prediction:** Arab. التقدّم بالقضية · Maimonides, *Šarḥ fuṣūl Abūqrāṭ* · trans. Anonymous (*Pirqei Abuqraṭ*), 2.19 (71): אמר אבוקרט: ההקדמה לגזור בחליים החדים למות או לחיים לא תהיה בתכלית הדקדוק. → NM 3:69.

• **הקדמת ההכרה** • I. **prediction:** Hippocrates, *Aphorisms* · trans. Hillel ben Samuel, 2.19 (71) (fol. 10ª): א"א: הקדמת ההכרה בחלאים החדים בכלם אינה אמיתית הן לא מהבריאות ולא מהמות. → NM 3:69.

• II. **prognosis:** Arab. تقدمة المعرفة · Maimonides, *K. al-fuṣūl fī al-ṭibb* · trans. Zeraḥyah Ḥen (*Sefer ha-Peraqim*), 6.94: ותנהיג זה הפרק בהשגחה גדולה כי הוא יספיק על חלקים הרבה מהקדמת ההכרה. → NM 1:140.

• **הקדמת הידיעה** • **prognosis:** Arab. تقدمة المعرفة · Maimonides, *K. al-fuṣūl fī al-ṭibb* · trans. Nathan ha-Me'ati (*Sefer ha-Peraqim*), 2.4: בפירושו לשני בהקדמת הידיעה. → NM 2:41.

• **ההקדמה במשפט** • **prediction:** Arab. التقدّم بالقضية / Gr. προαγόρευσις · Maimonides, *Šarḥ fuṣūl Abūqrāṭ* · trans. Moses ibn Tibbon (*Pirqei Abuqraṭ*), 2.19 (71): אמר אבקראט: ההקדמה במשפט בחליים החדים הן למות הן לבריאות לא יהיה בתכלית הבטחון. → NM 3:68–9.

הַקָּעָה • **dislocation:** Arab. خَلْع · Ibn al-Jazzār, *Zād al-musāfir wa-qūt al-ḥādir* · trans. Moses ibn Tibbon (*Sefer Ṣedat ha-Derakhim*), bk. 7, 15.1: הנה כל מורסא תתחדש מהגרת

ליחה אל אבר מהאברים וסבות ההגרה מהם מתחילות באות מחוץ ומהם קודמות פנימיות והמתחילות כמו הכאה או נגע או ריצוץ או הקעה או שבר או סדק. → NM 1:55.

• הקעת הפרקים ‣ **dislocation**: Arab. زوال المفاصل · Ibn al-Jazzār, *Zād al-musāfir wa-qūt al-ḥāḍir* · trans. Moses ibn Tibbon (*Sefer Ṣedat ha-Derakhim*), introduction (fol. 4ᵇ): השער הכ״ה בשבר והקעת הפרקים. → NM 4:47–8.

הֶקֵּף • *Plur.* הקפים ‣ **cycles**: Arab. دور, *Plur.* أدوار / Gr. περίοδος, *Plur.* περίοδοι · Maimonides, *Šarḥ fuṣūl Abūqrāṭ* · trans. Moses ibn Tibbon (*Pirqei Abuqraṭ*), 4.59 (196): אמר אבקראט: השלישית היותר ארוכה תכלה בשבעה הקפים. → NM 3:69.

הַקְפָּאָה ‣ **catalepsy**: Arab. جمود · Maimonides, *K. al-fuṣūl fī al-ṭibb* · trans. Zeraḥyah Ḥen (*Sefer ha-Peraqim*), 23.59: בהתחזק הקרירות על המוח ויתערב בו לחות יתחדש ממנו השרסאם הקר והוא ליתרגיאה. וכשיתערב עם הקרירות יובש יתחדש ההקפאה. → NM 1:140.

הַקָּפָה • *Plur.* הקפות ‣ **cycles**: Lat. circuitus, *Plur.* circuitus · Hippocrates, *Aphorisms* · trans. Hillel ben Samuel, 1.12 (39) (fol. 3ᵇ): א״א: העונות והעתים מודיעים אותם החולאים ותקופות השנה ותוספת ההקפות מאחת לאחת או שתהיה בכל יום או בשלישי או ביום הרביעי וכן העניינים מבשרים מה שעתיד לבא. → NM 3:69–70.

הַר • צמוקי החר → צִמּוּק.

הֵרָאוּת • יום הראות → יוֹם.

הֶרְגֵּל ‣ I. **application; use**: Arab. استعمال · Al-Zahrāwī, *K. al-taṣrīf li-man ʿağiza ʿan at-ta'līf* · trans. Shem Tov ben Isaac (*Sefer ha-Shimmush*), bk. 27, fol. 133ᵇ, col. a: וסדר ההרגל החשוב יותר לבעלי החמימות לבשלם בחבושים או לתקנם במי רמונים קוססים. → NM 4:48.

‣ II. **physical exercise**: Arab. رياضة · Maimonides, *Šarḥ fuṣūl Abūqrāṭ* · trans. Anonymous (*Pirqei Abuqraṭ*), 5.7 (227): רצה באמרו ההעתקה הכלות בחולי וזה יהיה בתיקון התערובת הקרה במזגה המולידה לכפייה והוא לבני רטוב בהעתקת השנים אל היובש ובהרגל ובהנהגה המייבשת עם הסמנים הנאותים. → NM 3:70.

• *Plur.* הרגלים ‣ **mathematics**: Arab. رياضيات · Maimonides, *K. al-fuṣūl fī al-ṭibb* · trans. Zeraḥyah Ḥen (*Sefer ha-Peraqim*), 25.59: והוא בלא ספק כלומר גליאנוס הרגיל בהרגלים. → NM 1:140.

הֶרְגֵּשׁ • גידי החרגש → גִּיד.

הַרְגָּשָׁה ‣ **conjecture**: Arab. حدس · Maimonides, *K. al-fuṣūl fī al-ṭibb* · trans. Zeraḥyah Ḥen (*Sefer ha-Peraqim*), 11.1: זמני החולי הכוללים הם ארבעה: התחלה ותוספת ועמידה וירידה. ולפי עמוד על ידיעת הזמן ההווה מזמני החולי בהרגשה אמתית אי זה מזמניו הוא עתה. → NM 1:140–1.

הַרְדָּמָה ‣ **stupor**: Hippocrates, *Aphorisms* · trans. Judah Shalom, 7.14 (366) (fol. 115ᵇ): בהכאה בראש הרדמה או ערבוב השכל הוא רע. → NM 3:70.

הֵרָיוֹן ‣ **reproduction**: Arab. تناسل · Maimonides, *K. al-fuṣūl fī al-ṭibb* · trans. Zeraḥyah Ḥen (*Sefer ha-Peraqim*), 16.10: כל הגידים הדופקים ושאינם דופקים בכל הגוף מהזכרים והנקיבות הם על דמיון אחד לא במספר לבדו אלא ביצירתם ותכונתם ומקומם אבל ישתנו בכלי ההריון ויתבאר בניתוח כי כלי ההריון בזכרים ובנקבות זה נוכח זה בדמיון כי בזכרים יוצאים ובנקבות הם בפנים עד שהרחם אילו נתהפך שטחו הפנימי לחוץ היה דומה לכיס הביצים והביצים אשר בצדי הרחם יהיו בתוך כיס ויהיה צואר הרחם דומה לגיד. → NM 1:133.

הֲרָקָה • **הרקת הירוקה מלמעלה ומלמטה** · **cholera**: Gr. χολέρα · Hippocrates, *Aphorisms* · trans. Joseph Delmedigo, 3.30 (136): וליוצאים מאלו השנים יקרם קוצר הנשימה וחולי הצד ומורסת הריאה ותנומות ומורסות קרומי המוח וקדחות בוערות ושלשולי הבטן ארוכים והרקת הירוקה מלמעלה ומלמטה ושלשול הדם וחלקות הבטן והטחורים. → NM 3:70.

הֲשָׁבָה · **restoration**: Lat. restauratio · Bruno Longobucco, *Cyrurgia Magna* · trans. Hillel ben Samuel (*Sefer Keritut*), fol. 51[a]: באמת הרפואות שאנו רגילים בם אחר ההשבה מכל השברים ומן ההשמטות ומן העקומים הם אותם שמיבשות ומדביקות עם מעט חום. → NM 1:22.

• **השבת חשברים** · **setting of bones**: Arab. جَبْر · Al-Zahrāwī, *K. al-taṣrīf li-man ʿağiza ʿan at-taʾlīf* · trans. Shem Tov ben Isaac (*Sefer ha-Shimmush*), bk. 30, introduction (201[a]). → NM 1:88.

הֶשְׁבּוֹן · **restoration**: Lat. restauratio · Bruno Longobucco, *Cyrurgia Magna* · trans. Hillel ben Samuel (*Sefer Keritut*), fol. 32[b]: אמר הגופים שמקבלים בחבלותיהן ההשבון במהרה הם ממזג יותר טוב עם דם מובחר מבלתי לחות עודפת ולא יובש. → NM 1:22–3.

הַשְׁוָיוּת · **equality**: Arab. مساواة · Maimonides, *K. al-fuṣūl fī al-ṭibb* · trans. Zeraḥyah Ḥen (*Sefer ha-Peraqim*), 8.45: רוע המזג המתחדש בכל אחד מן האברים הוא חולי אשר באברים המתדמים החלקים וימנע וייצר בכח בלתי כח מכחות אותו האבר ויהיו הליחות מורקות בעבור זה בזמנים משתנים אל אברים משתנים על בלתי השווית ועל בלתי הסדר. → NM 1:141.

הַשְׁחָנָה · **ulceration**: Hippocrates, *Aphorisms* · trans. Judah Shalom, 4.81 (218) (fol. 74[a]): אם דם ישתין ומוגלא וקלפות והריח יהיה כבד מורה השחנת המקוה. → NM 3:71.

הַשְׁמָטָה · **dislocation**: Arab. خَلْع · Maimonides, *K. al-fuṣūl fī al-ṭibb* · trans. Zeraḥyah Ḥen (*Sefer ha-Peraqim*), 15.46: ועל זה המשל כשיקרה בפרק מן הפרקים הגדולים השמטה עם חבלה נרפא החבלה עד שתתרפא ואע״פ שאי אפשר דבקות ההשמטה אחר מכן כי אנו אם נחשוב להשיב ההשמטה עם החבלה ימצאהו כיווץ ברוב העניין. → NM 1:141.

• **השמטת המעים** · **lientery**: Hippocrates, *Aphorisms* · trans. Do'eg ha-Edomi (*Sefer Agur*), 6.43 (335) (fol. 106[a]): מאריך להזיל הזלת הבטן עם דם ולו כובד הטחול סופו לבוא לחולי המים הרעים או להשמטת המעיים. → NM 3:71.

• *Plur.* **השמטות** · **dislocations**: Lat. dislocationes · Bruno Longobucco, *Cyrurgia Magna* · trans. Hillel ben Samuel (*Sefer Keritut*), fol. 51[a]: באמת הרפואות שאנו רגילים בם אחר ההשבה מכל השברים ומן ההשמטות ומן העקומים הם אותם שמיבשות ומדביקות עם מעט חום. → NM 1:23.

הַשְׁמָעוּת · **susceptibility**: Lat. obedientia · Bruno Longobucco, *Cyrurgia Magna* · trans. Hillel ben Samuel (*Sefer Keritut*), fol. 52[b]: ועוד מתהפך השבר לפי ההשמעות ובלתי ההשמעות מן המיתוח ומן ההשבה. → NM 1:23.

הַשְׁפָּעָה · **flow of menstrual blood; menstrual bleeding**: Arab. نَزْف · Al-Zahrāwī, *K. al-taṣrīf li-man ʿağiza ʿan at-taʾlīf* · trans. Shem Tov ben Isaac (*Sefer ha-Shimmush*), bk. 27, fol. 142[a], col. b: והקלפות הדקות אשר על הפרי עצמו מבפנים הנקראות בלשון הגרי ג׳פת אל בלוט קביצותם יותר חזקה מן הבטנים ולכן הם מועילים מרקיקת הדם וההשפעה אשר תקרה לנשים. → NM 4:48.

הַשְׁקָטָה · **treatment that consists of alleviating [remedies]**: Arab. تسكين · Maimonides, *Šarḥ fuṣūl Abūqrāṭ* · trans. Moses ibn Tibbon (*Pirqei Abuqraṭ*), 6.38 (330): אמר המפרש:

ר״ל בנסתר אשר יהיה בעומק הגוף ולא יהיה נראה או יהיה נגלה ולא יהיה נגע ור״ל בעזיבת הרפואה מין החתוך או הכויה לא ההשקטה. → NM 3:71.

הַשְׁקָעָה · **torpor**: Arab. استغراق · a) Maimonides, *K. al-fuṣūl fī al-ṭibb* · trans. Zeraḥyah Ḥen (*Sefer ha-Peraqim*), 23.64: ביטול הדמיון נקרא ההשקעה וההקפאה והגרת האף נקרא ערבוב. → NM 1:141–2.

b) Maimonides, *K. al-fuṣūl fī al-ṭibb* · trans. Nathan ha-Me'ati (*Sefer ha-Peraqim*), 23.68: כשירבה במוח ליחה לבניית עבה קרה אם לא נתעפשה עדיין יחדש כאב ראש מהתרדמה הנשקעת מבלי קדחת והוא הנקרא תרדמה והשקעה וקפאון. → NM 2:41.

הִשְׁתַּדְּלוּת • השתדלות הרפואה · ***De methodo medendi*** **(*On the Method of Healing*)**: Arab. حيلة البرء · Maimonides, *K. al-fuṣūl fī al-ṭibb* · trans. Zeraḥyah Ḥen (*Sefer ha-Peraqim*), 25.55: מקום הקושיא היותו מבאר בהשתדלות הרפואה כי מזון הטחול יותר עב ממזון הכבד. → NM 1:142.

הִשְׁתּוֹמְמוּת · **anxiety**: Arab. توحّش · Ibn Sīnā, *K. al-adwiya al-qalbiya* · trans. Anonymous (*Sammim Libbiyim*), fols. 123[a–b]: עוד תועלת השלשול בהשתוממות למה שיש בו מנקוי הרוח יותר מתועלתו בחולשת הלב. → NM 4:48.

• **ההשתוממות השחורי** · **atrabilious anxiety (anxiety caused by black bile)**: Arab. التوحّش السوداوي · Ibn Sīnā, *K. al-adwiya al-qalbiya* · trans. Anonymous (*Sammim Libbiyim*), fol. 133[b]: הסכנגנין אשר חברתיו לבעלי ההשתוממות השחורי והכפייה ינקה העלה לעט. → NM 4:48–9.

הַשְׁתָּנָה • השתנת הדם · **urinating blood (hematuria)**: Arab. بول الدم · Ibn al-Jazzār, *Zād al-musāfir wa-qūt al-ḥādir* · trans. Moses ibn Tibbon (*Sefer Ṣedat ha-Derakhim*), introduction (fol. 3[b]): השער הט״ו בהשתנת הדם. → NM 4:49.

• קֹשִׁי → קושי ההשתנה.

הִשְׁתַּתְּפוּת · **affinity; interrelationship; sympathetic affection**: Arab. مشاركة · Maimonides, *Šarḥ fuṣūl Abūqrāṭ* · trans. Anonymous (*Pirqei Abuqraṭ*), 5.37 (257): אמר המפרש: ידוע הוא השתתפות השדים לרחם וכאשר צומקה זה ראיה על מיעוט המזון המגיע אליהם וכאשר ימעט המזון המגיע לרחם גם כן תפיל העובר. → NM 3:71–2.

הִתְאַבְּקוּת · **disturbance (agitation)**: Arab. اضطراب / Gr. ταραχή · Galen, *De diebus decretoriis* · trans. Shimshon ben Shlomo (*Qibbuṣei Ma'amarei Galenus bi-Yemei ha-Buḥran*), 1: אם כן הבחראן הוא ההתהפכות מהיר חד יחדש בחולה קשי והתאבקות. → NM 2:172.

הִתְגַּבְּרוּת · **boiling; bubbling; simmering**: Arab. فوران · Ibn al-Jazzār, *Zād al-musāfir wa-qūt al-ḥādir* · trans. Moses ibn Tibbon (*Sefer Ṣedat ha-Derakhim*), bk. 1, ch. 18 (fol. 26[a]): ויקרה לחולה עם עלות החולי וקרוב חזקתו מקרים מפחידים כמו צמא חזק ונגוב פה ושעירות לשון ושחרותה וסער ודפיקת לב ושלא יראה ועלוף ושינוי תמונת הפנים מן הענין הטבעי אל ענין יוצא מהטבע אם אל האדמימות אם היתה סבת החולי רתיחת דם הלב והתגברותו או אל הכרכומות אם היתה סבת החולי התלהבות מרה כרכומית בגבול המוח. → NM 4:49.

הִתְגַּעֲשׁוּת · **disturbance**: Arab. اضطراب / Gr. ταραχή · Maimonides, *K. al-fuṣūl fī al-ṭibb* · trans. Nathan ha-Me'ati (*Sefer ha-Peraqim*), 6.86: היציאה אשר בה קצף מורה על אחד משני דברים: אם על חום מופלג ממיס הגוף ומחדש הקצף מפני הדבר הרותח מלחויות הגוף אשר

המיס אותו החום המופלג ואם על התגעשות מתחלפת מפני התקוממות רוחות עבות ללחותה. → NM 2:41.

הִתְחַכְּכוּת · **crepitus**: Lat. crepitatio · Bruno Longobucco, *Cyrurgia Magna* · trans. Hillel ben Samuel (*Sefer Keritut*), fol. 55^b–6^a: כשיבוא לצלעות השבר הזה אינו נעלם במישוש הידים בעבור שיש שעירות שם וחוש לא ימצא שם בשוה ולפעמים ישמע התחככות שברי העצם זה בזה. → NM 1:23–4; corr. 4:229.

הִתְחַמְּמוּת · **fomentation**: Hippocrates, *Aphorisms* · trans. Judah Shalom, 6.31 (323) (fol. 103^a): כאבי העינים ית⟨י⟩כם יין בלתי מזוג או המרחץ או ההתחממות או ההרקה או ההקזה. → NM 3:72.

הִתְחַנְּקוּת • התחנקות הרחם · **hysterical suffocation**: Arab. اختناق الرحم · Maimonides, *Šarḥ fuṣūl Abūqrāṭ* · trans. Anonymous (*Pirqei Abuqraṭ*), 5.35 (255): אמר המפרש: כי האשה כשתתבטל נשימתה בחולי הרחם הנקרא התחנקות הרחם והעטוש מורה על התעוררות הטבע לפעול פעולתו. → NM 3:72.

הִתְיַצְּבוּת · **orthopnea**: Arab. انتصاب · Maimonides, *K. al-fuṣūl fī al-ṭibb* · trans. Nathan ha-Me'ati (*Sefer ha-Peraqim*), 24.38: מצאתי בקצת העתים אדם מפורסם במלאכת הרפואה ומששתי עורקיו ומצאתי בו כל מין ממיני ההתחלפות מבלי קדחת ולא יורגש בנשימתו דבר כלל. ואמרתי לו: אני רואה ההתחלפות יהיה מלחיצה וצרות יהיה בעורקים הדופקים אשר בריאה אם בסבת סתימה מליחות עבות דבקות או מהולד המורסא הנקראת יציאה שלא נתבשלה ואמר לי אם כן היה ראוי שהיה בו ההתיצבות הבא מן הגניחה ואמרתי לו שההתיצבות יהיה בעת התקבצות הליחה העבה הדבקה בחלקי קנה הריאה לא בעת התקבצותה בעורקים הדופקים. → NM 2:42.

הִתְיַתְּרוּת · **stretching**: Arab. توتّر · Maimonides, *K. al-fuṣūl fī al-ṭibb* · trans. Zeraḥyah Ḥen (*Sefer ha-Peraqim*), 1.70: ואמנם המושקולי שלחזה ולבטן הוא הפך למושקולי של הידים והרגלים כי כשיתיתר יתרחב כי ימצא תחתיו גופות חלקים יכפפו לו בזמן התיתרותו. → NM 1:142.

הַתָּכָה · **marasmus**: Arab. ذبول · Maimonides, *K. al-fuṣūl fī al-ṭibb* · trans. Zeraḥyah Ḥen (*Sefer ha-Peraqim*), 8.58: ואני מכיר אדם אחד הלך למרחץ אחד מאילו המימות המעורבות מלח או ניטרי או גפרית כדי שיריק גופו. והיה עם זה הנהיג לצד הרקת המרות ולא היה יודע שהיה ראוי שיכניס על כל איכות גובר ויצא מהעניין המבעי הפרו ושזה יותר טוב מן ההרקה ולא קיבל מי שהודיעו בזה והביאו זה אל יובש גדול באיבריו השרשיים עד שמצאו ההתכה והטיסיש ואחר כך מת. → NM 1:142–3.

• התכת נפש · **fainting**: Arab. ذبول نفس / Gr. λειποψυχία · Maimonides, *Šarḥ fuṣūl Abūqrāṭ* · trans. Moses ibn Tibbon (*Pirqei Abuqraṭ*), 7.8 (360): אמר אבקראט: כאשר נפתחה היציאה לפנים יתחדש מזה נפילת כח וקיא והתכת נפש. → NM 3:72–3.

הַתְּכִי · **wasting**: Arab. ذوباني · Maimonides, *K. al-fuṣūl fī al-ṭibb* · trans. Zeraḥyah Ḥen (*Sefer ha-Peraqim*), 7.11: ועצם האברים יהיה ניתך או באורך חליים ארוכים או בחידוד חליים חדים או בקדחות התכיות. → NM 1:143.

הִתְלַבְּדוּת · **granulation**: Arab. تلبّد · Al-Zahrāwī, *K. al-taṣrīf li-man ʿağiza ʿan at-ta'līf* · trans. Shem Tov ben Isaac (*Sefer ha-Shimmush*), bk. 30, 2.86 (fol. 225^b): והיא להסתכל ואם יהיה הגרגתני נכר קרוב ובמקום בטוח רחוק מפרק או מעצב או מוריד או מגיד נח או אחד מן המקומות אשר זכרתי ראוי לבקעו על מה שקדם מן המלאכה ולהסיר מה שיש בו מן ההתלבדות. → NM 1:88.

הִתְלַהֲבוּת ‣ I. **burn**: Hippocrates, *Aphorisms* · trans. Judah Shalom, 7.13 (365) (fol. 115[b]): ובהתלהבויות החזקים הכווץ והמשיכה הוא רע. → NM 3:73.

‣ II. **heat**: Arab. التهاب · Maimonides, *Šarḥ fuṣūl Abūqrāṭ* · trans. Moses ibn Tibbon (*Pirqei Abuqraṭ*), 4.65 (202): אמר אבקראט: כשתהיה בקדחת התלהבות גדול באצטו׳ ודפיקה במוראה הנה זה אות רע. → NM 3:73.

‣ III. **inflammation**: a) Arab. التهاب · i. Al-Zahrāwī, *K. al-taṣrīf li-man ʿağiza ʿan at-taʾlīf* · trans. Shem Tov ben Isaac (*Sefer ha-Shimmush*), bk. 30, 2.74 (221[a]): ראוי להתבונן ואם יהיה כאב הצמח בתחלתו חם עם דפיקה והתלהבות וקדחת ויהיה אדום אין ראוי למהר לדקרו. → NM 1:89.

· ii. Ibn al-Jazzār, *Zād al-musāfir wa-qūt al-ḥādir* · trans. Moses ibn Tibbon (*Sefer Ṣedat ha-Derakhim*), bk. 7, 12.1: אולם הצרעה והדבורים הנה ארסם חם חד ובעבור זה יקרה ממנו כאב חזק והתלהבות ונקודות קטנות שחורות. → NM 1:55.

b) Arab. تلهّب · Maimonides, *K. al-fuṣūl fī al-ṭibb* · trans. Nathan ha-Me'ati (*Sefer ha-Peraqim*), 21.7: המים אינם משקיטים השעול ולא עוזרים על הרקיקה ומעוררים הצמא ומשתנים אל המררות ומחלישים הגופים אם ישתו על ריקות נפש ומוסיפים בגודל הכבד והטחול כשיהיה בהם התלהבות. → NM 2:42.

הִתְמַגְּלוּת ‣ I. **empyema**: Arab. تقيّح · Hippocrates, *Aphorisms* · trans. Nathan ha-Me'ati, 5.8 (228) (fol. 87[b]): אמר אבוקר׳: מי שימצאהו בעלת הצד ולא ינקה בי״ד יום הנה ענינו פונה אל ההתמגלות. → NM 3:73.

‣ II. **purulence**: Lat. saniatio · Arnau de Vilanova, *Medicationis Parabole* · trans. Abraham Avigdor (*Pirqei Arnauṭ de Vilanova*), 5.89 (108): התמגלות הפצעים מצד היותו בסבת חולשת הכח המשנה אינו מן הראָוי אל הרופא שישתדל בהגעתו. → NM 4:49.

‣ III. **suppuration**: Arab. تقيّح · Hippocrates, *Aphorisms* · trans. Nathan ha-Me'ati, 7.20 (372): ומהמורסא הנקראת חמרה העפוש וההתמגלות הוא רע. → NM 3:73.

הִתְנַעֲרוּת • **התנערות ללכת** ‣ **standing up**: Arab. نهوض · Ibn Sīnā, *K. al-Qānūn fī al-ṭibb* · trans. Nathan ha-Me'ati (*Sefer ha-Qanun*), bk. 1 (fol. 41[b]): ושם ישיגה הכבדות בעת ההתנערות ללכת והכריעה על הברכים. → NM 4:49.

הִתְנַצְּלוּת ‣ **recovery**: Arab. سلامة · Maimonides, *Šarḥ fuṣūl Abūqrāṭ* · trans. Anonymous (*Pirqei Abuqraṭ*), 7.45 (397): אמר המפרש: כשהיתה המוגלא בקרום ובגוף הכבד ינצל והוא אפשר ההתנצלות. → NM 3:73–4.

הִתְנַשְּׁמוּת ‣ **exhalation**: Lat. expiratio / Arab. تنفّس · Galen, *De inaequali intemperie* · trans. David Caslari (*Sefer Roʿa Mezeg Mitḥallef*), 4.3: כי עיפוש ממה שאין לו התנשמות נקל מאד וממהר וזה נמצא בדברים הפנימיים והחיצוניים. → NM 2:166.

הִתְעוֹרְרוּת • **עורר התעוררות** → [עור].

הִתְעַסְּקוּת • **התעסקות הרפואה** ‣ **treatment**: Arab. علاج · Maimonides, *K. al-fuṣūl fī al-ṭibb* · trans. Nathan ha-Me'ati (*Sefer ha-Peraqim*), 8.46: הרפואות המחממות חמום חזק מרפות הכח רפיון חזק פתאם ויחלש הגוף ולא יהיה אפשר בו לסבול התעסקות הרפואה. → NM 2:43.

הִתְעַתְּדוּת ‣ **disposition**: Arab. استعداد · Ibn Sīnā, *K. al-Qānūn fī al-ṭibb* · trans. Nathan ha-Me'ati (*Sefer ha-Qanun*), bk. 1 (fol. 38[a]): וזנאד העליון מעוקם כאלו לוקח מן הצד הפנימי ונוטה מעט אל החיצוני בקפול והתועלת בזה טוב ההתעתדות לתנועת הקפול והעקום. → NM 4:50.

הִתְפּוֹצְצוּת ‣ **shattering:** Arab. تفتّت · Al-Zahrāwī, *K. al-taṣrīf li-man ʿağiza ʿan at-taʾlīf* · trans. Shem Tov ben Isaac (*Sefer ha-Shimmush*), bk. 30, 3.15 (235[b]): פלך הארכובה לא יקרה בו שבר אלא על המעט אבל יקרה לו הריסוק ואם יקרה לו שבר אולם יהיה בקוע או התפוצצות. → NM 1:89.

הִתְפַּשְּׁטוּת • התפשטות הדפק ‣ **dilation of the pulse:** Arab. انبساط النبض · Ibn al-Jazzār, *Zād al-musāfir wa-qūt al-ḥādir* · trans. Moses ibn Tibbon (*Sefer Ṣedat ha-Derakhim*), bk. 1, ch. 20 (fol. 30[a]): ויהיו עיני בעליו בעבור זה עמוקים ממהרי התנועה בעבור סער הנפש במחשבה ותשוקתה להשיג מי שישתוקק אליו ויהיו עפעפיו כבדות ומראהו כרכומי לתנועת המרה האדומה בנדוד השינה ויהיה דפק עורקיו חזק לא ימצא בו התפשטות הדפק הטבעי ולא ישפל הכאתו. → NM 4:50.

הִתְקַבְּצוּת ‣ I. **contraction:** Arab. انقباض · Ibn Sīnā, *K. al-Qānūn fī al-ṭibb* · trans. Nathan ha-Meʾati (*Sefer ha-Qanun*), bk. 1 (fol. 52[a]): ומהם שישענו הטרפשות ועוזרים אצל הנפיחה לבעל ההתקבצות. → NM 4:50.

‣ II. **flexion:** Arab. انقباض · Ibn Sīnā, *K. al-Qānūn fī al-ṭibb* · trans. Nathan ha-Meʾati (*Sefer ha-Qanun*), bk. 1 (fol. 51[a]): והנה הושם הבהן מסתפק בהתקבצות על עצל אחד. → NM 4:50.

הִתְקַשְּׁרוּת ‣ I. **coagulation:** Arab. انعقاد · Maimonides, *K. al-fuṣūl fī al-ṭibb* · trans. Nathan ha-Meʾati (*Sefer ha-Peraqim*), 8.62: מדרגות היובש הם ארבעה ... והמדרגה השלישית הוא שיגיע היובש לכלות לחות האברים אשר הם מעצם לח קרוב ההתקשרות והקפיאה כמו השומן והבשר כשימסו ויזולו. → NM 2:43.

‣ II. **compactness; firmness; solidity:** Arab. متانة · Ibn Sīnā, *K. al-adwiya al-qalbiya* · trans. Anonymous (*Sammim Libbiyim*), fol. 123[b]: הסמים הקובצים והמטיחים יכנסו ברפואות הלב להקנות עצם הרוח התקשרות והתדבקות נאות. → NM 4:51.

‣ III. **consolidation; strengthening:** Arab. تمتين · Ibn Sīnā, *K. al-adwiya al-qalbiya* · trans. Anonymous (*Sammim Libbiyim*), fols. 130–131[a]: סוסן אראה: אותו קרוב הטבע מן הזעפראן קרוב המשפט ממשפטיו (ו)אבל הוא יותר חסר החום והיובש וזה יותר נאות לחיזוק הלב וזה ג״כ להיותו שמח כי בחוזק מהתקישרות הרוח קרוב ממה שהוא בזעפראן ואין בו התפשטות חזק והנעה מופלגת לרוח אל חוץ כמו שהוא בזעפראן. → NM 4:51.

הַתָּרָה ‣ I. **diarrhea:** Arab. استطلاق · Ibn al-Jazzār, *Zād al-musāfir wa-qūt al-ḥādir* · trans. Moses ibn Tibbon (*Sefer Ṣedat ha-Derakhim*), bk. 7, 8.5: וכאשר עברו על החולה שבעה ימים ראוי לו להזהר ממה שירכך הטבע כלל כי ההתרה מדרכה לבוא בקדחת הזאת מעצמה ויטה ההנהגה אל מה שיעצור הטבע. → NM 1:55.

‣ II. **flux (diarrhea):** Lat. fluxus / Arab. سيلان · Hippocrates, *Aphorisms* · trans. Hillel ben Samuel, 7.16 (368) (fol. 45[b]): א״א: ברקיקת המוגלא תתחדש הטיסיס וההתרה וכשיעצר הרוק ימותו. → NM 3:74.

• **התרת הבטן** ‣ I. **diarrhea:** Arab. الاستطلاق · Maimonides, *K. al-fuṣūl fī al-ṭibb* · trans. Zeraḥyah Ḥen (*Sefer ha-Peraqim*), 7.42: חולשת הכח שהוא סבת הרעש אינו סבה אחת אבל סבותיו מרובות. יוכל להיות בסבת המזון כמו שיהיה בשלשול הנק׳ איניישטיאון והתרת הבטן הגדולה. → NM 1:143.

‣ II. **looseness of the bowels:** Arab. استطلاق البطن · Maimonides, *Šarḥ fuṣūl*

Abūqrāṭ · trans. Moses ibn Tibbon (*Pirqei Abuqraṭ*), 2.14 (66): אמר אבקראט: עם התרת הבטן פעמים יועיל בהתחלף מראות הצואה כשלא יהיה השתנותו אל מינים רעים ממנו. → NM 3:74.

• **התרת הדבקות** · **dissolution of continuity**: Lat. solutio continuitatis · Bruno Longobucco, *Cyrurgia Magna* · trans. Hillel ben Samuel (*Sefer Keritut*), fol. 15[a]: אמר גלינו ושאר החכמים התרת הדבקות בגידים מרוב הרגשתם והדבקתם במוח ממהרות להביא הקיוץ. → NM 1:24.

• **התרת השתן** · **polyuria**: Arab. استطلاق البول · a) Maimonides, *K. al-fuṣūl fī al-ṭibb* · trans. Zeraḥyah Ḥen (*Sefer ha-Peraqim*), 24.39: התרת השתן והוא הנקרא דיאביטיס והצמא החזקה הוא החולי שאינו נמצא כי אם בזמן מועט ולא לעתים רחוקים כי אני עד היום הזה לא ראיתיהו אלא שני פעמים לבד. → NM 1:143.

b) Maimonides, *K. al-fuṣūl fī al-ṭibb* · trans. Nathan ha-Me'ati (*Sefer ha-Peraqim*), 24.39: התרת השתן והוא דיאביטס הנקרא הצמא החזק היא עלה שימעט מציאותה אלא בפליאה הנה אני עדין לא ראיתיה אלא פעמים. → NM 2:43.

הִתְרַחֲבוּת · **dilatation of the palpebral membrane**: Arab. انتشار · Maimonides, *K. al-fuṣūl fī al-ṭibb* · trans. Nathan ha-Me'ati (*Sefer ha-Peraqim*), 22.40: הכחילה במשקה וורדים סוכרי מחזק הראות ויבריא התמדת זה מההתרחבות. → NM 2:43.

ו

ודאג • הודאג הנגלה · **the external jugular vein**: Arab. الوداج الظاهر · Ibn Sīnā, *K. al-Qānūn fī al-ṭibb* · trans. Nathan ha-Me'ati (*Sefer ha-Qanun*), bk. 1 (fol. 65ᵃ): ואמנם הודאג הנגלה אחר התערב נפרדיו הנה מתחלק לשנים ונכנס בפנים חלק ממנו. → NM 4:51.

וַדַּאי · **[marker of the apodosis]**: a) Arab. -ف · Maimonides, *Šarḥ fuṣūl Abūqrāṭ* · trans. Anonymous (*Pirqei Abuqraṭ*), 2.32 (84): אמר אבוקרט: ברוב העתים כל מי שעניינו ברע ויקח מן המאכלים ולא יתוסף גופו כלל הנה באחריתו באשר לא ⟨יקח⟩ מן המאכלים. ואמנם מי שנמנע מתחלת ענינו הלקיחה מהמאכלים מניעה חזקה ואחר כך יקבל ממנו באחרונה ודאי ענינו יהיה יותר טוב. → NM 3:74.

b) Arab. فإنّه · Maimonides, *Šarḥ fuṣūl Abūqrāṭ* · trans. Anonymous (*Pirqei Abuqraṭ*), 3.1 (107): אמר המפרש: ר״ל שנוי טבעי הפרקים כמו שהיה פרק הסתיו חם או פרק הקיץ קר וכיוצא בהם. וכן שנוי העת האחד ממזגו כשהיה חזק ואע״פ ששאר הפרקים לא נשתנו ודאי יוליד תחלואים. → NM 3:74–5.

וורוס · **poisonous liquid**: Lat. virus · Bruno Longobucco, *Cyrurgia Magna* · trans. Hillel ben Samuel (*Sefer Keritut*), fol. 30ᵇ: עוד אמר שאותן שהן מעפוש דק נקראות וורוס ומעפוש עב נקראות שורדיציאיש. → NM 1:43.

ויאולש • סוכר ויאולש → **סֻכָּר**.

וינטוסי · **cupping glasses**: Lat. ventose · Bruno Longobucco, *Cyrurgia Magna* · trans. Hillel ben Samuel (*Sefer Keritut*), fol. 19ᵃ: ואם הרצוץ יהיה עמוק והדם קפוי או אין ההקזה מספקת ואז צריך הוינטוסי עם שריטה והעלוקות. → NM 1:43.

ויתן • *Plur.* ויתנים · **arteries**: Lat. arteriae · Bruno Longobucco, *Cyrurgia Magna* · trans. Hillel ben Samuel (*Sefer Keritut*), fol. 7ᵇ: וזה מנוסח דברי גליני׳ באמרו רבים חשב⟨ו⟩ שיהיה מן הנמנע שעצם הויתנים יתחבר אם יותר. → NM 1:24.

וֶסֶת • *Plur.* וסתות • וסתות הקדחת · **the paroxysms of the fever**: Arab. نوائب الحمّى · Maimonides, *Šarḥ fuṣūl Abūqrāṭ* · trans. Anonymous (*Pirqei Abuqraṭ*), 4.30 (167): אמר המפרש: מבואר כי כשהיינה וסחות הקדחת כולם יבאו על עת אחת בהתחלתה ותכליתה זה ראיה על אורך. → NM 3:75.

וֶרֶד • הורד הסוכרי · **rose syrup**: Lat. sirupum rosatum (Honofredi) · Ibn Zuhr, *Regimen of Health* · trans. Jacob ibn Tibbon (*Hanhagat ha-Beri'ut le-Abu 'Ali ben Zuhr*), ch. 10: ומשקה הורד הסוכרי ומשקה לינגא אלובין ההנדי מועילים ושומרים הבריאות. → NM 4:51.

• ***Plur.* ורדים • מי ורדים ⟨בו⟩ כלי שעושים** → **כְּלִי**.

וְרִיד · **artery**: Arab. شريان · Al-Zahrāwī, *K. al-taṣrīf li-man ʿağiza ʿan at-taʾlīf* · trans. Shem Tov ben Isaac (*Sefer ha-Shimmush*), bk. 30, 1.4 (204ᵃ): ועתיד אני עוד להביא זכרון הנהגת הרעיפה אשר תקרה מן הוריד. → NM 1:89.

• **הוריד הדופק** · **arterial vein (pulmonary artery)**: Arab. الوريد الشرياني · Ibn Sīnā, *K. al-Qānūn fī al-ṭibb* · trans. Zeraḥyah Ḥen (*Sefer ha-Qanun*), bk. 1 (fol. 32ᵃ): ואמנם הוריד הדופק אשר אנו זוכרים אותו ואע״פ שהוא שכן לריאה אבל יעבור ממנו מאחורו מקום שהוא סמוך לגב. → NM 4:52.

• **הוריד הזקני** · **sacral vein**: Arab. الوريد العجزي · Ibn Sīnā, *K. al-Qānūn fī al-ṭibb* ·

trans. Zeraḥyah Ḥen (*Sefer ha-Qanun*), bk. 1 (fol. 34[a]): וכת יורד תחת המושקולו הישר ויתחלק מהם שעיף וסופם מתדבק בחלקים העולים מן הוריד הזקני אשר אנו עתידים לזכרו. → NM 4:52.

• **הוריד החלול** · **vena cava**: Arab. الوريد الأجوف · Ibn Sīnā, *K. al-Qānūn fī al-ṭibb* · trans. Zeraḥyah Ḥen (*Sefer ha-Qanun*), bk. 1 (fol. 32[a]): ועל כן נקרא הגיד הורידי. אמנם נברא מקרום אחד למען היותו יותר לח ויותר משועבד לפשיטות ולקביצות ולמען היות משועבד להזיע מה שיזיע ממנו אל הריאה מן הדם הדק העשני הניאות בעצם הריאה הקרוב לבשול השלם בלב ואינו צריך למותר בשול כצורך הדם ההולך בוריד החלול. → NM 4:52–3.

• **הוריד הנבוב** · **vena cava**: Arab. الوريد الأجوف · Ibn Sīnā, *K. al-Qānūn fī al-ṭibb* · trans. Nathan ha-Me'ati (*Sefer ha-Qanun*), bk. 1 (fol. 60[b]): ולכן נקרא השריין הורידי. אמנם נברא מעור אחד שיהיה יותר רך ורפה ויותר נשמע להתפשטות והתקבצות ויותר נשמע להתדיית מה שיתדיית ממנו אל הריאה מן הדם הדק האדיי הנאות לעצם הריאה אשר כבר קדם לשלמות הבשול בלב ולא יצטרך ליתרון בשול כצורך הדם העובר בוריד הנבוב. → NM 4:53.

• **הוריד העגזי** · **sacral vein**: Arab. الوريد العجزي · Ibn Sīnā, *K. al-Qānūn fī al-ṭibb* · trans. Nathan ha-Me'ati (*Sefer ha-Qanun*), bk. 1 (fol. 64[b]): וכת יורד תחת העצלים הישרים ומתפרד מהם שריגים ואחריתם מתחברים בחלקים העולים מן הוריד העגזי אשר נזכירהו. → NM 4:53.

• **הוריד אשר על פי הטבעת** · **sacral vein**: Arab. الوريد العجزي · Ibn Sīnā, *K. al-Qānūn fī al-ṭibb* · trans. Joseph Lorki (*Sefer ha-Qanun*), bk. 1 (fol. 19[a]): וכת יורד תחת העצל הישר ומתפזרים בו שריגים וסופם דבק בחלקים העולים מן הוריד אשר על פי הטבעת אשר נזכר אותו. → NM 4:52.

• **הוריד הפנימי** · **vena cava**: Arab. الوريد الأجوف · Ibn Sīnā, *K. al-Qānūn fī al-ṭibb* · trans. Joseph Lorki (*Sefer ha-Qanun*), bk. 1 (fol. 18[a]): ועל כן נקרא הגיד הדופק בהיותו יותר לח ויותר רך ויותר נקל אל הפשיטה והקבוץ ולהיותו יותר נקל להטיב מה שנוסף ממנו אל הריאה מהדם הדקיק הקטורי הנאות לעצם הריאה אשר קרב בהשלמת הבשול בלב ואינו צריך ליתרון בשול כמו צורך הדם בוריד הפנימי. → NM 4:53–4.

• **הוריד הפנימי היורד** · **the inferior vena cava**: Arab. الأجوف النازل · Ibn Sīnā, *K. al-Qānūn fī al-ṭibb* · trans. Joseph Lorki (*Sefer ha-Qanun*), bk. 1 (fol. 19[b]): פרק ה׳ בנתוח הוריד הפנימי היורד כבר השלמנו מאמרינו בחלק העולה הפנימי והוא היותר קטן שבחלקיו. → NM 4:54.

• **הוריד השרייני** · **arterial vein (pulmonary artery)**: Arab. الوريد الشرياني · Ibn Sīnā, *K. al-Qānūn fī al-ṭibb* · trans. Nathan ha-Me'ati (*Sefer ha-Qanun*), bk. 1 (fol. 60[b]): ואמנם הוריד השרייני אשר נזכירהו אע״פ שהוא שכן לריאה אמנם הוא עובר ממנו מאחורו במה שנלוה לשדרה. → NM 4:54.

• *Plur.* **ורידים** • **ורידי הרחם** **פיות ורידי הרחם** → **פֶּה**.

וְרִידִי • **הגיד הורידי** → **גִּיד**.

• **הגיד הדופק הורידי** → **גִּיד**.

• **השריין הורידי** → **שריין**.

וֶשֶׁט · **throat**: Arab. حلقوم · Ibn Sīnā, *K. al-Qānūn fī al-ṭibb* · trans. Zeraḥyah Ḥen (*Sefer ha-Qanun*), bk. 1 (fol. 25[b]): המושקלו של הושט. אמנם הושט כולו יש לו שתי זוגות ימשכוהו למטה. → NM 4:54.

ותיקה · pulmentum spissius (anything dense eaten with bread); pultes (a thick pap or pottage): Arab. عصيدة · Al-Zahrāwī, *K. al-taṣrīf li-man ʿağiza ʿan at-taʾlīf* · trans. Shem Tov ben Isaac (*Sefer ha-Shimmush*), bk. 27, fol. 124[b], col. 1: הותיקה העשויה מן הגריסין היא קרובה להוליד החלט העב והסתומים והרטט. → NM 4:54–5.

ז

זְאֵב • **הורג הזאב** → הוֹרֵג.

• **חולי הזאב** → חֹלִי.

• **ממית הזאב** → [מות].

זֶבֶל • **זבל שטן** · **asafetida**: *Anonymous Glossary*, Ms. Leiden, Universiteitsbibliotheek, Cod. Or. 4732/1, fol. 7ª: מילשא היא גומ׳ והוא זבל שטן. → NM 4:55.

זָהָב • **דבקות הזהב** → דְּבֵקוּת.

• **מדביק הזהב** → [דבק].

• **סיג הזהב** → סִיג.

זָהוּב · I. **aureus**: Lat. aureus / Arab. مثقال · Ibn Sīnā, *K. al-adwiya al-qalbiya* · trans. Anonymous (*Sefer ha-Refu'ot ha-Libbiyot*), fol. 252ª: והרופאים הסכלים עדיין חושבים שיש למטרודיטוס ולתריאק חום גובר ומפני זה בורחים לתת ממנה שיעור חצי זהוב. → NM 4:55.

· II. ***mithqāl*** **(i.e., 4.46 grams)**: Arab. مثقال · Al-Zahrāwī, *K. al-taṣrīf li-man ʿağiza ʿan at-taʾlīf* · trans. Shem Tov ben Isaac (*Sefer ha-Shimmush*), bk. 27, fol. 136ª, col. b: ואם יקרה מאכילת המין הרע מהם קצת מה שזכרתי בפטריות מן החניקה והגנוח ראוי לשתות אחריהם מיד מים שנתבשל בהם שבת עם חמאת בקר או שמן שומשמין או לקחת מצואת התרנוגלות משקל שני זהובים ולצרף אותה באישרוב אסיטוס ומים חמין ולשתותם. → NM 4:55–6.

[זהם] • *Part. Hifʿil* **מַזְהִים** · **heavy [on the stomach]; indigestible**: Arab. وخم · Al-Rāzī, *K. al-Manṣūrī* · trans. Shem Tov ben Isaac (*Sefer Almansur*), Ayin 5 (62): ענאב: חם בשווי מרכך הגרון ומזכך הדם מזהים מתעכב הירידה מהאצטומכה. → NM 2:14.

זֻהֲמָה • **זוהמת הכוורת** · **bee glue**: Arab. وسخ الكور / Gr. πρόπολις · Maimonides, *K. al-fuṣūl fī al-ṭibb* · trans. Nathan ha-Me'ati (*Sefer ha-Peraqim*), 15.33: אמנם רפואות חבורות העצבים אני הייתי עושה בהם הגפרית שלא מצאו אש עם שמן עד שישוב בעובי זוהמת המרחץ. ולפעמים יעשה בגופות הנערים וכיוצא בהם עלך אלבטם לבדו או עם פרביון בגופות היבשים. וכן יעשה זוהמת הכוורת לבדה או עם פרביון מולש בשמן ישן. → NM 2:43–4.

• **זוהמת המרחץ** · **bath sordes**: Arab. وسخ الحمّام / Gr. γλοιός · Maimonides, *K. al-fuṣūl fī al-ṭibb* · trans. Nathan ha-Me'ati (*Sefer ha-Peraqim*), 15.33: אמנם רפואות חבורות העצבים אני הייתי עושה בהם הגפרית שלא מצאו אש עם שמן עד שישוב בעובי זוהמת המרחץ. ולפעמים יעשה בגופות הנערים וכיוצא בהם עלך אלבטם לבדו או עם פרביון בגופות היבשים. וכן יעשה זוהמת הכוורת לבדה או עם פרביון מולש בשמן ישן. → NM 2:44.

• **זוהמת הצמר** · **wool grease**: *Anonymous Glossary*, Ms. Vatican, Biblioteca Apostolica, ebr. 361, fol. 177ᵇ: זופ⟨ט⟩א רטב הוא אישוף לח יקראו זוהמת הצמר. → NM 4:56.

זוֹב · **fluid; liquid; moisture**: Lat. humor · Al-Rāzī, attr., *On the Treatment of Small Children* · trans. Anonymous, ch. 15: מקיא הילד. יקרה לילדים בפרק ראשון מן השנים קיא לסבות רבות או בעבור ריבוי חלב יותר מאשר יוכל לסבול או בעבור לחות החלב או בעבור הפסדו וכל שכן אם יהיה הילד מהאסטומ׳ לחה וחלושה. והנהגתו הוא שתמנע ריבוי החלב. ואחר כן הבט בקיא אם יורגש ממנו ריח חמוץ ויהיו בו זובים לחים ולבנים. → NM 2:178.

• **זוב דם הנחירים** · **nosebleed**: Hippocrates, *Aphorisms* · trans. Do'eg ha-Edomi (*Sefer

Agur), 3.27 (133) (fol. 57[b]): רבו התחלואים בהגיעם לבגר והם עת צמיחת השיער ויצמחו הקדחות הארוכות וזוב דם הנחירים. → NM 3:75.

• זוב הנחירים › I. **catarrh:** Hippocrates, *Aphorisms* · trans. Do'eg ha-Edomi (*Sefer Agur*), 7.38 (390) (fol. 117[a]): סבב זוב הנחירים לרדת אל הקרב העליון יכלה וישוב להיות עב טיט עד עשרים יום. → NM 3:76.

› II. **rheuma:** Hippocrates, *Aphorisms* · trans. Do'eg ha-Edomi (*Sefer Agur*), 3.23 (129) (fol. 55[b]): צרות יום הקור הם כאב הצדדים ותחת הצלעות והריאה וזוב הנחירים והשזרה סתימת המקורות ותרדמת הגוף. → NM 3:75–6.

זוג › **zygomatic arch:** Arab. زوج · Ibn Sīnā, *K. al-Qānūn fī al-ṭibb* · trans. Nathan ha-Me'ati (*Sefer ha-Qanun*), bk. 1 (fol. 30[a]): ובכל אחד משני צדי הצדעים שתי עצמות קשות מסתירות העצבים העוברים בצדעים והנחתם באורך הצדע באלכסון ונקראים הזוג. → NM 4:56.

זוהמה → זֻהֲמָה.

[זור] • *Part. Hif'il* **מֵזִיר** • *Plur.* **המזירים** › I. **repercussive remedies:** Lat. repercussiva · Bruno Longobucco, *Cyrurgia Magna* · trans. Hillel ben Samuel (*Sefer Keritut*), fol. 79[b]: ועם כל זה שים המזירים עליו בהתחלה. → NM 1:24.

› II. **restraint (i.e., restraining ingredients):** Lat. refrenatio · Bruno Longobucco, *Cyrurgia Magna* · trans. Hillel ben Samuel (*Sefer Keritut*), fol. 78[a]: וזה יעשה בדברים מרכבים ומתירים וקלים ועם כל זה תמיד תקדים המזירים. → NM 1:24.

זורקי › **navicular or scaphoid [bone]:** Arab. زورقي · Ibn Sīnā, *K. al-Qānūn fī al-ṭibb* · trans. Nathan ha-Me'ati (*Sefer ha-Qanun*), bk. 1 (fol. 41[b]): עצמות כף הרגל ששה ... וזורקי שבו יהיה החלל. → NM 4:56–7.

זְחִילָה • זחילת הבטן › **diarrhea:** Lat. fluxus ventris · Al-Rāzī, attr., *On the Treatment of Small Children* · trans. Anonymous, ch. 13: ואולי תקרה לקצת מהם קדחת וזחילת הבטן או עיצור. → NM 2:178.

זִיו • זיו האדם › **external condition:** Arab. سحنة · Maimonides, *K. al-fuṣūl fī al-ṭibb* · trans. Zeraḥyah Ḥen (*Sefer ha-Peraqim*), 12.3: לא יקיז הנער קודם י״ד שנה ולא אחר השבעים שנה ולא ישמור אל מספר השנים לבד אבל ישמור עם זה בזיו האדם. → NM 1:143–4.

זיכום › **defluxion:** Arab. زكام · Al-Zahrāwī, *K. al-taṣrīf li-man ʿağiza ʿan at-taʾlīf* · trans. Shem Tov ben Isaac (*Sefer ha-Shimmush*), bk. 30, 2.86 (fol. 225[a]): ידוע שכל חבורה או מורסא כשתתישן וארך זמנה ושבה שחין ולא הגלידה והיה יוצא ממנה מוגלא תמיד בלי הפסד תקרא על הכלל גרגתני באיזה אבר שתהיה ואני קראתיה זיכום. → NM 1:89.

זִינָה › **nourishment; nutriment:** Lat. nutrimentum · Bruno Longobucco, *Cyrurgia Magna* · trans. Hillel ben Samuel (*Sefer Keritut*), fol. 32[a]: אמר ואין צריך שתניח שם רפואה מצמחת עד שתטהר תחילה החבלה או שימשך שם הזינה אם יהיה שם חסרון באיזה מקום שיהיה. → NM 1:25.

זִיעָה • טהרת זיעה → טָהֳרָה.

• זיעה שלמה › **paroxysm:** Hippocrates, *Aphorisms* · trans. Do'eg ha-Edomi (*Sefer Agur*), 2.13 (65) (fol. 36[a]): דת הזיעה השלמה בהתנהג החולי בכבידות לפניה יום או לילה. → NM 3:76.

זיפק › **peritoneum:** Lat. siphac / Arab. صفاق · Bruno Longobucco, *Cyrurgia Magna* ·

trans. Hillel ben Samuel (*Sefer Keritut*), fol. 13[b]: וכשתשיב המעים מבפנים תאחוז החבלה באצבעותיך והזיפק יתפור ככתוב. → NM 1:43.

זירבאג׳ · ***zīrbāğa* (a kind of broth)**: Arab. زيرباج / Lat. species cibi iusculenti · Al-Zahrāwī, *K. al-taṣrīf li-man ʿağiza ʿan at-ta'līf* · trans. Shem Tov ben Isaac (*Sefer ha-Shimmush*), bk. 27, fol. 148[a], col. b: והרוצה להשוות המזג ולהשקיט חמימות האסטומ׳ ראוי לבשלם תבשיל זירבאג׳. → NM 4:57.

זירבו · **omentum**: Lat. zirbus · Bruno Longobucco, *Cyrurgia Magna* · trans. Hillel ben Samuel (*Sefer Keritut*), fol. 12[b]: שער הרביעי להשיב המעים והזירבו. → NM 1:43.

זְכוֹכִית • **כלי זכוכית** → כְּלִי.

• **עשב הזכוכית** → עֵשֶׂב.

זַכּוּת · **acumen**: Arab. ذكاء · Maimonides, *K. al-fuṣūl fī al-ṭibb* · trans. Zeraḥyah Ḥen (*Sefer ha-Peraqim*), 25.59: ובטוב שכלו וזכותו אשר שימש ברפואות והיותו מצא מה שידעו הוא בקצת מיני הדפק והניתוח והתועלות והפעולות יותר אמת מאשר שזכרו אריסטו׳ בספריו בלא ספק לפי דעת מי שיודה על האמת והביאו אותו המאמר לדבר בעניינים שהוא בהם קצר מאד וישמש זריזותו בהן. → NM 1:144.

זְלוּף • **זלוף הדם מן החוטם** · **nosebleed**: Judah ben Jacob, *Sefer Hanhagat ha-Beri'ut*, 8.5: וצריך להקיז מיד ויוציא מן הדם כפי השיעור הצריך שאם ימנע מהקיז תאחזהו הקדחת התמידית וחולי הצלעות וזלוף הדם מן החוטם והמות הפתאומית והרבה חליים מלבד אלה. → NM 4:57–8.

זלק • **הלקות המעים הוא זלק אלמעא** → חֲלָקוּת.

זְמוֹרָה · **varix**: Arab. دالية / Gr. κιρσός · Al-Zahrāwī, *K. al-taṣrīf li-man ʿağiza ʿan at-ta'līf* · trans. Shem Tov ben Isaac (*Sefer ha-Shimmush*), bk. 30, 2.64 (fol. 220[a]): הזמורה היא צמח נפתל קצת פיתול דומה לאשכול עם רפיון הבצים ותקשה על החולה התנועה והטיול וההליכה. → NM 1:89–90.

• *Plur.* **זמורות** · **varicose veins**: Arab. دوال · Al-Zahrāwī, *K. al-taṣrīf li-man ʿağiza ʿan at-ta'līf* · trans. Shem Tov ben Isaac (*Sefer ha-Shimmush*), bk. 27, fol. 127[a], col. a: הלחם העשוי מן העדשים יתילד מן ההתמדה עליו חליים שחורים כגון השטות והסרטנים והזמורות והטחורים והבהק השחור והספחת והדומה להם מן החליים. → NM 4:58.

זְמוֹרִי • **האשך הזמורי** → אֶשֶׁךְ.

זְמַן · **age**: Lat. etas · Bruno Longobucco, *Cyrurgia Magna* · trans. Hillel ben Samuel (*Sefer Keritut*), fol. 92[b]: ואז תשגיח בגודל השבר וישנו וזמן החולה. → NM 1:25.

• **זמן הקור** · **winter**: Arab. شتاء · Maimonides, *Šarḥ fuṣūl Abūqrāṭ* · trans. Zeraḥyah Ḥen (*Pirqei Abuqraṭ*), 3.2 (108): אמר בקראט: כי יש מן הטבעים שיהיה עניינו בקייץ יותר טוב ובקור יותר רע. ויש מהם שיהיה עניינו בזמן הקור יותר טוב ובקייץ יותר רע. → NM 3:76.

זנאד • **הזנאד העליון** · **radius**: Arab. الزند الأعلى · Ibn Sīnā, *K. al-Qānūn fī al-ṭibb* · trans. Nathan ha-Me'ati (*Sefer ha-Qanun*), bk. 1 (fol. 38[a]): אמנם פרק המרפק הנה הוא מחובר מן פרק הזנאד העליון ופרק הזנאד התחתון עם הזרוע. → NM 4:58.

• **הזנאד התחתון** · **ulna**: Arab. الزند الأسفل · Ibn Sīnā, *K. al-Qānūn fī al-ṭibb* · trans. Nathan ha-Me'ati (*Sefer ha-Qanun*), bk. 1 (fol. 38[a]): אמנם פרק המרפק הנה הוא מחובר מן פרק הזנאד העליון ופרק הזנאד התחתון עם הזרוע. → NM 4:58.

זָנָב • **חלל הזנב** → חָלָל.

• **זנב העין** ‧ **the outer corner of the eye**: Arab. ذنب العين ‧ Al-Zahrāwī, *K. al-taṣrīf li-man ʿağiza ʿan at-taʾlīf* ‧ trans. Shem Tov ben Isaac (*Sefer ha-Shimmush*), bk. 30, 1.13 (fol. 204[b]): והרוצה להוסיף יוכל לכוות כויה אחת בכל צד מזנב העין על קצות גב העין במכוה קטן. → NM 1:90.

• *Plur.* **זנבות** ‧ **the canthi (inner and outer angles) of the eyes**: Arab. مآقان ‧ Al-Zahrāwī, *K. al-taṣrīf li-man ʿağiza ʿan at-taʾlīf* ‧ trans. Shem Tov ben Isaac (*Sefer ha-Shimmush*), bk. 27, fol. 136[b], cols. a–b: וסחיטתו כשיוכחל בו העינים תחזק בת העין ותפסיק הלחויות העבות אשר בעפעפים ותועיל מגסות העין ומן החכוך אשר בראשי העינים וזנבותיהם. → NM 4:58–9.

זנד • *Plur.* **זנדים** • **שני הזנדים** ‧ **the two bones of the forearm (i.e., radius and ulna)**: Arab. الزندان ‧ Ibn Sīnā, *K. al-Qānūn fī al-ṭibb* ‧ trans. Nathan ha-Me'ati (*Sefer ha-Qanun*), bk. 1 (fol. 38[a]): הקנה מחוברת משני עצמים מדובקים באורך ונקרא שני הזנדים. → NM 4:59.

זֵעָה • **הסם המגיר לזיעה** → **סַם**.

• **הסם המתיר הזיעה** → **סַם**.

זֶפֶת • **זפת גריקא** ‧ **colophonia (i.e., Greek pitch (resin))**: Lat. colophonia, id est pix Greca ‧ Bruno Longobucco, *Cyrurgia Magna* ‧ trans. Hillel ben Samuel (*Sefer Keritut*), fol. 24[b]. → NM 1:45.

זָקוּף (*Pass. Part.*) → **זָקַף**.

זְקִיפָה • **זקיפת האמה** ‧ **satyriasis**: Lat. sathiriasis ‧ Hippocrates, *Aphorisms* ‧ trans. Judah Shalom, 3.26 (132) (fol. 77[b]): ובהיותם יותר גדולים יקרה להם מורסת הגרון ודחית חוליות הצואר לפנים ואשמא ואבן ותולעים עגולים והדלועיים והיבלות וזקיפת האמה וחזירים וצמחים אחרים ויותר נזכרים. → NM 3:77.

[זקן] • *Hifʿil* **הִזְקִין** ‧ **to become chronic**: Lat. veterasco ‧ Hippocrates, *Aphorisms* ‧ trans. Hillel ben Samuel, 3.28 (134) (fol. 19[a]): אבל איזה מהם שלא יתרפא בנערים בבגרות או בנשים כשיצא להן הגרת הנדות מנהגן להזקין עמם. → NM 3:77.

זָקָן ‧ **chin**: Arab. ذقن ‧ Ibn Sīnā, *K. al-Qānūn fī al-ṭibb* ‧ trans. Nathan ha-Me'ati (*Sefer ha-Qanun*), bk. 1 (fol. 31[a]): ואמנם הלחי התחתון הנה צורת עצמיו ותועלתו ידוע כי הוא משחי עצמות יחבר ביניהם תחת הזקן פרק מהודק. → NM 4:59.

• **שבולת הזקן** → **שִׁבֹּלֶת**.

• **הזקן התחתון** ‧ **pubes**: Arab. العانة ‧ Al-Zahrāwī, *K. al-taṣrīf li-man ʿağiza ʿan at-taʾlīf* ‧ trans. Shem Tov ben Isaac (*Sefer ha-Shimmush*), bk. 30, 2.54 (fol. 217[b]): ואחר כך להסתכל ואם יהיה התילד השקוי מצד המעי ראוי להרחיק הביקוע מן הטיבור שעור שלש אצבעות מלמטה עד למעלה מן הזקן התחתון. → NM 1:90.

• **זקן התיש** ‧ **goatsbeard** [***Tragopogon porrifolius***]: Arab. لحية التيس ‧ Al-Rāzī, *K. al-Manṣūrī* ‧ trans. Shem Tov ben Isaac (*Sefer Almansur*), He 5 (30): היופסטידאס איבוקושטידום ויקרא זקן התיש: קר קובץ ראוי להרגילו כשיביא הצורך לעצור ולקבוץ. → NM 2:12.

זָקֵן ‧ **sacrum**: Arab. عجز ‧ Ibn Sīnā, *K. al-Qānūn fī al-ṭibb* ‧ trans. Zeraḥyah Ḥen (*Sefer ha-Qanun*), bk. 1 (fol. 20[a]): הפרק האחד עשר בנתוח העצם הנקרא הזקן. → NM 4:59.

זקני • **הוריד הזקני** → **וְרִיד**.

זָקַף • *Pass. Part.* **זָקוּף** • **המעי הזקוף** → **מְעִי**.

זָר • אש זרה → אֵשׁ.

זְרוֹעַ · I. **humerus; upper arm**: Arab. عضد · Ibn Sīnā, *K. al-Qānūn fī al-ṭibb* · trans. Nathan ha-Me'ati (*Sefer ha-Qanun*), bk. 1 (fol. 37[a]): ונוטה אל הצד החיצוני ומחוברת בראש הכתף ונקשרת בה הכתף ובהם יחדו נקשר הזרוע. → NM 4:59–60.

· II. **the inner side [of the arm]**: Arab. مأبض · Maimonides, *K. al-fuṣūl fī al-ṭibb* · trans. Zeraḥyah Ḥen (*Sefer ha-Peraqim*), 25.53: במאמר החמישי מהתחבולה אמר בהתחילו לספר איך ירופא רקיקת הדם מן הריאה אמר מאמר זה לשונו: וצוה לחולה שלא יתנפש ניפוש חזק ושיעשה המנוחה והשלווה תמיד ויקיז מיד גיד הזרוע. → NM 1:144.

• דבוקי הזרוע → דִּבּוּק.

• חבל הזרוע → חֶבֶל.

• פרק קנה הזרוע הסמוך ליד → פֶּרֶק.

• קשר הזרוע → קֶשֶׁר.

• קשרי הזרועות → קֶשֶׁר.

זָרוּת · **coercion**: Arab. استكراه · Maimonides, *Šarḥ fuṣūl Abūqrāṭ* · trans. Moses ibn Tibbon (*Pirqei Abuqraṭ*), 2.42 (94): ואם מנע השתוק תנועת החזה הנה זה יותר גדול ויותר מסוכן שיהיה מהם וכאשר יתנשם ביותר גדול שיהיה מן הזרות הנה שתוקו חזק גם כן. → NM 3:77–8.

זְרִיקָה • *Plur.* זריקות · **syringes**: Arab. زراقة, *Plur.* زراقات · Ibn Sīnā, *K. al-adwiya al-qalbiya* · trans. Anonymous (*Sammim Libbiyim*), fol. 122[a]: ויספיק בזה המשך המימות המתאחרות בעת הזלת הקודמות וכן הרוחות וכן העורות בכוסות המציצה והמימות בזריקות. → NM 4:60.

זֶרַע • הגרת הזרע מבלי רצון → הֲגָרָה.

• *Plur.* זרעים • זרעים קרים · **counterfeit dishes; simulated dishes**: Arab. مزوّرات · Ibn al-Jazzār, *Zād al-musāfir wa-qūt al-ḥādir* · trans. Moses ibn Tibbon (*Sefer Ṣedat ha-Derakhim*), bk. 2, ch. 1 (fol. 41[a]): ויהיה מאכלו זרעים קרים ויהיה משתהו מים ערבים צלולים. → NM 4:60.

זֵרְעוֹן • *Plur.* זרעונים · **chickpeas [*Cicer arietinum* and var.]**: Arab. حمّص · Ibn al-Jazzār, *Zād al-musāfir wa-qūt al-ḥādir* · trans. Moses ibn Tibbon (*Sefer Ṣedat ha-Derakhim*), bk. 7, 16.3: ואמר דיאסקורידוס כי יאמרו אנשים כי הזרעונים יבריאו מן היבלות הקשות כשיקח מהזרעונים וישים אחד אחד מהם על אחת אחת מן היבלות וזה יעשה ביום הראשון מן החודש ואחר כן יקבץ הזרעונים ויקשרם בצרור בגד וישליך אותם לאחוריו. → NM 1:71.

ח

[חבא] • *Part. Nif'al* נֶחְבָּא • **congested:** Arab. محتقن · Maimonides, *K. al-fuṣūl fī al-ṭibb* · trans. Zeraḥyah Ḥen (*Sefer ha-Peraqim*), 9.54: תתחדש כמו כן תאות המשקים הרעים כמו שיתחדש זה למזונות הרעים כי בהיות ליחה רעה נחבאת בתוך קרומותיה או שתהיה הליחה מלוחה או מרירייה. → NM 1:169–70.

חִבּוּר • **פירוק חבור** → פֵּרוּק.

• *Plur.* **חיבורים** • **joints:** Lat. iuncturae · Al-Rāzī, attr., *On the Treatment of Small Children* · trans. Anonymous, ch. 24: וקודם שיינק הילד יושם במרחץ ומשח את חיבוריו משמן קושטיי או משמן קשטוריאו. → NM 2:178.

חֲבוּרָה • **מקום החבורה** → מָקוֹם.

חָבוּשׁ • *Plur.* **חבושים** • **מרקחת חבושים** → מִרְקַחַת.

חִבּוּשׁ • I. **the application [of a poultice]:** Arab. تضميد · Maimonides, *K. al-fuṣūl fī al-ṭibb* · trans. Zeraḥyah Ḥen (*Sefer ha-Peraqim*), 15.51: המורסא הנקראת חמרה תקררנה בתחלת העניין וככלות חומו ונתבטלה רתיחתו אז תועילנו השריטה והחיבוש בתחבושת יהיה נעשה בקמח השעורים מחומם. → NM 1:144–5.

• II. **fomentation; fomenting:** Arab. تكميد / Gr. πυρία · Maimonides, *Šarḥ fuṣūl Abūqrāṭ* · trans. Moses ibn Tibbon (*Pirqei Abuqraṭ*), 5.28 (248): אמר אבקראט: החבוש בסמנים מושך הדם אשר יבוא מן הנשים והנה יהיו מקבלים תועלת בו במקומות רבים אחרים לולי שהוא יחדש בראש כבדות. → NM 3:78.

• III. **setting (of bones):** Arab. جبر · Al-Zahrāwī, *K. al-taṣrīf li-man ʿağiza ʿan at-taʾlīf* · trans. Shem Tov ben Isaac (*Sefer ha-Shimmush*), bk. 27, fol. 143[b], col. b: הראש הוא בכלל עב מחמם רב המזון ... ועוזר על חבוש שבירת העצמות. → NM 4:60.

• IV. **setting (of a fracture):** Arab. جَبْر · a) Al-Zahrāwī, *K. al-taṣrīf li-man ʿağiza ʿan at-taʾlīf* · trans. Shem Tov ben Isaac (*Sefer ha-Shimmush*), bk. 30, 3.0 (fol. 232[a]): זה החלק גם כן גדול הצורך והתועלת במלאכה והוא חבוש השבר והשמיטה המתחדשים בעצמות. → NM 1:90.

b) Al-Rāzī, *K. al-Manṣūrī* · trans. Shem Tov ben Isaac (*Sefer Almansur*), Bet 10 (20): באן ובלעז ישמין: ירכך המורסא הגסה ויתיכה ויסיר הנתק כשיוטח בו הפנים ושמנו טוב לעובי הנשאר מרושם החיבוש. → NM 2:12.

• V. **treatment:** Arab. علاج · Al-Zahrāwī, *K. al-taṣrīf li-man ʿağiza ʿan at-taʾlīf* · trans. Shem Tov ben Isaac (*Sefer ha-Shimmush*), bk. 30, 3.2 (fol. 233[a]): וחבוש השבר הוא להסתכל בתחלה אל מקרי החולה. → NM 1:90.

חֲבִישָׁה • **setting (of bones):** Arab. جَبْر · Maimonides, *K. al-fuṣūl fī al-ṭibb* · trans. Nathan ha-Me'ati (*Sefer ha-Peraqim*), 15.63: העצמות בבחורים יחבשו קודם שיחבשו בנערים כי הנערים יצטרכו לליחה שיגדילו בה ולהחליף מה שנתך מהם. וזכר זה אסקלפיוס במאמר הראשון מפירושו בספר החבישה. → NM 2:44.

• *Plur.* **חבישות** • **trusses:** Arab. جبائر · Maimonides, *K. al-fuṣūl fī al-ṭibb* · trans. Nathan ha-Me'ati (*Sefer ha-Peraqim*), 15.69: ואם כן יהיה כל מה שמקיף באבר ארבע דברים: הקשירה הנוגעת האבר והרפידות והקשירה אשר עליהן והחבישות. → NM 2:44.

[חבל]¹ • *Pi'el* **חִבֵּל** ‣ **to ulcerate:** Arab. قرّح · Maimonides, *K. al-fuṣūl fī al-ṭibb* · trans. Zeraḥyah Ḥen (*Sefer ha-Peraqim*), 23.46: הסרטן שני מינים והוא מורסא נולדת מהמרה השחורה ובהשתפך המרה השחורה אל הבשר ותהיה נושכת תאכל כל העור אשר סמוך לה ותחבלנו והוא הסרטן המתחבל ובהיותה ממוצעת תחדש סרטן בלתי מתחבל. → NM 1:145.

• *Hitpa'el* **הִתְחַבֵּל** ‣ **to develop an ulcer:** Arab. قرح · Maimonides, *K. al-fuṣūl fī al-ṭibb* · trans. Zeraḥyah Ḥen (*Sefer ha-Peraqim*), 6.72: כשיתחבל מעי מן המיעים מן המרה השחורה לא יהיה לו רפואה. → NM 1:145.

[חבל]² • *Hitpa'el* **הִתְחַבֵּל** ‣ **to exercise one's skill:** Arab. احتال · Maimonides, *K. al-fuṣūl fī al-ṭibb* · trans. Zeraḥyah Ḥen (*Sefer ha-Peraqim*), 15.17: כשתקרה עקיצה בעצב מן העצבים על כל פנים יכאב כאב מרובה מפני חוש העצב. על כן תתחבל לשכך הכאב ולמנוע ככל יכולתך שלא תתחדש שם מורסא. → NM 1:145.

חֶבֶל • **חבל הזרוע** ‣ I. **cord of the arm (i.e., the vena cephalica pollicis and the vena cephalica antibrachii):** Arab. حبل الذراع · Al-Zahrāwī, *K. al-taṣrīf li-man 'ağiza 'an at-ta'līf* · trans. Shem Tov ben Isaac (*Sefer ha-Shimmush*), bk. 30, 2.95 (fol. 230ᵃ): והקזת חבל הזרוע יוקז תמורת גיד האכחל והבאסליק כשלא ימצאו או כשיהיו נעלמים כי הוא מורכב מהם. → NM 1:90–1; corr. 4:229.

‣ II. **funis brachii, the median cephalic vein of the arm:** Arab. حبل الذراع · Ibn Sīnā, *K. al-Qānūn fī al-ṭibb* · trans. Nathan ha-Me'ati (*Sefer ha-Qanun*), bk. 1 (fol. 65ᵇ): ואחר בקרוב מפרק המרפק מתחלק לשלשה חלקים אחד מהם חבל הזרוע. → NM 4:60.

חֵבֶל • *Plur.* **חבלים** ‣ I. **colic:** Arab. مغص · Hippocrates, *Aphorisms* · trans. Nathan ha-Me'ati, 5.41 (261) (fol. 96ᵃ): אמר בקראט: אם חפצת לדעת האשה הרה או לא תשקה אותה כשהיא רוצה לישן מי הדבש ואם ימצאוה חבלים בבטנה אז היא הרה ואם לא ימצאוה זה אז היא אינה הרה. → NM 3:78.

‣ II. **wounds:** Arab. جراحات · Maimonides, *K. al-fuṣūl fī al-ṭibb* · trans. Zeraḥyah Ḥen (*Sefer ha-Peraqim*), 15.33: אמנם רפואת חבלי העצבים אני עושה בה הגפרית אשר לא נגעהו אש עם השמן עד שובו עבה כטיט כתלי המרחץ. → NM 1:145–6.

• **צירים וחבלים** → **צִיר**.

חַבָלָה • *Plur.* **חבלות** ‣ I. **ulcers:** a) Lat. ulcera · Bruno Longobucco, *Cyrurgia Magna* · trans. Hillel ben Samuel (*Sefer Keritut*), fol. 31ᵃ: אחר כן אומר לפי דברי ב״צ שהחבלות אותן נראות או הן נעלמות. → NM 1:25.

b) Arab. قروح · Maimonides, *K. al-fuṣūl fī al-ṭibb* · trans. Zeraḥyah Ḥen (*Sefer ha-Peraqim*), 3.76: החליים הארוכים כמו צרות הניפוש והחול והטחורים באף והחבלות הרעות ודומיהם כי רוב אילו הכאבים אשר יתילדו לנערים ולילדים יתרפאו עד מ׳ יום או לז׳ חדשים או לז׳ שנים. → NM 1:146.

‣ II. **wounds:** Arab. جراحات · Maimonides, *K. al-fuṣūl fī al-ṭibb* · trans. Zeraḥyah Ḥen (*Sefer ha-Peraqim*), 12.32: הרפואה היותר מועילה לחבלות העצבים והיותר מתקנת להם הוא מה שהוא מייבש והוא במעט חמימות ותהיה חמימותו מספיק ומייבש עם כל זה. → NM 1:146.

• **החבלות הגממיות** ‣ **concave wounds:** Lat. vulnera concava · Bruno Longobucco,

Cyrurgia Magna · trans. Hillel ben Samuel (*Sefer Keritut*), fol. 23b: וענין אימון הרפואה בדברים הנזכרים היא שבחבלות הגוממיות שבהן חסרון בשר וכן בחבלות העמוקות שנאבד משם עצם הבשר תניח תחילה מן המולידות בשר. → NM 1:19.

• **החבלות המתפשטות** · **herpes**: Arab. القروح التي تسعى / Gr. ἑρπητές · Maimonides, *Šarḥ fuṣūl Abūqrāṭ* · trans. Zeraḥyah Ḥen (*Pirqei Abuqraṭ*), 5.22 (242): אמר בקראט: החם מביא המוגלא אבל לא בכל מוגלא וזה כי רוב הסימנים מורים על הבטחון והאמונה ויבשל המוגלא ויחליק העור ויפחות היזק הקרירות הנק׳ נאפץ והקיווץ וההמשכה ויתיר הכבידות הקורה בראש והוא מן היותר נאות לשברון העצמות וכל שכן לאצטומ׳ ולעצמות הראש ולכל מה שהמיתו הקרירות או חבל אותו ולחבלות המתפשטות והמתאכלות ולפי הטבעת ולחבלות שברחם ולשלפוחית כי החמימות לבעלי אילו החליים מועיל ומרפא והקור להם מזיק וממית. → NM 3:79.

[חבר] • *Part. Pi'el* **מְחַבֵּר** • **רפואה מחברת** → **רְפוּאָה**.

• *Part. Pu'al* **מְחֻבָּר** · **compounded**: Arab. مؤلّف · Maimonides, *K. al-fuṣūl fī al-ṭibb* · trans. Zeraḥyah Ḥen (*Sefer ha-Peraqim*), 13.13: כשתרצה להריק הגוף ממה שיש בו מן הליחות ותנקה הראש עמו עד שלא ירד ממנו קטרא ראוי לך שתהיה הרפואה מחוברת מרפואה משונה בכחותיה כמו הגרעינים אשר חברנו אנחנו. → NM 1:161.

חָבַשׁ · **to apply a fomentation; to apply a warm pack; to foment; to make a warm poultice**: Arab. كمّد · Ibn al-Jazzār, *Zād al-musāfir wa-qūt al-ḥāḍir* · trans. Moses ibn Tibbon (*Sefer Ṣedat ha-Derakhim*), bk. 2, ch. 1 (Ms. Oxford, Bodleian Library, Poc. 353, Uri Heb. 314, fol. 11b): ואם היה הכאב חזק ראוי שיחבוש העין במי בשול קורונא ריאל ופנגריג. → NM 4:61.

• *Nif'al* **נֶחְבַּשׁ** · **to heal**: Arab. انجبر · Maimonides, *K. al-fuṣūl fī al-ṭibb* · trans. Nathan ha-Me'ati (*Sefer ha-Peraqim*), 15.63: העצמות בבחורים יחבשו קודם שיחבשו בנערים כי הנערים יצטרכו לליחה שיגדילו בה ולהחליף מה שנתך מהם. וזכר זה אסקלפיוס במאמר הראשון מפירושו בספר החבישה. → NM 2:44.

• *Pi'el* **חִבֵּשׁ** · I. **to make firm; to strengthen**: Lat. consolido / Arab. متّن · Ibn Sīnā, *K. al-adwiya al-qalbiya* · trans. Anonymous (*Sefer ha-Refu'ot ha-Libbiyot*), fol. 247b: ולו עפיצות מעט ומפני זה מחבש עצם רוח הלב. → NM 4:61.

· II. **to repair**: Arab. جبّر · a) Al-Zahrāwī, *K. al-taṣrīf li-man ʿağiza ʿan at-ta'līf* · trans. Shem Tov ben Isaac (*Sefer ha-Shimmush*), bk. 30, 1.13 (fol. 232b): וזאת התחבושת אין בה כח לחבש. → NM 1:91.

b) Al-Zahrāwī, *K. al-taṣrīf li-man ʿağiza ʿan at-ta'līf* · trans. Shem Tov ben Isaac (*Sefer ha-Shimmush*), bk. 30, 1.13 (fol. 232b): תאר תחבושת מחבשת העצמים הנשברים. → NM 1:91.

• *Part. Pi'el* **מְחַבֵּשׁ** · **bonesetter**: Arab. مجبّر · Al-Zahrāwī, *K. al-taṣrīf li-man ʿağiza ʿan at-ta'līf* · trans. Shem Tov ben Isaac (*Sefer ha-Shimmush*), bk. 30, 3.3 (fol. 233b): וזכרו קצת המחבשים מן הראשונים לבלול הפתילות בחמאה ולהחליפן בכל יום ואין נכון אצלי לעשות כן. → NM 1:101.

• *Hitpa'el* **הִתְחַבֵּשׁ** · **to mend**: Arab. انجبر · Al-Zahrāwī, *K. al-taṣrīf li-man ʿağiza ʿan at-ta'līf* · trans. Shem Tov ben Isaac (*Sefer ha-Shimmush*), bk. 30, 3.12 (fol. 235b): וידוע ששבר הזרוע יתחבש בשלשים יום או בשנים ושלשים על הרוב ואפשר שיחבש לפעמים בשמנה ועשרים יום. → NM 1:91.

חִגֵּר • שב חגר → [שוב].

חִגְּרוּת • **lameness**: Arab. عَرَج • Maimonides, *Šarḥ fuṣūl Abūqrāṭ* • trans. Moses ibn Tibbon (*Pirqei Abuqraṭ*), 6.60 (352): אמר המפרש: התנגב הליחה ההיא המדובקת בכויה וכאשר לא יתנגב הליחה ההיא בכויה יתחדש החגרות ולא ילך הרגל כמנהגו ויצמק. → NM 3:80.

חַד • חוליים חדים → חֹלִי.

[חדד] • *Part. Pu'al* **מְחֻדָּד** • I. **acute**: Hippocrates, *Aphorisms* • trans. Do'eg ha-Edomi (*Sefer Agur*), 1.24 (51) (fol. 31ᵇ): תשקה סובלי מדוה מחודד משקה משלשל בראשיתם כדת הראויה להם. → NM 3:126–7.

• II. **conic**: Arab. مخروط • a) Maimonides, *K. al-fuṣūl fī al-ṭibb* • trans. Zeraḥyah Ḥen (*Sefer ha-Peraqim*), 4.44: לא תדמה תנועת הדפק בשלשה קצוותיו כתנועתו בגוף המרובע או המחודד וזולתם אלא תחשוב שהיא תנועה אחת והקפה אחת כתנועת הכדור כי תנועת הגיד תתבאר לחוש עגולה מאד. → NM 1:161.

b) Maimonides, *K. al-fuṣūl fī al-ṭibb* • trans. Nathan ha-Me'ati (*Sefer ha-Peraqim*), 4.44: לא תדמה תנועת העורק בשלשת קטריו כתנועה בגשם המרובע או המחודד הנקרא החרוט וזולתם. → NM 2:57–8.

חִדּוּשׁ • **freshness**: Arab. طراوة • Al-Zahrāwī, *K. al-taṣrīf li-man ʿağiza ʿan at-taʾlīf* • trans. Shem Tov ben Isaac (*Sefer ha-Shimmush*), bk. 27, fol. 144ᵇ, col. b: ולפעמים ישתנה החלב בפעולתו וכחו כפי מזג הבעל חיים אשר הוא ממנו ושניו ומדת זמן החלב מישנותו וחדושו. → NM 4:61.

חֶדֶר • **cavity**: Arab. فضاء • Maimonides, *Šarḥ fuṣūl Abūqrāṭ* • trans. Anonymous (*Pirqei Abuqraṭ*), 7.38 (390): אמר המפרש: הגוף העליון הוא חדר החזה אשר בו הריאה ויום העשרים הוא יום הגבול להיותו סוף השבוע השלישי. → NM 3:80.

• רוחב החדר → רֹחַב.

• *Plur.* **חדרים** • **ventricles (of the brain, heart)**: Arab. بطن • Ibn Sīnā, *K. al-Qānūn fī al-ṭibb* • trans. Nathan ha-Me'ati (*Sefer ha-Qanun*), bk. 1 (fol. 56ᵃ): הנה יצמח מן המוח מן העצביים ⟨שבעה⟩ זוגות הזוג הראשון התחלתו מעומק שני החדרים המוקדמים מן המוח אצל שכונת שתי התוספות הדומות לשתי פטומות. → NM 4:61.

• **חדרי הבטן** • **the internal parts (of the body)**: Hippocrates, *Aphorisms* • trans. Do'eg ha-Edomi (*Sefer Agur*), 4.48 (185) (fol. 70ᵃ): סערת קדחת מחודדת בוערה בחדרי הבטן ושטח הגוף קר מחוץ וצמאון מתמיד הוא אות מות. → NM 3:80–1.

חָדָשׁ • I. **fresh; green**: Arab. أخضر • Al-Zahrāwī, *K. al-taṣrīf li-man ʿağiza ʿan at-taʾlīf* • trans. Shem Tov ben Isaac (*Sefer ha-Shimmush*), bk. 27, fol. 126ᵃ, col. a: הפול: יש ממנו חדש אשר לא נגמר בשולו ויש ממנו יבש והחדש הלח קר באמצע המעלה הראשונה לח בסופה. → NM 4:61–2.

• II. **young man**: Arab. حَدَث / Gr. νέος • Maimonides, *Šarḥ fuṣūl Abūqrāṭ* • trans. Moses ibn Tibbon (*Pirqei Abuqraṭ*), 2.45 (97): אמר אבקראט: בעל חולי הנופל כשיהיה חדש הנה רפואתו תהיה לבד בהעתקו בשנים והארץ וההנהגה. → NM 3:81.

חוּג • **dizziness**: Arab. دوار • Al-Zahrāwī, *K. al-taṣrīf li-man ʿağiza ʿan at-taʾlīf* • trans. Shem Tov ben Isaac (*Sefer ha-Shimmush*), bk. 27, fol. 132ᵃ, col. b: והחוג והרעישה וכבדות כל הגוף וצרות הנשימה הממית בעליו באורך הזמן. → NM 4:62.

• גרם חוג → גָּרֶם.

חוֹזֵר (*Part.*) → חָזַר.

חוּט · I. **fiber:** Arab. ليف · Maimonides, *K. al-fuṣūl fī al-ṭibb* · trans. Zeraḥyah Ḥen (*Sefer ha-Peraqim*), 1.12: אלו השלשה כלים והם העצב והיתר והקישור כלם הם לבנים ומעשה מקשה נעדרים מהדם וכשתתירם יותרו אל חוט הולך אל האורך מלבד מה שיהיה מן הקישורים קשה מאד כי אי אפשר שיתיר וישוב חוט. NM 1:146.

· II. **(lit., line; streak; stripe); h.l., cerebral (longitudinal) fissure:** Arab. خطّ / Lat. linea · Ibn al-Jazzār, *Zād al-musāfir wa-qūt al-ḥādir* · trans. Moses ibn Tibbon (*Sefer Ṣedat ha-Derakhim*), bk. 1, ch. 11 (fol. 18[b]): המוח יחלק תחלה באורך לשני חלקים: ימין ושמאל וביניהם חוט נמשך באמצע המוח מבדיל בין מדוריו. → NM 4:62.

• **חוט השדרה** · **spinal chord:** Arab. نخاع الفقار · Ibn al-Jazzār, *Zād al-musāfir wa-qūt al-ḥādir* · trans. Moses ibn Tibbon (*Sefer Ṣedat ha-Derakhim*), bk. 1, ch. 23 (fol. 33[b]): ואם יהיה הסתום באחד מפלחי חוט השדרה ימין ושמאל יהיה הפלג במה שלמטה מן הצואר מן הפלח ההוא האטום. → NM 4:62.

• *Plur.* **חוטים** · **fibers:** Arab. شظايا · Maimonides, *K. al-fuṣūl fī al-ṭibb* · trans. Zeraḥyah Ḥen (*Sefer ha-Peraqim*), 1.74: החוטים בכל אחד מן המעים הם עגולים יכרכו ברוחב בשתי כרומות כלם כי המעים אמנם יקיפו על מה שבהם לבד ויאספהו ולא ימשכו שום דבר מן הדברים. → NM 1:146.

• **חוטי הבצים** · **spermatic cords:** Judah ben Jacob, *Sefer Hanhagat ha-Beri'ut*, 10.2: צריך אדם להזהר אם רצה לחיות בטובה שלא יבעול אלא כשימצא גופו בריא וחזק והוא מתקשה מאליו שלא מדעתו וימצא כובד ממתניו ולמטה כאילו חוטי הבצים נמשכים למטה. → NM 4:62.

• **החוטים הנתלים** · **suspensor:** Arab. معلاق · Al-Zahrāwī, *K. al-taṣrīf li-man ʿağiza ʿan at-ta'līf* · trans. Shem Tov ben Isaac (*Sefer ha-Shimmush*), bk. 30, 2.63 (fol. 219[b]): וזה המין לפעמים יתכן לבקע עליו ועל יתר מיני הבשר והוא לבקע עור הבצים ואחר כך למשוך הביצה למעלה ולהוציאה מן הקרום הלבן ולהפריד החוטין הנתלין מן הכיסים ולקשור הכיסים ולחתך החוטין אחר הפרדם מכל צד מצדי הביצה. → NM 1:91.

חוטם → חֹטֶם.

חוֹל · **stone(s):** Arab. حصاة · Maimonides, *K. al-fuṣūl fī al-ṭibb* · trans. Zeraḥyah Ḥen (*Sefer ha-Peraqim*), 3.76: החליים הארוכים כמו צרות הניפוש והחול והטחורים באף והחבלות הרעות ודומיהם כי רוב אילו הכאבים אשר יתילדו לנערים ולילדים יתרפאו עד מ׳ יום. → NM 1:146–7.

חוּלָב • *Plur.* **חולבים** • **החולבים** · **the [two] renal veins:** Arab. الطالعان (read: الحالبان) · Ibn Sīnā, *K. al-Qānūn fī al-ṭibb* · trans. Nathan ha-Me'ati (*Sefer ha-Qanun*), bk. 1 (fol. 66[b]): ואחר יתענף מהם שני עורקים גדולים נקראים החולבים פונים אל הכליות לזכך מימיות הדם. → NM 4:62–3.

• **שני החולבים** · **groins:** Arab. الحالبان · Maimonides, *K. al-fuṣūl fī al-ṭibb* · trans. Nathan ha-Me'ati (*Sefer ha-Peraqim*), 10.15: העפוש לפעמים יהיה בעורקים כלם בשוה ולפעמים יהיה ביותר גדול שבהם והנכבד שבהם והם העורקים שהם בין שני החולבים והאצילים. → NM 2:45.

חוּלָה • האלם לשון החולה → [אלם].

חוּלִי → חֳלִי.

חוליא → חֲלְיָה.
חוליה → חֲלְיָה.
חולשה → חֻלְשָׁה.
חום → חֹם.
חומר → חֹמֶר.
חומש → חֹמֶשׁ.
חוֹצֵץ (*Part.*) → חָצַץ.
חוּשׁ • **בטול החוש** → **בִּטּוּל**.
• **תרדמת החוש** → **תַּרְדֵּמָה**.
חוֹתֵךְ (*Part.*) → **חָתַךְ**.
חָזֶה • **אמצע החזה** → **אֶמְצַע**.
• **ארון החזה** → **אָרוֹן**.
• **מוגלת החזה** → **מֻגְלָא**.
• **למטה משחוס החזה** → **מַטָּה**.
• **עצם החזה** → **עֶצֶם**.
• **צלעות אמצע החזה** → **צֶלַע**.
חִזּוּק · **fibrous tissue; ligament**: Arab. عَقَب / Lat. nervi seu tendines, quibus chordae conficiuntur · Ibn Sīnā, *K. al-Qānūn fī al-ṭibb* · trans. Joseph Lorki (*Sefer ha-Qanun*), bk. 1 (fol. 13[b]): ועל כן חשב הבורא והצמיח מהעצמות דבר דומה בעצב נקרא חזוק וקשרים והוא נאסף מהעצב ונסתבך בו כדבר אחד. → NM 4:64.
חֲזִירִי • **צמח חזירי** → **צֶמַח**.
[חזק] • *Pi'el* **חִזֵּק** · **to protect**: Arab. وقى · Maimonides, *K. al-fuṣūl fī al-ṭibb* · trans. Zeraḥyah Ḥen (*Sefer ha-Peraqim*), 1.44: חוט של שדרה כלומר הגוף החלק אשר יצא מן המוח בחליות השדרה כלה יקיף בו אותן הקרומות בעצמן המקיפין במוח ואחד משתי הקרומות דבק באחר ויקיף בהם קרום כרוך עליהם מנראיהם כמו קרום שלישי חזק קשה מסוג העצבים לחזקו מפני חוזק תנועתו וכחו וקשייו. → NM 1:147.
• *Part. Pi'el* **מְחַזֵּק** • **הסם המחזק** → **סַם**.
• *Hif'il* **הֶחְזִיק** · **to surround**: Arab. حوى · Maimonides, *Šarḥ fuṣūl Abūqrāṭ* · trans. Moses ibn Tibbon (*Pirqei Abuqraṭ*), 7.24 (376): אמר המפרש: יאמר כי כאשר נחתך עצם הראש עד שיגיע החתך למקום הפנוי המחזיק למוח יתחדש ערבוב השכל. → NM 3:81.
• *Part. Hof'al* **מֻחְזָק** · **protected**: Arab. موقاة · Maimonides, *K. al-fuṣūl fī al-ṭibb* · trans. Zeraḥyah Ḥen (*Sefer ha-Peraqim*), 1.18: וכל העצבים והיתרים והגידים המוגבלים מן העצם מוחזק מכוסה בקרומות חזקים. → NM 1:161.
חָזְקָה · **burning heat**: Arab. وهج / Lat. fumus · Ibn al-Jazzār, *Zād al-musāfir wa-qūt al-ḥādir* · trans. Moses ibn Tibbon (*Sefer Ṣedat ha-Derakhim*), bk. 1, ch. 18 (fol. 26[a]): ותתילד משתי סבות אחת מהן התלהבות מרה כרכומית והתלקח בחלקי המוח והאחרת מרתיחת דם הלב והתגברו כי דם הלב כשירתח ויתלהב בחום מרה אדומה יתגבר ויעלה חזקתו אל הראש. → NM 4:64–5.
חָזַר • *Part.* **חוֹזֵר** • **העצב החוזר** → **עָצָב**.
• **העצב החוזר למפרע** → **עָצָב**.

• *Hif'il* הֶחֱזִיר · **to cause a relapse:** Hippocrates, *Aphorisms* · trans. Judah Shalom, 2.12 (64) (fol. 18[b]): הדברים שישארו בחלי‹י›ם אחרי הגבול מחזירים. → NM 3:81.

• *Part. Hif'il* מַחֲזִיר • **העצל המחזיר לאחור** → עָצֵל.

• *Part. Hof'al* מֻחְזָר · **repeated:** Arab. مكرّر · Maimonides, *Šarḥ fuṣūl Abūqrāṭ* · trans. Anonymous (*Pirqei Abuqraṭ*), introduction (13): ואלו פרקי אבוקרט מהם פרקים יצטרכו אל פירוש ומהם מבוארים בעצמם ומהם מוחזרים ומהם מה שאין בו תועלת במלאכת הרפואה ומהם טעות גמור. → NM 3:127.

חָח · **hook:** Arab. صنّارة / Gr. ἄγκιστρον · Al-Zahrāwī, *K. al-taṣrīf li-man ʿağiza ʿan at-taʾlīf* · trans. Shem Tov ben Isaac (*Sefer ha-Shimmush*), bk. 30, 2.6 (fol. 209[b]): ואם יצא החצץ במלקחים טוב ואם לא צריך להשתדל להוציאו בחח דק כפוף מעט. → NM 1:92.

[חטא] • *Part. Hif'il* מַחְטִיא • **הליחה המחטיאה** → לֵחָה.

חִטָּה • **גריש החטה** → גְּרִישׁ.

• **חלב החטה** → חֵלֶב.

• *Plur.* **חטים** · **tonsils:** Arab. لوزتان · Ibn al-Jazzār, *Zād al-musāfir wa-qūt al-ḥādir* · trans. Moses ibn Tibbon (*Sefer Ṣedat ha-Derakhim*), introduction (fol. 3[a]): השער הג׳ בכאיבי האונקלי והשפוי כובע והחטים. → NM 4:65.

• **שני החטים** · **tonsils:** Arab. اللوزتان · Al-Zahrāwī, *K. al-taṣrīf li-man ʿağiza ʿan at-taʾlīf* · trans. Shem Tov ben Isaac (*Sefer ha-Shimmush*), bk. 30, 2.43 (fol. 215[b]): אבל אשר יש להם צמח חם בפה או בגרון או בשני החטים כשלא יהיה חולי בקנה מחייב לבקע השפוי כובע פחד החניקה. → NM 1:92.

חֹטֶם • **זלוף הדם מן החוטם** → זִלּוּף.

• **עוקץ החוטם** → עֹקֶץ.

• **עריפת דם החוטם** → עֲרִיפָה.

• **קנה החוטם** → קָנֶה.

• **רעיפת דם מן החוטם** → רְעִיפָה.

חַי • **גפרית חי** → גָּפְרִית.

• **היין החי** → יַיִן.

• **הסיד החי** → סִיד.

• **הרוח החיה** → רוּחַ.

חיבור → חִבּוּר.

חיבוש → חִבּוּשׁ.

חימוץ → חִמּוּץ.

חִיצוֹנִי • **הקנה החיצוני** → קָנֶה.

חֵיק • **חיק העין** · **orbit:** Arab. شحمة العين · Al-Zahrāwī, *K. al-taṣrīf li-man ʿağiza ʿan at-taʾlīf* · trans. Shem Tov ben Isaac (*Sefer ha-Shimmush*), bk. 30, 2.93 (fol. 228[a]): והוצאתי חץ אחר ליהודי שכבר נפל לו בחיק עינו תחת העפעף השפל. → NM 1:92; corr. 4:229.

[חכך] • *Part. Pi'el* מְחַכֵּךְ • **הסם המחכך** → סַם.

[חכם] • *Part. Pu'al* מְחֻכָּם · **firm; precise; solid:** Arab. محكم · Ibn al-Jazzār, *Zād al-musāfir wa-qūt al-ḥādir* · trans. Moses ibn Tibbon (*Sefer Ṣedat ha-Derakhim*), bk. 7, 10.2: וראוי להתחיל ברפואתו בקשור למעלה ממקום הנשיכה קשירה מחוכמת כדי שלא יעבור הארס בעורקים אל האברים הראשים וימית. → NM 1:59.

חֶלְאָה · **foam**: Arab. رغوة · Al-Zahrāwī, *K. al-taṣrīf li-man ʿağiza ʿan at-taʾlīf* · trans. Shem Tov ben Isaac (*Sefer ha-Shimmush*), bk. 27, fol. 127[a], col. b: וכשיקרבו השעורים אל הבשול וישגו ויתפחו להסיר חלאתם ולרחצם במים חמין. → NM 4:66.

• **חלאת הים** · **(lit., filth of the sea); sea foam**: Lat. spuma maris / Gr. ἁλκυόνιον · Bruno Longobucco, *Cyrurgia Magna* · trans. Hillel ben Samuel (*Sefer Keritut*), fol. 86[b]. → NM 1:25.

חָלָב • **החלב החמוץ** · **sour buttermilk**: Arab. الدوغ · Al-Zahrāwī, *K. al-taṣrīf li-man ʿağiza ʿan at-taʾlīf* · trans. Shem Tov ben Isaac (*Sefer ha-Shimmush*), bk. 27, fol. 147[a], col. a: החלב החמוץ הנקרא אלדוע׳ קר יבש קשה להתעכל רחוק לרדת כבד על האצטומ. → NM 4:66.

• **מי החלב** → מַיִם.

• **מיץ (ה)חלב** → מִיץ.

• **החלב המשוכשך** · **buttermilk**: Arab. مخيض · Maimonides, *K. al-fuṣūl fī al-ṭibb* · trans. Nathan ha-Me'ati (*Sefer ha-Peraqim*), 23.107: בשמות מיני החלב כשישוכשך ויוסר ממנו חמאתו יקרא מה שישאר מכיץ כלומר החלב המשוכשך ונקרא אלדוג. → NM 2:63.

• **החלב הקרוש** · **thick curdled milk**: Arab. اللبن الرائب · Al-Zahrāwī, *K. al-taṣrīf li-man ʿağiza ʿan at-taʾlīf* · trans. Shem Tov ben Isaac (*Sefer ha-Shimmush*), bk. 27, fol. 147[a], col. a: החלב הקרוש הנקרא אלראיב יותר קר מן החמוץ ויותר נאות אל האצטומ׳ החמה ולבעלי החמימות. → NM 4:66.

חֵלֶב · **omentum**: Arab. ثرب · a) Maimonides, *K. al-fuṣūl fī al-ṭibb* · trans. Zeraḥyah Ḥen (*Sefer ha-Peraqim*), 9.102: אבל תראה ותדע כי הכיס אשר ירד בו הקרום אשר על האסטומכא והמיעים והוא החלב הוא חולי גדול וחזק אע״פ שמקומו אינו גדול. → NM 1:147.

b) Maimonides, *K. al-fuṣūl fī al-ṭibb* · trans. Nathan ha-Me'ati (*Sefer ha-Peraqim*), 1.60: החלב הוא מן האברים אשר אינם הכרחיים במציאות בעלי חיים. → NM 2:45.

• **חלב החטה** · **starch**: Arab. نشاء الحنطة وهو النشاستج / Gr. ἄμυλον · Al-Zahrāwī, *K. al-taṣrīf li-man ʿağiza ʿan at-taʾlīf* · trans. Shem Tov ben Isaac (*Sefer ha-Shimmush*), bk. 27, fol. 124[b], col. 1: חלב החטה קר ויבש והראיה על קרירותו החמיצות המועטת אשר בו והמזון המתילד ממנו יש בו חלוקה ולפי כך יועיל מנחרת החזה והריאה ועיצום המעים והפשטתם ומשחין כיס מקוה המים. → NM 4:66–7.

• **ידיעת החלב** → יְרִיעָה.

• **כיס החלב** → כִּיס.

• **חלב הכרס** · **omentum**: Gr. ἐπίπλοος · Hippocrates, *Aphorisms* · trans. Joseph Delmedigo, 7.55 (407): למי שכבדם מלא מים ויבקע משם אל חלב הכרס יתמלא בטנם וימות. → NM 3:82.

• **החלב המכסה** · **omentum**: Arab. ثرب · Maimonides, *K. al-fuṣūl fī al-ṭibb* · trans. Nathan ha-Me'ati (*Sefer ha-Peraqim*), 1.55: החלב המכסה הוא מחובר משני עורות גסים אחד מהם דבוק באחר ומעורקים דופקים ובלתי דופקים ושומן שאיננו מועט. → NM 2:46.

• **החלב המכסה (את) הקרב** · **omentum**: Arab. ثرب · a) Al-Zahrāwī, *K. al-taṣrīf li-man ʿağiza ʿan at-taʾlīf* · trans. Shem Tov ben Isaac (*Sefer ha-Shimmush*), bk. 30, 1.45 (fol. 207[b]): כשיקרה בתק בעקרי הירכים ויתגללו קצת המעים או החלב המכסה את הקרב אל האשכים. → NM 1:92.

b) Maimonides, *K. al-fuṣūl fī al-ṭibb* · trans. Zeraḥyah Ḥen (*Sefer ha-Peraqim*), 1.60: החלב המכסה הקרב הוא אחד מן האברים שאינם מוכרחים במציאות הבעל חיים ותועלתו בגוף מעוטה. → NM 1:147.

• **החלב אשר על הקרב** · **omentum**: Arab. ثرب · Al-Zahrāwī, *K. al-taṣrīf li-man ʿağiza ʿan at-taʾlīf* · trans. Shem Tov ben Isaac (*Sefer ha-Shimmush*), bk. 30, fol. 217ª. → NM 1:92.

חֲלוּדָה · I. **filth**: Lat. sordicies (Honofredi) · Ibn Zuhr, *Regimen of Health* · trans. Jacob ibn Tibbon (*Hanhagat ha-Beriʾut le-Abu ʿAli ben Zuhr*), ch. 20: ואמרו חכמי׳: כאשר ירחץ הבלן הגוף במרחץ בדבש יוציא מן הגשם מה שהוא דבק בין עור ובשר מן המותרות הלחות העשניות ויפתח הסתומים וימרק מה שעליו מן החלודה והדומה אליו. → NM 4:67.

· II. **fluid, watery moisture**: Arab. صديد · Maimonides, *K. al-fuṣūl fī al-ṭibb* · trans. Nathan ha-Meʾati (*Sefer ha-Peraqim*), 15.54: יולד בגופים שני מותרים בהכרח: אחד מהם דק נתך מן הגוף בהתכה נסתרת והשני עב והוא הזוהמא המתקבצת על הגוף. ואותו הדק בשחין יקרא חלודה ואותו העב בשחין יקרא מלוכלך. → NM 2:46.

· III. **viscous matters**: Lat. limositas, *Plur.* limositates · Hippocrates, *Aphorisms* · trans. Hillel ben Samuel, 4.53 (190) (fol. 26ᵇ): א״א: כל אותם שיש להם קדחת אם על השנים יעשה להם חלודה הקדחת נעשת יותר ארוכה ויותר חזקה. → NM 3:82.

חלודיי · **serous**: Arab. صديدي · Maimonides, *K. al-fuṣūl fī al-ṭibb* · trans. Nathan ha-Meʾati (*Sefer ha-Peraqim*), 6.78: וכשיהיה הדם רקיק וחלודיי מורה שהכבד יחלש מעשה הדם. → NM 2:46.

חלוחלת · I. **buttocks**: Arab. مقعدة · Ibn al-Jazzār, *Zād al-musāfir wa-qūt al-ḥāḍir* · trans. Moses ibn Tibbon (*Sefer Ṣedat ha-Derakhim*), introduction (fol. 3ᵇ): השער הכ׳ ברפיון החלוחלת ויציאתה. → NM 4:67.

· II. **rectum**: Arab. سرم · Ibn Sīnā, *K. al-Qānūn fī al-ṭibb* · trans. Nathan ha-Meʾati (*Sefer ha-Qanun*), bk. 1 (fol. 40ᵇ): וגם הונחו על העצם הזה איברים נכבדים כמו המקוה והרחם וכלי הזרע מן הזכרים והשת והחלוחלת. → NM 4:67–8.

חָלוּל • **החלול** · **vena cava**: Arab. الأجوف · Ibn Sīnā, *K. al-Qānūn fī al-ṭibb* · trans. Zeraḥyah Ḥen (*Sefer ha-Qanun*), bk. 1 (fol. 31ᵇ): הפרק החמישי בניתוח החלול היורד הוה חתמנו המאמר בחלק העולה מן החלול והוא היותר קטן שבחלקיו. → NM 4:68.

• **הוריד החלול** → **וָרִיד**.

• **החלול היורד** · **the inferior vena cava**: Arab. الأجوف النازل · Ibn Sīnā, *K. al-Qānūn fī al-ṭibb* · trans. Zeraḥyah Ḥen (*Sefer ha-Qanun*), bk. 1 (fol. 34ᵇ): הפרק החמישי בניתוח החלול היורד הנה חתמנו המאמר בחלק העולה מן החלול והוא היותר קטן שבחלקיו. → NM 4:68.

• *Plur.* **חלולים** · **the ventricles (of the heart)**: Arab. تجاويف · Maimonides, *K. al-fuṣūl fī al-ṭibb* · trans. Zeraḥyah Ḥen (*Sefer ha-Peraqim*), 4.18: וכן הלב בעצמו יזדמן כמה פעמים שיהיה הלב בעצמו יותר קר ממזגו הטבעי ויהיה העצם אשר יקיף עליו חלוליו יותר חד או בהפך. → NM 1:148.

חָלוֹם • *Plur.* **חלומות** • **שני החלומות** → **שֵׁן**.

חָלוּק · **viscous**: Arab. لزج · Al-Zahrāwī, *K. al-taṣrīf li-man ʿağiza ʿan at-taʾlīf* · trans. Shem Tov ben Isaac (*Sefer ha-Shimmush*), bk. 27, fol. 124ᵇ, col. 1: סובין של חטה חמים יבשים מעטי המזון מאד ומנגבים ולוטשים לטישה רבה יותר מלטישת קמח החטה וכשיעשה מהם שרף ימהר לרדת מן האסטומ׳ ולוטש מה שיש בחזה והריאה מהלחויות החלוקות. → NM 4:68.

חִלּוּק • ידיעת החלוק → יְדִיעָה.

חלוקה → חֲלֻקָּה.

חִלְחוּל · **rarefaction**: Arab. تخلخل · Maimonides, *K. al-fuṣūl fī al-ṭibb* · trans. Nathan ha-Me'ati (*Sefer ha-Peraqim*), 23.99: הרפיון והחלחול הם שני שמות נרדפים. → NM 2:47.

חלחולת → חַלְחֹלֶת.

[חלחל] • *Pi'el* חִלְחֵל · **to loosen**: Arab. خلخل · Maimonides, *K. al-fuṣūl fī al-ṭibb* · trans. Nathan ha-Me'ati (*Sefer ha-Peraqim*), 13.19: ראוי לרחוץ קודם לקיחת הרפואה המשלשלת יום או יומים או שלשה ימים רצופים כי הרחיצה ממיסה הליחות. ואם יהיה בגוף מקום שנתקשה ונמתח ירפהו ויחלחלהו ויתעתד הגוף שיזולו ממנו מה שיזול בנקלה. → NM 2:47.

• *Part. Pi'el* מְחַלְחֵל • **סמים מרפים ומחלחלים** → סַם.

• *Part. Pu'al* מְחֻלְחָל · **porous**: Arab. متخلخل · Maimonides, *K. al-fuṣūl fī al-ṭibb* · trans. Nathan ha-Me'ati (*Sefer ha-Peraqim*), 1.61: גרם הטחול רפה ומחולחל ורך דומה לספוג. → NM 2:58.

• *Part. Hitpa'el* מִתְחַלְחֵל · **porous**: Arab. متخلخل · Al-Zahrāwī, *K. al-taṣrīf li-man 'ağiza 'an at-ta'līf* · trans. Shem Tov ben Isaac (*Sefer ha-Shimmush*), bk. 30, 2.96 (fol. 231[a]) (2.97, Ms. Paris, BN, héb. 1163): כי מי שיהיה רך הבשר מתחלחל הנקבים ראוי לשרטו שריטה אחת לא יותר פן יתבעבע המקום. → NM 1:93.

חַלְחֹלֶת → חלוחלת.

חֳלִי · **harm**: Arab. آفة · Maimonides, *K. al-fuṣūl fī al-ṭibb* · trans. Zeraḥyah Ḥen (*Sefer ha-Peraqim*), 25.72: והפלאו קהל בעלי העיון איך נוכל להאמין בזה הספור עם האמיננו לו במה שזכר בפרק חמישי מההכרות והוא האמת והוא אומרו שם כי על כל פנים יבוא ללב חולי בבוא המות. → NM 1:148.

• **חולי האריה** · **leontiasis**: Arab. داء الأسد · Ibn al-Jazzār, *Zād al-musāfir wa-qūt al-ḥādir* · trans. Moses ibn Tibbon (*Sefer Ṣedat ha-Derakhim*), bk. 7, 17.1: והוא מתחלק לארבעה חלקים אחד מהם המתילד מן הדם ויקרא חולי השועל הנקרא אלופיציא והשני המתילד מליחת מרה כרכומית ויקרא חולי האריה הנקרא לאוניאה והשלישי המתילד מליחה מרה שחורה ויקרא חולי הפיל והרביעי מתילד מליחת הליחה הלבנה ויקרא חולי הנחש. → NM 1:56.

• **בא לו חולי חרגלים** → [בוא].

• **חולי הגרון** · **angina**: Hippocrates, *Aphorisms* · trans. Do'eg ha-Edomi (*Sefer Agur*), 7.49 (401) (fol. 119[a]): אמר אפוקרט: קרהו חולי הגרון וצמח צמח בחזה אות טוב הוא כי נטה החולי לצאת החוצה. → NM 3:83.

• **חולי הדאגה** · **delirium**: Arab. وسواس · Maimonides, *Šarḥ fuṣūl Abūqrāṭ* · trans. Anonymous (*Pirqei Abuqraṭ*), 1.12 (39): והשקוי וחולי הדאגה וחולי מיעים והכלית והוא נגע הריאה הם חליים ישנים. → NM 3:83.

• **חולי הזאב** · **lupus**: Lat. lupus · Arnau de Vilanova, *Medicationis Parabole* · trans. Abraham Avigdor (*Pirqei Arnauṭ de Vilanova*), 5.96 (110): הנגעים המתאכלים אשר יתרחבו ויתפשטו אל העומק מעצמם ראוי לרפאם עם דברים קובצים ומיבשים בלתי עוקצים ואם יהיו ארסיים כמו חולי הזאב יצטרך שיהיו בזהריים. → NM 4:55.

• **החולי חיבש** · **phthisis**: Hippocrates, *Aphorisms* · trans. Do'eg ha-Edomi (*Sefer Agur*), 3.29 (135) (fol. 58[a]): אמר אפוקרט: תכונת הבחורים מעשרים שנה ומעלה לחול עליהם החולי היבש ולרוק דם וקדחת מחודדת ומחלת הנפילה ורבים מהמדוים הנזכרים למעלה. → NM 3:83.

• **חולי מכרס הבטן** ‹ **hypochondriac illness**: Arab. مرض مراقّ البطن · Maimonides, *K. al-fuṣūl fī al-ṭibb* · trans. Nathan ha-Me'ati (*Sefer ha-Peraqim*), 23.65: מן הערבוב השחורי יש מין יהיה התחלתו מן האסטו' ורבים מן הקדמונים יקראו זאת העלה חולי מכרס הבטן וחולי נופח ויאמר לו גם כן המראקי כלו' הכרסיי והנופח. → NM 2:54–5.

• **חולי המים הרעים** ‹ **dropsy**: Hippocrates, *Aphorisms* · trans. Do'eg ha-Edomi (*Sefer Agur*), 6.43 (335): מאריך להזיל הזלת הבטן עם דם ולו כובד הטחול סופו לבוא לחולי המים הרעים או להשמטת המעיים. → NM 3:84.

• **מנוחת החולי** → **מְנוּחָה**.

• **חולי מעים** ‹ I. **colic**: Arab. قولنج · Maimonides, *Šarḥ fuṣūl Abūqrāṭ* · trans. Anonymous (*Pirqei Abuqraṭ*), 3.22 (128): אמר אבוקרט: ואמנם בחורף יקרה הרבה מתחלואי הקיץ וקדחת רביעית ארוכה ומעורבת והטחול והשקוי והטפת השתן ושלשול הדם וחלקת המעים וכאב הירכים והאסכרה ונזילה על הריאה וחולי מעים החזק אשר יקראוהו היונים איליאוש והכפיה והדאגה השחורי והשטות. → NM 3:84.

‹ II. **diarrhea**: Hippocrates, *Aphorisms* · trans. Do'eg ha-Edomi (*Sefer Agur*), 5.34 (254) (fol. 86[b]): מאשה הרה אם תתחל⟨ה⟩ בחולי מעים לאות כי תפיל. → NM 3:84.

• **החולי המפיל** ‹ **epilepsy**: Hippocrates, *Aphorisms* · trans. Do'eg ha-Edomi (*Sefer Agur*), 3.22 (128): אמר אפוקרט: פגרי החורף להביא על הגופים קצת המדוים אשר באו עליו בימי הקייץ פרצת קדחת רביעית נפח טחול אפיסת המים הרעים החולי היבש יציאת השתן במכאוב הזלת הבטן והדם וכאב הירכים פוקות מיני השעול וכאב המעי הגדול והחולי המפיל רעת הליחה השחורה וכאב הגרון. → NM 3:84–5.

• **החולי הנופל** ‹ **epilepsy**: a) Hippocrates, *Aphorisms* · trans. Do'eg ha-Edomi (*Sefer Agur*), 2.45 (97) (fol. 46[a]): אמר אפוקרט: רעת החולי הנופל בהיותו חדש והסובל נער ומזג מקומו והנהגותיו טובים יכול להרפא. → NM 3:85.

b) Arab. صرع · Ibn al-Jazzār, *Zād al-musāfir wa-qūt al-ḥādir* · trans. Moses ibn Tibbon (*Sefer Ṣedat ha-Derakhim*), introduction (Ms. Oxford, Bodleian Library, Poc. 353, Uri Heb. 314, fol. 1[b]): השער הכ״ב בחולי הנופל. → NM 4:68.

• **חולי הנחש** ‹ **ophiasis**: Arab. داء الحية · a) Ibn al-Jazzār, *Zād al-musāfir wa-qūt al-ḥādir* · trans. Moses ibn Tibbon (*Sefer Ṣedat ha-Derakhim*), bk. 7, 17.1: והוא מתחלק לארבעה חלקים אחד מהם המתילד מן הדם ויקרא חולי השועל הנקרא אלופיציא והשני המתילד מליחת מרה כרכומית ויקרא חולי האריה הנקרא לאוניאה והשלישי המתילד מליחה מרה שחורה ויקרא חולי הפיל והרביעי מתילד מליחת הליחה הלבנה ויקרא חולי הנחש. → NM 1:56; corr. 2:198.

b) Maimonides, *K. al-fuṣūl fī al-ṭibb* · trans. Nathan ha-Me'ati (*Sefer ha-Peraqim*), 23.53: חולי השועל וחולי הנחש הם עלה אחת ואמנם נתחלפו שמותיהם למקום התבנית כי המקום שיוסר השער בחולי הנחש יהיה על משל הנחש בעת הלוכו. → NM 2:47.

• **הניצול מן החולי** → **נִצּוֹל**.

• **הנמלט מחולי** → [**מלט**].

• **חלי הנפילה** ‹ **epilepsy**: Hippocrates, *Aphorisms* · trans. Do'eg ha-Edomi (*Sefer Agur*), 5.7 (227) (fol. 80[b]): אמר אפוקראט: גזור על סובל חולי הנפילה אם לא הביאה שתי שערות תמהר רפואתו. → NM 3:85–6.

• **הנקי מן החולי** → **נָקִי**.

• **חולי הפיל** · **elephantiasis**: Arab. داء الفيل · Ibn al-Jazzār, *Zād al-musāfir wa-qūt al-ḥādir* · trans. Moses ibn Tibbon (*Sefer Ṣedat ha-Derakhim*), bk. 7, 17.1: והוא מתחלק לארבעה חלקים אחד מהם המתילד מן הדם ויקרא חולי השועל הנקרא אלופיציא והשני המתילד מליחת מרה כרכומית ויקרא חולי האריה הנקרא לאוניאה והשלישי המתילד מליחה מרה שחורה ויקרא חולי הפיל והרביעי מתילד מליחת הליחה הלבנה ויקרא חולי הנחש. → NM 1:56; corr. 2:198.

• **חולי הצד** · **pleurisy**: Arab. ذات الجنب / Gr. πλευριτικός · a) Maimonides, *Šarḥ fuṣūl Abūqrāṭ* · trans. Moses ibn Tibbon (*Pirqei Abuqraṭ*), 5.8 (228): אמר אבקראט: מי שמצאהו חולי הצד ולא ינקה בארבעה עשר יום הנה יגיע עניינו לעשות מוגלא. → NM 3:86.

b) Maimonides, *K. al-fuṣūl fī al-ṭibb* · trans. Zeraḥyah Ḥen (*Sefer ha-Peraqim*), 4.42: איני יודע ששום אדם ימלט מחולי הצד בהיות דפק בעליו קשה בתכלית הקושי קטון ומתואתר מאד. → NM 1:148.

• **הקם מן החולי** → [קום].

• **חולי הריאה** · **pneumonia**: Hippocrates, *Aphorisms* · trans. Do'eg ha-Edomi (*Sefer Agur*) (fol. 112[b]), 7.11 (363): אמר אפוקרט: החל לבוא אחרי חולי כאב הצד היא פליורשין חולי הריאה היא פריפליומוניאה אות רע הוא. → NM 3:86.

• **חולי הרגלים** · **gouty affections**: Gr. ποδαγρικὰ νοσήματα · Hippocrates, *Aphorisms* · trans. Joseph Delmedigo, 6.49 (341): למי שבא לו חולי הרגלים אחר שתשכך הלהבה ינוח בתוך ארבעים יום. → NM 3:86.

• **חולי השועל** · **alopecia**: Arab. داء الثعلب · a) Ibn al-Jazzār, *Zād al-musāfir wa-qūt al-ḥādir* · trans. Moses ibn Tibbon (*Sefer Ṣedat ha-Derakhim*), bk. 7, 17.1: והוא מתחלק לארבעה חלקים אחד מהם המתילד מן הדם ויקרא חולי השועל הנקרא אלופיציא והשני המתילד מליחת מרה כרכומית ויקרא חולי האריה הנקרא לאוניאה והשלישי המתילד מליחה מרה שחורה ויקרא חולי הפיל והרביעי מתילד מליחת הליחה הלבנה ויקרא חולי הנחש. → NM 1:56.

b) Maimonides, *K. al-fuṣūl fī al-ṭibb* · trans. Nathan ha-Me'ati (*Sefer ha-Peraqim*), 23.53: חולי השועל וחולי הנחש הם עלה אחת ואמנם נתחלפו שמותיהם למקום התבנית כי המקום שיוסר השער בחולי הנחש יהיה על משל הנחש בעת הלוכו. → NM 2:47–8.

• **חולי השחורה** · **melancholic delusion; melancholy**: Gr. μελαγχολιά · Hippocrates, *Aphorisms* · trans. Joseph Delmedigo, 3.14 (120): ואם יהיה החורף צפוניי ונעדר המטר יהיה נאות למי שטבעו רטוב ולנשים אבל לשאר אנשים יקרם להבת העינים יבשה וקדחות חדות וארוכות ולקצתם חולי השחורה. → NM 3:87.

• *Plur.* **חוליים** • **חוליים חדים** · **acute diseases**: Arab. أمراض حادّة · Maimonides, *K. al-fuṣūl fī al-ṭibb* · trans. Nathan ha-Me'ati (*Sefer ha-Peraqim*), 7.11: ועצם האברים נתך אם באורך חליים נושנים או בחדות חליים חדים או בקדחות שהם מהמס האברים. → NM 2:44–5; corr. 4:229.

חֲלְיָה (also: **חֲלְיָא**) • **חולית הארכובה** · **patella**: Arab. رضفة · Ibn Sīnā, *K. al-Qānūn fī al-ṭibb* · trans. Joseph Lorki (*Sefer ha-Qanun*), bk. 1 (fol. 16[a]): ולו שתי ראשים האחד מהם בשרי וידבק בחולית הארכובה קודם שישוב יתר והאחר קרומי דבק בקצה השמאלי מקצוי הירך. → NM 4:63.

• **החוליא החולכת באורך** · **the longitudinal suture**: Arab. الدرز الطولي · Ibn Sīnā, *K. al-*

Qānūn fī al-ṭibb · trans. Zeraḥyah Ḥen (*Sefer ha-Qanun*), bk. 1 (fol. 17[a]): ותהיה החוליא ההולכת ברוחב באמצע הרחב מן האוזן אל האוזן כמו שהחוליא ההולכת באורך הוא באמצע האורך. → NM 4:63.

• **החוליא ההולכת ברוחב** · **the transverse suture:** Arab. الدرز العردي · Ibn Sīnā, *K. al-Qānūn fī al-ṭibb* · trans. Zeraḥyah Ḥen (*Sefer ha-Qanun*), bk. 1 (fol. 17[a]): ותהיה החוליא ההולכת ברוחב באמצע הרחב מן האוזן אל האוזן כמו שהחוליא ההולכת באורך הוא באמצע האורך. → NM 4:63.

• **החוליה הקלפית** · **the squamosal suture:** Arab. الدرز القشري · Ibn Sīnā, *K. al-Qānūn fī al-ṭibb* · trans. Zeraḥyah Ḥen (*Sefer ha-Qanun*), bk. 1 (fol. 17[b]): ושני השרשים שהם ימין ושמאל הם שתי העצמות אשר בהם האזנים ונקראות שתי האבנים מפני קשים כאבן וגבול כל אחד מהם מלמעלה לחוליה הקלפית. → NM 4:64.

• *Plur.* **חליות** · **cranial sutures:** Arab. شأن, *Plur.* شؤون · Ibn Sīnā, *K. al-Qānūn fī al-ṭibb* · trans. Zeraḥyah Ḥen (*Sefer ha-Qanun*), bk. 1 (fol. 17[a]): ולכמו זאת הצורה שלשה חליות אמתיות ושני חליות כוזביות. → NM 4:63.

חֲלִימָה · **intelligence; understanding; wisdom:** Arab. حِلْم · Ibn Sīnā, *K. al-Qānūn fī al-ṭibb* · trans. Nathan ha-Me'ati (*Sefer ha-Qanun*), bk. 1 (fol. 31[b]): והקצויות יצמחו ברוב באמצע זמן הגדול והוא אחר ההמרצה אל ההעמדה וזה כי ההעמדה קרובה מל׳ שנה ולכן נקראים שני אלחלם כלומ׳ החלימה. → NM 4:68–9.

• **שני החלימה** → שֵׁן.

• **שני אלחלם כלומר החלימה** → שֵׁן.

חֲלִיקוּת • **חליקות המעים** · **lientery:** Arab. زلق الأمعاء · Maimonides, *Šarḥ fuṣūl Abūqrāṭ* · trans. Anonymous (*Pirqei Abuqraṭ*), 3.30 (136): אמר אבוקרט: מי שעבר אלו השנים יקרה לו נזילה על הריאה וחולי הצד וחולי הריאה ושכחה והקדחת אשר תהיה עמה התעורה והקדחת אשר יהיה עמה ערבוב השכל וקדחת השורפת ושלשול היוצא הקיא ושלשול הארוך וגרידת המעים וחליקות המעים והתפתח פיות העורקים ממטה. → NM 3:87.

חָלָל · I. **cavity:** Arab. جوف · Maimonides, *Šarḥ fuṣūl Abūqrāṭ* · trans. Moses ibn Tibbon (*Pirqei Abuqraṭ*), 7.38 (390): אמר אבקראט: הירידות אשר ירדו אל החלל העליון יעשה חוולא בעשרים יום. → NM 3:87.

· II. **concave [part]:** Arab. مقعّر · Maimonides, *K. al-fuṣūl fī al-ṭibb* · trans. Zeraḥyah Ḥen (*Sefer ha-Peraqim*), 7.57: הצמא הגדולה שתהיה נעדרת מהתרת הבטן סבתו הראשונה רוע מזג חם או יבש או שניהם יחד יתחדש באסטומכא ובייחוד פיה. וסבתו השנית אחר האסטומכא כשיתחדש בה רוע מזג בכבד וכל שכן בחללו. → NM 1:148–9.

· III. **intestines:** Arab. أحشاء · Al-Zahrāwī, *K. al-taṣrīf li-man ʿağiza ʿan at-taʾlīf* · trans. Shem Tov ben Isaac (*Sefer ha-Shimmush*), bk. 27, fol. 129[a], col. a: ויזיקו למי שיש בתוך חללו מורסא. → NM 4:69.

· IV. **ventricle:** Arab. تجويف · Maimonides, *K. al-fuṣūl fī al-ṭibb* · trans. Nathan ha-Me'ati (*Sefer ha-Peraqim*), 1.53: החלל הימין משני חללי הלב אמנם נברא למקום הריאה. → NM 2:48.

• **חלל הזנב** · **the last vertebra of the tail:** Arab. عجز الذنب · Al-Zahrāwī, *K. al-taṣrīf li-man ʿağiza ʿan at-taʾlīf* · trans. Shem Tov ben Isaac (*Sefer ha-Shimmush*), bk. 30, 1.47

אמנם אם הגדמות כבר נתפרסם על החולה ויראה ראייה מבוארת ראוי אז לכוותו אלו :(208[a])
הכויות הנזכרות בראש ... וכויה אחת גדולה על העצה אצל חלל הזנב. → NM 1:93.

• **המקום החלל** → מָקוֹם.

• **חלל העורף** › **nape of the neck**: Arab. نقرة القفا · Al-Zahrāwī, *K. al-taṣrīf li-man ʿağiza ʿan at-taʾlīf* · trans. Shem Tov ben Isaac (*Sefer ha-Shimmush*), bk. 30, 1.47 (fol. 208[a]): והרוצה לכוותו צריך להתבונן אם בתחלת הגדמות רפאוה במה שזכרתי במאמר החלוקה ולא כהה הנגע ויש חשש על החולה שמא ישלוט ההפסד על כל מזגו ראוי לכוותו על הראש חמש כויות האחת באמצע הראש המפורסמת והשנית למטה ממנה לעמת המצח במקום הנחת תפלין ושתי כויות על שני הקרנים ואחת מאחוריו בחלל העורף. → NM 1:93–4.

• *Plur.* **חללים** › **cavities**: Arab. فضاء / Gr. κοιλία · Maimonides, *Šarḥ fuṣūl Abūqrāṭ* · trans. Moses ibn Tibbon (*Pirqei Abuqraṭ*), 7.54 (406): אמר אבקראט: מי שתהיה נבוכה בו הליחה הלבנה במה שבין האצטו׳ והמסך והתחדש בו כאב כשלא יהיה לה מעבר לאחד מן החללים הנה הליחה ההיא כשתלך בעורקים אל המקוה יתך ממנו חליו. → NM 3:87–8.

חֲלָלוּת › I. **cavity**: a) Hippocrates, *Aphorisms* · trans. Judah Shalom, 7.51 (403) (fol. 123[b]): העטוש יהיה מהראש ממוח מחומם או מלחלוח אשר בחללות הראש ירד האויר אשר הוא בתוך ויעשה קול בעבור כי המוצא הוא צר אליו. → NM 3:88.

b) Arab. تجويف · Ibn Sīnā, *K. al-adwiya al-qalbiya* · trans. Anonymous (*Sammim Libbiyim*), fol. 120[b]: והפותח הוא אשר יניע החומר אשר נופל בחללות המעברים ויוציאהו לא בפיותיהם לבד. → NM 4:69.

› II. **concavity**: Arab. تقعير · Al-Zahrāwī, *K. al-taṣrīf li-man ʿağiza ʿan at-taʾlīf* · trans. Shem Tov ben Isaac (*Sefer ha-Shimmush*), bk. 30, 3.31 (fol. 238[b]): פרק כף הירך ופרק השכם אמנם תקרה להם השמיטה בלבד ולא יקרה להם מה שיקרה ליתר הפרקים מן ההסרה המעוטה והחללות. → NM 1:94.

[חלף] • *Part. Hitpaʿel* **מִתְחַלֵּף** › **contrary**: Arab. مخالف · Maimonides, *K. al-fuṣūl fī al-ṭibb* · trans. Nathan ha-Meʾati (*Sefer ha-Peraqim*), 9.8: הניצוץ והברק אשר יראה האדם בפני עיניו הוא מן הליחות שעצמם ומראיהם מתחלף לליחות הבציית מתקבצת בין הגלדיית והקרניית. → NM 2:64.

[חלץ] • *Hifʿil* **הֶחֱלִיץ** › **to invigorate; to strengthen**: Judah ben Jacob, *Sefer Hanhagat ha-Beriʾut*, 4.5: ולפיכך ראוי לאדם שלא ישתה ממנו לתענוג ולשעשוע כדרך הסובאים אלא כדי להבריא גופו ולהחליץ אבריו. → NM 4:69.

חָלָץ • *Plur.* **חלצים** › **costal cartilages**: Arab. شراسيف · Ibn al-Jazzār, *Zād al-musāfir wa-qūt al-ḥādir* · trans. Moses ibn Tibbon (*Sefer Ṣedat ha-Derakhim*), bk. 1, ch. 18 (fol. 26[b]): הדרך הראשון כשיהיה החולי משוקע במוח עצמו והשני כשיהיה באסטו׳ ומה שקרוב ממנה כמו חולי החלצים הנפוחים אשר צבותם מן המרה השחורה והשלישי כשיבא מן הידים והרגלים. → NM 4:69.

• **מה שלמטה מן החלצים** → מִטָּה.

• **עצם החלצים** → עֶצֶם.

• **תחת החלציים** → תַּחַת.

• **מתחת החלצים** → תַּחַת.

[חלק] • *Hifʿil* **הֶחֱלִיק** › **to be loose (of bowels)**: Arab. لان · Maimonides, *Šarḥ fuṣūl*

Abūqrāṭ · trans. Zeraḥyah Ḥen (*Pirqei Abuqraṭ*), 4.27 (164): אמר בקראט: מי שיצא ממנו דם הרבה מאי זה מקום שיהיה הגרתו כי הוא בקחתו המזון יחליק בטנו ביותר מהשיעור. → NM 3:89.

• **החליק הבטן** · **to prescribe laxatives**: Arab. إلانة البطن · Maimonides, *K. al-fuṣūl fī al-ṭibb* · trans. Zeraḥyah Ḥen (*Sefer ha-Peraqim*), 12.8: אבל באדם אחר נקצר ויספיק לנו למנוע ממנו המאכל. ובאדם אחר יספיק לנו למעט לו המאכל ובאדם אחר יספיק לך שתחליק בטנו או שתשלשלהו או שתרבה לו להכניסו במרחץ או שיספיק לו הטורח לבדו או שתעשה החפיפה המרובה. → NM 1:149–50.

• **החליק לטבע** · **to soften the stools**: Arab. ليّن الطبيعة · Maimonides, *K. al-fuṣūl fī al-ṭibb* · trans. Zeraḥyah Ḥen (*Sefer ha-Peraqim*), 17.33: ראוי להקדים תחילה מכל מה שהאדם אוכל ושותה מה שיהיה מחליק לטבע כמו היינות המתוקים והירקות המחליקות הנעשות עם השמן והכותח. → NM 1:150.

• *Part. Hif'il* **מַחְלִיק** • **חסם המדביק או המחליק** → סַם.

• **דברים מחליקים** → דָּבָר.

• **רפואה מחליקה** → רְפוּאָה.

חָלָק · **soft**: Arab. ليّن · Maimonides, *K. al-fuṣūl fī al-ṭibb* · trans. Zeraḥyah Ḥen (*Sefer ha-Peraqim*), 1.9: היתרים יותר הם חלקים מן הקשרים ויותר הם קשים מן העצבים. → NM 1:149.

חֵלֶק • *Plur.* **חלקים** • **מקובץ החלקים** → קָבַץ.

חֲלֻקָּה · I. **evenness**: Arab. تناسب · Maimonides, *K. al-fuṣūl fī al-ṭibb*· trans. Nathan ha-Me'ati (*Sefer ha-Peraqim*), 12.12: כשיהיו הכימוסים נוספים כפי החלוקה אז תריק כלם בשוה. → NM 2:46–7.

· II. **glutinous property**: Arab. لزوجة · Al-Zahrāwī, *K. al-taṣrīf li-man ʿağiza ʿan at-taʾlīf* · trans. Shem Tov ben Isaac (*Sefer ha-Shimmush*), bk. 30, 3.1 (fol. 232[a]): וכשיתחיל העצם הנשבר להרפא ראוי ליזון במזונות זנין מזון עב שיש בו חלוקה. → NM 1:92–3.

· III. **viscosity**: Arab. لزوجة · Al-Zahrāwī, *K. al-taṣrīf li-man ʿağiza ʿan at-taʾlīf* · trans. Shem Tov ben Isaac (*Sefer ha-Shimmush*), bk. 27, 124[b], cols. 1–2: הדיסא היא גם כן מזה המין והיא בטבעה עבה וחלוקה ומתאחרה להתעכל ומולידה סתומים כהולדת הגריסין אלא שהיא כשתתעכל בגופי הבריאים תוליד דם יש בו לחות וחלוקה ותזון מזון רב. → NM 4:70.

חֲלָקוּת (also: **חַלְקוּת**) · I. **detergence**: Lat. abstersio · Bruno Longobucco, *Cyrurgia Magna* · trans. Hillel ben Samuel (*Sefer Keritut*), fol. 22[a]: כמו שנאמר בחלקות גם כן שלא תהיה חזקה אבל מעוטה בכמות מספקת לטהר העפוש בלי נשיכה. → NM 1:26.

· II. **softening effect**: Arab. تليين · Maimonides, *K. al-fuṣūl fī al-ṭibb* · trans. Zeraḥyah Ḥen (*Sefer ha-Peraqim*), 9.72: קושי הכבד ראוי שתהיה הרפואה המחליקה ברפואותיה חלושה מאד ויגבר בהם הדברים אשר יחממו וידקדקו יותר ממה שיגבר ברפואת קושי שאר האברים כי גוף הכבד אמנם הוא כמו לחות נקפא ואם החליקנו חלקות חזק יתכו כחותיו. → NM 1:150.

· III. **softness**: Arab. لين · Maimonides, *K. al-fuṣūl fī al-ṭibb* · trans. Zeraḥyah Ḥen (*Sefer ha-Peraqim*), 1.11: הקרומות כלם הם בתכלית הדקות והחלקות. → NM 1:150.

• **חלקות הבטן** · I. **lientery**: Hippocrates, *Aphorisms* · trans. Judah Shalom, 3.30 (136) (fol. 49[b]): ובאותם אשר על אלו השנים יקרה אשמא ופלברשין ומורסת הריאה ופרנשין ושכחה וקבשו׳ ואדומה ודיאריה ארוכה וזחיר וחלקות הבטן וטחורים. → NM 3:89.

‣ II. **looseness of bowels:** Arab. لين البطن · Maimonides, *Šarḥ fuṣūl Abūqrāṭ* · trans. Zeraḥyah Ḥen (*Pirqei Abuqraṭ*), 3.31 (137): אמר בקראט: אמנם הזקנים יקרה להם רוע הניפוש והנזל אשר עמו השעול וטיפות השתן ועוצר השתן וכאבי הפרקים וכאבי הכליות והגלגול בראש והשתוק והחבלות הרעות וחיכוך הגוף והתעורה וחלקות הבטן ולחות העיניים והאף ואפילת הראות וכובד השמיעה. → NM 3:89.

• **חלקות הבני מעים** ‣ **lientery:** Hippocrates, *Aphorisms* · trans. Joseph Delmedigo, 6.43 (335): חולי הטחול שנאחזים משלשול דם לאלו אם יאריך שלשול הדם יבוא שקוי או חלקות הבני מעים וימותו. → NM 3:89–90.

• **חלקות המעים** ‣ **lientery:** Arab. زلق الأمعاء · a) Maimonides, *K. al-fuṣūl fī al-ṭibb* · trans. Zeraḥyah Ḥen (*Sefer ha-Peraqim*), 23.50. → NM 1:150.

b) Maimonides, *Šarḥ fuṣūl Abūqrāṭ* · trans. Anonymous (*Pirqei Abuqraṭ*), 6.1 (293): אמר אבוקרט: כשנתחדש הגיהוק החמוץ במדוה הנקרא חלקות המעים אחרי שנתארך ולא היה זה לו מקודם זה אות משובח. → NM 3:90.

• **חלקות המעים הוא זלק אלמעא** ‣ **lientery:** Arab. زلق الأمعاء · Ibn al-Jazzār, *Zād al-musāfir wa-qūt al-ḥādir* · trans. Moses ibn Tibbon (*Sefer Ṣedat ha-Derakhim*), introduction (fol. 3[b]): השער הי״ד בחלקות המעים הוא זלק אלמעא. → NM 4:70.

חֲלַקְלַקּוּת • **חלקלקות המעים** ‣ **lientery:** Arab. زلق الأمعاء · Hippocrates, *Aphorisms* · trans. Nathan ha-Me'ati, 3.30 (136) (fol. 56[b]): אמר אבוקרט: ואמנם מי שיעבור אלו השנים יקרה להם הגניחה הוא רבו ובעלת הצד ובעלת הריאה וקדחת שיהיה עמה התעורה והקדחת שיהיה עמה בלבול השכל והדלקת והיצא הוא שלשול וקיא יחדו ושלשול ארוך הפשט המעים וחלקלקות המעים ונפיחת פיות העורקים מלמטה. → NM 3:90.

חֲלָשָׁה ‣ **pain:** Arab. كلال · Maimonides, *Šarḥ fuṣūl Abūqrāṭ* · trans. Zeraḥyah Ḥen (*Pirqei Abuqraṭ*), 4.44 (181): אמר בקראט: מי שמצאו קדחת ארוכה יקרה לו או צמחים או חולשה בפרקיו. → NM 3:90–1.

• **הפסד וחולשה** → הֶפְסֵד.

• **חלשת הנפש** ‣ **fainting:** Lat. defectio animi / Arab. ذبول نفس · Hippocrates, *Aphorisms* · trans. Hillel ben Samuel, 7.8 (360) (fol. 44[b]): א״א: בגלל שבר המורסא בפנים יעשה קיא וחלשת הנפש. → NM 3:91.

חַם • **הנחה חמה** → הֲנָחָה.

• **לט בבגד חם** → [לוט].

• **המים החמים** → מַיִם.

• **מרקחים חמים** → מֶרְקָח.

• **צבות חמה** → צְבוּת.

חֹם ‣ **fomentation; fomenting:** Lat. calefactio · Hippocrates, *Aphorisms* · trans. Hillel ben Samuel, 5.28 (248): א״א: דם הנדות יעוררוהו חום העניינים הריחניים וכמו כן יועילו לו דברים אחרים אם לא יעשו כאב הראש. → NM 3:91.

• **החום הטבעי** ‣ **innate heat:** Arab. الحرارة الغريزيّة / Gr. τὸ ἔμφυτον θερμόν · Maimonides, *Šarḥ fuṣūl Abūqrāṭ* · trans. Moses ibn Tibbon (*Pirqei Abuqraṭ*), 1.14 (41): אמר אבקראט: מה שהיה מן הגופות בגדול הנה החום הטבעי בו בתכלית מה שיהיה מן הרבוי. → NM 3:91.

• חום יסודי · **innate heat:** Lat. innatus calor · Hippocrates, *Aphorisms* · trans. Hillel ben Samuel, 1.14 (41) (fol. 4[b]): א״א: אותם שגדלים יש להם חום יסודי רב. → NM 3:91.

• חום נכרי · **unnatural heat:** Judah ben Jacob, *Sefer Hanhagat ha-Beri'ut*, 2.1: ומן הראיות הגדולות על זה כי כשיצא החום הטבעי מן הקו האמצעי באיכותו או בכמותו ויתערב עמו חום נכרי תראה הרגשת הראות והרגשת השמע ושאר ההרגשות משובשות. → NM 4:70–1.

חמאיי · **buttery:** Arab. سمني · Al-Zahrāwī, *K. al-taṣrīf li-man ʿağiza ʿan at-taʾlīf* · trans. Shem Tov ben Isaac (*Sefer ha-Shimmush*), bk. 27, fol. 146[b], col. a: חלב הבקר יותר עב מכל החלבים ויותר רחוק מן העכול והירידה ויותר כבד על האסטומ׳ ושלשולו הבטן יותר מועט אלא שהוא זן יותר מכל החלבים מפני שהוא יותר גביני ויותר חמאיי ועל כן חלבם מועיל מן השלשול המררי והעיצום הכרכומי. → NM 4:71 (corr.).

חִמּוּם · I. **bathing:** Arab. استحمام · Maimonides, *Šarḥ fuṣūl Abūqrāṭ* · trans. Zeraḥyah Ḥen (*Pirqei Abuqraṭ*), 7.42 (394): אמר המפרש: גאלנוס יאמר כי כוונתו באמרו קדחתו שאינה מן המרות אינו קדחת עיפוש אבל קצת ממיני קדחת יום ואין ספק שהחימום בה מועיל ובו יתר הקדחת. → NM 3:92.

· II. **fomentation; fomenting:** Hippocrates, *Aphorisms* · trans. Judah Shalom, 5.28 (248) (fol. 82[a]): החמום אשר עם הריחניים מביא דם הנדות ופעמים רבות יהיה מועיל בדברים אחרים אם לא יעשו כובד הראש. → NM 3:92.

חָמוּץ • החלב החמוץ → חָלָב.

• הירק החמוץ → יָרָק.

• התבשיל החמוץ → תַּבְשִׁיל.

חִמּוּץ • חימוץ האתרוגים · **the acidic inner part of the lemon:** Arab. حمّاض الأترجّ · Maimonides, *K. al-fuṣūl fī al-ṭibb* · trans. Zeraḥyah Ḥen (*Sefer ha-Peraqim*), 22.52: חימוץ האתרוגים יסיר הצמא והוא חזק בהסרת הקולורא מחזק לנפש. → NM 1:150.

חֲמִיצוּת • חמיצות האתרוג · **citron pulp:** Arab. حماض الأترج · Ibn al-Jazzār, *Zād al-musāfir wa-qūt al-ḥāḍir* · trans. Moses ibn Tibbon (*Sefer Ṣedat ha-Derakhim*), bk. 1, ch. 19 (fol. 29[b]): ויהיה מזונו פיישאן הנקרא בערב׳ דראג׳ ותרנוגלים קטנים ומאכלים חמוצים עשויים בקני הלגלווות ומי בוסר ומי חמיצות האתרוג. → NM 4:71.

[חמם] • *Part. Puʿal* מְחֻמָּם · **suffering from a fever:** Arab. محموم / Gr. πυρεταίνων · Maimonides, *Šarḥ fuṣūl Abūqrāṭ* · trans. Moses ibn Tibbon (*Pirqei Abuqraṭ*), 1.16 (43): אמר אבקראט: המזונות הלחים יאותו לכל המחוממים כל שכן הנערים ומי שכבר הרגיל שיאכל המזונות הלחים. → NM 3:128–9.

• *Hitpaʿel* הִתְחַמֵּם · **to suffer from fever:** Arab. حُمَّ · Maimonides, *Šarḥ fuṣūl Abūqrāṭ* · trans. Moses ibn Tibbon (*Pirqei Abuqraṭ*), 1.17 (44): ואולם החורף מי שיתחמם בו יצטרך אל תוספת משבעת המזון טוב להפסד הליחות בזמן ההוא. → NM 3:92.

[חמץ] • *Hifʿil* הֶחְמִיץ • הלחם השרוי במים עד שיחמיץ → לֶחֶם

חֹמֶר · **element:** Arab. عنصر · Maimonides, *Šarḥ fuṣūl Abūqrāṭ* · trans. Moses ibn Tibbon (*Pirqei Abuqraṭ*), 1.1 (21): ובכלל הקדמת הידיעה במה שיהיה הנה זה קשה במלאכת הרפואה מאד להגרת החומר ומיעוט קיומו על עניין אחד. → NM 3:92.

חֲמְרָה (also: חֶמְרָה) · **erysipelas:** Arab. حمرة · Maimonides, *K. al-fuṣūl fī al-ṭibb* · trans. Nathan ha-Me'ati (*Sefer ha-Peraqim*), 9.106: הרפואות המונחות על החמרה והנמלה אלא

אם תהיה מתאכלת הם אלו: חזרת ומטה הרועה וטחלב ונילופר וזרע קטונא ולגלוגות והנדבי וחי לעולם וכן ענבי השועל. → NM 2:48.

חֲמַרְמַר · **to be abraded:** Arab. سحج · Maimonides, *Šarḥ fuṣūl Abūqrāṭ* · trans. Moses ibn Tibbon (*Pirqei Abuqraṭ*), 4.24 (161): אמר המפרש: כאשר התחיל יציאת המרה האדומה וחמרמרו ממנה המעים ונתנגעו ובא הדם אחר כן הנה אפשר להרפא החמרמרות. → NM 3:93.

חֲמַרְמָרוּת · **abrasion:** Arab. سحج · Ibn al-Jazzār, *Zād al-musāfir wa-qūt al-ḥādir* · trans. Moses ibn Tibbon (*Sefer Ṣedat ha-Derakhim*), bk. 7, 29.1: ואם יהיה חמרמרות מבלתי נפח ומורסא יקח מן התחתון מן המנעל וישרפהו וישחקהו ויזרהו על החמרמרות. → NM 1:56.

• **חמרמרות המעיים** · **abrasion of the intestines:** Arab. سحج الأمعاء · Maimonides, *Šarḥ fuṣūl Abūqrāṭ* · trans. Moses ibn Tibbon (*Pirqei Abuqraṭ*), 6.3 (295): אמר המפרש: שלשול הדם כאשר היה עם חמרמרות המעיים וארך עמידתו יתוספו החפירות בעומק האיברים וישובו נגעים בהם עפוש ותכאב האצטו' בשותפות וישיג בשולה הנזק. → NM 3:93.

חֹמֶשׁ · **hypochondrium:** Arab. خاصرة · Al-Zahrāwī, *K. al-taṣrīf li-man ʿağiza ʿan at-taʾlīf* · trans. Shem Tov ben Isaac (*Sefer ha-Shimmush*), bk. 30, 1.33 (fol. 206[a]): ואם תראינה הלחויות רבות והחולה סובל הכויה ראוי לכוותו על הזקן התחתון כויה אחת וכויה אחרת על כל חומש. → NM 1:91–2.

חנגרי · **xiphoid [cartilage]:** Arab. خنجري · Ibn Sīnā, *K. al-Qānūn fī al-ṭibb* · trans. Nathan ha-Me'ati (*Sefer ha-Qanun*), bk. 1 (fol. 52[b]): וקצה שנים האחרים אצל החנגרי. → NM 4:71.

חִנּוּק · **suffocation:** Arab. اختناق / Gr. πνίξ · Maimonides, *Šarḥ fuṣūl Abūqrāṭ* · trans. Anonymous (*Pirqei Abuqraṭ*), 4.34 (171): אמר אבוקרט: מי שהכשילו קדחת ואין בגרונו נפח וקרה לו חנוק בפתע פתאום זהו מאותות מות. → NM 3:93–4.

חֲנִיקָה · **quinsy:** Arab. خوانيق / Gr. κυνάγχη · Al-Zahrāwī, *K. al-taṣrīf li-man ʿağiza ʿan at-taʾlīf* · trans. Shem Tov ben Isaac (*Sefer ha-Shimmush*), bk. 30, 2.95 (fol. 229[a]): ושני הגידים אשר תחת הלשון תועלת הקזתם אחר הקזת גיד הראש אל החניקה אשר תהיה בגרון וחלי ערלתו ותחלאי הפה. → NM 1:94.

• **חניקת האם** · **hysterical suffocation:** Maimonides, *Šarḥ fuṣūl Abūqrāṭ* · trans. Anonymous (*Pirqei Abuqraṭ*), 5.35 (255) (Ms. Oxford, Bodleian Library, Opp. 685, fol. 86[b], anonymous marginal variant reading): בעבור שתנועת העטוש תחמם הגוף שנתקרר בחניקת האם או האיפילינסיאה. → NM 3:94.

• **חניקת הרחם** · **hysterical suffocation:** Arab. اختناق الرحم · Maimonides, *Šarḥ fuṣūl Abūqrāṭ* · trans. Zeraḥyah Ḥen (*Pirqei Abuqraṭ*), 5.35 (255): אמר המפרש: ירצה לומר בחולי הרחם חניקת הרחם והעיטוש יורה על הערת הטבע שיפעל פעולתו והוא כמו כן סבה לנקות האיברים ממה שדבק בהם ונשתבך מן הליחות המזיקות ובזה הצד ינקה העיטוש השונגלוצו. → NM 3:94.

[חנק] • *Inf. Nifʿal* הֵחָנֵק • **החנק הרחם** · **hysterical suffocation:** Arab. اختناق الرحم · Maimonides, *Šarḥ fuṣūl Abūqrāṭ* · trans. Moses ibn Tibbon (*Pirqei Abuqraṭ*), 5.35 (255): אמר המפרש: ירצה בחולי הרחם החנק הרחם והעיטוש אות על התעוררות הטבע שיעשה פעולותיו. → NM 3:94.

חֶנֶק · **angina:** a) Arab. خوانيق · Maimonides, *K. al-fuṣūl fī al-ṭibb* · trans. Zeraḥyah Ḥen

(*Sefer ha-Peraqim*), 25.11: ומפני זה העיקר הגדול בתועלת יצוינו גליאנוס שנקיז גיד הראש הנקרא קיפאל בחוליי העין החזקים ובחנק ודומהו. → NM 1:150–1; corr. 4:229.

b) Arab. ذبحة · Maimonides, *Šarḥ fuṣūl Abūqrāṭ* · trans. Zeraḥyah Ḥen (*Pirqei Abuqraṭ*), 1.12 (39): אמר המפרש: מטבע החולי בעצמו תוכל לדעת אם קצו מהר או מאוחר כי חולי הצד וחולי הריאה והשרסאם חליים חדים והחנק והשלשול הנקרא היצה והקווץ הם חליים חדים מאד. → NM 3:94–5.

חֲסְפְּנִיתָא (*Aram.*) · **heat rash; miliaria:** Arab. حصف · Ibn al-Jazzār, *Zād al-musāfir wa-qūt al-ḥādir* · trans. Moses ibn Tibbon (*Sefer Ṣedat ha-Derakhim*), bk. 7, 24.3: והחספניתא אמנם תצא בקיץ כשיתחזק החום עם רוב הזיעה והיותו מחומר ידמה המותר אשר מדרכו שיתך בכל יום מן הגופות וכאשר יתעבה יום אחר יום על נשומי הגוף ונקבי העור יסתמם ויהיה עליו כגלד והקלפה ולכלוך ויביא זה לחספניתא ואל כנים וחכוך ואם יארך זה ישוב גרב גמור. → NM 1:57.

[חסר] • *Pi'el* **חִסֵּר** • **חיסר הרוח** · **to cause fainting:** Lat. defectiones spiritus ... facere · Hippocrates, *Aphorisms* · trans. Hillel ben Samuel, 5.16 (236) (fol. 31b): א"א: החום המחודד מרפה הבשר ומחליש העצבים ומבלבל הדעת ומגיר הדם ומחסר הרוח ותבא מזה המות. → NM 3:95.

חֶסְרוֹן • **חסרון הכח** · **fainting:** Hippocrates, *Aphorisms* · trans. Judah Shalom, 7.8 (360) (fol. 114b): בפתיחת מורסא בפנים יתחדש התרה קיא וחסרון הכח. → NM 3:95.

• **חסרון נשימה** · **fainting:** Arab. ذبول نفس · Hippocrates, *Aphorisms* · trans. Nathan ha-Me'ati, 7.8 (360) (fol. 128a): אמר אבקראט: כשיבקע יציאה מבפנים יתחדש מזה נפילת כח וקיא וחסרון נשימה. → NM 3:95.

• **חסרון הרוח** · **fainting:** Hippocrates, *Aphorisms* · trans. Judah Shalom, 5.16 (236) (fols. 78a–b): החום מזיק למרגילים אותו תמיד אלו ההזקים נקביות הבשר ובלתי קיום העצבים והרדמת השכל והגרת דם וחסרון הרוח אשר מאלו תמשך המות. → NM 3:95.

חפור → חָפֹר.

חָפַז · **to become urgent:** Arab. حفز · Maimonides, *K. al-fuṣūl fī al-ṭibb* · trans. Zeraḥyah Ḥen (*Sefer ha-Peraqim*), 8.41: המקרים המזיקים בכח אשר ראוי לכוין להם כשהם חופזים מאד. → NM 1:151.

חֲפִיפָה · **massage:** a) Arab. غمز · Ibn al-Jazzār, *Zād al-musāfir wa-qūt al-ḥādir* · trans. Moses ibn Tibbon (*Sefer Ṣedat ha-Derakhim*), bk. 7, 14.1: ותהיה החפיפה לאלו האברים באלו השמנים בנחת ומצוע ויכנסו במרחץ ממוצע החום. → NM 1:57.

b) Arab. دلك · i. Maimonides, *Šarḥ fuṣūl Abūqrāṭ* · trans. Moses ibn Tibbon (*Pirqei Abuqraṭ*), 1.20 (47): אמר המפרש: אמרו יבא אליהם ר"ל שהוכנו סיבותיו ונראו אותואיו והוא מזומן שיהיה ואמרו ולא בזולתה מן התנועות כמו הרחיצה וההזעה והגרת השתן או דם הנדות והחפיפה. → NM 3:95–6.

· ii. Maimonides, *K. al-fuṣūl fī al-ṭibb* · trans. Zeraḥyah Ḥen (*Sefer ha-Peraqim*), 8.12: הרקת הגוף כולו יהיה בהוצאת הדם או ברפואה המתירה לבטן או ברפואה המקיאה או בחפיפה המרובה. → NM 1:151.

· iii. Maimonides, *K. al-fuṣūl fī al-ṭibb* · trans. Nathan ha-Me'ati (*Sefer ha-Peraqim*), 8.12: הרקת הגוף כלו יהיה בהוצאת הדם או ברפואות המתירות הבטן או

ברפואות המקיאות או בחפיפה הרבה ובכל תנועה גם כן או ברחיצה במרחץ וביחוד מה שיהיה ממנו מתיך וברפואות החדות אם ירטו על הגוף. → NM 2:48.

חֲפִירָה · **cavity**: Ibn Zuhr, *Regimen of Health* · trans. Jacob ibn Tibbon (*Hanhagat ha-Beri'ut le-Abu 'Ali ben Zuhr*), ch. 28: ואם תרצה שלא יהיה בשיניך חפירה ולא שנוי יהיה חכוכך בעץ האפרסק. → NM 4:71.

• *Plur.* **חפירות** · **emaciation**: Arab. حفر · Maimonides, *Šarḥ fuṣūl Abūqrāṭ* · trans. Moses ibn Tibbon (*Pirqei Abuqraṭ*), 6.3 (295): אמר המפרש: שלשול הדם כאשר היה עם חמרמרות המעיים וארך עמידתו יתוספו החפירות בעומק האיברים וישובו נגעים בהם עפוש ותכאב האצטו' בשותפות וישיג בשולה הנזק. → NM 3:96.

[חפף] • *Pi'el* **חִפֵּף** · **to massage**: Arab. دلك · Maimonides, *K. al-fuṣūl fī al-ṭibb* · trans. Nathan ha-Me'ati (*Sefer ha-Peraqim*), 8.60: האברים החלושים בעת הבריאות ראוי שיחופפו יותר ממה שתחפף שאר האברים וכל שכן החפיפה היבשה. → NM 2:49.

• *Pu'al* **חֻפַּף** · **to get a massage**: Maimonides, *K. al-fuṣūl fī al-ṭibb* · trans. Nathan ha-Me'ati (*Sefer ha-Peraqim*), 8.60: האברים החלושים בעת הבריאות ראוי שיחופפו יותר ממה שתחפף שאר האברים וכל שכן החפיפה היבשה. → NM 2:49; corr. 4:229.

חֵפֶץ • **חפץ מאכל** · **appetite**: Lat. appetitus (Honofredi) · Ibn Zuhr, *Regimen of Health* · trans. Jacob ibn Tibbon (*Hanhagat ha-Beri'ut le-Abu 'Ali ben Zuhr*), ch. 10: ואמר אריסטו: בלקיחת המרקחות מן הליגנא אלובין וריברברי ד' דרה' בכל יום ברקות האצטו' יחזק החם אשר בה העוזר לעכול ויתיך הבלגם מפיה ויתן חפץ מאכל ויסיר הרוח אשר בה. → NM 4:71–2.

• **חפץ הקיא** · **nausea**: Arab. غثيان · Maimonides, *K. al-fuṣūl fī al-ṭibb* · trans. Nathan ha-Me'ati (*Sefer ha-Peraqim*), 9.55: יקשה רפואת חולשת פי האסטומכה ומהירות חפץ הקיא עם עוצר הבטן כי כל מה שיתיר הבטן מעורר אסטנסות ומהפך הנפש ומה שמחזק פי האסטו' עוצר הבטן. → NM 2:49.

חֵפֶר · **emaciation**: Arab. حفر · Maimonides, *Šarḥ fuṣūl Abūqrāṭ* · trans. Zeraḥyah Ḥen (*Pirqei Abuqraṭ*), 6.3 (295): אמר המפרש: שינוי הדם בהיותו עם שלשול המעיים הנק' סחג' פונט ויאריך יוסיף לחפור בעומק האיברים וישוב נגע בעל עיפוש והכאב האצטומ' עם השיתוף ויקח בה ההזק. ובעלות החולי לפי האצטומ' תסור תאוות המזון ממנה ויהיה זה ראייה על שהחולי נאחז והמשך ריעותו. → NM 3:96.

[חפש] • *Part. Pi'el* **מְחַפֵּשׂ** · I. **explorer**: Arab. مدس · Al-Zahrāwī, *K. al-taṣrīf li-man 'ağiza 'an at-ta'līf* · trans. Shem Tov ben Isaac (*Sefer ha-Shimmush*), bk. 30, 2.45 (fol. 216[a]): וראוי למתחיל ברפואת האגודה לבדוק אותה ולחפשה בתחלה במחפש. → NM 1:101.

· II. **probe**: Arab. مسبار · Al-Zahrāwī, *K. al-taṣrīf li-man 'ağiza 'an at-ta'līf* · trans. Shem Tov ben Isaac (*Sefer ha-Shimmush*), bk. 30, 2.46 (fol. 216[a]): וזאת צורות מחפשים. → NM 1:101.

חֵץ • **התוספות שהם כמו החץ** → **תּוֹסֶפֶת**.

• *Plur.* **חצים** • **התוספות הדומות לחצים** → **תּוֹסֶפֶת**.

חִצִּי · **sagittal**: Arab. سهمي · Ibn Sīnā, *K. al-Qānūn fī al-ṭibb* · trans. Nathan ha-Me'ati (*Sefer ha-Qanun*), bk. 1 (fol. 29[a]): ושלב מחלק לאורך הראש ישר יאמר לו לבדו חציי וכשיחקר מצד חבורו עם הכלילי אז יאמר לו שפודיי. → NM 4:72.

• קדחת חצי שלישית → קַדַּחַת.

• התוספות החיציות → תּוֹסֶפֶת.

חציי → חֵצִי.

חָצַץ • *Part.* חוֹצֵץ › spine of the scapula: Arab. حاجز · Ibn Sīnā, *K. al-Qānūn fī al-ṭibb* · trans. Nathan ha-Me'ati (*Sefer ha-Qanun*), bk. 1 (fol. 49[a]): וחמשה עצלים צמיחתם מעצמות הכתף מהם עצל תולדתו מעצם הכתף ומתחבר מה שבין החוצץ והצלע העליון לכתף. → NM 4:64.

חָצֵר • חצר הכבד › diaphragm: Lat. dyaphragma · Hippocrates, *Aphorisms* · trans. Hillel ben Samuel, 4.18 (155) (fol. 21[b]): הכאבים אשר מחצר הכבד ולמעלה מורים שצריך רפואה מנקה מלמעלה ואותם שמחצר הכבד ולמטה מורים שצריך רפואה מנקה מלמטה. → NM 3:96.

חַרְטוֹם • החרטום הנק׳ מנקאר › the [coracoid] process: Arab. منقار / Gr. κορακοειδής · Ibn Sīnā, *K. al-Qānūn fī al-ṭibb* · trans. Nathan ha-Me'ati (*Sefer ha-Qanun*), bk. 1 (fol. 49[b]): ולמקבצים יש זוג שאחד נפרדין והוא היותר גדול מקבץ עם נטיה לפנים וזה כי צמיחתו מן הזר התחתון מן הכתף ומן החרטום הנק׳ מנקאר. → NM 4:72.

• חרטום העורב › (lit., crow's beak); coracoid process: Arab. منقار الغراب · Ibn Sīnā, *K. al-Qānūn fī al-ṭibb* · trans. Nathan ha-Me'ati (*Sefer ha-Qanun*), bk. 1 (fol. 37[a]): ויש לה שתי תוספות אחת מהן למעלה ומאחור ונקרא אלגזם וחרטום העורב ובה קשורי הכתף עם התרקוה. → NM 4:72–3 (corr.).

חֲרִיכוּת › burning: Arab. حرقة · Al-Zahrāwī, *K. al-taṣrīf li-man 'ağiza 'an at-ta'līf* · trans. Shem Tov ben Isaac (*Sefer ha-Shimmush*), bk. 30, 2.87 (fol. 226[b]): ואני מודיע בדמיון שקרה לאדם ברגלו זה המקרה בעצמו אשר אגיד וזה כי נתחדש ברגלו שחרות עם חריכות דומה לשרפת האש. → NM 1:94–5.

חָרִיצוּת › intuition: Arab. حدس · Maimonides, *Šarḥ fuṣūl Abūqrāṭ* · trans. Moses ibn Tibbon (*Pirqei Abuqraṭ*), 1.7 (21): ולכן יצטרך אל שמוש ארוך בראיית הראיות הפרטיות ואז יוכל לשפוט על מה שיתחדש בחריצות טוב יהיה קרוב מן האמת. → NM 3:97.

חֶרֶס › dandruff: Arab. إبرية · Al-Zahrāwī, *K. al-taṣrīf li-man 'ağiza 'an at-ta'līf* · trans. Shem Tov ben Isaac (*Sefer ha-Shimmush*), bk. 27, fol. 134[b], col. b: ומסגולתה עוד כי הלוקח מסחיטתה ורוחץ בה הראש חוקה החרס וביצי הכנים ממנו ותאריך השער. → NM 4:73.

חָשַׁב › I. to call for; to seek; to strive: Arab رام · Maimonides, *K. al-fuṣūl fī al-ṭibb* · trans. Zeraḥyah Ḥen (*Sefer ha-Peraqim*), 8.43: הדרך אשר תלך בו תמיד הוא שתחשוב להריק ולהתיר מה שהוא חוץ מהטבע ואם לא יהיה יכול להשלים זה בעבור טבע האבר או בסבת שהחולי לא יקח בו רפואה תשים ידך לעפש אותו הדבר שהוא חוץ מהטבע ולהביאו לידי מוגלא. → NM 1:151.

› II. to be determined: Arab. عزم · Maimonides, *Šarḥ fuṣūl Abūqrāṭ* · trans. Moses ibn Tibbon (*Pirqei Abuqraṭ*), 4.73 (210): ובמי שיש בו קדחת לבד יהיה בטוח באלו האותות וידע כי הטבע כבר חשב לדחות הדבר המזיק ולהוציאו בשתן או בצואה. → NM 3:97.

› III. to have doubts: Arab. اتّهم · Maimonides, *K. al-fuṣūl fī al-ṭibb* · trans. Zeraḥyah Ḥen (*Sefer ha-Peraqim*), introduction: ובהיותו חושב שום אדם לשון אותו הפרק או ענינו ישוב לאותו המאמר בנקלה. → NM 1:151.

› IV. to imagine: Arab. أوهم أنّ · Maimonides, *K. al-fuṣūl fī al-ṭibb* · trans. Zeraḥyah Ḥen (*Sefer ha-Peraqim*), 9.57: מי שיהיה מן הממולאים וזולתם ימצא באסטומכתו שרפה

חזקה עד שתחשוב שיהיה שם מורסא חמה הצרוטו העשוי בשמן ורדים או בשמן חבושים יועיל לו. → NM 1:151–2.

‣ v. to pretend: Arab. ادّعى · Maimonides, *K. al-fuṣūl fī al-ṭibb* · trans. Zeraḥyah Ḥen (*Sefer ha-Peraqim*), 25.61: ולא עמד על כל זה הגדר אלא מחוזק הנאתו במה שנראה לו מקצת תועלת האברים חשב להתנבאות ואמר כי מלאך בא אליו מאת השם ולמדהו כך וצווהו כך. → NM 1:152.

‣ vi. to want: Arab. رام · Maimonides, *Šarḥ fuṣūl Abūqrāṭ* · trans. Zeraḥyah Ḥen (*Pirqei Abuqraṭ*), introduction (3): והסבה השנית שעזב הקדמות הספר והוא שהמחבר חבר ספרו והיה סומך שהמעיין קדמה לו ידיעה באותן ההקדמות הפלוניות וכאשר יחשוב להבין אותו הספר מי שאין לו חכמה באותן ההקדמות לא יבין בו שום דבר. → NM 3:97.

• *Nif'al* **נֶחְשַׁב** • **נחשב ש-** ‣ **almost**: Arab. كاد · Maimonides, *K. al-fuṣūl fī al-ṭibb* · trans. Nathan ha-Me'ati (*Sefer ha-Peraqim*), 10.18: ולא יאות להם לבד ההרקה בחפיפה החזקה אשר יחשב שתחדש כדמות היגיעה בשביל רצוץ הבשר ורסוקו ברוב החפיפה. → NM 2:49.

• **לא נחשב ש-** ‣ **hardly**: Arab. لا يكاد · Maimonides, *K. al-fuṣūl fī al-ṭibb* · trans. Nathan ha-Me'ati (*Sefer ha-Peraqim*), 3.88: לא יחשב שיהיה בכבד ובחזה מורסא לבנית. → NM 2:49.

חָשׁוּךְ ‣ **livid**: Gr. πελιδνός · Hippocrates, *Aphorisms* · trans. Joseph Delmedigo, 4.47 (184): בקדחות הבלתי פוסקות רקיקות חשוכות ודמיות ומוסרחות ומרירות כלן רעות. → NM 3:97.

• **חשוך המראה** ‣ **livid**: Arab. كمد · Maimonides, *Šarḥ fuṣūl Abūqrāṭ* · trans. Moses ibn Tibbon (*Pirqei Abuqraṭ*), 4.47 (184): אמר אבקראט: בקדחות שלא יפסקו הרקיקה חשוכת המראה והדומה בדם והמוסרחת ואשר היא מסוג המרה האדומה כולם רעות. → NM 3:98.

חשוכי • **סבוב חשוכי** → **סִבּוּב**.

חֲשִׁיבוּת ‣ **virtue**: Arab. فضيلة · Maimonides, *Šarḥ fuṣūl Abūqrāṭ* · trans. Anonymous (*Pirqei Abuqraṭ*), introduction (8): וכל זה להפך אחר זכות ואע"פ שהיה אבוקרט מגדולי חשובי הרופאים בלא ספק אך הנה רדיפת הזכות בדברי שקר אינו חשיבות ואפילו היה זה בחק החשוב. → NM 3:98.

חֲשֵׁיכוּת ‣ **dizziness:** Hippocrates, *Aphorisms* · trans. Judah Shalom, 4.17 (154) (fol. 56[b]): בלא מוקדח בהיות ניעול המאכלים ונשיכת הלב וחשיכות והפה מר יורה שיצטרך הרקה מלמעלה. → NM 3:98.

חֲשֵׁכוּת (also: **חֲשְׁכוּת**) → **חֲשֵׁיכוּת**.

חֲשֶׁל ‣ **feebleness; weakness:** Arab. ضعف · Ibn Sīnā, *K. al-Qānūn fī al-ṭibb* · trans. Nathan ha-Me'ati (*Sefer ha-Qanun*), bk. 1 (fol. 39[a]): ונסתפק בעצמות שלשה כי אם היה נוסף מספרם והיה מקנה זה תוספת מספר תנועות היה בלי ספק מוריש חולשה וחשל באחיזת מה שיהיה צריך לאחוז אל תוספת החזקה בחוזק. → NM 4:73.

חִתּוּךְ ‣ **supination**: Arab. بَطْح · Ibn Sīnā, *K. al-Qānūn fī al-ṭibb* · trans. Zeraḥyah Ḥen (*Sefer ha-Qanun*), bk. 1 (fol. 27[a]): ואלו הקובצים והפושטים הם בעצמם יפעלו הקיבוב והחיתוך. → NM 4:73.

חָתוּם (*Pass. Part.*) → **חָתַם**.

חִתּוּם ‣ **growing together (of fractured parts)**: Arab. إلحام · Ibn al-Jazzār, *Zād al-musāfir wa-qūt al-ḥādir* · trans. Moses ibn Tibbon (*Sefer Ṣedat ha-Derakhim*), bk. 7, 25.2: ואחר כך נכון בסוף להולדת החתום. → NM 1:57.

חֲתִימָה · **cicatrization:** Arab. خَتْم · Maimonides, *K. al-fuṣūl fī al-ṭibb* · trans. Nathan ha-Me'ati (*Sefer ha-Peraqim*), 23.44: כל שחין יקשה הבראתו וחתימתו מפני לחויות יורדות אליו אם רבים ואם חמים מבלי שיגמר רוע מזג האבר אשר בו השחין הנה אנחנו נקראהו קשה ההבראה. → NM 2:49–50.

חָתַךְ • *Part.* **חוֹתֵךְ** • **הסם החותך** → **סַם**.

• *Nif'al* **נֶחְתַּךְ** · **to stop:** Arab. تقطّع · Maimonides, *K. al-fuṣūl fī al-ṭibb* · trans. Zeraḥyah Ḥen (*Sefer ha-Peraqim*), 24.24: אשה הרה אחר ההריון בקצת חדשים ראתה תחלה דם ואחר כן טרי רקיק מוסרח ואחר האריך בה הזמן הפילה ואחר מכן הוציאה מן השילייא בכל יום מעט כי השילייא נתעפשה בפנים. ואחר שנחתכה מה שנשאר מן השלייא חשבו המילדות וכל הרופאים זולתי שהאשה נקתה לגמרי. → NM 1:152.

• *Part. Pi'el* **מְחַתֵּךְ** • **הסם המחתך** → **סַם**.

[חתל] • *Pu'al* **חֻתַּל** · **to be applied as a poultice:** Arab. ضُمِّدَ · Al-Zahrāwī, *K. al-taṣrīf li-man 'ağiza 'an at-ta'līf* · trans. Shem Tov ben Isaac (*Sefer ha-Shimmush*), bk. 27, fol. 124[b], col. a: וכשיבושלו ביין ומים ויחותלו בהם השדים אשר נקפא בהם החלב יתיכוהו. → NM 4:73–4.

חָתַם · **to cicatrize:** Arab. خَتَم · Maimonides, *K. al-fuṣūl fī al-ṭibb* · trans. Zeraḥyah Ḥen (*Sefer ha-Peraqim*), 9.95: כשתגיע מורסא בכליות ותתבשל וישתין החולה טרי יגיע ריחו מהרעי אבל על כאב מחבלת הכליות. ותשמור עצמך שלא תאחר מחתום אותה החבלה. → NM 1:152–3.

• *Pass. Part.* **חָתוּם** • **טירה חתומה** → **טִירָה**.

• *Nif'al* **נֶחְתַּם** · **to be regenerated:** Arab. تجبّر · Maimonides, *Šarḥ fuṣūl Abūqrāṭ* · trans. Moses ibn Tibbon (*Pirqei Abuqraṭ*), 4.26 (163): אמר המפרש: כי זה ראיה על שקיעת הנגע במעים עד אשר יחתוך גרמם ואי אפשר להחתם הבשר ההוא. → NM 3:98–9.

• *Hitpa'el* **הִתְחַתֵּם** · I. **to be closed up:** Arab. التحم · Ibn al-Jazzār, *Zād al-musāfir wa-qūt al-ḥāḍir* · trans. Moses ibn Tibbon (*Sefer Ṣedat ha-Derakhim*), bk. 7, 25.1: וכאשר הותרו החתולים והקשרים ביום השביעי או קרוב ממנו תעיין בו ואם ראית האבר בריא מן הנפח או ראית אותו קטן ממה שהיה לפנים בעת בריאותו שים רווחך להחתים העצם ושים עליו המחתימים כדי שיצמח הבשר אשר יתחתם בו ויקשרהו. → NM 1:58.

· II. **to be mended:** Arab. جُبِر · Ibn al-Jazzār, *Zād al-musāfir wa-qūt al-ḥāḍir* · trans. Moses ibn Tibbon (*Sefer Ṣedat ha-Derakhim*), bk. 7, 25.2: וזה כי מזון מימי אי אפשר שיתילד ממנו בשר אשר יתחתם בו העצם אבל במזון עב אשר אין בו דבקות. → NM 1:58.

• *Hif'il* **הֶחְתִּים** · I. **to close up:** Arab. ألحم · Ibn al-Jazzār, *Zād al-musāfir wa-qūt al-ḥāḍir* · trans. Moses ibn Tibbon (*Sefer Ṣedat ha-Derakhim*), bk. 7, 25.1: וכאשר הותרו החתולים והקשרים ביום השביעי או קרוב ממנו תעיין בו ואם ראית האבר בריא מן הנפח או ראית אותו קטן ממה שהיה לפנים בעת בריאותו שים כונתך להחתים העצם ושים עליו המחתימים כדי שיצמח הבשר אשר יתחתם בו ויקשרהו. → NM 1:57.

· II. **to mend; to set:** Arab. جبر · Ibn al-Jazzār, *Zād al-musāfir wa-qūt al-ḥāḍir* · trans. Moses ibn Tibbon (*Sefer Ṣedat ha-Derakhim*), bk. 7, 25.5: ומזה תאר טיחה מחתימה העצמות והפרקים. → NM 1:58.

· III. **to scar over (heal):** Arab. اندمل · Maimonides, *Šarḥ fuṣūl Abūqrāṭ* · trans.

Moses ibn Tibbon (*Pirqei Abuqraṭ*), 6.8 (300): אמר המפרש: הנגעים לא יחתימו עד שיתנגבו נגוב שלם ולא יקל זה במזג בעלי השקוי. → NM 3:99.

• *Part. Hifʿil* **מַחְתִּים** • *Plur.* **מחתימים** · **splints:** Arab. جبائر · Ibn al-Jazzār, *Zād al-musāfir wa-qūt al-ḥādir* · trans. Moses ibn Tibbon (*Sefer Ṣedat ha-Derakhim*), bk. 7, 25.1: וכאשר הותרו החתולים והקשרים ביום השביעי או קרוב ממנו תעיין בו ואם ראית האבר בריא מן הנפח או ראית אותו קטן ממה שהיה לפנים בעת בריאותו שים כונתך להחתים העצם ושים עליו המחתימים כדי שיצמח הבשר אשר יתחתם בו ויקשרהו. → NM 1:59–60.

ט

טִבּוּל · **the application of a hot compress:** Arab. تكميد · Maimonides, *K. al-fuṣūl fī al-ṭibb* · trans. Zeraḥyah Ḥen (*Sefer ha-Peraqim*), 9.81: רפואת חולי הצד בהקזה ובטיבול וחלקות הבטן. → NM 1:153.

• *Plur.* **טיבולים** · **fomentations:** Arab. نطولات · Maimonides, *K. al-fuṣūl fī al-ṭibb* · trans. Zeraḥyah Ḥen (*Sefer ha-Peraqim*), 8.2: הדברים אשר יעזרו על בשול הליחות הם כל הדברים אשר יחממו במיצוע קצתם הם מזון וקצתם הם משקים וקצתם טיבולים וקצתם תחבושות. → NM 1:153.

טַבּוּר • **תחת הטבור** → תַּחַת.

טָבַל · I. **to apply a compress:** Arab. كمّد · Maimonides, *K. al-fuṣūl fī al-ṭibb* · trans. Zeraḥyah Ḥen (*Sefer ha-Peraqim*), 9.22: ראוי שתרחץ העין באספוג במים שנתבשל בו האזמרינו ופינוגרקו ואם היה הכאב נקל תמשחנו פעם או פעמים ביום אחד. ואם היה הכאב חזק תטבלנו פעמים רבות וכל שכן בימים הארוכים. → NM 1:153–4.

· II. **to foment:** Arab. نطل · Maimonides, *K. al-fuṣūl fī al-ṭibb* · trans. Zeraḥyah Ḥen (*Sefer ha-Peraqim*), 9.6: בהיות המותרות הניגרים מן האף מימיות בלתי מבושלים היותינו מתקנים אותם יהיה בדברים אשר תטבול הראש כדי שיחמם המוח ועם הדברים אשר תשאף ואשר יריק באוזן. → NM 1:153.

טֶבַע · **bowels:** Arab. بطن / Gr. κοιλία · Maimonides, *Šarḥ fuṣūl Abūqrāṭ* · trans. Moses ibn Tibbon (*Pirqei Abuqraṭ*), 3.31 (137): אמר אבקראט: ואולם הישישים הנה יקרה להם רוע הנשימה והירידה אשר יקרה עמה השעול וטפטוף השתן ועצירתו וכאבי הפרקים וכאבי הכליות והסבוב והשתוק והנגעים הרעים וחכוך הגוף והיקיצה ורכות הטבע ולחות בעינים והנחירים וחושך הראות ולובן העינים וכבדות השמע. → NM 3:99.

• **החליק לטבע** → [חלק].

טִבְעִי • **החום הטבעי** → חֹם.

טַבַּעַת • **הוריד אשר על פי הטבעת** → וָרִיד.

• **קצה פי הטבעת** → קָצֶה.

טָהֳרָה • **טהרת זיעה** · **crisis:** Hippocrates, *Aphorisms* · trans. Do'eg ha-Edomi (*Sefer Agur*), 2.23 (75) (fol. 39[a]): אמר אפוקרט: טהרת זיעה מדוה מחודד תבוא בעת ארבעה עשר יום. → NM 3:99–100.

טוֹב • **קנה הטוב** → קָנֶה.

• **שמן טוב** → שֶׁמֶן.

[טוח] • **טח בדבקות** · **to agglutinate:** Arab. غرّى · Maimonides, *K. al-fuṣūl fī al-ṭibb* · trans. Nathan ha-Me'ati (*Sefer ha-Peraqim*), 13.43: החוקן שיעשה לנגעי המעים יחובר מענינים קובצים ומנקים ומבשלים ומרדימים החוש וטחים בדבקות הנקראים גלודטינאש. → NM 2:50.

• *Hif'il* **הֵטִיחַ** · **to dirty; to foil; to rub; to smear; to stain:** Arab. لطخ · Al-Zahrāwī, *K. al-taṣrīf li-man ʿağiza ʿan at-taʾlīf* · trans. Shem Tov ben Isaac (*Sefer ha-Shimmush*), bk. 27, fol. 144[a], col. a: המוח חם לח מוליד דם קר חלוק רע אל האסטומ׳ מטיח אותה בלחותו קשה להתעכל וגורם אסטניסות ומסיר תאות המאכל. → NM 4:74.

• *Part. Hif'il* **מַטִּיחַ** • **הסם המטיח** → סַם.

טוֹחֵן (*Part.*) → טָחַן.

טורח → טֹרַח.

טָחוּל · **spleen patient**: Arab. مطحول · Maimonides, *K. al-fuṣūl fī al-ṭibb* · trans. Zeraḥyah Ḥen (*Sefer ha-Peraqim*), 23.89: הרופאים באמרם טחולים ירצו לומר במי שיקרה בטחולו קושי ואבנינות מבלתי מורסא. → NM 1:154.

• **בעל הטחול** → בַּעַל.

טָחוֹר • *Plur.* **טחורים** · **polyps**: Arab. بواسير / Gr. πολύπους · Al-Rāzī, *K. al-Manṣūrī* · trans. Shem Tov ben Isaac (*Sefer Almansur*), Qof 9 (70): קלקנת: אוכל חם יש בו קביצות יסיר הטחורים מן האף. → NM 2:12.

טְחִינָה · **digestion**: Arab. استمراء · Al-Zahrāwī, *K. al-taṣrīf li-man ʿağiza ʿan at-taʾlīf* · trans. Shem Tov ben Isaac (*Sefer ha-Shimmush*), bk. 27, fol. 123b, col. 2: ולמי שחלשה טחינתו מן הזקנים והנמלטים מן החליים. → NM 4:74.

[טחל] • *Part. Hofʿal* **מֻטְחָל** · **someone suffering from an illness of the spleen**: Arab. مطحول · Hippocrates, *Aphorisms* · trans. Nathan ha-Me'ati, 6.43 (335) (fol. 120a): אמר אבוקרט: כשימצא המוטחל שלשול דם ויארך בו יתחדש בו שקוי או המעדת המעים וימות. → NM 3:129–30.

טָחַן • *Part.* **טוֹחֵן** • **הכח הטוחן** → כֹּחַ.

טיבול → טִבּוּל.

טִיּוּל · **physical exercise**: Arab. رياضة · Al-Zahrāwī, *K. al-taṣrīf li-man ʿağiza ʿan at-taʾlīf* · trans. Shem Tov ben Isaac (*Sefer ha-Shimmush*), bk. 27, fol. 123b, col. 2: הרביכות: הרביכה זנה מועט וממהרת להתעכל ולרדת מן האסטומ׳ יותר מן הלחם הטבול במרק ולפי כך ראוי להנזר מן הרביכות בעלי היגיעה והטיול והרוצה להנעים גופו. → NM 4:74–5.

טִיחָה · I. **agglutination**: Arab. تغرية · Ibn Sīnā, *K. al-adwiya al-qalbiya* · trans. Anonymous (*Sammim Libbiyim*), fol. 128a: טין מכתום: הוא שוה המזג בחום והקור מתדמה למזג האדם אלא שיבשו יותר רב מלחותו ויש בו לחות חזק המזג ביובש ולזה יש בו דבקות וטיחה. → NM 4:75.

· II. **liniment**: Arab. طلاء · a) Al-Zahrāwī, *K. al-taṣrīf li-man ʿağiza ʿan at-taʾlīf* · trans. Shem Tov ben Isaac (*Sefer ha-Shimmush*), bk. 30, 3.1 (fol. 232b). → NM 1:95.

b) Ibn al-Jazzār, *Zād al-musāfir wa-qūt al-ḥādir* · trans. Moses ibn Tibbon (*Sefer Ṣedat ha-Derakhim*), bk. 7, 18.3: וכאשר עשינו בנקוי הגוף והוצאת החומר הנפסד ממנו נשוב אל הטיחות מחוץ. → NM 1:58.

· III. **poultice**: Arab. لطوخ · Al-Zahrāwī, *K. al-taṣrīf li-man ʿağiza ʿan at-taʾlīf* · trans. Shem Tov ben Isaac (*Sefer ha-Shimmush*), bk. 30, 2.20 (fol. 211b): ואחר לתת על העין טיחה עשויה מאקקיא ואילווא ולבונה וכרכום. → NM 1:95.

· IV. **salve**: Arab. لطوخ · Ibn al-Jazzār, *Zād al-musāfir wa-qūt al-ḥādir* · trans. Moses ibn Tibbon (*Sefer Ṣedat ha-Derakhim*), bk. 7, 16.3: והנה יעשו מן המירא וקשיא ליניאה ודבש טיחות ליבלות. → NM 1:58.

טִיט • **בלוי הטיט** → בְּלוֹי.

• **בלוי עב טיט** → בְּלוֹי.

• **הטיט הנאכל** · **edible earth**: Arab. الطين المأكول · Ibn Sīnā, *K. al-adwiya al-qalbiya*

· trans. Anonymous (*Sammim Libbiyim*), fol. 221[a]: והסותם הוא הסם אשר כאשר עבר במעברם התגבר על הכח המניע לדחותו ועמד נגד כל מציק ומלא את החלל כמו הטיט הנאכל. → NM 4:75.

• קִבּוּץ עב טיט → קִבּוּץ.

טיסיס · **phthisis**: Lat. ptisis · Bruno Longobucco, *Cyrurgia Magna* · trans. Hillel ben Samuel (*Sefer Keritut*), fol. 18[a]: ואני אומר שחבלת הריאה תילקח על שני פנים או מעילה חיצונית או מעילה פנימית. הפנימית נקראה טיסיס ואינה מקבלת רפואה. → NM 1:43–4.

טירה • טירה חתומה · **sigillate earth**: Lat. terra sigillata · Bruno Longobucco, *Cyrurgia Magna* · trans. Hillel ben Samuel (*Sefer Keritut*), fol. 15[a]. → NM 1:45.

טנטא · **probe**: Lat. tenta · Bruno Longobucco, *Cyrurgia Magna* · trans. Hillel ben Samuel (*Sefer Keritut*), fol. 29[a]: וצריך שתשים עוד הטנטא בחבלה למען תכיר בעבור הדרך שלקח לו החץ. → NM 1:44.

טִפָּה • *Plur.* **טיפות • טיפות השתן** · **strangury**: Arab. تقطير البول / Gr. στραγγουρία · Maimonides, *Šarḥ fuṣūl Abūqrāṭ* · trans. Zeraḥyah Ḥen (*Pirqei Abuqraṭ*), 3.31 (137): אמר בקראט: אמנם הזקנים יקרה להם רוע הניפוש והנזל אשר עמו השעול וטיפות השתן ועוצר השתן וכאבי הפרקים וכאבי הכליות והגלגול בראש והשתוק והחבלות הרעות וחיכוך הגוף והתעורה וחלקות הבטן ולחות העיניים והאף ואפילת הראות וכובד השמיעה. → NM 3:100.

[טפח] • *Hif'il* הִטְפִּיחַ · **to foment**: Arab. نطل · Al-Zahrāwī, *K. al-taṣrīf li-man ʿağiza ʿan at-ta'līf* · trans. Shem Tov ben Isaac (*Sefer ha-Shimmush*), bk. 30, 2.1 (fol. 209[a]): ואחר הבקיעה ראוי להוציא הלחות כלו ולהדק הבקיעות בבגדים וכלונסות ואחר להטפיחם ממעלה ביין ושמן עד היום החמישי. → NM 1:95.

טִפְטוּף · **strangury**: Hippocrates, *Aphorisms* · trans. Judah Shalom, 3.31 (137) (fol. 50[b]): וביותר זקנים יקרה דישמא ואשמא ונזילה ושעול וטפטוף ועצירת השתן וכאב הפרקים ונפרישין וסבוב ראש ושתוק ורועקניה(?) וחכוך כל הגוף והיקיצה ולחות הבטן והעינים והנחירים וחשיכות ולכלוכם וכובד השמע. → NM 3:100.

• טפטוף השתן · **strangury**: Arab. تقطير البول · Maimonides, *Šarḥ fuṣūl Abūqrāṭ* · trans. Moses ibn Tibbon (*Pirqei Abuqraṭ*), 3.31 (137): אמר אבקראט: ואולם הישישים הנה יקרה להם רוע הנשימה והירידה אשר יקרה עמה השעול וטפטוף השתן ועצירתו וכאבי הפרקים וכאבי הכליות והסבוב והשתוק והנגעים הרעים וחכוך הגוף והיקיצה ורכות הטבע ולחות בעינים והנחירים וחושך הראות ולובן העינים וכבדות השמע ואלזרקה פירו׳ מראה החשמל. → NM 3:101.

טָפֵל • הגבנה הטפלה בבצק → גְּבִנָּה.

טרגאאלי · **arytenoid [cartilage of the larynx]**: Arab. طرجهالي, read طرجهاري / Gr. ἀρυταινοειδής · Ibn Sīnā, *K. al-Qānūn fī al-ṭibb* · trans. Nathan ha-Me'ati (*Sefer ha-Qanun*), bk. 1 (fols. 46[b]–47[a]): והשפוי כובע צריך אל עצלים יאחזו הציניי אל אותו שאין שם לו ועצלים יאחזו הטרגאאלי בו ויקיפוהו ועצלים ירחיקו הטרגאאלי מן האחרים ויפתחו השפוי כובע. → NM 4:75.

טרוחמטרא (*Aram.*) · **trochanter**: Arab. طروخانطير / Gr. τροχαντήρ · Ibn Sīnā, *K. al-Qānūn fī al-ṭibb* · trans. Nathan ha-Me'ati (*Sefer ha-Qanun*), bk. 1 (fol. 53[a]): ומהם עצל צמיחתו מכל חיצוני עצמות הכסל ומתחבר בעליוני התוספת הגדול הנקרא טרוחמטרא הגדול. → NM 4:76.

טָרַח · **to exercise**: Arab. ارتاض · Maimonides, *K. al-fuṣūl fī al-ṭibb* · trans. Zeraḥyah Ḥen

(*Sefer ha-Peraqim*), 12.7: הגוף אשר יהיה הדם הטוב בו מעט והליחות הנאות הרבה מאד אין ראוי שיתנועע בשום דבר כלל ולא יכנס למרחץ מפני שההקזה תוציא הדם הטוב ותמשוך הדם הרע המקובץ בעורקים הראשונים אשר בכבד וישלחהו בגוף כולו. אבל הרפואה המשלשלת יחדש לבעלי זה העניין נשיכה ועקיצה והתעלפות ולא ישלשלנו דבר בעל שיעור. והליחות בעבור עבים יתקדמו ויסתמו המעברות ומפני זה אין ראוי שיטרח ולא יכנס למרחץ. → NM 1:154–5.

• *Hif'il* הִטְרִיחַ · **to cause pain**: Arab. أتعب · Maimonides, *Šarḥ fuṣūl Abūqrāṭ* · trans. Zeraḥyah Ḥen (*Pirqei Abuqraṭ*), 4.33 (170): אמר בקראט: ואם כמו כן הקדים והטריח אבר מן האיברים קודם שיחלה בעליו באותו האבר יתאחז החולי. → NM 3:101.

טֹרַח · I. **exercise**: Arab. رياضة · Maimonides, *K. al-fuṣūl fī al-ṭibb* · trans. Zeraḥyah Ḥen (*Sefer ha-Peraqim*), 3.11: ובתנאי שישגיחו בהגרת המותרות מגופותם בטורח. → NM 1:154.

· II. **pain**: Lat. labor · Hippocrates, *Aphorisms* · trans. Judah Shalom, 2.1 (52) (fol. 16[a]): איזה חולי שיהיה השינה עושה טורח היא אות מות ואם השינה תועיל אינה אות מות. → NM 3:101.

• **בטורח** · **rarely**: Lat. raro · Bruno Longobucco, *Cyrurgia Magna* · trans. Hillel ben Samuel (*Sefer Keritut*), fol. 82[a]: ודע כי המורסות בעלות הליחה הפשוטות בטורח יבואו לידי עפוש → NM 1:26.

טַרְחָן • *Plur.* **טרחנים** · **wrestlers**: Arab. مصارع, *Plur.* مصارعون · Maimonides, *Šarḥ fuṣūl Abūqrāṭ* · trans. Anonymous (*Pirqei Abuqraṭ*), 1.3. (30): אמר המפרש: ירצה בבעלי התנועה הטרחנים ודומיהם ממי שלקח התנועה המתמדת לו לאומנות. → NM 3:101–2.

טַרְחָנִי • *Plur.* **טרחניים** · **wrestlers**: Arab. صريع, *Plur.* صريعون · Maimonides, *Šarḥ fuṣūl Abūqrāṭ* · trans. Anonymous (*Pirqei Abuqraṭ*), 1.15 (42): אמר אבוקרט: הגופים בסתיו ובאביב הם יותר חמים מכל מה שיהיה בטבע והשינה יותר ארוכה ממה שיהיה ויצטרך באלו העתים שיהיה מה שינתן להם מן המזונות הרבה וזה כי החום היסודי בגופים באלו שני הזמנים הרבה ולזה צריכים אל מזון רב והראיה על זה השנים והטרחניים. → NM 3:102.

טריאקי • **הסם הטריאקי** → סַם.

טריאקיות · **having theriacal (antidotal) property**: Arab. ترياقيّة · Ibn Sīnā, *K. al-adwiya al-qalbiya* · trans. Anonymous (*Sammim Libbiyim*), fol. 124[a]: הסמים המחזקים אשר להם טריאקיות יכנסו כלם ברפואות חלב לפי שהם נאותים בטבע האדם בסגולה. → NM 4:76.

טְרִיּוּת · **freshness**: Arab. طراوة · Al-Zahrāwī, *K. al-taṣrīf li-man ʿağiza ʿan at-taʾlīf* · trans. Shem Tov ben Isaac (*Sefer ha-Shimmush*), bk. 27, bk. 27, fol. 147[a], col. b: ומולידה החצץ בכליות אע״פ שתשתנה כפי מיניה וסוגי בעלי חיים שלה וטריותה וישנותה ומצועה. → NM 4:76 (corr.).

טַרְפָּשָׁה · **pleura**: Arab. حجاب · Al-Zahrāwī, *K. al-taṣrīf li-man ʿağiza ʿan at-taʾlīf* · trans. Shem Tov ben Isaac (*Sefer ha-Shimmush*), bk. 30, 2.92 (fol. 228[a]): ואם יפול החץ על הטרפשה אשר בחזה יהיה קרוב מן הצלעות הקטנות. → NM 1:95–6.

טשטי · **lints (for dressing wounds)**: Ital. tessuti / Lat. licinia · Bruno Longobucco, *Cyrurgia Magna* · trans. Hillel ben Samuel (*Sefer Keritut*), fols. 14[b], 27[b]: ויזרה מזה במספיק על המכה ויבלול הטשטי באבק זה בעבור שזה האבק מופלא. → NM 1:44.

יַבֶּלֶת · wart: Arab. ثآلول / Gr. ἀκροχορδών · Ibn al-Jazzār, *Zād al-musāfir wa-qūt al-ḥāḍir* · trans. Moses ibn Tibbon (*Sefer Ṣedat ha-Derakhim*), bk. 7, ch. 16.1: היבלת הוא בשר יצמח עגול חזק קשה יצא בכל הגוף וכל שכן בידין והרגלים. → NM 4:76–7.

יָבֵשׁ • **החולי היבש** → **חֹלִי**.

יְגִיעָה · pain: Hippocrates, *Aphorisms* · trans. Judah Shalom, 2.6 (58) (fol. 17b): מי שיהיו יגעים כפי קצת הגוף ולא יחושו חוזק היגיעה הנה הידיעה חולה באלו. → NM 3:102.

יָגַע · to suffer from pain: Arab. تعب / Gr. πονέω · Maimonides, *Šarḥ fuṣūl Abūqrāṭ* · trans. Moses ibn Tibbon (*Pirqei Abuqraṭ*), 4.33 (170): ואם היה ג״כ כבר קדם ויגע אבר מן האיברים קודם שיחלה בעליו הנה באבר ההוא ישתקע החולי. → NM 3:102–3.

יָד • **בית יד** → **בַּיִת**.
- • **דבק היד** → **דֶּבֶק**.
- • **מסרק היד** → **מַסְרֵק**.
- • **פרק היד** → **פֶּרֶק**.
- • **פרק קנה הזרוע הסמוך ליד** → **פֶּרֶק**.
- • *Dual* **יָדַיִם** • **המישמוש בידים** → **מִשְׁמוּשׁ**.

יָדוּעַ (*Pass. Part.*) → **יָדַע**.

יְדִיעָה • **הקדמת הידיעה** → **הַקְדָּמָה**.
- • **ידיעת החלוק** · anatomy: Arab. علم التشريح · Maimonides, *Šarḥ fuṣūl Abūqrāṭ* · trans. Moses ibn Tibbon (*Pirqei Abuqraṭ*), 1.1 (15): הראשון מה שיתלה ברופא מידיעת נושא מלאכתו והוא גוף האדם וזהו ידיעת החלוק. → NM 3:103.

יָדַע • *Pass. Part.* **יָדוּעַ** • **באין סבה ידועה אליו** → **סִבָּה**.
- • *Part. Nif'al* **נוֹדָע** • **לא נודע אליה סבה** · spontaneous: Arab. لا يعرف له سبب · Maimonides, *Šarḥ fuṣūl Abūqrāṭ* · trans. Moses ibn Tibbon (*Pirqei Abuqraṭ*), 2.5 (57): אמר אבקראט: היגיעה אשר לא נודע אליה סבה מורה בחולי. → NM 3:167.

יווני ← **יְוָנִי**.

יוֹם • **יום דין** · a day of prognostic indication: Hippocrates, *Aphorisms* · trans. Do'eg ha-Edomi (*Sefer Agur*), 2.24 (76) (fol. 39b): אמר אפוקר׳: יום שבעה עשר הוא יום דין והוא רביעי לארבעה עשר והיום השביעי לאחד עשר. → NM 3:103.
- • **יום ההבטה** · a day of prognostic indication: Arab. يوم إنذار · Maimonides, *Šarḥ fuṣūl Abūqrāṭ* · trans. Anonymous (*Pirqei Abuqraṭ*), 2.24 (76): אמר אבוקרט: הרביעי מביט בשביעי ותחלת השבוע השני הוא היום השמיני והמביט בי״ד הוא יום הי״א כי הוא הרביעי מן השבוע השני והיום הי״ז גם כן הוא יום ההבטה כי הוא הרביעי מן הי״ד והיום השביעי מן הי״א. → NM 3:103.
- • **יום הוראה** · a day of prognostic indication: Arab. يوم إنذار · Maimonides, *Šarḥ fuṣūl Abūqrāṭ* · trans. Moses ibn Tibbon (*Pirqei Abuqraṭ*), 2.24 (76): אמר אבקראט: הרביעי מורה לשביעי וראשית השבוע השני היום השמיני והמורה ליום הארבעה עשר יום האחד עשר כי הוא הרביעי מן השבוע השני ויום השבעה עשר גם כן יום הוראה כי הוא היום הרביעי מיום הארבעה עשר והיום השביעי מן היום האחד עשר. → NM 3:104.

• **יום הראות** · **a day of prognostic indication**: Arab. يوم إنذار · Maimonides, *Šarḥ fuṣūl Abūqrāṭ* · trans. Zeraḥyah Ḥen (*Pirqei Abuqraṭ*), 2.24 (76): אמר בקראט: היום הרביעי יורה על היום השביעי ותחילת השבוע השני הוא היום השמיני והמורה בי״ד הוא היום הי״א כי הוא הרביעי מן השבוע השנית. והיום הי״ז כמו כן יום הראות כי הוא היום הרביעי מיום הי״ד והיום הז׳ מן היום הי״א. → NM 3:104.

• **יום מבשר** · **a day of prognostic indication**: Arab. يوم إنذار · Hippocrates, *Aphorisms* · trans. Nathan ha-Me'ati, 2.24 (76) (fol. 30b): אמר אבקראט: הרביעי מבשר בשביעי ותחלת השבוע השני הוא השמיני והמבשר לארבעה עשר יום אחד עשר כי הוא הרביעי מהשבוע השני והיום שבעה עשר ג״כ יום מבשר ⟨ליום העשרים⟩ כי הוא יום ד׳ מהארבעה עשר יום והיום השביעי מהאחד עשר. → NM 3:104.

• **הקדחת הבאה בכל יום** → קַדַּחַת.

• **קדחת יום** → קַדַּחַת.

• **הקדחת העונה בכל יום** → קַדַּחַת.

• **הקדחת שעונתה בכל יום** → קַדַּחַת.

• *Plur.*[1] **ימים** • **ימי הבשורה** · **the days of warning; the indicator days**: Arab. الأيّام المنذرة · Galen, *De diebus decretoriis* · trans. Shimshon ben Shlomo (*Qibbuṣei Ma'amarei Galenus bi-Yemei ha-Buḥran*), 13: ויקראו אלו הימים שיראו בם אותם האותות ימי הבשורה וימי המבט. → NM 2: 172.

• **ימי המבט** · **the days to be watched**: Galen, *De diebus decretoriis* · trans. Shimshon ben Shlomo (*Qibbuṣei Ma'amarei Galenus bi-Yemei ha-Buḥran*), 13: ויקראו אלו הימים שיראו בם אותם האותות ימי הבשורה וימי המבט. → NM 2:172.

• **ימי הקור** · **winter**: Arab. شتاء · Maimonides, *Šarḥ fuṣūl Abūqrāṭ* · trans. Zeraḥyah Ḥen (*Pirqei Abuqraṭ*), 1.17 (44): אבל אמצע הזמן הנקרא וֶיר ובערבי אלרַבִיע כשיתקרב מן הקיץ ראוי שיפרנס במזון מועט בין שעות ארוכים כי זה העת אפשר שיהיו הגופות בו מלאים כי הכימוסים אשר היו נקפאים בימי הקור יתכו ויזובו. → NM 3:105.

• *Plur.*[2] **ימות** • **ימות הגשמים** · **winter**: Arab. شتاء · Maimonides, *Šarḥ fuṣūl Abūqrāṭ* · trans. Zeraḥyah Ḥen (*Pirqei Abuqraṭ*), 1.17 (44): אבל העת כן הראיה לפי הכח והחולי. והשנים והמנהג ודומהו על זה המשל: הקייץ יהיה ראוי בו להאכיל לפעמים רבות ומעט בכל פעם ופעם ובימות הגשמים ראוי להרבות המזון ולמעט הפעמים. → NM 3:104.

יָוָנִי • *Plur.* **יוונים** • **העצם הדומה ללמד בכתיבת היוונים** → עֶצֶם.

יוֹצֵא (*Part.*) → יָצָא.

יוֹקֶדֶת · **fuel**: Arab. وقود · Maimonides, *Šarḥ fuṣūl Abūqrāṭ* · trans. Zeraḥyah Ḥen (*Pirqei Abuqraṭ*), 1.14 (41): אמר אבקראט: מה שיהיה מן הגופות בגידול החום הטבעי בהם בתכלית הריבוי וצריך ליוקדת יותר ממה שצריכים אליו שאר הגופות. → NM 3:105.

יוֹרֵד (*Part.*) → יָרַד.

יותרת → יֹתֶרֶת.

יִחוּד · **specific property**: Arab. خاصّية · Maimonides, *Šarḥ fuṣūl Abūqrāṭ* · trans. Zeraḥyah Ḥen (*Pirqei Abuqraṭ*), 1.1 (27): ודע ששם רפואה תהיה פעולתה בגופותינו הנמשך אחר החומר שלה הוא הנראה המבואר ופעולתה הנמשכת אחר צורתה לא ישוער בה כרוב הרפואות אשר לא יתואר אליהם יחוד ולא סגולה בפעולה. → NM 3:106.

יָחִיד · **unmixed:** Arab. صرف · Maimonides, *Šarḥ fuṣūl Abūqrāṭ* · trans. Zeraḥyah Ḥen (*Pirqei Abuqraṭ*), 7.23 (375): אמר בקראט: ומהיציאה היחידה עירוב הדם. → NM 3:106.

[יחס] • *Part. Pu'al* מְיֻחָס • האיברים המיוחסים → אֵבֶר.

יַיִן • יין הדבש השרוי · **wine prepared from dried macerated grapes sweetened with honey:** Arab. شراب العسل النقيع · Al-Zahrāwī, *K. al-taṣrīf li-man ʿağiza ʿan at-ta'līf* · trans. Shem Tov ben Isaac (*Sefer ha-Shimmush*), bk. 27, fol. 131^{b}, col. a: יין הדבש השרוי חמומו ונגובו יותר מעטים מן המבושל ולפיכך הוא יותר נאות אל בעלי החמימות ובזמן הסתו. → NM 4:77.

• (ה)יין (ה)חי · **pure, unmixed wine:** a) Arab. شراب صرف · Ibn al-Jazzār, *Zād al-musāfir wa-qūt al-ḥādir* · trans. Moses ibn Tibbon (*Sefer Ṣedat ha-Derakhim*), bk. 7, 11.1: או יקח שרש זעפראן גנים הוא אלקרטם או פריו או עלהו ויכתשהו עם מעט פלפל וישתהו ביין חי. → NM 1:55–6.

b) Arab. الخمر الصرف · Maimonides, *K. al-fuṣūl fī al-ṭibb* · trans. Nathan ha-Me'ati (*Sefer ha-Peraqim*), 9.4: העם אשר ימצאם כאב חזק כפלות הראש וכיוצא בו מעובי הדם או מקור בפנים יועילם שתית היין החי אחר המאכל או עם המאכל תועלת מבוארת וישקיט כאבם בחמום היין ודקדוקו. → NM 2:45.

c) Arab. الشراب الصرف / Gr. ἀκρατοποσία · Maimonides, *Šarḥ fuṣūl Abūqrāṭ* · trans. Moses ibn Tibbon (*Pirqei Abuqraṭ*), 6.31 (323): אמר אבקראט: כאיבי העינים יתיכו אותם שתית היין החי או המרחץ והרטיה או הקזת העורק או שתית המשלשל. → NM 3:82.

• יין מבושל עד ששב כדבש · **grape juice (must) boiled down to a syrup:** Arab. ربّ العنب · Ibn al-Jazzār, *Zād al-musāfir wa-qūt al-ḥādir* · trans. Moses ibn Tibbon (*Sefer Ṣedat ha-Derakhim*), bk. 2, ch. 17 (fol. 58^{a}): ואם תהיה המורסה קשה יעשה גרגור בחלב שנחלב מיד או בחלב אתון או ביין מבושל עד ששב כדבש. → NM 4:77.

[ילד] • *Hif'il* הוֹלִיד • הוליד תולדות · **to draw conclusions:** Arab. نتج نتائج · Maimonides, *Šarḥ fuṣūl Abūqrāṭ* · trans. Moses ibn Tibbon (*Pirqei Abuqraṭ*), introduction (7): וכן גם כן אלו אשר יולידו תולדות מדברי אדם אחד ויקראו זה פירוש. → NM 3:106.

יֶלֶד • *Plur.* ילדים • אם הילדים → אֵם.

יַלֶּפֶת · **dandruff:** Arab. إبرية / Lat. furfures capitis · Al-Rāzī, *K. al-Manṣūrī* · trans. Shem Tov ben Isaac (*Sefer Almansur*), Zayin 9 (34): זכוכית: יש לו סגולה יפרד בה החצץ המתילד בביס מקוה המים ויסיר הילפת כשרוחצין בו הראש. → NM 2:12–3.

יָם • חלאת הים → חֶלְאָה.

• סוס הים → סוּס.

• קצף הים → קֶצֶף.

יַמִּי • הארנבת הימית → אַרְנֶבֶת.

יְמָנִי • הקנה הימני → קָנֶה.

יְסוֹדִי • חום יסודי → חֹם.

[יסף] • *Part. Nif'al* נוֹסָף · **residue:** Hippocrates, *Aphorisms* · trans. Do'eg ha-Edomi (*Sefer Agur*), 1.2 (29): אמר אפוקרט: בבא הזלת הבטן והקיא מן הנוסף הוא אות מרפא וחיים ומזולתו יהיה ההפך. → NM 3:151–2.

• בשר נוסף → בָּשָׂר.

יַעֲרָה • יערת הדבש ‣ **honeycomb**: Arab. شهدة · Maimonides, *K. al-fuṣūl fī al-ṭibb* · trans. Zeraḥyah Ḥen (*Sefer ha-Peraqim*), 23.54: בעור הראש תתחדש חולי מסוג המורסא יהיה בה חורים קטנים מליאים לחות רקיק ויסקוסו יאמר לו האלצעפא. ויתחדש בעור הראש חולי דומה לאילו בראייה ונקביו יותר גדולים ויותר רחבים מנקבי האלצעפא והם מליאים מלחות דומה ביערת הדבורים וזה נקרא יערת הדבש. → NM 1:155.

יָצָא ‣ **to exfoliate**: Arab. تبيّن / Gr. ἀφίσταμαι · Maimonides, *Šarḥ fuṣūl Abūqrāṭ* · trans. Moses ibn Tibbon (*Pirqei Abuqraṭ*), 6.45 (337): אמר אבקראט: כאשר עבר על הנגע שנה או זמן יותר גדול מזה יתחייב בהכרח שיצאו ממנו עצמות ושיהיה מקום הנגע אחר החתמו עמוק. → NM 3:107.

• *Inf.* **צֵאת • אחרי צאת המאכל מן האצטומכא** → אַחֲרֵי.

• **צאת דם הנחירים** ‣ **nosebleed**: Arab. رعاف / Gr. ἐκ ῥινῶν αἵματος ῥύσιες · Maimonides, *Šarḥ fuṣūl Abūqrāṭ* · trans. Moses ibn Tibbon (*Pirqei Abuqraṭ*), 3.27 (133): אמר אבקראט: ואולם מי שעבר אלו השנים וקרב שיצמח לו השער סביב הערוה הנה יקרו לו רבים מאלו החליים וקדחות יותר ארוכות וצאת דם הנחירים. → NM 3:191.

• *Part.* **יוֹצֵא** ‣ I. **exterior**: Arab. خارج · Maimonides, *K. al-fuṣūl fī al-ṭibb* · trans. Zeraḥyah Ḥen (*Sefer ha-Peraqim*), 1.56: על האסטומכא קרום יקיף בבשר היוצא וזה הקרום יקשרנו עם הגב. → NM 1:155.

‣ II. **external**: Arab. خارج / Gr. ἔξω · Maimonides, *Šarḥ fuṣūl Abūqrāṭ* · trans. Moses ibn Tibbon (*Pirqei Abuqraṭ*), 7.36 (388): אמר אבקראט: מי שהיה בכוליתו חולי וקרה לו אלו המקרים שקדם זכרם והתחדש בו כאב בגיד הגב הנה אם היה הכאב במקומות היוצאים יפחד מיציאה תבא בו מחוץ. → NM 3:105.

• **שלשול היוצא הקיא** → שִׁלְשׁוּל.

• *Hif'il* **הוֹצִיא** ‣ **to translate**: Arab. أخرج · Maimonides, *K. al-fuṣūl fī al-ṭibb* · trans. Zeraḥyah Ḥen (*Sefer ha-Peraqim*), 24.1: ספר כאבי הנשים לאבקראט הוציאו חונין וביארו גליאנוס ונמצא תוספת באותו הספר הוציאו זולתי חונין וביארו זולתי גליאנוס. → NM 1:155.

• **הוציא ביציאה** ‣ **to defecate**: Arab. تبرّز · Maimonides, *K. al-fuṣūl fī al-ṭibb* · trans. Nathan ha-Me'ati (*Sefer ha-Peraqim*), 9.64: דיות הדם הוא מפתיחת עורקים קטנים או הרקת מימיות הדם כמו שיקרה ביחוד בחולשת הכבד והכליות כי בעל העלה הזאת יקרה לו פעמים רבות שישתין או יוציא ביציאה מימיות הדם. → NM 2:50.

יְצִיאָה ‣ I. **abscess**: Arab. خراج · Maimonides, *K. al-fuṣūl fī al-ṭibb* · trans. Nathan ha-Me'ati (*Sefer ha-Peraqim*), 8.53: לפעמים יתחדש בשול חלקיי לא תבטח בו כמו שתבושל היציאה שתחת האזנים ותחשוב שחחולה כבר נתרפא והוא ימות כי הליחות אשר בתוך העורקים לא נתבשלו והם סבת החולי. → NM 2:50.

‣ II. **excrements**: Arab. براز · Maimonides, *K. al-fuṣūl fī al-ṭibb* · trans. Nathan ha-Me'ati (*Sefer ha-Peraqim*), 5.1: וכשיהיה החולי בבטן ויהיה עמו קדחה אז תעיין תחילה ביציאה ואחר תעיין בשתן ואם לא יהיה שם קדחת אז תבדוק היציאה לבדה. → NM 2:50.

‣ III. **stools**: Lat. secessus · Hippocrates, *Aphorisms* · trans. Hillel ben Samuel, 4.83 (220) (fol. 30ᵃ): א״א: מי שמשתין הרבה בלילה הנה תמעט יציאתו. → NM 3:107.

• **הוציא ביציאה** → יָצָא.

• **יציאת דם הנחירים** ‣ **nosebleed**: Arab. رعاف · Maimonides, *Šarḥ fuṣūl Abūqrāṭ* · trans.

Moses ibn Tibbon (*Pirqei Abuqraṭ*), 5.33 (253): אמר אבקראט: כשיפסק דם הנדות הנה יציאת דם הנחירים טוב. → NM 3:107.

• **יציאת מורסא** › **abscess:** Arab. خراج · Maimonides, *K. al-fuṣūl fī al-ṭibb* · trans. Nathan ha-Me'ati (*Sefer ha-Peraqim*), 11.28: הימים אשר יעברו הארבעים יום לא יחשב שיהיה בהם בחראן שיודע ולא במין ממיני ההרקה כלל אך כלות החולי אם שיבושל מעט מעט או ביציאת מורסא. → NM 2:51.

• **קשי יציאת השתן** → קֹשִׁי.

• **יציאת השתן במכאוב** › **strangury:** Hippocrates, *Aphorisms* · trans. Do'eg ha-Edomi (*Sefer Agur*), 3.22 (128) (fol. 55[b]): אמר אפוקרט: פגרי החורף להביא על הגופים קצת המדוים אשר באו עליו בימי הקייץ פרצת קדחת רביעית נפח טחול אפיסת המים הרעים החולי היבש יציאת השתן במכאוב הזלת הבטן והדם וכאב היריכים פוקות מיני השעול וכאב המעי הגדול והחולי המפיל רעת הליחה השחורה וכאב הגרון. → NM 3:107–8.

• *Plur.* **יציאות** › **abscesses:** Arab. خراجات · Ibn al-Jazzār, *Zād al-musāfir wa-qūt al-ḥāḍir* · trans. Moses ibn Tibbon (*Sefer Ṣedat ha-Derakhim*), bk. 7, 23.2: פתילות ליציאות ולחזירים ואלרישה. → NM 1:58.

יְצִיקָה • *Plur.* **יציקות** › I. **embrocations:** Lat. embroca · Bruno Longobucco, *Cyrurgia Magna* · trans. Hillel ben Samuel (*Sefer Keritut*), fol. 84[b]: ראוי שתניח היציקות מקמח חיטים עם דבש ומיץ כרפס אפיאו. → NM 1:26.

› II. **fomentations:** Arab. نطولات · Maimonides, *K. al-fuṣūl fī al-ṭibb* · trans. Nathan ha-Me'ati (*Sefer ha-Peraqim*), 8.2: הדברים העוזרים לבשול הליחות הם כל הדברים המחממים בשווי הנה קצתם הם מאכלים וקצתם משקים וקצתם יציקות וקצתם החבושות. → NM 2:51.

[יצע] • *Part. Hifʿil* **מֵצִיעַ** › **writer [of books]:** Arab. واضع · Maimonides, *Šarḥ fuṣūl Abūqrāṭ* · trans. Anonymous (*Pirqei Abuqraṭ*), introduction (1): אמר השר משה בן עבד האלהי' הקרטובי הישראלי לא אחשוב אחד מן החכמים אשר חברו ספרים חבר ספר במין ממיני החכמות והוא יכוון שלא יובן מה שיכללהו ספרו עד שיפורש. ואלו כיון כן אחד ממציעי הספרים היה כבר בטל תכלית חבור ספרו כי המחבר לא יחבר חיבורו להבין עצמו מה שיכללהו החיבור ההוא. → NM 3:137.

• *Part. Hofʿal* **מֻצָּע** › **composed:** Arab. موضوع · Maimonides, *Šarḥ fuṣūl Abūqrāṭ* · trans. Anonymous (*Pirqei Abuqraṭ*), 1.1 (17): וידוע כי ידיעת זה החלק השביעי כלו ושמירתם מן הספרים המוצעים לכל חלק מהם לא יגיע אליו תכלית פעולת הרופא ולא ישיג לזה החכם השלם במלאכה עד שישמש את האנשים בענין בריאותם וענין חוליהם. → NM 3:137.

יְקִידָה › **fuel:** Arab. وقود / Gr. ὑπέκκαυμα · Maimonides, *Šarḥ fuṣūl Abūqrāṭ* · trans. Zeraḥyah Ḥen (*Pirqei Abuqraṭ*), 1.14 (41): אבל הזקנים חמימותם מועטת ומפני זה לא יצטרכו יקידה אלא הדבר המועט כי חומם תכבה מרוב ימיהם. → NM 3:108.

יָקַע › **to be dislocated:** Arab. انخلع / Gr. ἐξίσταμαι · Maimonides, *Šarḥ fuṣūl Abūqrāṭ* · trans. Moses ibn Tibbon (*Pirqei Abuqraṭ*), 6.59 (351): אמר אבקראט: מי שהיה בו כאב גיד הנשה ותקע יריכו ואחר תשוב הנה התחדש בה לחות דומה כדמות הליחה היוצאת מן הנחירים. → NM 3:108–9.

יָרֵא › **to be careful:** Lat. vereor / Arab. توقّى / Gr. εὐλαβέομαι · Hippocrates, *Aphorisms* ·

trans. Hillel ben Samuel, 4.1 (138) (fol. 19[b]): אמר אפוקרט: אם צריך לנקות ההרה תתנקה מן החדש הרביעי עד השביעי אמנם באלה מעט אבל בקודמים לאלה והבאים אחר אלה ראוי לירוא. → NM 3:109.

יָרַד • ירד ב- · **to affect; to afflict**: Arab. نزل ب- · Maimonides, *K. al-fuṣūl fī al-ṭibb* · trans. Nathan ha-Me'ati (*Sefer ha-Peraqim*), 15.6: הכויה בברזל מלובן או ברפואות השורפות ראוי שתעשה במקומות אשר ירד בהם מן העלות דבר גדול מרוב הליחות ורעתם כמו מה שיהיה בשחינים הרעים. → NM 2:51.

• *Part.* **יוֹרֵד • הוריד הפנימי היורד** → וְרִיד.

• **החלול היורד** → חָלוּל.

• **הנבוב היורד** → נָבוּב.

• **הקצוות אשר הדמע יורד מהן** → קָצֶה.

• *Hif'il* **הוֹרִיד** · **to supply**: Arab. أورد · Maimonides, *K. al-fuṣūl fī al-ṭibb* · trans. Nathan ha-Me'ati (*Sefer ha-Peraqim*), 7.15: אמר משה: החזק שבפנים בשמירה מנפילת העלוף הוא שתשים כל כונתך ומגמתך בכל חולי בשלשת האברים הראשיים ובפי האסטומכה לגודל השתוף אשר בינו ובין האברים הראשים. ושתשמור על אלו האברים כחותיהם וזה בשווי מזגם במה שתורידהו על הגוף ובמה שתשים על האבר מחוץ. → NM 2:51–2.

יְרוּקָה • הרקת הירוקה מלמעלה ומלמטה → הֲרָקָה.

יְרִידָה · I. **catarrh**: Arab. نزل / Gr. κατάρροια · Maimonides, *Šarḥ fuṣūl Abūqrāṭ* · trans. Moses ibn Tibbon (*Pirqei Abuqraṭ*), 3.31 (137): אמר אבקראט: ואולם הישישים הנה יקרה להם רוע הנשימה והירידה אשר יקרה עמה השעול וטפטוף השתן ועצירתו וכאבי הפרקים וכאבי הכליות והסבוב והשתוק והנגעים הרעים וחכוך הגוף והיקיצה ורכות הטבע ולחות בעינים והנחירים וחושך הראות ולובן העינים וכבדות השמע ואלזרקה פירו׳ מראה החשמל. → NM 3:110–1.

· II. **decline (of a disease)**: Arab. إنحطاط · Maimonides, *Šarḥ fuṣūl Abūqrāṭ* · trans. Moses ibn Tibbon (*Pirqei Abuqraṭ*), 2.1 (53): והעתים אשר תועיל בהם השינה הוא אחר הכלות התחלת העונה או המורסא וכל שכן בעת התכלית. והיותר מועלה שתהיה השינה עת הירידה. → NM 3:110.

· III. **relaxation**: Arab. إنحطاط / Gr. ὑποκαταβαίνειν · Maimonides, *Šarḥ fuṣūl Abūqrāṭ* · trans. Moses ibn Tibbon (*Pirqei Abuqraṭ*), 1.7 (34): אמר אבקראט: וכאשר היה החולי חד מאד הנה הכאבים אשר בתכלית האחרון יבואו בו בתחילה וראוי בהכרח שתעשה בו ההנהגה אשר בתכלית האחרון מן הדקות. וכאשר לא יהיה כן אבל יהיה סובל מן ההנהגה מה שהוא יותר עב מזה הנה ראוי שתהיה הירידה לפי רפיון החולי וחסרונו מן התכלית האחרון. → NM 3:109–10.

• **ירידת המים** · **cataract**: a) Al-Rāzī, *K. al-Manṣūrī* · trans. Shem Tov ben Isaac (*Sefer Almansur*), Mem 17 (54): מראיר וב״מ מררות: כלם חמים לוטשים חשכת העין ומונעים ירידת המים בהם. → NM 2:13.

b) Arab. نزول الماء · Maimonides, *K. al-fuṣūl fī al-ṭibb* · trans. Nathan ha-Me'ati (*Sefer ha-Peraqim*), 7.69: הלחות הבציית אשר בעין בהיותה יותר או פחות על הראוי תזיק בראות. וכשתתעבה יחסר יציאת הראות עד שלא יראה הדברים הרחוקים ולא יבאר הדברים הקרובים. וכשתתעבה בתכלית העובי כמו מה שיקרה בירידת המים שיצר הראות. → NM 2:52.

• ירידת המים בעין · **cataract**: a) Arab. نزول الماء · Maimonides, *K. al-fuṣūl fī al-ṭibb* · trans. Zeraḥyah Ḥen (*Sefer ha-Peraqim*), 7.69: הלחות הלבנית אם היא יותר או פחות מן הראוי תזיק בראות העין. ואם יתעבה תחסר הראות עד שלא יראה הדברים הרחוקים ולא יתבאר הדברים הקרובים. ואם יתעבה בתכלית כמו שיקרה בירידת המים בעין ימנע הראות. → NM 1:155–6; corr. 4:229.

b) Lat. descensus aque ad oculos; fluxum reumatis ad oculos (Honofredi) · Ibn Zuhr, *Regimen of Health* · trans. Jacob ibn Tibbon (*Hanhagat ha-Beri'ut le-Abu 'Ali ben Zuhr*), ch. 28: ונאמר שכאב הראש כאשר התמיד והתחזק והשקיקה גם כן כאשר התמיד יקרה ממנו ירידת המים בעין ונשירת שער העפעפים. → NM 4:77.

יְרִיעָה • יריעת החלב · **omentum**: Hippocrates, *Aphorisms* · trans. Do'eg ha-Edomi (*Sefer Agur*), 6.58 (350) (fol. 110ª): שברה ונפסקה יריעת החלב תדין כי באמת יתעפש החלב ההוא. → NM 3:111.

• היריעה הלבנה · **conjunctiva**: Arab. الحجاب الملتحم · Ibn al-Jazzār, *Zād al-musāfir wa-qūt al-ḥāḍir* · trans. Moses ibn Tibbon (*Sefer Ṣedat ha-Derakhim*), bk. 2, ch. 1 (fol. 40ᵇ): ואולם הסבה מבפנים הוא מותר יטה אל היריעה הלבנה וינפחה כמו שיקרה לשאר האברים. → NM 4:77.

יָרֵךְ • כף הירך → **כַּף**.

• פחד הירך → **²פַּחַד**.

• *Dual* יְרֵכַיִם • עיקרי הירכים → **עִקָּר**.

• פחדי הירכים → **²פַּחַד**.

• ראשי הירכים → **רֹאשׁ**.

יָרָק • הירק החמוץ · **(lit., the sour plant); prob., a kind of sorrel**: Arab. البقلة الحامضة · Al-Zahrāwī, *K. al-taṣrīf li-man ʿağiza ʿan at-taʾlīf* · trans. Shem Tov ben Isaac (*Sefer ha-Shimmush*), bk. 27, fol. 136ª, col. b: ירקי שדה מיניה רבים והם כלם בכלל ובפרט מולידים מרה שחורה והם רחוקים ממזג האדם ואין ראוי לזון בהם אלא בעת הצורך כירק הססי והירק החמוץ. → NM 4:78.

• הירק הססי · **field mustard [*Sinapis arvensis* L.]**: Arab. البقلة الحرشا · Al-Zahrāwī, *K. al-taṣrīf li-man ʿağiza ʿan at-taʾlīf* · trans. Shem Tov ben Isaac (*Sefer ha-Shimmush*), bk. 27, fol. 136ª, col. b: ירקי שדה מיניה רבים והם כלם בכלל ובפרט מולידים מרה שחורה והם רחוקים ממזג האדם ואין ראוי לזון בהם אלא בעת הצורך כירק הססי והירק החמוץ. → NM 4:78.

יַרְקָנוּת · **greenness**: Arab. خضرة · Maimonides, *K. al-fuṣūl fī al-ṭibb* · trans. Zeraḥyah Ḥen (*Sefer ha-Peraqim*), 15.50: המורסות הבאות מסבת דם המתחדשות מבלתי סבה מבחוץ כשתשרטנו תביא על בעליהם רעה רבה וכל שכן אם תרצה לעשותה בתחילת החולי. אבל כשהחולי יאריך אינו רע שתשרטנו. וכן המורסא הנקראת ריזיפילא בערבי חמרה כשתגיע עניינה לשחרות או למראה העופרת או לירקנות טוב לשרט. → NM 1:156.

יְרַקְרַקּוּת · **jaundice**: Arab. يرقان / Gr. ἴκτερος · Maimonides, *Šarḥ fuṣūl Abūqrāṭ* · trans. Anonymous (*Pirqei Abuqraṭ*), 4.62 (199): אמר אבוקרט: כשקרה הירקרקות בקדחת לפני יום השביעי הוא סימן רע. → NM 3:111.

[ירש] • *Hifʿil* הוֹרִישׁ · **to cause**: Arab. أورث · Maimonides, *K. al-fuṣūl fī al-ṭibb* · trans.

Nathan ha-Me'ati (*Sefer ha-Peraqim*), 20.51: והפירות הרטובים כלם רעים הכימוס ואם יפסדו באסטו' יורישו ארס כסמי המות. → NM 2:52.

[ישן][1] • *Part. Pi'el* מְיַשֵּׁן • *Plur.* **מישנים** • **soporifics**: Arab. منوّمات • Maimonides, *K. al-fuṣūl fī al-ṭibb* • trans. Nathan ha-Me'ati (*Sefer ha-Peraqim*), 8.38: הרפואות המשקיטות הכאבים והם אותם אשר יעורב בהם המרדימים החוש והמישנים אין ראוי שיוקחו אלא במקום שהכאבים הם חזקים וקשים. → NM 2:59.

[ישן][2] • *Hitpa'el* הִתְיַשֵּׁן • **to become chronic**: Arab. أزمن • Al-Zahrāwī, *K. al-taṣrīf li-man 'ağiza 'an at-ta'līf* • trans. Shem Tov ben Isaac (*Sefer ha-Shimmush*), bk. 30, 2.81 (fol. 223[b]): והפלחים יקרו הרבה מצד נגוב הצואה ואומץ המעים וכשיתישנו ולא יועיל בהם סם ראוי לגרדם בפי המסמר גרע. → NM 1:96.

יָשָׁר • **moderate**: Arab. معتدل • Maimonides, *K. al-fuṣūl fī al-ṭibb* • trans. Zeraḥyah Ḥen (*Sefer ha-Peraqim*), 8.2: הדברים אשר יעזרו על בשול הליחות הם כל הדברים אשר יחממו במיצוע קצתם הם מזון וקצתם הם משקים וקצתם טיבולים וקצתם תחבושות והחפיפה הישרה והמרחץ הממוצע הוא מזה הסוג. → NM 1:156.

• **האברים הישרים** → **אֵבֶר**.

• **המעי הישר** → **מְעִי**.

• **העצל הישר מעצלי הבטן** → **עָצָל**.

יְתֵדִי • **sphenoid [bone]**: Arab. وتدي • Ibn Sīnā, *K. al-Qānūn fī al-ṭibb* • trans. Nathan ha-Me'ati (*Sefer ha-Qanun*), bk. 1 (fol. 29[b]): אמנם מושב וכן המוח הוא העצם אשר יסבול וישא שאר העצמות ויאמר לו היתדי. → NM 4:78.

[יתר] • *Part. Pu'al* מְיֻתָּר • **tense**: Arab. موتّر • Maimonides, *K. al-fuṣūl fī al-ṭibb* • trans. Zeraḥyah Ḥen (*Sefer ha-Peraqim*), 1.24: כל מיני תנועות המושקולי ארבעה וזה או שיתקבץ או שיתפשט או שיתעקם או שישאר נמשך מיותר. → NM 1:162.

• *Hitpa'el* הִתְיַתֵּר • **to become tense**: Arab. توتّر • Maimonides, *K. al-fuṣūl fī al-ṭibb* • trans. Zeraḥyah Ḥen (*Sefer ha-Peraqim*), 1.25: אמר משה זה שגמר דעתו במאמרו באלו הארבעה תנועות הוא שהרצון כשישלח הכח הנפשיי בעצבים נוכח מושקולו מן המושקולי כשירצה להכפיל בהם אותו האיבר לצד התחלתו יכפול האבר ההוא. וכן כשירצה להשאיר האבר נמשך תפשוט הרצון אותו המושקולי עם המושקולי שהוא נכחו ויתיתרו יחד. → NM 1:156–7.

יֶתֶר • *Plur.* **יתרים** • **tendons**: Arab أوتار • Maimonides, *K. al-fuṣūl fī al-ṭibb* • trans. Zeraḥyah Ḥen (*Sefer ha-Peraqim*), 1.7: הקשרים העגולים והיתרים יחשוב מי שאין לו עיון בניתוח שהן עצבים ולא היינו כמו כן מכירים אחד מהם לולי רפואת הניתוח. → NM 1:157.

יְתֵרוּת • **stretching**: Arab. توتّر • Maimonides, *Šarḥ fuṣūl Abūqrāṭ* • trans. Zeraḥyah Ḥen (*Pirqei Abuqraṭ*), 5.49 (269): אמר המפרש: כי יחדש בבטן המשכה ויתרות ויעזור על השליה שתהיה נופלת. → NM 3:111.

יֹתֶרֶת • **diaphragm**: Arab. حجاب • Maimonides, *Šarḥ fuṣūl Abūqrāṭ* • trans. Moses ibn Tibbon (*Pirqei Abuqraṭ*), 4.18 (155): אמר אבקראט: הכאבים אשר יהיו למעלה מהיותרת יורו על שההרקה ברפואה מלמעלה והכאבים אשר מלמטה מן היותרת יורו על שההרקה ברפואה מלמטה. → NM 3:105–6.

כ

כְּאֵב • כאב המוח · **coma; faint; swoon; unconsciousness**: Arab. إغماء · Galen, attr., *Prohibition of Burial* · trans. Judah al-Ḥarizi (*Sefer Issur ha-Qevurah le-Galienus*), par. 1: אני הנחתי ספר בד׳ מאמרים. הראשון מי שיקבר ועודנו חי מפני כאב המוח. → NM 4:78.

• **כאב המעי** · **colic**: Hippocrates, *Aphorisms* · trans. Do'eg ha-Edomi (*Sefer Agur*), 3.22 (128) (fol. 55[b]): אמר אפוקרט: פגרי החורף להביא על הגופים קצת המדוים אשר באו עליו בימי הקייץ פרצת קדחת רביעית נפח טחול אפיסת המים הרעים החולי היבש יציאת השתן במכאוב הזלת הבטן והדם וכאב היריכים פוקות מיני השעול וכאב המעי הגדול והחולי המפיל רעת הליחה השחורה וכאב הגרון. → NM 3:111–2.

• **כאב מעים** · **colic**: Arab. مغس · Maimonides, *K. al-fuṣūl fī al-ṭibb* · trans. Nathan ha-Me'ati (*Sefer ha-Peraqim*), 12.7: ואמנם הרפואה המשלשלת מחדשת לבעל הענין הזה כאב מעים ועקיצה ועלוף ולא יורק דבר שיהיה לו שעור. → NM 2:52–3.

• **כאב המעיים הדקים** · **severe colic**: Gr. εἰλεοί · Hippocrates, *Aphorisms* · trans. Joseph Delmedigo, 3.22 (128): ובחורף יקרו רוב חולאי הקיץ וקדחות רביעיות מעורבבת ועובי הטחול והשקוי והשדפון וטפטוף השתן וחלקות הבטן ושלשול הדם וכאב גיד הנשה ואסכרה וגניחה וכאב המעים הדקים והכפיון והשוטות והשחורה. → NM 3:112.

• **כאב הצדדים** · **pleurisy**: Hippocrates, *Aphorisms* · trans. Do'eg ha-Edomi (*Sefer Agur*), 3.23 (129) (fol. 55[b]): צרות יום הקור הם כאב הצדדים ותחת הצלעות והריאה וזוב הנחירים והשזרה סתימת המקורות ותרדמת הגוף. → NM 3:112.

• **כאב הקיבה** · **cholera**: Arab. هيضة · Maimonides, *Šarḥ fuṣūl Abūqrāṭ* · trans. Anonymous (*Pirqei Abuqraṭ*), 1.12 (39): אמר המפרש: מטבע החולי עצמו תדע האם קצהו ימהר או יאחר. כי מדוה הצד ומדוה הריאה ומדוה הטרפש הם חליים חדים והאסכרה וכאב הקיבה וחולי הקווץ הם חליים חדים מאד. → NM 3:113.

• **כאב קשרי העצמות** · **gout**: Hippocrates, *Aphorisms* · trans. Do'eg ha-Edomi (*Sefer Agur*), 6.49 (341) (fol. 107[b]): ספור זמן רפואת צמח הצומח במי שסובל כאב קשרי העצמות לסוף מ׳ יום. → NM 3:113.

• **כאב הראות** · **ophthalmia**: Hippocrates, *Aphorisms* · trans. Do'eg ha-Edomi (*Sefer Agur*), 3.21 (127) (fol. 55[a]): ערך ימי הקייץ להוליד הקדחת מחודדת גם שלישית והקיא ואפיסת הלב כאב הראות והשמע חבורות הפה ומיני השחין הדק. → NM 3:113–4.

• **כאב הריאה** · **pneumonia**: Hippocrates, *Aphorisms* · trans. Do'eg ha-Edomi (*Sefer Agur*), 3.23 (129) (fol. 55[b]): צרות יום הקור הם כאב הצדדים ותחת הצלעות והריאה וזוב הנחירים והשזרה סתימת המקורות ותרדמת הגוף. → NM 3:113.

• **כאב תחת הצלעות** · **pleurisy**: Hippocrates, *Aphorisms* · trans. Do'eg ha-Edomi (*Sefer Agur*), 5.8 (228) (fol. 81[a]): גדל כאב תחת הצלעות אם לא יתרפא עד י״ד יום לאות כי יקבץ שם עב טיט ויעבר עליו לחולי אחר. → NM 3:114.

[כאה] • *Nif'al* **נִכְאָה** · **to be emaciated**: Arab. انتهك · Maimonides, *Šarḥ fuṣūl Abūqrāṭ* · trans. Zeraḥyah Ḥen (*Pirqei Abuqraṭ*), 2.35 (87): אמר המפרש: המוֹתֶן במה שבין הערוה והטבור יהיו חלקי הבטן שלשה המקומות אשר תחת החלצים וסמוך לטבור והמותן ובהיות אותם המקומות יותר עבים הוא יותר טוב. ובהיותם כחושים העניין יותר רע וזה כי הוא סימן רע ⟨...⟩ ושהוא יורה על חולשת אותם האיברים אשר נכאו ונתכו. → NM 3:114.

• *Part. Nif'al* נִכְאָה • **emaciated**: Arab. منهوك / Gr. ἐκτετηκός · Maimonides, *Šarḥ fuṣūl Abūqrāṭ* · trans. Zeraḥyah Ḥen (*Pirqei Abuqraṭ*), 2.35 (87): אמר בקראט: היותר טוב בכל חולי הוא שיהיה מה שסמוך לטבור ולעצם שלערוה לו עובי וכשיהיה רקיק מאד נכאה זה רע ובהיות זה כמו כן השלשול בזה פחד. → NM 3:155–6.

כָּבֵד¹ • **חצר הכבד** → **חָצֵר**.

כָּבֵד² • *Plur.* **כבדים** • **כבדי הלשון** • **people who lisp**: Gr. τραυλοί · Hippocrates, *Aphorisms* · trans. Joseph Delmedigo, 6.32 (324): כבדי הלשון לרוב הם נאחזים משלשול בטן ארוך. → NM 3:115.

• **כבדי הפה** • **people who lisp**: Hippocrates, *Aphorisms* · trans. Do'eg ha-Edomi (*Sefer Agur*), 6.32 (324) (fol. 103[b]): כבדי הפה הנקראים טרבולי בסגולה טפלים בדיאריאה ארוכה ונקראים בלבי ונעשה או מרוב לחות המוח או מרטיבות הלשון או שניהם יחד. → NM 3:115.

כֹּבֶד • **כובד חולת השתן** • **strangury**: Hippocrates, *Aphorisms* · trans. Do'eg ha-Edomi (*Sefer Agur*), 3.16 (122) (fol. 53[b]): אמר אפוקרט: כח יבשות האויר בהמנע הגשם יוליד תחלואי העיניים כאב קשרי הדבקים כובד הזלת השתן ונזילת דם. → NM 3:115.

כִּבּוּס • *Plur.* **כיבוסים** • **evacuation; purgation**: Hippocrates, *Aphorisms* · trans. Do'eg ha-Edomi (*Sefer Agur*), 4.4 (141) (fol. 59[b]): אמר אפוקרט: בימי הקייץ תרגיל רוב כיבוסיך למעלה ובימי הקור למטה. → NM 3:115–6.

[כבס] • *Part. Pu'al* **מְכֻבָּס** • **clean**: Hippocrates, *Aphorisms* · trans. Do'eg ha-Edomi (*Sefer Agur*), 2.10 (62) (fol. 35[b]): גוף אשר אינו מכובס אם ירבה לאכל יזיק אליו ויוסיף חולי. → NM 3:130.

כַּד • **blunt**: Arab. أفطس · Al-Zahrāwī, *K. al-taṣrīf li-man ʿağiza ʿan at-taʾlīf* · trans. Shem Tov ben Isaac (*Sefer ha-Shimmush*), bk. 30, 2.85 (fol. 224[b]): וזאת צורת הכלי יהיה קצהו האחד הכפוף חד והקצה האחר בלתי חד והקצה הדק לא יהיה בדקות מסמר הגרע אבל יהיה כד מעט. → NM 1:96.

כובד → **כֹּבֶד**.

כּוֹבַע • **שפוי כובע** → **שִׁפּוּי**.

כָּוָה • *Part.* **כּוֹוֶה** • **הסם הכווה** → **סַם**.

כּוֹוֶה (*Part.*) → **כָּוָה**.

כִּוּוּץ (see also: קִוּוּץ) • I. **contraction**: Arab. تقلّص · Maimonides, *K. al-fuṣūl fī al-ṭibb* · trans. Zeraḥyah Ḥen (*Sefer ha-Peraqim*), 1.71: לתנועות כל המושקולי צד אחד והוא הכווץ והקבוץ אל התחלתו. → NM 1:157.

• II. **spasm**: Arab. تشنّج · Al-Zahrāwī, *K. al-taṣrīf li-man ʿağiza ʿan at-taʾlīf* · trans. Shem Tov ben Isaac (*Sefer ha-Shimmush*), bk. 30, 1.6 (fol. 204[a]): וראוי להזהר שלא לכוות כלל הנטייה המתחדשת מן הנגוב וכווץ העצב. → NM 1:96.

כוורת → **כַּוֶּרֶת**.

כּוֹזֵב (*Part.*) → **כָּזַב**.

כוח → **כֹּחַ**.

כּוּלְיָא (*Aram.*) • **kidney**: Arab. كلية · a) Al-Zahrāwī, *K. al-taṣrīf li-man ʿağiza ʿan at-taʾlīf* · trans. Shem Tov ben Isaac (*Sefer ha-Shimmush*), bk. 30, 1.37 (fol. 206[b]): כשיתחדש בכליות כאב מרוח עבה או קרירות ויחסר בסבתם המשגל ראוי לכוותו במתניו על עצם הכליות כויה אחת על כל כוליא וכוליא במכוה המסמרי אשר קדם זכרו. → NM 1:96.

b) Maimonides, *K. al-fuṣūl fī al-ṭibb* · trans. Nathan ha-Me'ati (*Sefer ha-Peraqim*), 1.62: הכוליא הימנית יותר גבוהה עד שבקצת בעלי החיים נוגעת לכבד. → NM 2:53.

[כון] • *Pi'el* **כִּוֵּן** · **to advise:** Arab. أرشد · Maimonides, *K. al-fuṣūl fī al-ṭibb* · trans. Nathan ha-Me'ati (*Sefer ha-Peraqim*), 21.67: לכן אכוין לשמור טבעי הסמים המורגלים להעשות הרבה בכל מקום מפורסמים שמותיהם היורדים בתוך הגוף. → NM 2:53.

• *Part. Pu'al* **מְכֻוָּן** • **השיעור המכוון** → **שִׁעוּר**.

כּוֹס • *Plur.* **כוסות** • **הכוסות המוצצים** · **cupping glasses:** Arab. المحاجم · Maimonides, *K. al-fuṣūl fī al-ṭibb* · trans. Nathan ha-Me'ati (*Sefer ha-Peraqim*), 9.119: הרקת ארס בעלי החיים מן העקוץ ברפואות המושכות משיכה חזקה וישנוהו ויעתיקוהו ממה שהוא עליו אם ברפואות משנות איכות הארס או ברפואות משנות עצמיותו. ומה שמושך משיכה חזקה מבלי חמום קרני המציצה החלולים והכוסות המוצצים. → NM 2:53.

• **כוסות הרחם** · **cotyledons:** Gr. κοτυληδών, *Plur.* κοτυληδόνες · Hippocrates, *Aphorisms* · trans. Joseph Delmedigo, 5.45 (265): והממוצעות בבשר עם (*אם) מפילות בחדש השני או השלישי בלי סבה מבוארת תדע שכוסות הרחם מליאים מליחה דבקיית ואינן יכולים להחזיק העובר מפני הכובד וקשורי השוליא נפרקים. → NM 3:116.

כּוּפְּרָא (*Aram.*) • *Plur.* **כופרי** · **envelope, spathe of the palm flower:** Arab. جفرّى ; كفرّى · Al-Zahrāwī, *K. al-taṣrīf li-man 'ağiza 'an at-ta'līf* · trans. Shem Tov ben Isaac (*Sefer ha-Shimmush*), bk. 27, fol. 140[a], col. a: הכופרי והוא לולבי הדקל הרך הנקרא בלשונם אלג'פרי קודם יביא פריו קרוב מטבע הקור של דקל. → NM 4:78–9.

כַּוֶּרֶת • **זוהמת הכוורת** → **זֻהֲמָה**.

כּוֹרֵת • *Plur.* **כורתים** · **surgeons:** Lat. cyrurgici · Bruno Longobucco, *Cyrurgia Magna* · trans. Hillel ben Samuel (*Sefer Keritut*), fol. 4[b]: כונת הכורתים צריך שיהיה על ג' מינים: האחד הדבקת החלקים שנפרדו. → NM 1:26–7.

כּוּתָּח · **garum:** Arab. مرّي · Maimonides, *K. al-fuṣūl fī al-ṭibb* · trans. Zeraḥyah Ḥen (*Sefer ha-Peraqim*), 17.33: ראוי להקדים תחילה מכל מה שהאדם אוכל ושותה מה שיהיה מחליק לטבע כמו היינות המתוקים והירקות המחליקות הנעשות עם השמן והכותח. → NM 1:157.

כָּזַב • *Part.* **כּוֹזֵב** • **עלעות כוזבות** → **צֶלַע**.

כֹּחַ • **חסרון הכח** → **חֶסְרוֹן**.

• **הכח הטוחן** · **the digestive faculty:** Judah ben Jacob, *Sefer Hanhagat ha-Beri'ut*, 8.1: והשלישי הכח הטוחן והוא אשר יבשל המאכלים הנמשכים ויטחון אותם. → NM 4:79.

• **הכח המפרנס** · **the nutritive faculty:** Arab. القوة الغاذية · Maimonides, *K. al-fuṣūl fī al-ṭibb* · trans. Zeraḥyah Ḥen (*Sefer ha-Peraqim*), 1.72: והכח אשר יפרנס האבר עד שיצמח ויגדל או שיחליף עליו מה שהותך ממנו הוא הכח המפרנס. → NM 1:164–5.

• **הכח המשליך** · **the expulsive faculty:** Judah ben Jacob, *Sefer Hanhagat ha-Beri'ut*, 8.1: והרביעי הכח המשליך והוא אשר ישליך הפסולת הנותר מן המאכלים אחר קחת האברים מהם כל צרכם. → NM 4:79.

• **נפילת כח** → **נְפִילָה**.

• **הכח העוצר** · **the retentive faculty:** Judah ben Jacob, *Sefer Hanhagat ha-Beri'ut*, 8.1: והשני הכח העוצר והוא המעכב אותם ומונע יציאתם עד שתפעל בם התולדה מפעלה. → NM 4:79.

כָּחוּשׁ (*Pass. Part.*) → **כָּחַשׁ**.

כָּחַל · **to apply as a collyrium:** Arab. اكتحل · Ibn al-Jazzār, *Zād al-musāfir wa-qūt al-ḥāḍir* · trans. Moses ibn Tibbon (*Sefer Ṣedat ha-Derakhim*), bk. 2, ch. 4 (fol. 45[a]): ויעשה ממנו גרגרים קטנים ויקח ממנו אחת וישרה אותה במי מטר ויטיף ממנו בעין או תחכך אותה על המשחזת ויכחול בו. → NM 4:79–80.

• *Hofʿal* **הֻכְחַל** · **to be used as a collyrium:** Arab. اكتحل · Ibn Sīnā, *K. al-adwiya al-qalbiya* · trans. Anonymous (*Sammim Libbiyim*), fol. 125[a]: ולא יופשט חזקו ברוח זולת רוח אבל הוא נאות לעצם הרוח כלו עד שהוא יועיל לרוח אשר במוח למה שנתפרסם ממנו מחזוק הראות כאשר יוכחל בו. → NM 4:80.

כָּחַשׁ • *Pass. Part.* **כָּחוּשׁ** · **dry:** Arab. قحل / Gr. καρφαλέος · Maimonides, *Šarḥ fuṣūl Abūqrāṭ* · trans. Moses ibn Tibbon (*Pirqei Abuqraṭ*), 5.71 (291): אמר אבקראט: מי שהיה עורו נמשך כחוש קשה הנה הוא ימות מבלתי זיעה ומי שהיה עורו רפה ספוגי הנה הוא ימות עם זיעה. → NM 3:116–7.

כַּחַשׁ • **קדחות חצמוק והכחש** → קַדַּחַת.

כיבוס → כִּבּוּס.

כִּיּוֹר • **צנור הכיור** → צִנּוֹר.

כִּיס · **hernia:** Arab. قيلة · Maimonides, *K. al-fuṣūl fī al-ṭibb* · trans. Zeraḥyah Ḥen (*Sefer ha-Peraqim*), 9.102: ויש חולי קטון ומקומו גדול והכיס אשר ירדו בו מעט מן המעים יותר גדול ויותר חזק וכן בשאר החליים. → NM 1:158.

• **כיס הבשר** · **sarcocele:** Arab. قيلة اللحم · Maimonides, *K. al-fuṣūl fī al-ṭibb* · trans. Zeraḥyah Ḥen (*Sefer ha-Peraqim*), 23.57: קושי הבצים נקרא כיס הבשר כמו שנקרא הלחות המימיי המתקבץ בקרומות אשר סביבות הבצים כיס המים. אבל כיס החלב וכיס המעים והחולי המורכב מהם כלומר כיס החלב והמעים הם שמות בדויים מן הרופאים החדשים אשר קורין כל המורסות המתחדשות במה שסמוך הביצים כיס בערבי קילה. → NM 1:158.

• **חגרת הבשר בכיס** → חֲגֹרָה.

• **כיס החלב** · **epiplocele:** Arab. قيلة الثرب · Maimonides, *K. al-fuṣūl fī al-ṭibb* · trans. Zeraḥyah Ḥen (*Sefer ha-Peraqim*), 23.57: קושי הבצים נקרא כיס הבשר כמו שנקרא הלחות המימיי המתקבץ בקרומות אשר סביבות הבצים כיס המים. אבל כיס החלב וכיס המעים והחולי המורכב מהם כלומר כיס החלב והמעים הם שמות בדויים מן הרופאים החדשים אשר קורין כל המורסות המתחדשות במה שסמוך הביצים כיס בערבי קילה. → NM 1:159.

• **כיס הלב** · **pericardium:** Arab. غلاف القلب · Ibn Sīnā, *K. al-Qānūn fī al-ṭibb* · trans. Nathan ha-Me'ati (*Sefer ha-Qanun*), bk. 1 (fol. 64[a]): ואחד מנכח כיס הלב ומשלח אליו שריגים רבים מתחלקים כשער וזנין אותו. → NM 4:80.

• **כיס המים** · I. **hydrocele:** Arab. قيلة الماء · Maimonides, *K. al-fuṣūl fī al-ṭibb* · trans. Zeraḥyah Ḥen (*Sefer ha-Peraqim*), 23.57: קושי הבצים נקרא כיס הבשר כמו שנקרא הלחות המימיי המתקבץ בקרומות אשר סביבות הבצים כיס המים. אבל כיס החלב וכיס המעים והחולי המורכב מהם כלומר כיס החלב והמעים הם שמות בדויים מן הרופאים החדשים אשר קורין כל המורסות המתחדשות במה שסמוך הביצים כיס בערבי קילה. → NM 1:159.

· II. **urinary bladder:** Judah ben Jacob, *Sefer Hanhagat ha-Beri'ut*, 8.1: והכליות מושכות המים הרעים אשר בדם ומתפרנסות ממעט האדמימות הנשאר בו ושולחות המותר אל כיס המים והוא מזומן לקבלו ולהוציאו לחוץ על פי האבר הקטן והוא השתן. → NM 4:80.

• **כיס המעים** · **enterocele**: Arab. قيلة الأمعاء · Maimonides, *K. al-fuṣūl fī al-ṭibb* · trans. Zeraḥyah Ḥen (*Sefer ha-Peraqim*), 23.57: קושי הבצים נקרא כיס הבשר כמו שנקרא הלחות המימי המתקבץ בקרומות אשר סביבות הבצים כיס המים. אבל כיס החלב וכיס המעים והחולי המורכב מהם כלומר כיס החלב והמעים הם שמות בדויים מן הרופאים החדשים אשר קורין כל המורסות המתחדשות במה שסמוך הביצים כיס בערבי קילה. → NM 1:159.

• **כיס מקוה המים** · **urinary bladder**: Arab. مثانة · Al-Zahrāwī, *K. al-taṣrīf li-man ʿağiza ʿan at-taʾlīf* · trans. Shem Tov ben Isaac (*Sefer ha-Shimmush*), bk. 30, 1.38 (fol. 206[a]): כשיתחדש בכיס מקוה המים חולשה ורפיון מקרירות ולחויות עד שלא יוכל להחזיק השתן ראוי לכוותו כויה אחת למטה מן הטיבור על הכיס במקום שיתחיל שער הזקן התחתון. → NM 1:97.

• **כיס המרה** · **gallbladder**: Judah ben Jacob, *Sefer Hanhagat ha-Beriʾut*, 8.1: כי הטחול הוכן למשוך ממנה המרה השחורה וכיס המרה לטהר הדם ולנקותו. → NM 4:80–1.

• *Plur.* **כיסים** · **vessels (i.e., blood vessels)**: Arab. أوعية · a) Al-Zahrāwī, *K. al-taṣrīf li-man ʿağiza ʿan at-taʾlīf* · trans. Shem Tov ben Isaac (*Sefer ha-Shimmush*), bk. 30, 2.4 (fol. 209[b]): הכיסים היורדים מן הראש אל העינים. → NM 1:97.

b) Maimonides, *K. al-fuṣūl fī al-ṭibb*· trans. Zeraḥyah Ḥen (*Sefer ha-Peraqim*), 18.8: מי שהרבה במנוחה יוליד בגופו מזה שני מיני המילוי כולם כלומר המילוי אשר לפי הכיסים והמילוי אשר יהיה לפי הכח. → NM 1:158.

כַּךְ • *Plur.* **ככים** · **gums**: Arab. لثة · Ibn al-Jazzār, *Zād al-musāfir wa-qūt al-ḥādir* · trans. Moses ibn Tibbon (*Sefer Ṣedat ha-Derakhim*), bk. 2, ch. 18 (fol. 59[a]): ומהם מקרים נסתרים כמו שירגיש החולה בתוך שניו דפיקה וכאב חזק ויראה גלויה כאלו אין בה חולי ואולם יקרה להם זה מפני רבוי המותרות והגרתם בהם מן הראש או מן האצטו׳ או מחדוד מותרות נפסדות נוטות אשר הם נמשכות אל הככים ר״ל מושבי השנים. → NM 4:81.

כֶּלֶב • **כלב שוטה** · **a mad dog**: Arab. الكَلْب الكَلِب · Ibn al-Jazzār, *Zād al-musāfir wa-qūt al-ḥādir* · trans. Moses ibn Tibbon (*Sefer Ṣedat ha-Derakhim*), bk. 7, cf. 13.1: והטובה שבראיות והאותות עליו גם כן לקחת פת לחם ולמשוח אותה מן הדם היוצא מן המקום הנשוך ואחר כן ישליכנה לכלבים ואם לא יאכלוה ידע כי הנשיכה נשיכת כלב שוטה ואם יאכלוה ידע כי הכלב אשר נשכו משאר הכלבים. → NM 1:59.

כַּלְבִּי • **השנים הכלביים** → שֵׁן.

• **התאוה הכלבית** → תַּאֲוָה.

כָּלָה · **to come to a crisis**: Arab. انقضى / Gr. κρίνομαι · Maimonides, *Šarḥ fuṣūl Abūqrāṭ* · trans. Moses ibn Tibbon (*Pirqei Abuqraṭ*), 4.59 (196): אמר אבקראט: השלישית היותר ארוכה שתהיה תכלה בשבעה סבובים. → NM 3:117.

כְּלוֹנָס • *Plur.* **כלונסות** · **pads**: Arab. رفائد · Al-Zahrāwī, *K. al-taṣrīf li-man ʿağiza ʿan at-taʾlīf* · trans. Shem Tov ben Isaac (*Sefer ha-Shimmush*), bk. 30, introduction (fol. 201[b]): וראיתי אחר מתעסק בזאת המלאכה בכדי חייו אצל קצת קציני ארצותינו ונתחדש לסריס שחור שנשבר שוקו קרוב מן הערקוב ונתחדשה בו חבורה ומהר הסכל בסכלותו והדק השבר על החבורה בכלונסות ובקשישים. → NM 1:97.

[כלח] • *Part. Hofʿal* **מֻכְלָח** · **old**: Arab. هرم · Al-Zahrāwī, *K. al-taṣrīf li-man ʿağiza ʿan at-taʾlīf* · trans. Shem Tov ben Isaac (*Sefer ha-Shimmush*), bk. 27, fol. 142[b], col. b: בשר הכבש המוכלח יותר רע מכל מיני בשר הצאן. → NM 4:81.

כַּלָחוּת · **old age**: Arab. هرم · Al-Zahrāwī, *K. al-taṣrīf li-man ʿağiza ʿan at-taʾlīf* · trans. Shem Tov ben Isaac (*Sefer ha-Shimmush*), bk. 27, fol. 143[a], col. a: ולאכול מבשר הצלעות ולבשלו אספידבאג'ה מתובלת בשווי או לבשלו בדבש וכל שכן הקרוב אל הכלחות. → NM 4:81–2.

כְּלִי • **כלי ברזל** · **knife (i.e., surgical knife)**: Arab. حديد · Al-Zahrāwī, *K. al-taṣrīf li-man ʿağiza ʿan at-taʾlīf* · trans. Shem Tov ben Isaac (*Sefer ha-Shimmush*), bk. 30, 2.74 (fol. 221[a]): וראוי לי שאזכור בזה המאמר הצמח החם אשר יקרה ברחם כשיהיה מן הצמחים המקבצים מוגלא איך תהיה דקירתו בכלי ברזל. → NM 1:97–8.

• **כלי זכוכית** · **cupping glass**: Arab. محجمة / Gr. σικύα · Maimonides, *Šarḥ fuṣūl Abūqrāṭ* · trans. Moses ibn Tibbon (*Pirqei Abuqraṭ*), 5.50 (270): אמר אבקראט: כשתרצה שיעצר דם הנדות שים בכל אחד משדיה כלי זכוכית מן היותר גדולים שיהיו. → NM 3:117.

• **כלי הממשש** · **probe**: Lat. tenta · Bruno Longobucco, *Cyrurgia Magna* · trans. Hillel ben Samuel (*Sefer Keritut*), fol. 37[a]: ואף על פי כן הנגע הבא אל הבשר אינו מכאיב כל כך כמו הבא אל הגיד ובסגולה כאשר יגע בעומקה בכלי הממשש הוא טנטא בלעז. → NM 1:27.

• **כלי המציצה** · **cupping glass**: Arab. محجمة · Ibn al-Jazzār, *Zād al-musāfir wa-qūt al-ḥāḍir* · trans. Moses ibn Tibbon (*Sefer Ṣedat ha-Derakhim*), bk. 1, ch. 10 (fol. 14[b]): ואולם כשיתחמם מחום השמש והאויר הנה הראש יתחמם וימשוך אליו המותרות מכל הגוף כמו שימשוך כלי המציצה. → NM 4:82.

b) Maimonides, *Šarḥ fuṣūl Abūqrāṭ* · trans. Anonymous (*Pirqei Abuqraṭ*), 5.50 (270): אמר אבוקרט: כשתרצה להפסיק דם נדות אשה תשים על כל אחד משדיה כלי המציצה מהגדול שאיפשר להמצ. → NM 3:117.

• **הכלי הנוקב** · **drill**: Arab. مثقب · Al-Zahrāwī, *K. al-taṣrīf li-man ʿağiza ʿan at-taʾlīf* · trans. Shem Tov ben Isaac (*Sefer ha-Shimmush*), bk. 30, 2.2 (fol. 332[b]): אמנם איכות הנקב סביב העצם הנשבר הוא לתת הכלי הנוקב על העצם ולסובבו עד שיודע שהעצם מפולש → NM 1:104 (s.v. מקבת).

• **כלי שעושים ⟨בו⟩ מי ורדים** · **(lit., a vessel for making rose water); alembic**: Arab. أنبيق · Ibn al-Jazzār, *Zād al-musāfir wa-qūt al-ḥāḍir* · trans. Moses ibn Tibbon (*Sefer Ṣedat ha-Derakhim*), bk. 1, ch. 4 (fol. 9[b]): וישים האלקנה בכלי שעושים מי ורדים. → NM 4:82.

כְּלָיָה · **phthisis**: Arab. سلّ · Maimonides, *Šarḥ fuṣūl Abūqrāṭ* · trans. Anonymous (*Pirqei Abuqraṭ*), 1.12 (39): והשקוי וחולי הדאגה וחולי מיעים והכליה והוא נגע הריאה הם חליים ישנים. → NM 3:117–8.

כִּלָּיוֹן · I. **dissipation**: Lat. resolutio / Arab. تحلّل · Galen, *De inaequali intemperie* · trans. David Caslari (*Sefer Roʿa Mezeg Mitḥallef*), 3.2: ואולם הבריאות היותר משובחת משני אלו היא אותה שהיא בכליון. → NM 2:166.

· II. **phthisis**: Arab. سلّ · Maimonides, *Šarḥ fuṣūl Abūqrāṭ* · trans. Anonymous (*Pirqei Abuqraṭ*), 3.29 (135): אמר אבוקרט: ואמנם הבחורים יקרה להם רקיקת דם וכליון וקדחות חדות וכפייה ושאר החליים אלא שרוב מה שיקרה להם הוא מה שזכרנו → NM 3:118.

כְּלִילִי · **coronal**: Arab. إكليلي · Ibn Sīnā, *K. al-Qānūn fī al-ṭibb* · trans. Nathan ha-Meʾati (*Sefer ha-Qanun*), bk. 1 (fol. 29[a]): ומן הראשונים שלב משותף עם המצח קשתי) ונקרא הכלילי כן. → NM 4:82.

כַּלָל • כלל העין · **eyeball:** Arab. مقلة · Ibn Sīnā, *K. al-Qānūn fī al-ṭibb* · trans. Nathan ha-Me'ati (*Sefer ha-Qanun*), bk. 1 (fol. 43[a]): הפרק הרביעי בנתוח עצלי כלל העין ואמנם העצלים המניעים לכלל העין הם עצלים ששה ארבעה מהם בצד הם הארבעה למעלה ולמטה בשתי קצוות העין הנקרא מאקים. → NM 4:82.

כָּמֵהַ (also: כְּמֵהָה) • *Plur.* **כמיהים** · **fungus:** Lat. fungus · Bruno Longobucco, *Cyrurgia Magna* · trans. Hillel ben Samuel (*Sefer Keritut*), fol. 89[b]: והיא מורסא בשרית גדולה ורכה ודומה לכמיהים פונגו בלעז. → NM 1:27.

כְּמֵהָה → כָּמֵהַ.

כַּמּוֹנִי • הכמוני · **the cumin [stomachic]:** Arab. الكموني · Ibn Sīnā, *K. al-adwiya al-qalbiya* · trans. Anonymous (*Sammim Libbiyim*), fol. 133[a]: עוד החולקים מן הרופאים יחשבו שיש מן הטריאק והמטרידיטוס חום עובר הגבול ויעמדו מלהשתמש בשעור חצי משקל ממנו ולא יעמדו מלהשתמש בארבעה משקלים הכמוני ומן הפלפליי. → NM 4:82–3.

כָּמָךְ · **fish brine:** Arab. صير · Al-Zahrāwī, *K. al-taṣrīf li-man ʿağiza ʿan at-taʾlīf* · trans. Shem Tov ben Isaac (*Sefer ha-Shimmush*), bk. 27, fol. 150, col. b: ואמנם הכמך העשוי ממנו חם יבש גורם צמא ולוטש האסטומכא מהליחה הלבנה העבה והתמדתו מפסדת הדם. → NM 4:83.

כֵּן¹ · **basis:** Arab. قاعدة · Ibn Sīnā, *K. al-Qānūn fī al-ṭibb* · trans. Nathan ha-Me'ati (*Sefer ha-Qanun*), bk. 1 (fol. 39[b]): ונבראו העצמות שהכנים שלהם יותר רחבים וראשיהם יותר דקים. → NM 4:83–4.

כֵּן² • *Plur.* **כנים • כיני הפיל** · **marking nut [*Semecarpus anacardium*]:** Arab. بلاذر · Ibn al-Jazzār, *Zād al-musāfir wa-qūt al-ḥādir* · trans. Moses ibn Tibbon (*Sefer Ṣedat ha-Derakhim*), bk. 1, ch. 14 (fol. 21[b]): והיותר מיוחד להועיל בו הרפואה העשויה בכיני הפיל הוא בלאדור כשישתה ממנו בכל יום מדרהם עד שקל במים חמים על צום הנפש. → NM 4:84.

כנדי (also: קנדי) • **סוכר כנדי** → סֻכָּר.

• **סוכרי קנדי** → סֻכָּר.

[כנס] • *Nifʿal* **נִכְנַס** · **to be firmly established:** Arab. تمكّن · Maimonides, *K. al-fuṣūl fī al-ṭibb* · trans. Zeraḥyah Ḥen (*Sefer ha-Peraqim*), 9.65: בכל מיני ההדרוקן הכבד בעצמו הוא אשר לא ישנה מה שיבואנו מן המזון אל הדם בסבת רוע מזג קר שולט על אחד מכלי המזון או אחד מכלי הניפוש וישוב ממנו אל מה שקרוב ממנו מן האברים עד שיגיע הקור בעצם הכבד בשיתוף הגידים והמחלה תכנס בכבד בעצמו ויתחדש ההדרוקן. → NM 1:159.

• *Part. Nifʿal* **נִכְנָס** · **internal:** Arab. داخل / Gr. ἔσω · a) Maimonides, *Šarḥ fuṣūl Abūqrāṭ* · trans. Moses ibn Tibbon (*Pirqei Abuqraṭ*), 7.36 (388): ואם היה הכאב ההוא במקומות הנכנסים הנה יותר קרוב שתהיה המורסא הנק׳ דבילה מב. → NM 3:156.

b) Maimonides, *K. al-fuṣūl fī al-ṭibb* · trans. Nathan ha-Me'ati (*Sefer ha-Peraqim*), 4.36: המנוחה הנכנסת אי אפשר שתדענה באמת בעת מן העתים אך תושג אם יהיה הדפק חזק מאד ותכבוש עליו בידך כבישה חזקה. → NM 2: 66–7.

כָּנָף · **(lit., wing); transverse process:** Arab. جناح / Gr. ἀπόφυσις ἐγκάρσια · Ibn Sīnā, *K. al-Qānūn fī al-ṭibb* · trans. Nathan ha-Me'ati (*Sefer ha-Qanun*), bk. 1 (fol. 32[a]): ומה שיהיה מאלו מונחים לאחור נקרא קוץ וסנסן ומה שיהיה מונח ימין ושמאל נקרא כנף. → NM 4:84.

[כסה] • *Part. Pi'el* **מְכַסֶּה** • **החלב המכסה** → **חֵלֶב**.

• **החלב המכסה (את) הקרב** → **חֵלֶב**.

• **המכסה המבדיל** › **diaphragm:** Lat. diafragma · Bruno Longobucco, *Cyrurgia Magna* · trans. Hillel ben Samuel (*Sefer Keritut*), fol. 5[a]: או שבמכסה המבדיל ונקרא שבר. → NM 1:29–30.

כִּסּוּי › **membrane:** Arab. غشاء · Maimonides, *Šarḥ fuṣūl Abūqrāṭ* · trans. Moses ibn Tibbon (*Pirqei Abuqraṭ*), 5.46 (266): אמר אבקראט: כשתהיה האשה על עניין יוצא מן הטבע בשמנות ולא תתעבר הנה הכסוי הפנימי מכסויי הבטן הנקרא החלב המכסה סותם לה פי הרחם ולא תתעבר עד שתכחיש. → NM 3:118.

כֶּסֶל • **עצם הכסל** → **עֶצֶם**.

• *Plur.* **כסלים** › **inward parts:** Arab. حشا, *Plur.* أحشاء · Al-Zahrāwī, *K. al-taṣrīf li-man ʿağiza ʿan at-taʾlīf* · trans. Shem Tov ben Isaac (*Sefer ha-Shimmush*), bk. 27, fol. 148[b], col. a: איברי העופות: כסלי העוף מיוחסים אל בשרו כיחס כסלי כל בעלי חיים ⟨מיוחסים⟩ אל בשרו. → NM 4:85.

• **מה שלמטה מצדי הכסלים** → **מַטָּה**.

• **תחת הכסלים** → **תַּחַת**.

כָּסַף › **to have appetite:** Arab. اشتهى · Maimonides, *Šarḥ fuṣūl Abūqrāṭ* · trans. Anonymous (*Pirqei Abuqraṭ*), 2.32 (84): וכאשר היה בתחלה לא יכסוף בעבור שהטבע מתעסק בבשול ומעת שמתחיל לכסוף תדע שכבר נתבשלו התערובות ודאי עניינו על הרוב לטוב. → NM 3:118–9.

כֶּסֶף • **סיג הכסף** → **סִיג**.

כַּף › **kneecap; patella:** Lat. rotula · Bruno Longobucco, *Cyrurgia Magna* · trans. Hillel ben Samuel (*Sefer Keritut*), fol. 63[b]: ומצד פנים לא תעשה השמטה בעבור הכף שמונעה. → NM 1:27.

• **כף הירך** › I. **the acetabulum of the femur:** Arab. حقّ الورك · Al-Zahrāwī, *K. al-taṣrīf li-man ʿağiza ʿan at-taʾlīf* · trans. Shem Tov ben Isaac (*Sefer ha-Shimmush*), bk. 27, fol. 231[b]. → NM 1:98.

› II. **hip joint:** Arab. ورك · Al-Zahrāwī, *K. al-taṣrīf li-man ʿağiza ʿan at-taʾlīf* · trans. Shem Tov ben Isaac (*Sefer ha-Shimmush*), bk. 30, 1.40 (fol. 203): לפעמים תשתפכנה לחויות עבות אל כף הירך ותהיינה סבה לצאתו ממקומו. → NM 1:98.

כָּפוּל (*Pass. Part.*) → **כָּפַל**.

כְּפוֹרִי • **הלחות הכפורית** → **לַחוּת**.

כִּפְיוֹן › **epilepsy:** Arab. صرع · a) Al-Zahrāwī, *K. al-taṣrīf li-man ʿağiza ʿan at-taʾlīf* · trans. Shem Tov ben Isaac (*Sefer ha-Shimmush*), bk. 27, fol. 132[a], col. a: והכווץ והמשיכה המביאים אל הכפיון. → NM 4:85.

b) Hippocrates, *Aphorisms* · trans. Nathan ha-Me'ati, 2.45 (97) (fol. 38[a]): אמר אבוקרט: בעל הכפיון אם יהיה בחור הנה רפואתו תהיה בייחוד בהעתקו בשנים והארצות וההנהגה. → NM 3:119.

כְּפִיפָה • **כפיפת הארכובה** › **the knee pit (popliteal fossa):** Arab. مثنى الركبة · Ibn Sīnā, *K. al-Qānūn fī al-ṭibb* · trans. Nathan ha-Me'ati (*Sefer ha-Qanun*), bk. 1, fol. 67[a]: והאמצעי נמתח בכפיפת הארכובה יורד. → NM 4:85.

• **כפיפת המרפק** › **the elbow pit (cubital fossa)**: Arab. معطف المرفق · Ibn Sīnā, *K. al-Qānūn fī al-ṭibb* · trans. Nathan ha-Me'ati (*Sefer ha-Qanun*), bk. 1 (fols. 65[b]–66[a]): והשני פונה אל מקום כפיפת המרפק בחיצוני הקנה ומתערב בעומק בשריג גם כן מן האצ⟨י⟩לי. → NM 4:85–6.

כָּפַל › **to be flexed**: Arab. انثنى · Maimonides, *K. al-fuṣūl fī al-ṭibb* · trans. Zeraḥyah Ḥen (*Sefer ha-Peraqim*), 1.25: אמר משה זה שגמר דעתו במאמרו באלו הארבעה תנועות הוא שהרצון כשישלח הכח הנפשיי בעצבים נוכח מושקולו מן המושקולי כשירצה להכפיל בהם אותו האיבר לצד התחלתו יכפול האבר ההוא. וכן כשירצה להשאיר האבר נמשך תפשוט הרצון אותו המושקולי עם המושקולי שהוא נכחו ויתיתרו יחד. → NM 1:160.

• *Pass. Part.* **כָּפוּל** › I. **flexed**: Arab. مثني · Maimonides, *K. al-fuṣūl fī al-ṭibb* · trans. Zeraḥyah Ḥen (*Sefer ha-Peraqim*), 1.25: ואמנם תנועת הפישוט היא רצונית והיא תנועת המושקולי במקרה כי הרצון כשירצה לפשוט האבר הכפול תבטל הכח הנפשיי מן המושקולי אשר נכפל מקווץ ושולח אותו הכח למושקולי הנכחי. → NM 1:159.

› II. **repeated**: Arab. مكرّر · Maimonides, *Šarḥ fuṣūl Abūqrāṭ* · trans. Moses ibn Tibbon (*Pirqei Abuqraṭ*), introduction (13): ופרקי אבקראט אלו יש מהם פרקים מסופקים צריכים לפירוש ומהם מבוארים בעצמם ומהם כפולים ומהם מה שלא יועיל במלאכת הרפואות ומהם רעיון פשוט נאמר בלי עיון. → NM 3:119.

• *Nif'al* **נִכְפַּל** › **to be flexed**: Arab. انثنى · Maimonides, *K. al-fuṣūl fī al-ṭibb* · trans. Zeraḥyah Ḥen (*Sefer ha-Peraqim*), 1.25: ואמנם תנועת הפישוט היא רצונית והיא תנועת המושקולי במקרה כי הרצון כשירצה לפשוט האבר הכפול תבטל הכח הנפשיי מן המושקולי אשר נכפל מקווץ ושולח אותו הכח למושקולי הנכחי. → NM 1:160.

• *Part. Nif'al* **נִכְפָּל** • **יותר נכפל** › **more frequent**: Arab. أكثر تكررا · Ibn Sīnā, *K. al-Qānūn fī al-ṭibb* · trans. Nathan ha-Me'ati (*Sefer ha-Qanun*), bk. 1 (fol. 44[b]): כי תנועות איברי הרקה והשפה יותר רבי המספר ויותר נכפלים ושוקדים. → NM 4:86.

• *Hif'il* **הִכְפִּיל** › **to flex**: Arab. ثنى · Maimonides, *K. al-fuṣūl fī al-ṭibb* · trans. Zeraḥyah Ḥen (*Sefer ha-Peraqim*), 1.25: אמר משה זה שגמר דעתו במאמרו באלו הארבעה תנועות הוא שהרצון כשישלח הכח הנפשיי בעצבים נוכח מושקולו מן המושקולי כשירצה להכפיל בהם אותו האיבר לצד התחלתו יכפול האבר ההוא. וכן כשירצה להשאיר האבר נמשך תפשוט הרצון אותו המושקולי עם המושקולי שהוא נכחו ויתיתרו יחד. → NM 1:160.

כֶּפֶל • **כפל הארכובה** › **the knee pit (popliteal fossa)**: Arab. مثنى الركبة · Ibn Sīnā, *K. al-Qānūn fī al-ṭibb* · trans. Zeraḥyah Ḥen (*Sefer ha-Qanun*), bk. 1 (fol. 35[a]): והאמצעי יתפשט במקום כפל הארכובה ויורד. → NM 4:86.

• **כפל הקובדי** › **the elbow pit (cubital fossa)**: Arab. معطف المرفق · Ibn Sīnā, *K. al-Qānūn fī al-ṭibb* · trans. Zeraḥyah Ḥen (*Sefer ha-Qanun*), bk. 1 (fol. 34[b]): והשני ישתלח אל כפל הקובדי בנראה של הזרוע ויתערבו בו שעיפים מן השחיי. → NM 4:86.

כְּרוּב • **תבשיל הכרוב** → **תַּבְשִׁיל**.

[כרח] • *Hif'il* **הִכְרִיחַ** › I. **to be most likely**: Arab. رجّح · Maimonides, *K. al-fuṣūl fī al-ṭibb* · trans. Nathan ha-Me'ati (*Sefer ha-Peraqim*), 16.17: והנה הכריח בזאת העלה שיהיה סבתו העצר הזרע באשה והפסדו שם ואריכות ביאור זה באחרית ההודעה. → NM 2:54.

› II. **to induce**: Arab. استدعى · Maimonides, *K. al-fuṣūl fī al-ṭibb* · trans. Nathan ha-Me'ati (*Sefer ha-Peraqim*), 10.70: ואמנם אם לא יתנועעו אל האסטומכה לא תכריח הקיא

ובחר מהרפואות אשר תפעל בהם אחד מן ההרקות מה שלא יחמם או שיחמם חמום מעט. → NM 2:54.

כְּרִיתָה • הכריתה בברזל · **cutting; surgery:** Lat. sectio · Arnau de Vilanova, *Medicationis Parabole* · trans. Abraham Avigdor (*Pirqei Arnauṭ de Vilanova*), 3.7 (44): כמו שהכויה והכריתה בברזל קשה לסבלם כן הרפואות החזקות יקשה ענינם אל הגופים או אל האיברים קלי ההפעלות. → NM 4:86.

כְּרִיתוּת · **surgery:** Lat. cyrurgia · Bruno Longobucco, *Cyrurgia Magna* · trans. Hillel ben Samuel (*Sefer Keritut*), fol. 3[a]: זה ספר כריתות אשר חברו מאשטרו ברונו בלשון נוצרי. → NM 1:27; cf. *Sefer ha-Yosher* (Ms. Oxford, Bodleian Library, Opp. 180 (cat. Neubauer 2134), fol. 19[a]): ואזכור עזרם בשער הכריתות.

כַּרְכֶּשֶׁה · **rectum:** Arab. مبعر · Al-Zahrāwī, *K. al-taṣrīf li-man ʿağiza ʿan at-taʾlīf* · trans. Shem Tov ben Isaac (*Sefer ha-Shimmush*), bk. 30, 2.80 (fol. 222[b]): ועוד יהיה ממיני הגרגתני מין מפולש אל הכרכשה ואל המעי או בלתי מפולש. → NM 1:98.

כֶּרֶם • תבשיל בסר הכרם → תַּבְשִׁיל.

כַּרְמֶל • גרש כרמל → גֶּרֶשׂ.

• **הכרמל המהובהב באש** · **green toasted wheat:** Arab. فريك · Al-Zahrāwī, *K. al-taṣrīf li-man ʿağiza ʿan at-taʾlīf* · trans. Shem Tov ben Isaac (*Sefer ha-Shimmush*), bk. 27, fol. 124[a], col. 1: הכרמל המהובהב באש העשוי מן השבלים אשר יש בהם מותר לחות ולא יגמר בשולם. → NM 4:87.

כֶּרֶס • חולי מכרס הבטן → חֹלִי.

• **חלב הכרס** → חֵלֶב.

כַּשִּׁיל · **pickax (i.e., a phlebotome):** Arab. فأس · Al-Zahrāwī, *K. al-taṣrīf li-man ʿağiza ʿan at-taʾlīf* · trans. Shem Tov ben Isaac (*Sefer ha-Shimmush*), bk. 30, 2.95 (fol. 229[a]): ואיכות הקזתו על מה שאגיד והוא להדק צואר החולה במצנפת עד שיראה הגיד ואחר לקחת הכלי הנקרא כשיל. → NM 1:98.

כַּת · **a detached or distinct part or portion; a piece or bit; [or somewhat] of a thing and of men (i.e., a class, division, party, or portion thereof):** Arab. طائفة · Ibn Sīnā, *K. al-Qānūn fī al-ṭibb* · trans. Nathan ha-Meʾati (*Sefer ha-Qanun*), bk. 1 (fol. 64[b]): ויצא לחוץ מהם כת אל העצל היוצא מן החזה. → NM 4:87.

• **הכת הקרניי** · **the horn-like tunic:** Arab. الطبقة القرنية · Maimonides, *K. al-fuṣūl fī al-ṭibb* · trans. Zeraḥyah Ḥen (*Sefer ha-Peraqim*), 3.52: הלחות הכפורי והביציי הזכוכיי וכן הכת הקרניי אין בו גידים בשום פנים. → NM 1:160.

• *Plur.* **כתות** · **layers:** Arab. طبقات · Maimonides, *K. al-fuṣūl fī al-ṭibb* · trans. Zeraḥyah Ḥen (*Sefer ha-Peraqim*), 1.43: וזאת השכבה היא כתות הרבה. → NM 1:160.

כְּתִיבָה • העצם הדומה ללמד בכתיבת היוונים → עֶצֶם.

כְּתִישָׁה · **crushing [of a limb]:** Arab. شَدْخ / Gr. ῥῆγμα · Maimonides, *Šarḥ fuṣūl Abūqrāṭ* · trans. Moses ibn Tibbon (*Pirqei Abuqraṭ*), 2.6 (58): אמר המפרש: רוצה בכאב בכאן סבת הכאב כמו שיהיה בחולה מורסא חמה או חומרא והנגע והרסוק והכתישה ומה שדומה לזה והיה בלתי מרגיש בו שכלו מעורבב. → NM 3:119.

כֶּתֶם • *Plur.* כתמים · **pustules:** Arab. بثور · Maimonides, *Šarḥ fuṣūl Abūqrāṭ* · trans. Anonymous (*Pirqei Abuqraṭ*), 6.9 (301): אמר אבוקרט: הכתמים הרחבים לא יתכן היות עמם חכוך. → NM 3:119.

כֻּתֹּנֶת • *Plur.* **כתנות** · **membranes; tunics:** a) Lat. tunicae · i. Bruno Longobucco, *Cyrurgia Magna* · trans. Hillel ben Samuel (*Sefer Keritut*), fol. 7[b]: שני הכתנות של וותנים. → NM 1:27.

· ii. Bruno Longobucco, *Cyrurgia Magna* · trans. Hillel ben Samuel (*Sefer Keritut*), fol. 67[a]: ועם כל זה פעולת הכריתות בעין מסוכנת מאד מפחד פן יגע בכתונת הנקרא קורניאה. → NM 1:27–8.

· iii. Al-Rāzī, attr., *On the Treatment of Small Children* · trans. Anonymous, 5: עיטוש הנער יקרה למוח ולכתנות שלו. → NM 2:178–9.

b) Arab. صفاقات · Maimonides, *K. al-fuṣūl fī al-ṭibb* · trans. Nathan ha-Me'ati (*Sefer ha-Peraqim*), 23.25: אמר משה: אלו המפרשים לספרי ג'אלינוס כבר בלבלו מקצת שמות ולכן ראוי שאעיר עליהם. וזה שכתנות האברים הפנימיים שנקראו בספר תועלות האברים ספאקאת כלומר קרומות. → NM 2:55.

כָּתֵף · **shoulder; shoulder blade (scapula):** Arab. كتف · Ibn Sīnā, *K. al-Qānūn fī al-ṭibb* · trans. Nathan ha-Me'ati (*Sefer ha-Qanun*), bk. 1 (fol. 37[a]): ונוטה אל הצד החיצוני ומחוברת בראש הכתף ונקשרת בה הכתף ובהם יחדו נקשר הזרוע. → NM 4:87.

• **עין הכתף** → **עַיִן**.

• **עצם הכתף** → **עֶצֶם**.

• **ראש הכתף** → **רֹאשׁ**.

כְּתֵפִי • **הכתפי** · **cephalic vein; vein of the shoulder:** Arab. الكتفي · Ibn Sīnā, *K. al-Qānūn fī al-ṭibb* · trans. Nathan ha-Me'ati (*Sefer ha-Qanun*), bk. 1 (fol. 65[b]): אמנם הכתפיי והוא הקיפאל הנה בתחלת מה שיתענף ממנו שריג מתפרק בעור בחלקים הנראים החיצונים מן העצלים. → NM 4:87.

כֶּתֶר • **כתר מלכות** · **king's clover; melilot** [*Melilotus officinalis*]: Arab. إكليل الملك · Ibn al-Jazzār, *Zād al-musāfir wa-qūt al-ḥādir* · trans. Moses ibn Tibbon (*Sefer Ṣedat ha-Derakhim*), bk. 1, ch. 17 (Ms. Munich, Bayerische Staatsbibliothek, Cod. hebr. 19, fol. 19[a]): ואם היתה התעורה מיובש המרה השחורה נצוה החולה לשפוך על ראשו מים שנתבשלו בהם קממילא וכתר מלכות ואניט וקליפת פאפויר וזרע מלוישקלי ומה שדומה להם. → NM 4:88.

ל

לב · **gromwell** [*Lithospermum officinale*]: Arab. قلّب · Al-Rāzī, *K. al-Manṣūrī* · trans. Shem Tov ben Isaac (*Sefer Almansur*), Qof 18 (72): קלב וב״מ לב הוא זרע לבן הודיי ונקרא כן מפני שהוא דומה ללב כל ב״ח: יגיר השתן ויפרך החצץ. → NM 2:13.

לֵב • **אפיסת הלב** → **אֲפִיסָה**.

• **דפיקת (ה)לב** → **דְּפִיקָה**.

• **כיס הלב** → **כִּיס**.

• **מכסה הלב** → **מִכְסֶה**.

• **נשיכת הלב** → **נְשִׁיכָה**.

• **נשיכה בלב** → **נְשִׁיכָה**.

• **עקיצה בלב** → **עֲקִיצָה**.

• **קרום הלב** → **קְרוּם**.

• **ראש הלב** → **רֹאשׁ**.

[לבד] • *Part. Hitpa'el* **מִתְלַבֵּד** · **compact**: Arab. متلبّد · Al-Zahrāwī, *K. al-taṣrīf li-man 'ağiza 'an at-ta'līf* · trans. Shem Tov ben Isaac (*Sefer ha-Shimmush*), bk. 30, 2.82 (fol. 223[b]): והנמלה היא גם כן גרגתני קטן מתלבד עב הגוף הולכת בעומק מאד. → NM 1:98.

לְבַד · **especially**: Arab. خاصّة · Maimonides, *Šarḥ fuṣūl Abūqrāṭ* · trans. Moses ibn Tibbon (*Pirqei Abuqraṭ*), 2.29 (81): אמר המפרש: הנה יתן סבת זה בפרק אשר אחריו. ואמרו אם ראית שיתנועע דבר הניע רוצה בו ההקזה לבד ופעמים יעשה השלשול גם כן. → NM 3:120.

לבוני → **לבני**.

לְבוּשׁ · **membrane**: Arab. لباس · Ibn al-Jazzār, *Zād al-musāfir wa-qūt al-ḥāḍir* · trans. Moses ibn Tibbon (*Sefer Ṣedat ha-Derakhim*), bk. 2, ch. 6 (fol. 46[a]): ויכחול ברפואות שיכנס בהם מי המררות וזה כי כל המררות יועילו מקבוץ המים בעין ויטהרו הראות ויסירו מותרי הלחות אשר יתקבץ בלבוש העין. → NM 4:88.

לָבָן · **phlegmatic**: Arab. بلغمي · Maimonides, *Šarḥ fuṣūl Abūqrāṭ* · trans. Moses ibn Tibbon (*Pirqei Abuqraṭ*), 3.53 (190): אלו הדבקיות אמנם יתחדשו מחום חזק פעלו בלחיות לבנות עד שנגבו אותם. → NM 3:120.

• **חירִיעה הלבנה** → **יְרִיעָה**.

• **המחיצה הלבנה** → **מְחִיצָה**.

לֹבֶן · **conjunctiva**: Arab. ملتحم · Ibn al-Jazzār, *Zād al-musāfir wa-qūt al-ḥāḍir* · trans. Moses ibn Tibbon (*Sefer Ṣedat ha-Derakhim*), bk. 2, ch. 3 (fol. 43[b]): הטרפא הוא דם ישפך בלובן מבקיעת הורידים אשר בה. → NM 4:88.

• **לובן הצפרנים** · **whiteness of the nails**: Arab. بياض الأظفار · Ibn al-Jazzār, *Zād al-musāfir wa-qūt al-ḥāḍir* · trans. Moses ibn Tibbon (*Sefer Ṣedat ha-Derakhim*), bk. 7, ch. 27.1: השער העשרים ושבעה בלובן הצפרנים ורפואת מוגלתם הנקרא גלאיי פעמים יקרה בצפרנים לובן וכאשר נרצה לרפאתו נבוא אליו באחת מאלו הרפואות הנזכרות לזה. → NM 4:89.

לְבָנָה · **phlegm**: Arab. بلغم · Maimonides, *K. al-fuṣūl fī al-ṭibb* · trans. Nathan ha-Me'ati (*Sefer ha-Peraqim*), 14.6: מי שיהיה באסטומכתו לבנה דבקה נחה בה ויהיה ממי שיקל עליו הקיא אין רוע אם יקיא בצנון עם סכנגבין. → NM 2:55.

לבני · **pertaining to frankincense**: Arab. لباني · Al-Zahrāwī, *K. al-taṣrīf li-man ʿağiza ʿan at-taʾlīf* · trans. Shem Tov ben Isaac (*Sefer ha-Shimmush*), bk. 27, fol. 138b, col. a: וראוי להנזר ממנו מי שירבו בו הרוחות וימהר אליו הגעש החמוץ ואם יגבר עליו יצרו ויאכל ממנו ראוי לשתות אחריו מיד מן היין החי או לאכול ממרקחת הכמון הלבן או מרקחת הלבוניי. → NM 4:89.

לֵדָה • **עוזר הלידה** → עֵצֶר.

[להב] • *Part. Nifʿal* **נִלְהָב** · **inflamed**: Arab. ملتهب · Maimonides, *K. al-fuṣūl fī al-ṭibb* · trans. Nathan ha-Meʾati (*Sefer ha-Peraqim*), 6.47: מי שכבדו נפוחה יהיה מראהו לבן וירוק ומראה מי שטחולו נפוח ירוק ושחור ומי שריאתו נפוחה יתראה מראהו לבן וכמוש. ואמנם יהיו מראיהם כן כשיהיו מורסותיהם ונפיחתם בלתי נלהבות. → NM 2:67.

• *Piʿel* **לִהֵב** · **to cause an inflammation; to make something inflamed**: Arab. ألهب · Al-Zahrāwī, *K. al-taṣrīf li-man ʿağiza ʿan at-taʾlīf* · trans. Shem Tov ben Isaac (*Sefer ha-Shimmush*), bk. 27, fol. 143b, col. a: בשר הגמל חזק החמימות מלהב עם עובי רב ומוליד מרה שחורה. → NM 4:89.

• *Part. Hitpaʿel* **מִתְלַהֵב** · **inflamed**: Arab. ملتهب · Al-Rāzī, *K. al-Manṣūrī* · trans. Shem Tov ben Isaac (*Sefer Almansur*), Ayin 4 (62): ענב אלתעלב ובלעז מברילה וב״מ ענב השועל: קר טוב לכבד המתלהבת. → NM 2:13.

לֶהָבָה · **inflammation**: Arab. التهاب · Al-Rāzī, *K. al-Manṣūrī* · trans. Shem Tov ben Isaac (*Sefer Almansur*), Ayin 1 (60): עצה אלראעי ובלעז וירגא פשטורא וב״מ מקל הרועה וב״ח חוטרא רעיא: קר טוב למורסות החמות ולהבת האצטומכה כשיחובש בו. → NM 2:13.

• **להבת העינים** · **ophthalmia**: Gr. ὀφθαλμία · Hippocrates, *Aphorisms* · trans. Joseph Delmedigo, 3.21 (127): ובקיץ יהיו קצת הנזכרים וקדחות תמידיות ושורפות ושלישיות רבות ורביעיות וקיא ושלשול ולהבת העינים וכאב האזנים ושחיני הפה ועפוש אברי ההולדה וצמחי הזיעה. → NM 3:120.

לובן → לֹבֶן.

לוּחַ • *Plur.* **לוחות** · **splints**: Lat. astellae · Bruno Longobucco, *Cyrurgia Magna* · trans. Hillel ben Samuel (*Sefer Keritut*), fol. 50: אמנם על הקשירות הנזכרות ישים לאלתר הלוחות הנקרא׳ שקלולי. → NM 1:28.

[לוט] • **לט בבגד חם** · **to foment**: Hippocrates, *Aphorisms* · trans. Doʾeg ha-Edomi (*Sefer Agur*), 6.31 (323) (fol. 103a): יכאבו העיניים כי יעביר כאבם שתיית היין הטוב או הכנסת המרחץ או ילוט אותם בבגד חם או הקזת דם או טהרת הגוף במשקה. → NM 3:120–1.

לוּלָב • **לולב הדקל** · **envelope, spathe of the palm flower**: Arab. كفرّى ; جفرّى · Al-Zahrāwī, *K. al-taṣrīf li-man ʿağiza ʿan at-taʾlīf* · trans. Shem Tov ben Isaac (*Sefer ha-Shimmush*), bk. 27, fol. 140a, col. a: הכופרי והוא לולבי הדקל הרך הנקרא בלשונם אלג׳פרי קודם יביא פריו קרוב מטבע הקור של דקל. → NM 4:89.

לופיני • **קמח לופיני** → קֶמַח.

לַח · **loose (of bowels)**: Arab. ليّن / Gr. ὑγρός · Maimonides, *Šarḥ fuṣūl Abūqrāṭ* · trans. Moses ibn Tibbon (*Pirqei Abuqraṭ*), 2.20 (72): אמר אבקראט: מי שהיה בטנו בבחרותו לח הנה הוא כאשר יהיה ישיש יבש בטנו ומי שהיה בבחרותו יבש הנה כאשר יהיה ישיש יתלחלח בטנו. → NM 3:121.

לֵחָה • **הליחה המחטיאה** · **peccant humor**: Lat. vitiosus humor · Arnau de Vilanova, *Med-*

icationis Parabole · trans. Abraham Avigdor (*Pirqei Arnauṭ de Vilanova*), 4.1 (48): רוע מזג אם יקרה בלי ליחה הנה יתוקן ענינו עם הדברים המשנים המזג אך אם יהיה עם ליחה לא יתוקן ענינו אלא עם נקוי הליחה המחטיאה. → NM 4:65.

• **רעת הליחה השחורה** → רָעָה.

לַחוּת • **הלחות הכפורית** · **the crystalline humor:** Arab. الرطوبة الجلدية · Ibn al-Jazzār, *Zād al-musāfir wa-qūt al-ḥāḍir* · trans. Moses ibn Tibbon (*Sefer Ṣedat ha-Derakhim*), bk. 2, ch. 2 (Ms. Oxford, Bodleian Library, Poc. 353, Uri Heb. 314, fol. 12ª): והלחות הכפורית אם היה דק הנה מי רושילש יסירהו ואם היה עב יצטרך אל מה שהוא יותר חזק. → NM 4:85.

• *Plur.* **לחויות** • **לחויות ממעידות** · **synovial fluids:** Arab. رطوبات مزلّقة · Al-Zahrāwī, *K. al-taṣrīf li-man ʿağiza ʿan at-taʾlīf* · trans. Shem Tov ben Isaac (*Sefer ha-Shimmush*), bk. 30, 1.25 (fol. 205ᵇ): כשישמט ראש פרק המרפק הנקרא בלשונם אל עצ׳ד בסבת לחויות ממעידות. → NM 1:104.

לְחִי • **מורסא לחיית** → מֻרְסָא.

[לחלח] • *Puʿal* **לֻחְלַח** · **to be loose (of bowels):** Hippocrates, *Aphorisms* · trans. Judah Shalom, 4.27 (164) (fol. 59ª): כל מי שבקדחות בחזרתו לקחת יוציא רבוי דם מאיזה מקום שיהיה ילוחלח הבטן בזה. → NM 3:121.

• *Hitpaʿel* **הִתְלַחְלֵחַ** · **to be loose (of bowels):** Arab. لان / Gr. ὑγραίνομαι · Maimonides, *Šarḥ fuṣūl Abūqrāṭ* · trans. Moses ibn Tibbon (*Pirqei Abuqraṭ*), 2.20 (72): אמר אבקראט: מי שהיה בטנו בבחרותו לח הנה הוא כאשר יהיה ישיש יבש בטנו ומי שהיה בבחרותו יבש הנה כאשר יהיה ישיש יתלחלח בטנו. → NM 3:121.

[לחם] • *Part. Nifʿal* **נִלְחָם** • *Plur.* **נלחמים** · **wrestlers:** Lat. athletae / Arab. صريعون · Hippocrates, *Aphorisms* · trans. Hillel ben Samuel, 1.15 (42) (fol. 5ª): הבטנים בסתיו ובאביב הם חמים בטבע וגם השינות ארוכות ע״כ באלו הזמנים צריך שינתן יותר מאכל בעבור שהחום היסודי רב ולכן צריכים מזון רב והאות על זה השנים והנלחמים. → NM 3:156–7.

• *Part. Hitpaʿel* **מִתְלַחֵם** · **interrupted:** Lat. offendens / Gr. προσκόπτος · Hippocrates, *Aphorisms* · trans. Judah Shalom, 4.68 (205) (fol. 69ª): בקדחות כאשר הרוח מתלחם רע כי יורה כווץ. → NM 3:148–9.

לֶחֶם • **הלחם האפוי באלפס** · **water bread:** Arab. خبز الماء · Al-Zahrawi, *K. al-taṣrīf li-man ʿağiza ʿan at-taʾlīf* · trans. Shem Tov ben Isaac (*Sefer ha-Shimmush*), bk. 27, fol. 125ª, col. a: הלחם האפוי באלפס יותר עב ויותר חזק הכח מלחם הפורני. → NM 4:90.

• **לחם ניקודים** · **biscuit:** Arab. بشماط · Al-Zahrāwī, *K. al-taṣrīf li-man ʿağiza ʿan at-taʾlīf* · trans. Shem Tov ben Isaac (*Sefer ha-Shimmush*), bk. 27, fol. 123ᵇ, col. a: הכעכין ולחם ניקודים יש בהם תוספת נגוב יוצא משווי הלחם והם מולידים חלט שחורי מאמץ המעים ומנגבים לחות האסטומ׳ והמעים ומולידים סתומים וחול בכליות ומזיקים לבעלי ההדרקון נזק מבואר. → NM 4:117.

• **לחם קיבר** · **bread from coarse meal:** Arab. الخبز الخشكار · Maimonides, *K. al-fuṣūl fī al-ṭibb* · trans. Nathan ha-Me'ati (*Sefer ha-Peraqim*), 15.52: ויאות גם כן במורסות האלו התחבשת הלקוח בתאנים והוא שיבושלו התאנים עד שישובו המים במעמד הדבש וערבהו פעם בקמח שעורים ופעם בלחם קיבר. → NM 2:81–2.

• **הלחם הרחוץ** · **washed bread:** Arab. الخبز المغسول · Al-Zahrāwī, *K. al-taṣrīf li-man ʿağiza*

ʿan at-taʾlīf · trans. Shem Tov ben Isaac (*Sefer ha-Shimmush*), bk. 27, fol. 125[a], col. 2: הלחם הרחוץ קר לח יאות לחליים החדים ויזיק לבעלי הלחה הלבנה והקרירות וכבר זכרתי רחיצתו במאמר מטעמי החולים. → NM 4:90.

• **חלחם השרוי במים עד שיחמיץ** · **bread soaked in water:** Arab. البريد · Al-Zahrāwī, *K. al-taṣrīf li-man ʿağiza ʿan at-taʾlīf* · trans. Shem Tov ben Isaac (*Sefer ha-Shimmush*), bk. 27, fol. 125[a], col. b: הלחם השרוי במים עד שיחמיץ הנקרא בלשונם אלבריד הוא רב הרוחות והנפח ומזיק אל האסטומ׳ בלתי מרפה המעים. → NM 4:90.

לְטִישָׁה · **a cleansing effect:** Arab. جلاء · Al-Zahrāwī, *K. al-taṣrīf li-man ʿağiza ʿan at-taʾlīf* · trans. Shem Tov ben Isaac (*Sefer ha-Shimmush*), bk. 27, fol. 124[b], col. a: סובין של חטה חמים יבשים מעטי המזון מאד ומנגבים ולוטשים לטישה רבה יותר מלטישת קמח החטה. → NM 4:90–1.

לָטַשׁ · **to cleanse; to clear:** Arab. جلا · a) Al-Zahrāwī, *K. al-taṣrīf li-man ʿağiza ʿan at-taʾlīf* · trans. Shem Tov ben Isaac (*Sefer ha-Shimmush*), bk. 27, fol. 124[b], col. a: סובין של חטה חמים יבשים מעטי המזון מאד ומנגבים ולוטשים לטישה רבה יותר מלטישת קמח החטה. → NM 4:91.

b) Al-Zahrāwī, *K. al-taṣrīf li-man ʿağiza ʿan at-taʾlīf* · trans. Shem Tov ben Isaac (*Sefer ha-Shimmush*), bk. 30, 3.2 (fol. 233[b]): ובכלל ראוי להרגיל מהם כל סם לוטש בלתי עוקץ. → NM 1:98–9.

c) Al-Rāzī, *K. al-Manṣūrī* · trans. Shem Tov ben Isaac (*Sefer Almansur*), Mem 17 (54): מראיר: וב״מ מררות: כלם חמים לוטשים חשכת העין ומונעים ירידת המים בהם. → NM 2:13–4.

לידה → לֵדָה.

ליחה → לֵחָה.

לֵילִית · **night blindness:** Arab. عشاء / Gr. νυκταλωπίασις · Ibn al-Jazzār, *Zād al-musāfir wa-qūt al-ḥāḍir* · trans. Moses ibn Tibbon (*Sefer Ṣedat ha-Derakhim*), bk. 2, ch. 5 (Ms. Oxford, Bodleian Library, Poc. 353, Uri Heb. 314, fol. 12[b]): השער הה׳ בלילית הוא בערבי עשא כאשר יקרה לאחד החולי הזה ואות ישלו כי בעליו לא יראה בלילה ראוי להקיזו בגיד העליון ולשלשל טבעו בגירא פיגרא או בגרגרי אצטמטיקון. → NM 4:91.

ליעוק → לעוק.

לִכְלוּךְ • **לכלוך העינים** · **cataract:** Hippocrates, *Aphorisms* · trans. Judah Shalom, 3.31 (137) (fol. 50[b]): וביותר זקנים יקרה דישמא ואשמא ונזילה ושעול וטפטוף ועצירת השתן וכאב הפרקים ונפרישין וסבוב ראש ושתוק ורועקניה(?) וחכוך כל הגוף והיקיצה ולחות הבטן והעינים והנחירים וחשיכות ולכלוכם וכובד השמע. → NM 3:122.

[לכלך] • *Piʿel* **לִכְלֵךְ** · **to spread:** Arab. لطخ · Al-Zahrāwī, *K. al-taṣrīf li-man ʿağiza ʿan at-taʾlīf* · trans. Shem Tov ben Isaac (*Sefer ha-Shimmush*), bk. 30, 2.13 (fol. 211[a]): ורטיית הדיאכילון נתכת עם מעט מן השמנים וללכלך בה הפתילה ולרפא בה. → NM 1:99.

לָמֶד · **hyoid [bone]; lamdoid [bone] (shaped like the letter *Lām*):** Arab. لامي / Gr. λαμβδοειδής (formed like a Λ) · Ibn Sīnā, *K. al-Qānūn fī al-ṭibb* · trans. Zeraḥyah Ḥen (*Sefer ha-Qanun*), bk. 1 (fol. 25[b]): הפרק הי״ג בניתוח המושקלו של הלמד. → NM 4:91.

• **העצם הדומה ללמד בכתיבת היוונים** → עֶצֶם.

למדי · I. **lamdoid (shaped like the letter *Lām*)**: Arab. لامي / Gr. λαμβδοειδής (formed like a Λ) · Ibn Sīnā, *K. al-Qānūn fī al-ṭibb* · trans. Nathan ha-Me'ati (*Sefer ha-Qanun*), bk. 1 (fol. 29[a]): והשלב השלישי הוא משותף בין הראש מאחור ובין תחתיתו והוא על תבנית זוית מתחברת בנקודתו קצה החציי ונקרא שלב הלמדי להתדמותו לאות למד יונית. → NM 4:91–2.

· II. **hyoid [bone]; lamdoid [bone] (shaped like the letter *Lām*)**: Arab. لامي · Ibn Sīnā, *K. al-Qānūn fī al-ṭibb* · trans. Nathan ha-Me'ati (*Sefer ha-Qanun*), bk. 1 (fol. 47[b]): הפרק שלשה עשר בנתוח עצלי הלמדי. → NM 4:92.

• **העצם הלמדי** → עֶצֶם.

לעוסה • *Plur.* **לעוסות** · **medicaments to chew**: Arab. مماضغ · Al-Zahrāwī, *K. al-taṣrīf li-man ʿağiza ʿan at-ta'līf* · trans. Shem Tov ben Isaac (*Sefer ha-Shimmush*), bk. 30, 1.10 (fol. 204[a]). → NM 1:99.

לעוק • *Plur.* **ליעוקים** · **linctuses**: Ibn Zuhr, *Regimen of Health* · trans. Jacob ibn Tibbon (*Hanhagat ha-Beri'ut le-Abu ʿAli ben Zuhr*), ch. 28: והלעיקה בכל יום מימי הסתו ג' ליעוקים דבש או ג' ליעוקים מן נופת ירחיק הברסאם. → NM 4:92.

לִפְלוּף · **pus; secretion**: Arab. رمص · a) Ibn al-Jazzār, *Zād al-musāfir wa-qūt al-ḥādir* · trans. Moses ibn Tibbon (*Sefer Ṣedat ha-Derakhim*), bk. 2, ch. 1 (fol. 41[a]): והמופת אשר תכיר בו המותר אשר נגר אל המחיצה הלבנה עד שיעשה מורסא הוא כי מי שקרה לו זה מפני מותר דמי ימצא בעיניו כבדות חזק ותראה העין אדומה נפוחה משלכת לפלוף ויכבד מצחו וירבו הדמעות. → NM 4:92.

b) Maimonides, *K. al-fuṣūl fī al-ṭibb* · trans. Nathan ha-Me'ati (*Sefer ha-Peraqim*), 6.13: מה שיתנגב מן הלפלוף בעין ועל הפנים מן הזיעה עד שישוב כאבק הוא מופת רע. → NM 2:55–6; corr. 3:268, 4:92.

• **לפלוף הוא קצידה** · **ophthalmia**: Arab. رمد · Maimonides, *Šarḥ fuṣūl Abūqrāṭ* · trans. Moses ibn Tibbon (*Pirqei Abuqraṭ*), 6.17 (309): אמר אבקראט: כשיהיה באדם לפלוף הוא קצידה וקרה לו שלשול הנה זה טוב. → NM 3:122.

לֶפֶת • **תבשיל הלפת** → תַּבְשִׁיל.

לצרטי · **(upper) arms**: Lat. lacertus, *Plur.* lacerti · Bruno Longobucco, *Cyrurgia Magna* · trans. Hillel ben Samuel (*Sefer Keritut*), fol. 18[b]: והחבלות הבאות בקצווי הלצרטי. → NM 1:44.

לָקַח · I. **to begin; to start**: a) Arab. أخذ · i. Ibn al-Jazzār, *Zād al-musāfir wa-qūt al-ḥādir* · trans. Moses ibn Tibbon (*Sefer Ṣedat ha-Derakhim*), bk, 2, ch. 13 (fol. 52[b]): ואם לא נראה בנחירים דבר ממה שזכרנו ידענו כי הוא מפני ליחה יורדת מוסרחת מלוחה ואז ראוי שנקח להריק הראש בגירש הגדולות. → NM 4:92.

· ii. Maimonides, *Šarḥ fuṣūl Abūqrāṭ* · trans. Moses ibn Tibbon (*Pirqei Abuqraṭ*), 1.17 (44): בעבור שנתן הדרך בכמות המזון תחלה ואחר כן באיכותו לקח לתת בכאן הדרך בצורת אכילתו. → NM 3:122.

· iii. Maimonides, *K. al-fuṣūl fī al-ṭibb* · trans. Zeraḥyah Ḥen (*Sefer ha-Peraqim*), 25.43: ואמר בזה המאמר בדברו על עניין זה האיש בעצמו זה המאמר אמר: אין ראוי שיהיה היובש נשאר כמו שהוא לבדו ויהיה החמימות והקרירות משתוים לא יחסר דבר כי האברים כשאינם מתפרנסים יתקררו בזמן קצר. זה לשונו כמו כן שם וזהו

האמת. ובזוכרו מה שקדם לו ממאמרו בזה האיש שהוא היה בין החמימות והקרירות בריא לקח להשיג זה בזה הלשון. → NM 1:160.

b) Lat. incipere · Al-Rāzī, attr., *On the Treatment of Small Children* · trans. Anonymous, ch. 3: אחר ילקח בהנהגתו עם הדברים אשר יוכנסו בנחירי הנער. → NM 2:179.

‣ II. **to prepare:** Arab. اتّخذ · Maimonides, *K. al-fuṣūl fī al-ṭibb* · trans. Nathan ha-Me'ati (*Sefer ha-Peraqim*), 23.106: פחות מזון שבכל מיני היינות הוא מה שיהיה מראהו לבן ועצמו רקיק ויהיה דומה למים. ומה שיהיה מן היין כך הנה הוא נאות ונכון למה שילקח ממנו מי הדבש הנקרא אידרומל. → NM 2:56.

• **לקח ראיה על** ‣ **to conclude to:** Arab. استدلّ على / Gr. τεκμαίρομαι · Maimonides, *Šarḥ fuṣūl Abūqrāṭ* · trans. Moses ibn Tibbon (*Pirqei Abuqraṭ*), 1.23 (50): אמר אבקראט: אין ראוי שתקח ראיה על השעור אשר ראוי שיורק מן הגוף מרבויו. → NM 3:123.

לָשׁוֹן • **האלם לשון החולה** → [אלם].

• **כבדי הלשון** → כָּבֵד².

• **לשון הצפרים** ‣ **European ash** [***Fraxinus excelsior*** **L.**]: *Anonymous Glossary*, Ms. Oxford, Bodleian Library, Mich. Add. 22, fol. 11b: לשון הצפרים לינגא פשארינאש. → NM 4:93.

• **שרש הלשון** → שֹׁרֶשׁ.

• *Plur.* **לשונים** • **לשוני הים** ‣ **lake:** Arab. بحيرة, *Plur.* بحيرات · Al-Zahrāwī, *K. al-taṣrīf li-man ʿağiza ʿan at-taʾlīf* · trans. Shem Tov ben Isaac (*Sefer ha-Shimmush*), bk. 27, fol. 129a, col. b: המים החמים מן השמש וזולתו וכל שכן כשיהיו מן המים העומדים בברכות ובלשוני הים הנחים מעפשים הד. → NM 4:93.

לָתַת ‣ **to mix; to stir:** Arab. لتّ · Ibn al-Jazzār, *Zād al-musāfir wa-qūt al-ḥāḍir* · trans. Moses ibn Tibbon (*Sefer Ṣedat ha-Derakhim*), bk. 1, ch. 23 (fol. 36b): יודקו הסמים וינופו ויחתך הסרפי לחלקים קטנים ויערב הכל וילתות אותו בשמן שקדים מתוקים. → NM 4:93.

מְ

מְאַדֵּם (*Part. Piʿel*) → [אדם].

מְאִיסוּת · **foulness**: Arab. نَتْن · Maimonides, *Šarḥ fuṣūl Abūqrāṭ* · trans. Anonymous (*Pirqei Abuqraṭ*), 5.11 (231): אמר המפרש: מאיסות הריח מורה על הפסד הליחות וחוזק עפושם ונפילת שער הראש הוא ממה שילקח ראיה על הפסד הליחה וגם כן יורה על העדר האיברים מן המזון. → NM 3:123.

מאירה → מְאֵרָה.

מַאֲכָל • **אחרי צאת המאכל מן האצטומכא** → אַחֲרֵי.

• **החמתנה מן המאכל** → הַמְתָּנָה.

• **חפץ מאכל** → חֵפֶץ.

• *Plur.* **מאכלים** • **ניעול המאכלים** → נִעוּל.

מְאַכֵּל (*Part. Piʿel*) → [אכל].

מְאֵרָה • *Plur.* **מאירות** · **cantharides (Spanish flies)**: Arab. ذراريح · Al-Zahrāwī, *K. al-taṣrīf li-man ʿağiza ʿan at-taʾlīf* · trans. Shem Tov ben Isaac (*Sefer ha-Shimmush*), bk. 27, fol. 146^{b}, col. a: חלב הנשים יותר שוה מכל החלבים ... ולפיכך הוא מועיל מן העקיצה אשר תקרה באסטומ׳ ומשחין הריאה והמעים ומשתיית הארנבת הימית ומשתית הסם הנודע בהורג הזאב ומשתית המאירות ועוד יועיל מאדמימות זנב העין. → NM 4:93.

מְבֹאָר (*Part. Puʿal*) → [באר].

מַבְדִּיל (*Part. Hifʿil*) → [בדל].

מבואר → מְבֹאָר.

מבולבל → מְבֻלְבָּל.

מְבוּשִׁים · **pudenda**: Arab. أنثيان · Al-Zahrāwī, *K. al-taṣrīf li-man ʿağiza ʿan at-taʾlīf* · trans. Shem Tov ben Isaac (*Sefer ha-Shimmush*), bk. 27, fol. 126^{b}, col. a: ומתועלות הפולים על דרך הסם כי המערב אותם בורדים ולבונה וחלבוני בצים יועילו מבליטת בת העין והמבשלם ונותנן על המבושים יתיכו נפחם. → NM 4:94.

מבושל → מְבֻשָּׁל.

מבחר • *Plur.* **מבחרים** • **ספר המבחרים** → סֵפֶר.

מַבָּט • **ימי המבט** → יוֹם.

מֻבְטָן (*Part. Hofʿal*) → [בטן].

מֵבִיא (*Part. Hifʿil*) → [בוא].

מְבֻלְבָּל (*Part. Puʿal*) → [בלבל].

מְבַשֵּׁל (*Part. Piʿel*) → [בשל].

מְבֻשָּׁל (*Part. Puʿal*) → [בשל].

מְבַשֵּׂר (*Part. Piʿel*) → [בשר].

מְגֻבָּן (*Part. Puʿal*) → [גבן].

מְגַדֵּל (*Part. Piʿel*) → [גדל].

מגובן → מְגֻבָּן.

מגולל → מְגֻלָּל.

מְגוּפָה · **lid**: Arab. غطاء · Al-Zahrāwī, *K. al-taṣrīf li-man ʿağiza ʿan at-taʾlīf* · trans. Shem

Tov ben Isaac (*Sefer ha-Shimmush*), bk. 30, 2.78 (fol. 222[b]): ואם לא ראוי לקחת קדרה ולהגיף אותה ולנקוב במגופה נקב ולתת בה העשבים הפותחים פי הרחם. → NM 1:99.

מַגְזֵר · **chisel:** Arab. مقطع · Al-Zahrāwī, *K. al-taṣrīf li-man ʿağiza ʿan at-taʾlīf* · trans. Shem Tov ben Isaac (*Sefer ha-Shimmush*), bk. 30, 3.2 (fol. 233[a]): וזה יהיה על אחד משני פנים מן המלאכה האופן האחד הוא לכרות העצם בתחלה במגזר דק צר הפה אשר זאת צורתו ואחר כך להרגיל מגזר אחר אחר זה המגזר יותר רחב ממנו מעט וזאת צורתו. → NM 1:100.

מַגְזֵרָה • *Plur.* **מגזרות** · **chisels:** Arab. مقاطع · Al-Zahrāwī, *K. al-taṣrīf li-man ʿağiza ʿan at-taʾlīf* · trans. Shem Tov ben Isaac (*Sefer ha-Shimmush*), bk. 30, 3.2 (fol. 233[a]): ומן הראוי להיות אצל הרופא מגזרות משתנות זאת מזאת וזה להיות קצתן יותר רחבות מקצתן וקצתן יותר קצרות מקצתן ולהיות פיותיהן בתכלית החדוד. → NM 1:100.

מַגִּיר (*Part. Hifʿil*) → [**נגר**].

[מגל] • *Piʿel* **מִגֵּל** · **to cause suppuration:** Arab. قيّح / Gr. ἐκπυέω · Hippocrates, *Aphorisms* · trans. Nathan ha-Meʾati, 5.22 (242) (fol. 90[b]): אמר אבוקרט: המים החמים ימגלו אך לא בכל שחין וזה מהיותר גדול שבאותות להורות על אמתות והבטחון. → NM 3:124.

מֻגְלָא (*Aram.*) · I. **empyema:** Arab. تقييح / Gr. ἐμπύημα · Maimonides, *Šarḥ fuṣūl Abūqrāṭ* · trans. Zeraḥyah Ḥen (*Pirqei Abuqraṭ*), 5.8 (228): אמר בקראט: מי שקרה לו חולי הצד ולא ינקה בי״ד ימים עניינו יבוא לידי מוגלא. → NM 3:125.

· II. **suppuration:** Arab. تقيّح · Maimonides, *Šarḥ fuṣūl Abūqrāṭ* · trans. Zeraḥyah Ḥen (*Pirqei Abuqraṭ*), 7.20 (372): אמר בקראט: ובעבור הרציפלא העיפוש והמוגלא. → NM 3:125.

• **המוגלא הבלויה** · **pus; sputum:** Arab. قيح · Ibn al-Jazzār, *Zād al-musāfir wa-qūt al-ḥādir* · trans. Moses ibn Tibbon (*Sefer Ṣedat ha-Derakhim*), introduction (fol. 3[a]): השער הי׳ ברקיקת המוגלא הבלויה. → NM 4:94.

• **בעלי מוגלא** → **בַּעַל**.

• **גמר מוגלא** → **גָּמַר**.

• **הוצאת מוגלא** → **הוֹצָאָה**.

• **מוגלת החזה** · **empyema:** Gr. ἐμπύημα · Hippocrates, *Aphorisms* · trans. Joseph Delmedigo, 5.8 (228): האחוזים מחולי הצד אם לא ינקו דרך רקיקה בארבעה עשר יום יתהפך בהם למוגלת החזה. → NM 3:125.

• **עשות מוגלא** → **עָשָׂה**.

• **עשיית המוגלא** → **עֲשִׂיָּה**.

מֻגְלִי · **serous:** Arab. صديدي · Maimonides, *K. al-fuṣūl fī al-ṭibb* · trans. Zeraḥyah Ḥen (*Sefer ha-Peraqim*), 6.78: ואם יהיה הדם אשר יצא דקיק מוגלי מורה על שהכבד יחלש ממנו מעשה הדם. → NM 1:160–1.

מְגֻלְגָּל (*Part. Puʿal*) → [**גלל**].

מָגֵן • **מגן הארכובה** · **patella:** Arab. عين الركبة · Ibn Sīnā, *K. al-Qānūn fī al-ṭibb* · trans. Nathan ha-Meʾati (*Sefer ha-Qanun*), bk. 1 (fol. 41[a]): והוכן בצמצום מקודם שלה ברצפה והוא מגן הארכובה. → NM 4:94.

מְגֵרָה • **גרר במגרה** → **גָּרַר**.

מַדְבִּיק (*Part. Hifʿil*) → [**דבק**].

מְדֻבָּק (*Part. Pu'al*) → [דבק].
מֻדְבָּק (*Part. Hof'al*) → [דבק].
מדובק → מְדֻבָּק.
מַדְוֶה • מדוה הגלגלת · **(lit., helmet disease); a headache that afflicts the whole head:** Arab. داء البيضة · Ibn al-Jazzār, *Zād al-musāfir wa-qūt al-ḥādir* · trans. Moses ibn Tibbon (*Sefer Ṣedat ha-Derakhim*), bk. 1, ch. 12 (fol. 19ᵃ): השער הי״ב בחולי הנקרא מדוה הגלגלת. פעמים יקרה בגלגלת כאב חזק מזיק קשה להרפא עד שהחולה ירגיש ממנו כמו שיוכה ראשו במהלומות ולא יוכל לסבול שישמע דבור חזק ולא קול הברה מדבר שיכה בדבר ולא יוכל להביט האורה. → NM 4:94–5.
• **מדוה הפיל** · **elephantiasis:** Arab. داء الفيل · Al-Rāzī, *K. al-Manṣūrī* · trans. Shem Tov ben Isaac (*Sefer Almansur*), Ḥet 5 (36): חם יבש דק חנטל ובלעז קולוקוינטידא וב״ח פקועות: ישלשל ליחה לבנה עבה וינקה הראש ויועיל ממכאובי העצבים וגיד הנשה והפדגרא הקרה ומדוה הפיל. → NM 2:14.
• **מדוה חצד** · **pleurisy:** Arab. ذات الجنب / Gr. πλευρῖτις · Maimonides, *Šarḥ fuṣūl Abūqrāṭ* · trans. Moses ibn Tibbon (*Pirqei Abuqraṭ*), 3.23 (129): אמר אבקראט: ואולם בסתו יקרה מדוה הצד ומדוה הריאה והרובמאס והבחוחה והשעול וכאבי הצדדים ושפל השדרה וכאב הראש והסבוב והשתוק. → NM 3:125.
• **מדוה הריאה** · **pneumonia:** Arab. ذات الرئة / Gr. περιπλευμονία · Maimonides, *Šarḥ fuṣūl Abūqrāṭ* · trans. Moses ibn Tibbon (*Pirqei Abuqraṭ*), 3.23 (129): אמר אבקראט: ואולם בסתו יקרה מדוה הצד ומדוה הריאה והרובמאס והבחוחה והשעול וכאבי הצדדים ושפל השדרה וכאב הראש והסבוב והשתוק. → NM 3:125–6.
• **מדוה השועל** · **alopecia:** Al-Rāzī, *K. al-Manṣūrī* · trans. Shem Tov ben Isaac (*Sefer Almansur*), Zayin 7 (34): כל מיני זרניך חמים שורפים מועילים מן הגרב והבהק ומדוה השועל. → NM 2:14.
מָדוֹר · **ventricle (h.l., hemisphere):** Arab. وعى · Ibn al-Jazzār, *Zād al-musāfir wa-qūt al-ḥādir* · trans. Moses ibn Tibbon (*Sefer Ṣedat ha-Derakhim*), bk. 1, ch. 11 (fol. 18ᵇ): המוח יחלק תחלה באורך לשני חלקים: ימין ושמאל וביניהם חוט נמשך באמצע המוח מבדיל בין מדוריו. → NM 4:95.
מדחה · **obturator:** Arab. مدفع · Al-Zahrāwī, *K. al-taṣrīf li-man ʿağiza ʿan at-taʾlīf* · trans. Shem Tov ben Isaac (*Sefer ha-Shimmush*), bk. 30, 2.6 (fol. 210ᵃ): והרוצה להיות המדחה אשר בתוך השפופרת של נחשת עשוי בחכמה הרשות בידו. → NM 1:100.
מדני • הגיד המדני → גִּיד.
מְדַקְדֵּק (*Part. Pi'el*) → [דקדק].
מַדְרֵגָה • *Plur.* **מדרגות • על מדרגות** · **gradually:** Arab. على تدريج · Ibn al-Jazzār, *Zād al-musāfir wa-qūt al-ḥādir* · trans. Moses ibn Tibbon (*Sefer Ṣedat ha-Derakhim*), bk. 1, ch. 22 (fol. 32ᵇ): ונתחיל בכל מה שזכרנו מן הרפואה ביותר קל ואחר כך נעלה אל תכליתו והיותר חזק על מדרגות. → NM 4:95.
מְהֻבְהָב (*Part. Pu'al*) → [הבהב].
מהובהב → מְהֻבְהָב.
מַהֲלָךְ • *Plur.* **מהלכים** · **passages [in the body]:** Arab. مجرى, *Plur.* مجار · Maimonides, *Šarḥ*

fuṣūl Abūqrāṭ · trans. Zeraḥyah Ḥen (*Pirqei Abuqraṭ*), 1.24 (51): ושיהיו המהלכים אשר יהיה עובר בהם השלשול רחבים פתוחים אין בהם שום סתימה. → NM 3:126.

מובטן → מֻבְטָן.

[מוג] • *Hitpaʿel* **הִתְמוֹגֵג** · **to dissolve:** Arab. انحلّ · Maimonides, *Šarḥ fuṣūl Abūqrāṭ* · trans. Anonymous (*Pirqei Abuqraṭ*), 2.26 (77): אמר המפרש: לא הקדחת הרביעית לבד תהיה בקיץ קצרה אכן גם שאר החליים כי הכימוסים יזובו ויתפשטו בכל הגוף ויתמוגגו. → NM 3:126.

מוגלא → מֻגְלָא.

מוגלי → מֻגְלִי.

מודבק → מֻדְבָּק.

מוח → מֹחַ.

מוחזר → מֻחְזָר.

מוחיות → מחיות.

מוטחל → מֻטְחָל.

מוכלח → מֻכְלָח.

מונח → מֻנָּח.

מוסקולו · **muscles:** Lat. musculi · Bruno Longobucco, *Cyrurgia Magna* · trans. Hillel ben Samuel (*Sefer Keritut*), fol. 18[b]: ודע כי אמרו גלינו ואלמנסור כי המוסקולו הם מורכבים מבשר וגידים ומקשרים. → NM 1:44.

מוסרח → מֻסְרָח.

מופשט → מֻפְשָׁט.

מוֹצָא · **anus:** Lat. anus · Bruno Longobucco, *Cyrurgia Magna* · trans. Hillel ben Samuel (*Sefer Keritut*), fols. 98[a–b]: והם על שני פנים או שיהיו בתוך המוצא ואז יוצא הדם מהם תמיד או שהם מחוץ לו. → NM 1:28.

מוצע → מֻצָּע.

מוֹצֵץ (*Part.*) → מָצַץ.

מוקץ → מֻקָּץ.

מוֹרָאָה • **דפיקה במוראה** → דְּפִיקָה.

• **נשיכה במוראה** → נְשִׁיכָה.

מורך → מֹרֶךְ.

מורסא → מֻרְסָא.

מוֹשָׁב · **basis:** Arab. قاعدة · Ibn Sīnā, *K. al-Qānūn fī al-ṭibb* · trans. Nathan ha-Me'ati (*Sefer ha-Qanun*), bk. 1 (fol. 2[b]): הנה יש לראש אחר זה גם כן חמשה עצמות כגדרות ואחד כמושב. → NM 4:96.

מושחת → מֻשְׁחָת.

מוֹשֵׁךְ (*Part.*) → מָשַׁךְ.

מוֹשֵׁל (*Part.*) → מָשַׁל.

[מות] • **מת מיתה משונה** · **to die during illness:** Arab. مات سقيما · Al-Zahrāwī, *K. al-taṣrīf li-man ʿağiza ʿan at-taʾlīf* · trans. Shem Tov ben Isaac (*Sefer ha-Shimmush*), bk. 27, fol. 132[b], col. b: ואני לא ראיתי מימיי מי שהרגיל השכרות ושתיית היין אחריו והתמדתו שלא מת מיתה משונה. → NM 4:98–9.

• *Part. Hif'il* מְמִית • ממית הזאב › **aconite**: Arab. قاتل الذئب · Maimonides, *K. al-fuṣūl fī al-ṭibb* · trans. Zeraḥyah Ḥen (*Sefer ha-Peraqim*), 23.101: הרפואה אשר תחמם ותלחלח עד שתפסיד מה שתמצא היא באמת הרפואה המעפשת. וכן נקראות כמו כן כל הרפואות החמות היבשות העבות בעצמותם בהיותם נושכים מעט או שורפות מעט מבלתי חדש כאב נקראות מעפשות כי הם יתיכו ויאכלו הבשר ויעשו בו מה שיעשה המעפשת באמת והם כמו הארסניק ודבקות הזהב והפיניי וממית הזאב. → NM 1:163.

• הסם הממית → סַם.

מָזַג › **to moderate**: Lat. contempero · Arnau de Vilanova, *Medicationis Parabole* · trans. Abraham Avigdor (*Pirqei Arnauṭ de Vilanova*), 4.34 (58): כאשר יהיה הדם עב יש לחוש שאם נקיז בעת הקור הגובר יורק הדם הרקיק וישאר העב ולזה אם יביאנו ההכרח להקיז בעת ההיא ראוי למזוג קור האיברים ולהשוותם לא עם חום האש אך עם תנועה שוה. → NM 4:96.

• *Pass. Part.* מָזוּג › **balanced**: Lat. moderatus / Arab. معتدل · Hippocrates, *Aphorisms* · trans. Hillel ben Samuel, 5.62 (282) (fol. 36[a]): כל אותם שהאם שלהם קרה וקשה לא תהרנה וכל אותם שהאם שלהם לחה לא תהרנה מפני שיעצר בה הזרע וכל שיש להם יבשות ודלקה באם לא תהרנה כי הזרע יפסד מחסרון המזון וכל אותם שמזוגות בשני הענינים מתעברות. → NM 3:126.

• *Pi'el* מִזֵּג › **to moderate**: Lat. tempero · Ibn Sīnā, *K. al-adwiya al-qalbiya* · trans. Anonymous (*Sefer ha-Refu'ot ha-Libbiyot*), fol. 281[b]: תמר אינדיש: קרים ויבשים בשלישית וחשבו בהם שהם מחזקים הלב אמנם נראה שזה בסגולה לאותם שיש להם רוע מזג נוטה לאדומה כי הוא ממזג בקורו ומנקה מהאדומה בכח המתיך שבו. → NM 4:96.

מֶזֶג • הפסד המזג → הֶפְסֵד.

מָזוּג (*Pass. Part.*) → מָזַג.

מָזוֹן • מיץ המזון → מִיץ.

מַזְלֵג › I. **hook**: Lat. uncinus · Bruno Longobucco, *Cyrurgia Magna* · trans. Hillel ben Samuel (*Sefer Keritut*), fol. 28[a]: וכשהדם יוצא מן הוותנים או מן הורידים הגדולים והדברים הנזכרים לא יועילו צריך שתאחוז במזלג אחד דק אותו הקצה מן הווייתן או אותו הוריד. → NM 1:29.

› II. **lancet**: Arab. نشل · Al-Zahrāwī, *K. al-taṣrīf li-man 'ağiza 'an at-ta'līf* · trans. Shem Tov ben Isaac (*Sefer ha-Shimmush*), bk. 30, 2.95 (fol. 229[a]): זה המזלג העשוי לבקע בו יש ממנו מין רחב ומין דק כפי רוחב הגידים וצרתם ותוקח ראיה מהם על זולתם והוא אצל הרופאים מפורסם. → NM 1:100.

מזלגי • המסמר המזלגי → מַסְמֵר.

מַזְרֵק • *Plur.* מזרקים › **passages (i.e., blood vessels)**: Arab. مجار · Al-Zahrāwī, *K. al-taṣrīf li-man 'ağiza 'an at-ta'līf* · trans. Shem Tov ben Isaac (*Sefer ha-Shimmush*), bk. 27, fol. 130[a], col. a: ומי שלא יוכל למצוא דרך לסננם מרוב טרדתו אם יהיה בדרך או בים צריך לקחת אחריהם דברים פותחים הסתומים ומנקים מזרקי הכבד והכליות וכיס מקוה המים. → NM 4:96–7.

מֹחַ • מוח הביצה › **eggyolk**: Arab. مخ البيض · Maimonides, *K. al-fuṣūl fī al-ṭibb* · trans. Zeraḥyah Ḥen (*Sefer ha-Peraqim*), 2.4: המרות העבות האדומות אשר אינם אדומות מאד הוא אשר יקראו קצת בני אדם במוח הביצה. → NM 1:161 (corr.).

• כאב המוח → כְּאֵב.

• מורסת המוח → מֻרְסָא.

• פלח המח → פֶּלַח.
• צמח במוח → צֶמַח.
• צמח אשר צמח במוח הראש → צֶמַח.
• קרומ(י) המוח → קְרוּם.

מחבוא · I. **sinuous ulcer:** Arab. مخبأ · Maimonides, *K. al-fuṣūl fī al-ṭibb* · trans. Nathan ha-Me'ati (*Sefer ha-Peraqim*), 15.45: הנה יעשה חוקן במורסא הנקר׳ מחבוא כשתהיה מלוכלכת מאד במי האפר והוא הנקר׳ אלקטאר או במים ודבש. → NM 2:57.

· II. **sinus:** Arab. مخبأ · Al-Zahrāwī, *K. al-taṣrīf li-man ʿağiza ʿan at-taʾlīf* · trans. Shem Tov ben Isaac (*Sefer ha-Shimmush*), bk. 30, 2.88 (fol. 226b): ומהנה נתחיב לקראו מחבוא ולא נקרא גרגתני. → NM 1:101.

מְחַבֵּר (*Part. Piʿel*) → [חבר].

מְחֻבָּר (*Part. Puʿal*) → [חבר].

מְחַבֵּשׁ (*Part. Piʿel*) → חָבַשׁ.

מְחֻדָּד (*Part. Puʿal*) → [חדד].

מחובר → מְחֻבָּר.

מָחוֹג • מחוג הראש · **dizziness:** Hippocrates, *Aphorisms* · trans. Do'eg ha-Edomi (*Sefer Agur*), 3.31 (137) (fol. 58b): חבורות רעות ותעורה כאב קשרי הדבקים והכליות ומחוג הראש. → NM 3:127.

מחודד → מְחֻדָּד.

מחוכם → מְחֻכָּם.

מחולחל → מְחֻלְחָל.

מחומם → מְחֻמָּם.

מַחֲזִיר (*Part. Hifʿil*) → חָזַר.

מְחַזֵּק (*Part. Piʿel*) → [חזק].

מָחְזָק (*Part. Hofʿal*) → [חזק].

מָחְזָר (*Part. Hofʿal*) → [חזר].

מַחַט • *Plur.* מחטים • התוספות הדומות למחטים → תּוֹסֶפֶת.

מַחְטִי • התוספות המחטייות → תּוֹסֶפֶת.

מַחְטִיא (*Part. Hifʿil*) → [חטא].

מחטיי → מַחְטִי.

מחיות • מוחיות השדרה · **spinal marrow:** Lat. spinalis medulla · Hippocrates, *Aphorisms* · trans. Judah Shalom, 5.18 (238) (fol. 78b): הקר שונא לעצבים ולעצמות ולשנים ולמוח ולמוחיות השדרה. → NM 3:127.

מחילה → מְחִלָּה.

מְחִיצָה • המחיצה הלבנה · **conjunctiva:** Arab. الحجاب الملتحم · Ibn al-Jazzār, *Zād al-musāfir wa-qūt al-ḥādir* · trans. Moses ibn Tibbon (*Sefer Ṣedat ha-Derakhim*), bk. 2, ch. 1 (fol. 41a): והמופת אשר תכיר בו המותר אשר נגר אל המחיצה הלבנה עד שיעשה מורסא הוא כי מי שקרה לו זה מפני מותר דמי ימצא בעיניו כבדות חזק ותראה העין אדומה נפוחה משלכת לפלוף ויכבד מצחו וירבו הדמעות. → NM 4:97.

מְחַכֵּךְ (*Part. Piʿel*) → [חכך].

מְחֻכָּם (*Part. Puʿal*) → [חכם].

מַחֲלָה • בשול המחלה → בִּשּׁוּל.

• **מחלת הדבקים וקשרי העצמות** · **gout**: Hippocrates, *Aphorisms* · trans. Do'eg ha-Edomi (*Sefer Agur*), 6.28 (320) (fol. 102[a]): טוב אל הסריסים אשר לא יקרה להם לעולם מחלת הדבקים וקשרי העצמות. → NM 3:128.

• **מחלת הנפילה** · **epilepsy**: Hippocrates, *Aphorisms* · trans. Do'eg ha-Edomi (*Sefer Agur*), 3.29 (135) (fol. 58[a]): אמר אפוקרט: תכונת הבחורים מעשרים שנה ומעלה לחול עליהם החולי היבש ולרוק דם וקדחת מחודדת ומחלת הנפילה ורבים מהמדוים הנזכרים למעלה. → NM 3:128.

• **מחלת קשרי העצמות** · **gout**: Hippocrates, *Aphorisms* · trans. Do'eg ha-Edomi (*Sefer Agur*), 6.29 (321) (fol. 102[b]): ימנעו פרחי הנשים מהם מחלת קשרי העצמות. → NM 3:128.

מְחִלָּה · **cavity**: Lat. caverna · Bruno Longobucco, *Cyrurgia Magna* · trans. Hillel ben Samuel (*Sefer Keritut*), fol. 32[a]: ובאמת החבלות העמוקות שיש בהן סתרים ומחילות לא ינקו ברפואות מצמיחות בשר. → NM 1:29.

מְחַלְחֵל (*Part. Piʿel*) → [חלחל].

מְחֻלְחָל (*Part. Puʿal*) → [חלחל].

מַחֲלִיק (*Part. Hifʿil*) → [חלק].

מְחֻמָּם (*Part. Puʿal*) → [חמם].

מַחֲנָק • מחנק הרחם · **hysterical suffocation**: Arab. اختناق الرحم · Maimonides, *K. al-fuṣūl fī al-ṭibb* · trans. Nathan ha-Me'ati (*Sefer ha-Peraqim*), 24.58: ויקרה לנשים אשר הן כן מחנק הרחם ויקרה אחר המחנק הפלאג מהרה. → NM 2:58.

מְחַפֵּשׂ (*Part. Piʿel*) → [חפש].

[מחץ] • *Nifʿal* **נִמְחַץ** · **to suffer pain**: Arab. كلّ / Gr. πονέω · Hippocrates, *Aphorisms* · trans. Nathan ha-Me'ati, 4.32 (169) (fol. 68[a]–68[b]): אמר אבוקרט: מי שיקום מחולי וימחץ ממנו מקום מגופו יתחדש בו באותו מקום יציאה. → NM 3:129.

מַחַץ · **pain**: Arab. كلال · Hippocrates, *Aphorisms* · trans. Nathan ha-Me'ati, 4.44 (181) (fol. 73[a]): אמר אבוקרט: מי שימצאהו קדחת ארוכה הנה יקרה לו אם יציאות אם מחץ בפרקיו. → NM 3:129.

[מחק] • *Nifʿal* **נִמְחַק** · **to be blended; to be steeped**: Lat. distemperor · Ibn Zuhr, *Regimen of Health* · trans. Jacob ibn Tibbon (*Hanhagat ha-Beri'ut le-Abu ʿAli ben Zuhr*), ch. 3: תשמר בריאות העין בעזוב האכילה בלילה והשינה על המלוי והתמדת הכחול אצל השינה באבק אנטימוני הנמחק במי הכמהין שמועיל בקיץ ובחורף. → NM 4:97.

מַחְשָׁבָה · I. **anxiety**: Arab. غمّ · Maimonides, *K. al-fuṣūl fī al-ṭibb* · trans. Zeraḥyah Ḥen (*Sefer ha-Peraqim*), 7.2: הדברים המחלישים הכח ויפסידו עליו הם שבע סבות: הראשונה הצום השנית התעורה השלישית המחשבה. → NM 1:162.

· II. **suspicion**: Arab. تهمة · Maimonides, *K. al-fuṣūl fī al-ṭibb* · trans. Zeraḥyah Ḥen (*Sefer ha-Peraqim*), 6.95: כשתקרה לבריאים תורה על החולי וכשתקרה לחולים תורה על בריאות. ותאות המזון החזקה כשתקרה לבריאים תהיה מקום מחשבה וראיה על חולי וכשתקרה לחולים תהיה ראיה טובה. → NM 1:162.

מְחַתֵּךְ (*Part. Piʿel*) → חָתַךְ.

מַטָּה • הניח למטה → [נוח].

• הרקת הירוקה מלמעלה ומלמטה → הֲרָקָה.

• מה שלמטה מן החלצים · hypochondrium: Arab. ما دون الشراسيف · Maimonides, *Šarḥ fuṣūl Abūqrāṭ* · trans. Moses ibn Tibbon (*Pirqei Abuqraṭ*), 1.24 (51): והנה ראוי שיעיין תחלה אם גוף החולה מזומן ומוכן לזה השלשול כי האנשים אשר יהיה תחלת חליים מהפסד בשול מאכלו באצטומכא הפסד גדול או ממאכלים דבקים עבים ואשר בהם במה שלמטה מן החלצים משיכה או נפח או חום חזק מופלג או שם בקצת הבני מעיים מורסא אין גוף אחד מהם מוכן לשלשול. → NM 3:88–9 (corr.).

• נפיחת פיות העורקים מלמטה → נְפִיחָה.

• מה שלמטה מצדי הכסלים · hypochondrium: Arab. ما دون الشراسيف · Maimonides, *K. al-fuṣūl fī al-ṭibb* · trans. Nathan ha-Me'ati (*Sefer ha-Peraqim*), 6.52: אותות הפרנשין הבא מן הכרס הנקרא מראק שימשך אחר לקיחת המאכל פהוק חמוץ הוא רט ורוק רטוב ורב השעור ושרפה במה שלמטה מצדי הכסלים וקרקורים בבטן לא יתחדשו אלא אחר לקיחת המאכל בשעה אחת. → NM 2:54.

• למטה משחוס החזה · hypochondrium: Arab. ما دون الشراسيف · Ibn al-Jazzār, *Zād al-musāfir wa-qūt al-ḥādir* · trans. Moses ibn Tibbon (*Sefer Ṣedat ha-Derakhim*), bk. 2, ch. 15: ואם לא יפסק הדם במה שזכרנו וירבה ההגרה נקשור הידים והרגלים מלמעלה למטה ונשים למטה משחוס החזה מצד הנחיר אשר נגר ממנו הדם כלי המציצה. → NM 4:201.

מַטֶּה • מטה הרועה · knotgrass [***Polygonum aviculare***]: Arab. عصا الراعي · Maimonides, *K. al-fuṣūl fī al-ṭibb* · trans. Nathan ha-Me'ati (*Sefer ha-Peraqim*), 9.106: הרפואות המונחות על החמרה והנמלה אלא אם תהיה מתאכלת הם אלו: חזרת ומטה הרועה וטחלב ונילופר וזרע קטונא ולגלוגות והנדבי וחי לעולם וכן ענבי השועל. → NM 2:58–9.

מִטָּה • השתין במטה → [שתן].

מֻטְחָל (*Part. Hofʿal*) → [טחל].

מיוחס → מְיֻחָס.

מיותר → מְיֻתָּר.

מְיֻחָס (*Part. Puʿal*) → [יחס].

מילוי → מִלּוּי.

מַיִם • אפיסת המים הרעים → אֲפִיסָה.

• מי האפר · lye from ashes: Arab. ماء الرماد · Maimonides, *K. al-fuṣūl fī al-ṭibb* · trans. Nathan ha-Me'ati (*Sefer ha-Peraqim*), 15.45: הנה יעשה חוקן במורסא הנקר׳ מחבוא כשתהיה מלוכלכת מאד במי האפר והוא הנקר׳ אלקטאר או במים ודבש → NM 2:59.

• מי הגבנה · whey: Arab. ماء الجبن · Maimonides, *K. al-fuṣūl fī al-ṭibb* · trans. Nathan ha-Me'ati (*Sefer ha-Peraqim*), 21.29: והגבנה עוצרת הבטן ומי הגבנה מתיר הבטן. → NM 2:59.

• המים הגפריתיים והבורקיים · thermal waters: Lat. aquae terminales · Arnau de Vilanova, *Medicationis Parabole* · trans. Abraham Avigdor (*Pirqei Arnauṭ de Vilanova*), 4.104: החלאים הנושנים הוא יעקר שרשם עם הכויות או עם המים הגפריתיים והבורקיים. → NM 4:97–8.

• הגרת המים → הַגָּרָה.

• ההדרוקן אשר בו המים כמי הנאד → הִידְרוֹקָן.

• חולי המים הרעים → חֳלִי.
• מי החלב ‹ whey: Arab. ماء الجبن · Maimonides, *K. al-fuṣūl fī al-ṭibb* · trans. Nathan ha-Me'ati (*Sefer ha-Peraqim*), 9.108: מזונות בעלי הצרעת הגדמית והסרטאן רובם מי כשך השעורים ומי החלב. → NM 2:59.
• המים החמים ‹ vapor bath: Gr. πυρία · Hippocrates, *Aphorisms* · trans. Joseph Delmedigo, 6.31 (323): כאבי העינים מתיר שתית היין או המרחץ או המים החמים על העינים או ההקזה או ההרקה. → NM 3:130.
• ירידת המים → יְרִידָה.
• ירידת המים בעין → יְרִידָה.
• כיס המים → כִּיס.
• כיס מקוה המים → כִּיס.
• כלי שעושים ⟨בו⟩ מי ורדים → כְּלִי.
• הלחם השרוי במים עד שיחמיץ → לֶחֶם.
• עדשי המים → עֲדָשָׁה.
• עשות מי רגלים → עָשָׂה.
• פחד המים → פַּחַד[2].
• המים הרעים ‹ dropsy: Hippocrates, *Aphorisms* · trans. Do'eg ha-Edomi (*Sefer Agur*), 4.11 (148) (fol. 61[a]): גזור על אשר רעמו מעיו וכאב רב על טבורו ועל תחתית שדרתו ולא יעבור בכבוס ולא ברפואה אחרת כי נכון הוא לסבול היבש מארבעת מיני המים הרעים. → NM 3:130.
• המים השורפים ‹ (lit., burning water); alcohol: Lat. aqua ardens · Arnau de Vilanova, *Medicationis Parabole* · trans. Abraham Avigdor (*Pirqei Arnauṭ de Vilanova*), 4.70 (70): כאשר יהיו החמרים מימיים או נגרים ראוי שנזהר מעשיית המבשלים בהם לחים בפועל, אם לא שיהיה להם כח להריק הליחה המחטיאה, כמו מי חלב העז לבעלי השקוי, או יהיה להם כח להתיך הליחה ולכלותה, כמו המים השורפים בבעלי הפלג. → NM 4:98.
• מי השעור ‹ barley groats: Arab. كشك الشعير · Maimonides, *K. al-fuṣūl fī al-ṭibb* · trans. Nathan ha-Me'ati (*Sefer ha-Peraqim*), 8.36. → NM 2:59.

מֵימִי • האשך המימי → אֶשֶׁךְ.

מֵימִיּוּת ‹ serum: Arab. مائية · Al-Zahrāwī, *K. al-taṣrīf li-man ʿağiza ʿan at-taʾlīf* · trans. Shem Tov ben Isaac (*Sefer ha-Shimmush*), bk. 30, 2.96 (fol. 231[a]): ואם יהיה בדם עובי ראוי לשרטו שתי פעמים בפעם הראשונה לפתוח דרך לדם הדק ומימיותו ובשנית לחטט אחר הוצאת הדם העב. → NM 1:101.

מִיץ • מיץ (ה)חלב ‹ I. buttermilk: Arab. مخيض · Al-Zahrāwī, *K. al-taṣrīf li-man ʿağiza ʿan at-taʾlīf* · trans. Shem Tov ben Isaac (*Sefer ha-Shimmush*), bk. 27, fol. 146[b], col. b–147[a], col. a: מיץ החלב אמנם כשתוסר שפותו והתחיל להחמיץ הוא טוב לשלשול המתהוה מן המרה הכרכומית עם כחשות הגוף וחולשתו. → NM 4:98.

‹ II. whey: Arab. ماء الجبن · Ibn al-Jazzār, *Zād al-musāfir wa-qūt al-ḥāḍir* · trans. Moses ibn Tibbon (*Sefer Ṣedat ha-Derakhim*), bk. 7, 9.7: וישתה אחר זה החלב שנחלב מיד כי תועלתו גדולה מאד או ישתה מיץ חלב או יין מבושל ישן. → NM 1:71.

• מיץ המזון ‹ the purified food: Arab. صفو الطعام · Maimonides, *K. al-fuṣūl fī al-ṭibb* ·

trans. Zeraḥyah Ḥen (*Sefer ha-Peraqim*), 3.34: מיץ המזון אשר יגיע מן האסטומכה אל הכבד ירתח ויתבשל בכבד וישתנה לדם. → NM 1:162.

מירכב → **מרכב**.

מירק · **abdomen; abdominal wall**: Lat. mirac(h) / Arab. مراقّ · Bruno Longobucco, *Cyrurgia Magna* · trans. Hillel ben Samuel (*Sefer Keritut*), fol. 13ᵇ: והטוב בתפירתו הוא כמו שלמדנו גלינו בספר תחבולות הבריאות שאמ׳ היה כונתך בשברון הבטן שהזיפק תתפור בתפירה מדבקת עם המירק. → NM 1:44.

מישוש → **מְשׁוּשׁ**.

מישמוש → **מְשְׁמוּשׁ**.

מְיַשֵּׁן (*Part. Pi'el*) → [ישן]¹.

מִיתָה • **מת מיתה משונה** → [מות].

מֵיתָר • *Plur.* **מיתרים** · **ligaments**: Arab. رباط · Ibn al-Jazzār, *Zād al-musāfir wa-qūt al-ḥāḍir* · trans. Moses ibn Tibbon (*Sefer Ṣedat ha-Derakhim*), bk. 2, ch. 19 (fol. 61ᵇ): ומאשר יקרה לשנים גם כן האיכול והנקוב ופעמים יתחדש בהם התולעת ופעמים ישתנו מראיהם ויהיו כרכומיות או ירוקות או שחורות. זה כלו מתחדש בהם מפני לחה מעופשת רעה מתילדת מהפסד המזון באצטו׳ וימשכו הליחות האלה וילכו בעצבי המיתרים המחזיקים השנים. → NM 4:99.

• **אבר שיש לו מתרים רבים** → **אֵבֶר**.

מְיֻתָּר (*Part. Pu'al*) → [יתר].

מַכְאוֹב • **יציאת השתן במכאוב** → **יְצִיאָה**.

מְכֻבָּס (*Part. Pu'al*) → [כבס].

מַכָּה • *Plur.* **מכות** · **ulcers**: Lati. ulcera · Bruno Longobucco, *Cyrurgia Magna* · trans. Hillel ben Samuel (*Sefer Keritut*), fol. 32ᵃ: וזאת היא חזקה אמנם המכות שהן מעופשות מעט לא יסבלוה. → NM 1:29.

מכובס → **מְכֻבָּס**.

מִכְוָה · **cautery**: Arab. مكواة · Al-Zahrāwī, *K. al-taṣrīf li-man ʿağiza ʿan at-taʾlīf* · trans. Shem Tov ben Isaac (*Sefer ha-Shimmush*), bk. 30, introduction (fol. 202ᵃ): והכויה בו יותר טובה ויותר חשובה מן הכויה בברזל כמו שאמרו אלא שהרופא כשיחמם מכוה הזהב לא תתבאר בו חמימותו על השעור המכוון. → NM 1:101.

• **מכות אש** · **cauterization**: Hippocrates, *Aphorisms* · trans. Do'eg ha-Edomi (*Sefer Agur*), 6.60 (352) (fol. 110ᵇ): תתארך המחלה על יריכו עם רקבון תדע כי הרגל כולו יחלה אם לא תעזור אליו במכות אש. → NM 3:130–1.

• **מכוה סכיני** · **knife-edged cautery**: Arab. مكواة سكّينيّة · Al-Zahrāwī, *K. al-taṣrīf li-man ʿağiza ʿan at-taʾlīf* · trans. Shem Tov ben Isaac (*Sefer ha-Shimmush*), bk. 30, 2.62 (fol. 219ᵇ): ויש שעושין רפואת זה האשך גם כן בכויה חלף מן הבקוע בכלי ברזל והוא לקחת מכוה סכיני דק ולבקע בו עור הבצים. → NM 1:102.

מכוון → **מְכֻוָּן**.

מְכֻוָּן (*Part. Pu'al*) → [כון].

מְכוֹנָה · **basis**: Arab. قاعدة · Ibn Sīnā, *K. al-Qānūn fī al-ṭibb* · trans. Zeraḥyah Ḥen (*Sefer ha-Qanun*), bk. 1 (fols. 17ᵇ–18ᵃ): והרכבת עצם משני עצמות כמו שני המשולשים יפגוש מהם שתי זויות והם מלמעלה ושתי המכונות הממששות בזוית ומתפרדות בשני זויות. → NM 4:99.

מִכְחוֹל · I. **probe**: a) Arab. مرود · Al-Zahrāwī, *K. al-taṣrīf li-man ʿağiza ʿan at-taʾlīf* · trans. Shem Tov ben Isaac (*Sefer ha-Shimmush*), bk. 30, 1.17 (fol. 205[b]): שעושין המכוה בעל שלשה שפודין ותהיה תבנית הכויה אז שש כויות ויהיו השפודין על דקות המכחל. → NM 1:102; corr. 2:198.

b) Arab. ميل · Maimonides, *K. al-fuṣūl fī al-ṭibb* · trans. Nathan ha-Meʾati (*Sefer ha-Peraqim*), 9.27: כבר ידעת בנסיון שאין ראוי שתגע נקב האזן בעת הכאב בדבר כלל אבל הטיף בו מה שתטיף שיהיה חם בשעור הסבל וידך תלויה באויר והרפואה נוזלת מקצה המכחול עד שיגיע אל תוך הנקב. → NM 2:60; corr. 4:229.

· II. **style**: Arab. ميل · Ibn al-Jazzār, *Zād al-musāfir wa-qūt al-ḥādir* · trans. Moses ibn Tibbon (*Sefer Ṣedat ha-Derakhim*), bk. 2, ch. 2 (fol. 43[b]): יודק הכל שחיקה מופלגת וינופה ויולש בלובן ביצה ויעשה ממנו גרגרים ויותך אחד במים ויושם במכחול בעין. → NM 4:99.

מכחל → מִכְחוֹל.

מֻכְלָח (*Part. Hofʿal*) → [**כלח**].

מְכַסֶּה (*Part. Piʿel*) → [**כסח**].

מִכְסֶה · **membrane**: Arab. غشاء / Gr. χιτών · Maimonides, *Šarḥ fuṣūl Abūqrāṭ* · trans. Moses ibn Tibbon (*Pirqei Abuqraṭ*), 7.45 (397): אמר אבקראט: מי שהיה בכבדו מוגלא ונכוה ויצא ממנו ליחה נקיה לבנה הנה הוא יהיה בבטח וזה כי הליחה ההיא בו במכסה הכבד ואם יצא ממנו בדמיון שמרי השמן ימות. → NM 3:131.

• **מכסה הבטן** · **hypogastrium**: Arab. مراقّ البطن · Al-Zahrāwī, *K. al-taṣrīf li-man ʿağiza ʿan at-taʾlīf* · trans. Shem Tov ben Isaac (*Sefer ha-Shimmush*), bk. 30, 2.62 (fol. 219[b]): ולהכניס בפלחים צמר מן הגזה טבול בשמן זית או בשמן ורד ולתת מחוץ צמר אחר טבול ביין ושמן ולהשטיח על הבצים ומכסה הבטן. → NM 1:102.

• **המכסה הבצלי** · **bulbar conjunctiva**: Arab. الغشاء البصلي / Lat. tunica conjunctiva bulbi · Ibn al-Jazzār, *Zād al-musāfir wa-qūt al-ḥādir* · trans. Moses ibn Tibbon (*Sefer Ṣedat ha-Derakhim*), bk. 2, ch. 1 (fol. 40[b]): הקצידא מורסא חמה תתחדש במכסה המלובש על לובן העין הנקראת הבצלי. → NM 4:100.

• **מכסה הלב** · **pericardium**: Arab. غلاف القلب · Ibn Sīnā, *K. al-Qānūn fī al-ṭibb* · trans. Joseph Lorki (*Sefer ha-Qanun*), bk. 1 (fol. 18[b]): ואחר כך הולכים כנגד מכסה הלב ומשלחים אליו שריגים רבים ישתרגו כמו השער וזנין אותו. → NM 4:100.

• **קרום מכסה** → קְרוּם.

[מלא] • *Part. Puʿal* **מְמֻלָּא** · **someone suffering from indigestion**: Arab. متخوم · Maimonides, *K. al-fuṣūl fī al-ṭibb* · trans. Zeraḥyah Ḥen (*Sefer ha-Peraqim*), 9.56: כשתרצה לחזק אסטומכת הממולאים ודומיהם ואפילו יהיה עמהם קדחת יום תשים הדברים המחזקים על האסטומכה. → NM 1:163.

• *Hitpaʿel* **הִתְמַלֵּא** · **to suffer from an indigestion**: Arab. تخم · Maimonides, *K. al-fuṣūl fī al-ṭibb* · trans. Zeraḥyah Ḥen (*Sefer ha-Peraqim*), 9.44: המחלה הנופחת ישים בעליה כואב ודואג רעת התוחלת מתיאש מהטובה ובכלל עניינה כעניין בעל השעמום המלינקוניקו בעבור שיתוף פי האסטומכא למוח ותתחזק חליים כשיתמלאו ורובם הם בעלי טחול. → NM 1:162–3.

מִלּוּי · I. **dyspepsia; indigestion**: Arab. تخمة · Maimonides, *K. al-fuṣūl fī al-ṭibb* · trans. Zeraḥyah Ḥen (*Sefer ha-Peraqim*), 9.47: המילוי אשר ישתלשל עמו הטבע עד שיתרבה ויחטוף

הכח תפרנסנו בדברים עוצרים בסדר והרבה פעמים תפול תאות המזון עם אחד ממיני השלשול הנק׳ דרב וצריך שיקח החולה מרקחת החבושים ודומיהו. → NM 1:163.

‣ II. **satiation**: Lat. plenitudo · Hippocrates, *Aphorisms* · trans. Hillel ben Samuel, 2.4 (56) (fol. 8ª): א״א: לא המלוי ולא הרעב ולא זולתם מן הענינים טוב כשיעבור השיעור הטבעי. → NM 3:131–2.

מֶלַח • מלח סדומי ‣ **salt of Sodom**: *Anonymous Glossary*, Ms. Leiden, Universiteitsbibliotheek, Cod. Or. 4732/1, fol. 2ᵇ: ארמונייקום הוא מלח סדומי חם מאד. → NM 4:100.

• פרח המלח → פֶּרַח.

[מלט] • *Part. Nif'al* **נִמְלָט • הנמלט מחולי** ‣ **convalescent**: Arab. الناقه · Maimonides, *K. al-fuṣūl fī al-ṭibb* · trans. Nathan ha-Me'ati (*Sefer ha-Peraqim*), 3.71: וכן אם יעבור חזקן והנמלט מחולי בכמות המאכל ובאיכותו העברה מעוטה יגיעהו מזה היזק גדול. → NM 2:67.

מָלִיחַ • הבשר המליח המתובל → בָּשָׂר.

מֶלֶךְ • עטרת המלך → עֲטָרָה.

מַלְכוּת • כתר מלכות → כֶּתֶר.

מֶלְקָחַיִם ‣ **forceps**: a) Lat. forceps · Bruno Longobucco, *Cyrurgia Magna* · trans. Hillel ben Samuel (*Sefer Keritut*), fol. 47ª: אם העצם נשבר ונפרד כלו במהרה תוכל להוציאו עם פיציקרולי או במלקחים והשמר מאד שלא תיגע הכתונת. → NM 1:30.

b) Arab. كلاليب · Al-Zahrāwī, *K. al-taṣrīf li-man ʿağiza ʿan at-ta'līf* · trans. Shem Tov ben Isaac (*Sefer ha-Shimmush*), bk. 30, 2.77 (fol. 222ª): תאר כלי אחר יותר נקל מזה ויותר דק עשוי מהבנים או מברוש על תבנית המלקחים. → NM 1:102.

מַלְתָּעָה → מתלעת.

מַלְתַּעַת → מתלעת.

ממולא → מְמֻלָּא.

ממוסך → מְמֻסָּךְ.

ממורסם → מְמֻרְסָם.

מֵמִית (*Part. Hif'il*) → **[מות]**.

מְמֻלָּא (*Part. Pu'al*) → **[מלא]**.

מְמֻסָּךְ (*Part. Pu'al*) → **[מסך]**.

מַמְעִיד (*Part. Hif'il*) → **[מעד]**.

מְמֻרְסָם (*Part. Pu'al*) → **[מרסם]**.

מְמָרֵק (*Part. Pi'el*) → **[מרק]**.

מַמָּשׁוּת ‣ **consistency**: Arab. قوام · Ibn Sīnā, *K. al-adwiya al-qalbiya* · trans. Anonymous (*Sammim Libbiyim*), fol. 120ª: המדקדק הוא הסם אשר מדרכו שישים ממשות הליחות יותר רקיק בהתכה חסרה בחום שוה. → NM 4:100.

ממשש ‣ **probe**: Lat. tenta · Bruno Longobucco, *Cyrurgia Magna* · trans. Hillel ben Samuel (*Sefer Keritut*), fol. 39ª: ואז צריך הממשש מן העופרת כשהוא יותר רך ונכפף. → NM 1:30.

מְנַגֵּעַ (*Part. Pi'el*) → **נָגַע**.

מְנֻגָּע (*Part. Pu'al*) → **נָגַע**.

מנוגע → מְנֻגָּע.

מְנוּחָה • מנוחת החולי · **the easing of the illness**: Lat. quies egritudinis / Arab. سكون الألم · Galen, *De inaequali intemperie* · trans. David Caslari (*Sefer Ro'a Mezeg Mitḥallef*), 3.4: אמנם התחלת מנוחת החולי בהם יהיה כשידמו האיברים אל העניין המתחלף ומשנה אותם. → NM 2:167.

מֻנָּח (*Part. Hof'al*) → [נוח].

מַנְהִיר (*Part. Hif'il*) → [נהר].

מָנַע · **to forbid**: Arab. نهى · Maimonides, *K. al-fuṣūl fī al-ṭibb* · trans. Zeraḥyah Ḥen (*Sefer ha-Peraqim*), 25.48: אמר משה: בני אדם מקשים לגליאנוס באומרו כי ההקזה היא טובה בכל הקדחות המעופשות והנה מנע ההקזה במאמרו שעשה בהקזות ובמקומות אחרים בקדחת הפליאומטיקה הפשוטה כיון שהליחות פגות. וכן ימנע ההקזה בקדחת הרביעית הפשוטה אלא אם היה נראה בו סימני הדם. → NM 1:163–4.

מְנַפֵּחַ (*Part. Pi'el*) → **נָפַח**.

מנקאר • החרטום הנק׳ מנקאר → **חַרְטוֹם**.

מְסַבֵּב (Part *Pi'el*) → [סבב].

[מסך] • *Part. Pu'al* **מְמֻסָּךְ** · **balanced**: Hippocrates, *Aphorisms* · trans. Do'eg ha-Edomi (*Sefer Agur*), 5.62 (282) (fol. 93[a]): תחפס לדעת אם רחם האשה קר או לח או חם ונלהב או יבש מאד כי כל אלה ימנעו ההריון והממוסך טוב ונכון. → NM 3:132.

מָסָךְ · **husk**: Arab. حجاب · Maimonides, *K. al-fuṣūl fī al-ṭibb* · trans. Zeraḥyah Ḥen (*Sefer ha-Peraqim*), 13.51: מדבריו: הקולוקוינטידא תיקונה יהיה בליבות הפסתק ואחריו לבות השקדים נתאמת זה בניסיון ארוך ומסך התורפיד פרח הנילופר ואם יחבר לו שמן השקדים היה זה טוב. → NM 1:164.

• **מורסת המסך** → **מֻרְסָא**.

• **המסך אשר בפנים** · **omentum**: Arab. الغشاء الباطن · Maimonides, *Šarḥ fuṣūl Abūqrāṭ* · trans. Moses ibn Tibbon (*Pirqei Abuqraṭ*), 7.55 (407): אמר אבקראט: כשנמלא הכבד ממים ואחר כן יצאו המים ההם אל המסך אשר בפנים ימלא בטנו ממים וימות. → NM 3:133.

• **המסך הפנימי** · **omentum**: Hippocrates, *Aphorisms* · trans. Judah Shalom, 7.55 (407) (fol. 125[a]): בכל מי שיהיה הכבד מלא מים וישבור אל המסך הפנימי הנה באלו ימלא הבטן מים וימות. → NM 3:133.

מַסְמֵר · **corn**: Arab. مسمار · Al-Zahrāwī, *K. al-taṣrīf li-man 'ağiza 'an at-ta'līf* · trans. Shem Tov ben Isaac (*Sefer ha-Shimmush*), bk. 30, 2.82 (fol. 223[b]): המסמר אמנם הוא דבר עגול על עין הגוף דומה לראש המסמר. → NM 1:103.

• **מסמר הגרע** · **scalpel**: Arab. مبضع · Al-Zahrāwī, *K. al-taṣrīf li-man 'ağiza 'an at-ta'līf* · trans. Shem Tov ben Isaac (*Sefer ha-Shimmush*), bk. 30, 1.3 (fol. 203[b]): ואחר לבקע מקום הכאב מן הצדע במסמר הגרע. → NM 1:103.

• **המסמר המזולגי** · **lancet**: Arab. المبضع النشل · Al-Zahrāwī, *K. al-taṣrīf li-man 'ağiza 'an at-ta'līf* · trans. Shem Tov ben Isaac (*Sefer ha-Shimmush*), bk. 30, 2.95 (fol. 229[b]): ולקשור הזרוע ולבקע הגיד בקוע בנטיה במסמר המזולגי כמו שאמרתי. → NM 1:103 (corr.).

• *Plur.* **מסמרים** · **(lit., nails); calluses; corns**: Arab. مسامير / Gr. ἧλοι · Ibn al-Jazzār, *Zād al-musāfir wa-qūt al-ḥāḍir* · trans. Moses ibn Tibbon (*Sefer Ṣedat ha-Derakhim*), bk. 7, ch. 16.0: השער הי״ו ביבלת והמסמרים. → NM 4:100–1.

מְסֻנֶּנֶת • **מסננת האף** · **lamina cribrosa (i.e., the cribriform plate of the ethmoid bone):** Lat. calami narium · Arnau de Vilanova, *Medicationis Parabole* · trans. Abraham Avigdor (*Pirqei Arnauṭ de Vilanova*), 5.22 (88): ההגרה הבלתי טבעית יאות להטותה אל מעבר טבעי, כמו הזלת הנצור אשר יהיה בדמע העין נטה אותו אל מסננת האף אם העצם כבר נתעפש. → NM 4:101.

מֻסְרָח (*Part. Hofʿal*) → [סרח].

מַסְרֵק · **metatarsus:** Arab. مشط · Ibn Sīnā, *K. al-Qānūn fī al-ṭibb* · trans. Nathan ha-Me'ati (*Sefer ha-Qanun*), bk. 1 (fol. 41[b]): וארבע עצמות הרסג במה שיתחבר במסרק. → NM 4:101.

• **מסרק היד** · **metacarpus:** Arab. مشط اليد · Al-Zahrāwī, *K. al-taṣrīf li-man ʿağiza ʿan at-ta'līf* · trans. Shem Tov ben Isaac (*Sefer ha-Shimmush*), bk. 30, 1.44 (fol. 207[b]): ואם ישארו מן המכאובים באצבעות ראוי לנקוד אותם על כל פרק ופרק נקודה אחת ועל מסרק היד. → NM 1:103.

• **מסרק הרגל** · **metatarsus:** Arab. مشط الرجل · Al-Zahrāwī, *K. al-taṣrīf li-man ʿağiza ʿan at-ta'līf* · trans. Shem Tov ben Isaac (*Sefer ha-Shimmush*), bk. 30, 2.86 (fol. 225[b]): ואם יהיה ההפסד במסרק היד או במסרק הרגל רפואתו קשה מאד. → NM 1:103.

מִסְתַּעֵר (*Part. Hitpaʿel*) → [סער].

מְעַבֶּה (*Part. Piʿel*) → [עבה].

מַעֲבָר • **מעבר השתן** · **urethra:** Arab. مجرى القضيب · Al-Zahrāwī, *K. al-taṣrīf li-man ʿağiza ʿan at-ta'līf* · trans. Shem Tov ben Isaac (*Sefer ha-Shimmush*), bk. 30, 2.80 (fol. 220[a]): ולפעמים יהיה מהם טחורים כשיהיו בבית הפרשות מפולשים אל כיס מקוה המים ואל מעבר השתן. → NM 1:103–4.

• *Plur.*[1] **מעברים** • **מעברי השמירה** · **the sensory channels:** Arab. مجاري الحسة · Galen, attr., *Prohibition of Burial* · trans. Judah al-Ḥarizi (*Sefer Issur ha-Qevurah le-Galienus*), fol. 136[b]: ואולם אחת מהעלות היא עלה תהיה בקרום המוח מן המותרות העבים הדבקים ירדו במעברים נקראים מעברי השמירה ויהיה מהם השעמום הדומה למות.

• *Plur.*[2] **מעברות** · **passages (in the body):** Hippocrates, *Aphorisms* · trans. Do'eg ha-Edomi (*Sefer Agur*), 4.34 (171) (fol. 66[b]): יש לפחד על סובל הקדחת ואין בגרונו נפח וצרו מעברותיו ולא יוכל להעביר האוכל גם נפשו תתעבנו ויחפוץ להקיא אות מות היא. → NM 3:134.

[מעד] • *Hifʿil* **הֶמְעִיד** · **to make smooth; to soften:** Arab. أزلق · Al-Zahrāwī, *K. al-taṣrīf li-man ʿağiza ʿan at-ta'līf* · trans. Shem Tov ben Isaac (*Sefer ha-Shimmush*), bk. 27, fol. 133[b], col. b: ואם יפגושו לחה לבנה יולידו שלשול וקיא יחד ויזיקו בעצבי האצטומ' ויחדשו רוחות פגות והברה וימעידו המזון. → NM 4:101.

• *Part. Hifʿil* **מַמְעִיד** • **לחויות ממעידות** → **לַחוּת**.

• **הסם הממעיד** → **סַם**.

מעוותת → **מְעֻוֶּתֶת**.

מעוכב → **מְעֻכָּב**.

מעולה → **מְעֻלֶּה**.

מעונג → **מְעֻנָּג**.

מעורב → **מְעֹרָב**.

מְעֻוָּת (*Part. Puʿal*) → [עות].

מעותד → מְעֻתָּד.

מַעֲטִישׁ (*Part. Hif'il*) → [עטש].

מְעִי • המעי האחרון ‣ **anus:** Lat. anus · Arnau de Vilanova, *Medicationis Parabole* · trans. Abraham Avigdor (*Pirqei Arnauṭ de Vilanova*), 5.60 (98): האבר אשר יצא מהנחתו הטבעית מבלי הפסד בתמונתו, הנה יתוקן ענינו עם דחייה, כמו המעי האחרון אם יצא מחוץ. → NM 4:101–2.

• **המעי הנקרא י״ב אצבעות** ‣ **duodenum:** Arab. المعى الاثنى عشر · Ibn Sīnā, *K. al-Qānūn fī al-ṭibb* · trans. Joseph Lorki (*Sefer ha-Qanun*), bk. 1 (fol. 18[b]): והאחד משני חלקים הקטנים ידבק במעי הנקרא י״ב אצבעות וימשך ממנו המזון. → NM 4:102.

• **המעי הזקוף** ‣ **rectum:** Arab. المعى المستقيم · Ibn Sīnā, *K. al-Qānūn fī al-ṭibb* · trans. Zeraḥyah Ḥen (*Sefer ha-Qanun*), bk. 1 (fol. 33[b]): והחלק השלישי מן הששה הראשונים יקח אל הצד השמאלי ויתפרד בתעלות של העורקים אשר סביב המעי הזקוף. → NM 4:102.

• **המעי הישר** ‣ **rectum:** Arab. المعى المستقيم · Ibn Sīnā, *K. al-Qānūn fī al-ṭibb* · trans. Nathan ha-Me'ati (*Sefer ha-Qanun*), bk. 1 (fol. 63[b]): והחלק השלישי מן הששה הראשונה לוקח אל הצד השמאלי ומתפרד בתעלות העורקים אשר סביב המעי הישר. → NM 4:102.

• **כאב המעי** → כְּאֵב.

• **המעי העור** ‣ **caecum:** Arab. المعى الاعور · Al-Zahrāwī, *K. al-taṣrīf li-man 'ağiza 'an at-ta'līf* · trans. Shem Tov ben Isaac (*Sefer ha-Shimmush*), bk. 27, fol. 141[b], col. a: והם מועילים אל המעי העור ואל המעי הצם. → NM 4:102.

• **המעי הצם** ‣ **jejunum:** Arab. المعى الصائم · Al-Zahrāwī, *K. al-taṣrīf li-man 'ağiza 'an at-ta'līf* · trans. Shem Tov ben Isaac (*Sefer ha-Shimmush*), bk. 27, fol. 141[b], col. a: והם מועילים אל המעי העור ואל המעי הצם. → NM 4:102–3.

• **המעי הנקרא שנים עשר** ‣ **duodenum:** Arab. المعى الاثنى عشر · Ibn Sīnā, *K. al-Qānūn fī al-ṭibb* · trans. Nathan ha-Me'ati (*Sefer ha-Qanun*), bk. 1 (fols. 63[a]–63[b]): והנה אחד משני החלקים מתחבר בחלק המעי הנקרא שנים עשר שימשוך ממנו המזון. → NM 4:102.

• **המעי התחתון** ‣ I. **anus:** Lat. anus · Bruno Longobucco, *Cyrurgia Magna* · trans. Hillel ben Samuel (*Sefer Keritut*), 83[a]: אמנם מאלה כלומר המורסות הנולדות במעי התחתון לא תאחר בהן הבקוע עד עת הבשול. → NM 1:30.

‣ II. **rectum:** Gr. ἀρχός · Hippocrates, *Aphorisms* · trans. Joseph Delmedigo, 5.58 (278): ממורסת הדם במעי התחתון וברחם וממוגלא בכליות יקרה טפטוף השתן וממורסת הכבד יקרה גיהוק. → NM 3:135.

• *Plur.* **מעים • אומץ המעים** → אֹמֶץ.

• **אמיץ המעים** → [אמץ]

• **אמיצות המעים** → אֲמִיצוּת.

• **גרידת המעים** → גְּרִידָה.

• **המעדת המעים** → הַמְעָדָה.

• **השמטת המעים** → הַשְׁמָטָה.

• **חולי מעים** → חֹלִי.

• **חליקות המעים** → חֲלִיקוּת.

• **חלקות הבני מעים** → חַלְקוּת.

- חלקות המעים → חֲלָקוֹת.
- חלקות המעים הוא זלק אלמעא → חֲלָקוֹת.
- חלקלקות המעים → חֲלַקְלַקּוֹת.
- חמרמרות המעיים → חֲמַרְמָרוֹת.
- כאב מעים → כְּאֵב.
- כאב המעיים הדקים → כְּאֵב.
- כיס המעים → כִּיס.
- מעידת המעים → מְעִידָה.
- עצור המעים → עִצּוּר.
- קלוח המעים → קִלּוּחַ.
- שלשול (ה)מעיים → שִׁלְשׁוּל.

מְעִידָה • **מעידת המעים** · lientery: Arab. زلق الأمعاء · Maimonides, *K. al-fuṣūl fī al-ṭibb* · trans. Zeraḥyah Ḥen (*Sefer ha-Peraqim*), 22.36: לשתות משקל תשעה גרעיני חיטה מהזמרד שחוק ומנופה יבלענו במים על הריקנות יפסיק שלשול הסמום ואם יתלנו על מי שיש בו שלשול או מעידת המעים ירפאנו. → NM 1:164.

מְעִיִּי • **האשך המעיי** → אֶשֶׁךְ.

מעיין → מְעַיֵּן.

מְעַיֵּן (*Part. Pi'el*) → עַיֵּן.

מְעֻכָּב (*Part. Pu'al*) → [עכב].

מְעַכֵּל (*Part. Pi'el*) → [עכל].

מַעְלָה • **הרקת הירוקה מלמעלה ומלמטה** → הֲרָקָה.

מְעֻלֶּה (*Part. Pu'al*) → [עלה].

מַעֲמָד · I. **consistency**: Arab. قوام · Maimonides, *K. al-fuṣūl fī al-ṭibb* · trans. Nathan ha-Me'ati (*Sefer ha-Peraqim*), 15.52: ויאות גם כן במורסות האלו התחבשת הלקוח בתאנים והוא שיבושלו התאנים עד שישובו המים במעמד הדבש. → NM 2:61.

· II. **culmination**: Lat. status · Hippocrates, *Aphorisms* · trans. Hillel ben Samuel, 2.30 (82) (fol. 12[b]): א״א: בעת ההתחלה והסוף כל המקרים הם חלשים אבל קרוב לעת המעמד הם חזקים יותר. → NM 3:135–6.

מְעֻנָּג (*Part. Pu'al*) → [ענג].

מְעַפֵּשׁ (*Part. Pi'el*) → [עפש].

מַעֲצוֹר · I. **abstention; abstinence**: a) Lat. abstinentia · Bruno Longobucco, *Cyrurgia Magna* · trans. Hillel ben Samuel (*Sefer Keritut*), fols. 89[a–b]: והמעצור משתיית המים ומכל מזונות הקרים ומן הקשים להתעכל. → NM 1:30.

b) Arab. إمساك · Maimonides, *K. al-fuṣūl fī al-ṭibb* · trans. Nathan ha-Me'ati (*Sefer ha-Peraqim*), 10.68: וכל מי שקדחתו מפני תעורה או דאגה או יגון או הפעלויות נפשיות הנה המעצור מאכילה הוא הדבר היותר מזיק להם. → NM 2:61.

· II. **diet**: Arab. حمية · Ibn al-Jazzār, *Zād al-musāfir wa-qūt al-ḥāḍir* · trans. Moses ibn Tibbon (*Sefer Ṣedat ha-Derakhim*), bk. 7, 17.5: ויתמיד השמירה ויעזוב התערובות במאכלים וכבר שאלו לגאליה מה היא הרפואה היותר גדולה? אמר המעצור. → NM 1:60.

מְעֹרָב • **קדחות מעורבות** → קַדַּחַת.

מְעָרָה · **fossa (depression, hollow (in the bone); h.l., pterygopalatine fossa)**: Arab. مغارة · Ibn Sīnā, *K. al-Qānūn fī al-ṭibb* · trans. Nathan ha-Me'ati (*Sefer ha-Qanun*), bk. 1 (fol. 45[a]): ושני אלו העצלים הם נעזרים בשני עצלים שיכניס בתוך הפה יורדים אל הלחי התחתון בהמערה. → NM 4:103.

מַעֲשֶׂה • **מקום המעשה** → **מָקוֹם**.

• *Plur.* **מעשים** · **observation**: Arab. مباشرة · Maimonides, *Šarḥ fuṣūl Abūqrāṭ* · trans. Zeraḥyah Ḥen (*Pirqei Abuqraṭ*), 1.1 (17): וכן יודע בנקלה באורך מעשיו עם האנשים ובאותם הצורות הרשומות בדעתו איך ישמש אותם הכלים כלומר המזונות והרפואות ושאר הכלים וזה צריך אל זמן ארוך מאד. → NM 3:136.

מְעֻתָּד (*Part. Puʿal*) → [**עתד**].

מפוזר → **מְפֻזָּר**.

מְפֻזָּר (*Part. Puʿal*) → [**פזר**].

מְפַחֵד (*Part. Piʿel*) → **פָּחַד**.

מֵפִיג (*Part. Hifʿil*) → [**פוג**].

מַפִּיל (*Part. Hifʿil*) → **נָפַל**.

מִפְצָל • *Plur.* **מפצלים** · **joints**: Arab. مفاصل · Al-Rāzī, *K. al-Manṣūrī* · trans. Shem Tov ben Isaac (*Sefer Almansur*), Bet 13: בזרקטונא ובלעז שליום וכשישתה באישרוב גלאבי תכבה החום ותשקיט הלהבה ותרכך החזה ותועיל מן העיצום אשר יהיה במעים והטורף אותה בחומץ ויחובש בה המפצלים כשיהיה בהם מורסות חמות תשקיט אותם ר״ל תשקיט כאבם. → NM 2:14–5.

מְפַרְנֵס (*Part. Piʿel*) → [**פרנס**].

מִפְרַע • **העצב החוזר למפרע** → **עָצָב**.

מֻפְשָׁט (*Part. Hofʿal*) → **פָּשַׁט**.

מָצָא · I. **to compose**: Arab. وضع · Ibn al-Jazzār, *Zād al-musāfir wa-qūt al-ḥāḍir* · trans. Moses ibn Tibbon (*Sefer Ṣedat ha-Derakhim*), bk. 1, ch. 20 (Ms. Oxford, Bodleian Library, Poc. 353, Uri Heb. 314, fol. 8[b]): וספר יעקב בן יצחק הכנדי כי אראקאוס אשר מצא הנגונים אמר המלכים יביאוני למושבם כדי שיתענגו בי וישמחו ממני. → NM 4:103.

· II. **to do the right thing**: Arab. أصاب · Maimonides, *K. al-fuṣūl fī al-ṭibb* · trans. Nathan ha-Me'ati (*Sefer ha-Peraqim*), 21.19: החומץ יש בו עם דקות חלקיו כח דוחה מונע אינו מועט. וכבר ימצאו אותו הרופאים לעשותו בהתחלת עלות המוח אחר שיעורב עמו שמן ורד. → NM 2:61

מַצָּב · **orthopnea**: Arab. انتصاب · Maimonides, *K. al-fuṣūl fī al-ṭibb* · trans. Zeraḥyah Ḥen (*Sefer ha-Peraqim*), 24.38: פגשתי יום אחד רופא אחד מפורסם במלאכת הרפואות ומששתי לו הדפק ומצאתי בו כל מין ממיני השינוי בלא קדחת ולא היה מרגיש בניפושו שום דבר כלל. ואמרתי לו אני רואה שזה השינוי יהיה מדוחק וצרות שיהיה בגידים אשר בריאה או בעבור סתימה מליחות עבות דבקות או מתולדת צמח שלא נתבשל. ואמר לי אם כן היה ראוי שהיה לי בניפוש מצב מרימפלי. ואמרתי לו כי המצב יהיה בהתקבץ הליחה הדבקה בחלקי קנה הריאה לא בהתקבצו בגידים הדופקים. → NM 1:165.

מצומק → **מְצֻמָּק**.

מָצוֹק · **colic**: Arab. مغس · Maimonides, *Šarḥ fuṣūl Abūqrāṭ* · trans. Anonymous (*Pirqei*

Abuqraṭ), 4.11 (148): אמר אבוקרט: מי שהיה בו מצוק ומכאובים סביב לטבור וכאב הכסלים תמיד ולא יותר לא בסם משלשל ולא בזולתו ודאי ענינו יגיע אל השקוי היבש. → NM 3:136.

מִצְטַעֵר (*Part. Hitpaʿel*) → [**צער**].

מַצִּיל (*Part. Hifʿil*) → [**נצל**].

מַצִּיעַ (*Part. Hifʿil*) → [**יצע**].

מְצִיצָה • **כלי המציצה** → **כְּלִי**.

• **קרני המציצה** → **קֶרֶן**.

מְצֻמָּק (*Part. Puʿal*) → [**צמק**].

מִצְנֶפֶת • *Plur.* **מצנפות** ‣ I. **bandages**: Arab. رباط · Ibn al-Jazzār, *Zād al-musāfir wa-qūt al-ḥādir* · trans. Moses ibn Tibbon (*Sefer Ṣedat ha-Derakhim*), bk. 7, 26.2: וראוי שתושם הרפואה הזאת על העורק עצמו אשר יגר ממנו הדם ואחר כן יושם ממנו הרבה על הנגע כלו ואחר כך יקשרהו במצנפות מבגד פשתן על הרפואה. → NM 1:60–1.

‣ II. **rags**: a) Arab. خِرَق · Ibn al-Jazzār, *Zād al-musāfir wa-qūt al-ḥādir* · trans. Moses ibn Tibbon (*Sefer Ṣedat ha-Derakhim*), bk. 7, 25.3: ואולם הקעת הפרקים הנה ראוי לשפוך עליו מים חמים ואחרי כן יושבו בדקות עד שישוב אל ענין השווי ויחותל במצנפות חתול שוה וישים עליו אחת מאלו הרפואות המורכבות המועילות. → NM 1:61.

b) Arab. رفائد · Ibn al-Jazzār, *Zād al-musāfir wa-qūt al-ḥādir* · trans. Moses ibn Tibbon (*Sefer Ṣedat ha-Derakhim*), bk. 7, 26.3: כבר זכר בן מאסויה בספר התועלת רפואה תפסיק הדם מן הנגעים וזה תארה: יקח אלובי אוקיא קלפת לבונה שתי אוקיות דם שני האחים וסרקא קולא מ״א שמונה שקלים וירדיט חמשה שקלים יודק וינופה ויושם על המקום בלובן ביצה ושער ארנבת ולחם שחוק ויחותל במצנפות. → NM 1:61.

מֻצָּע (*Part. Hofʿal*) → [**יצע**].

מצעת ‣ **sieve**: Arab. مصفاة · Maimonides, *K. al-fuṣūl fī al-ṭibb* · trans. Zeraḥyah Ḥen (*Sefer ha-Peraqim*), 1.42: אבל העצם אשר יגן בעד המוח סמוך לפנים ולחיך הוא חלול ובעלי הנתוח יקראוהו המצעת. → NM 1:165.

מָצָץ • *Part.* **מוֹצֵץ** • **הכוסות המוצצים** → **כּוֹס**.

מְקֻבָּץ (*Part. Puʿal*) → **קָבַץ**.

מַקֶּבֶת ‣ **drill**: Arab. مثقب · Al-Zahrāwī, *K. al-taṣrīf li-man ʿağiza ʿan at-taʾlīf* · trans. Shem Tov ben Isaac (*Sefer ha-Shimmush*), bk. 30, 2.94 (fol. 228[a]): ואם לא יצא אחר ימים ראוי לנקוב סביב החץ בעצם עצמו מכל צד במקבת דקה כדי להרחיב לחץ ואחר למשכו. → NM 1:104.

מַקְדֵּחַ ‣ **couching needle**: Arab. مقدح · Maimonides, *K. al-fuṣūl fī al-ṭibb* · trans. Nathan ha-Me'ati (*Sefer ha-Peraqim*), 15.30: המים אחר שירדו ויזלו בפני הרואה ראוי שתאחז המקדח זמן ארוך במקומות אשר ירצה שינוחו המים כדי שישתרגו בו. → NM 2:62.

מקובץ → **מְקֻבָּץ**.

מִקְוֶה ‣ **urinary bladder**: Arab. مثانة · Maimonides, *Šarḥ fuṣūl Abūqrāṭ* · trans. Moses ibn Tibbon (*Pirqei Abuqraṭ*), 1.21 (48): אמר ג׳אלינוס: הדברים אשר ראוי שיונקו הם הליחות המולידות החליים אשר בא בהם הנקיון בלתי שלם והמקומות אשר הם טובים לנקוי הם הבני מעים והאצטומכא והמקוה והרחם והעור. → NM 3:138.

מָקוֹם ‣ **size**: Arab. حجم · Maimonides, *K. al-fuṣūl fī al-ṭibb* · trans. Zeraḥyah Ḥen (*Sefer *ha-Peraqim*), 9.102: אל יפחדך במלאכת היד גודל החליים אבל תעיין בסכנתה וכוחה וחולשתה. מזה שאין ראוי שיפחדך גודל החולי ותחשבנו חולי חזק אבל תראה ותדע כי הכיס אשר ירד בו הקרום אשר על האסטומכא והמיעים והוא החלב הוא חולי גדול וחזק אע״פ שמקומו אינו גדול. → NM 1:165–6.

• **מקום הבטן** · **cavity**: Gr. κοιλία · Hippocrates, *Aphorisms* · trans. Joseph Delmedigo, 7.54 (406): למי שנסגרת ליחה בין הטרפש לקיבה וגורמת כאב אחר שאין לה יציאה אל אחד ממקומות הבטן אם תתהפך הליחה דרך הורידים אל המקוה נעשים היתר בחולי. → NM 3:138.

• **מקום שדופק** · **bregma; sinciput, spot of the anterior fontanel**: Arab. يأفوخ · Ibn al-Jazzār, *Zād al-musāfir wa-qūt al-ḥāḍir* · trans. Moses ibn Tibbon (*Sefer Ṣedat ha-Derakhim*), bk. 1, ch. 17 (fols. 24[b]–25[a]): ויחלוב על הראש במקום שדופק אחר שיעביר שער הראש חלב אשה או חלב אתון או חלב צאן. → NM 4:103.

• **מקום החבורה** · **scar**: Hippocrates, *Aphorisms* · trans. Do'eg ha-Edomi (*Sefer Agur*), 6.45 (337) (fol. 106[b]): נזק החבורה בעבור עליה זמן ארוך יאות להשמר פן ידבק בעצם וירקב או ישאר מקום החבורה עמוק. → NM 3:138.

• **המקום החלל** · **cavity**: Arab. الموضع الخالي · Maimonides, *Šarḥ fuṣūl Abūqrāṭ* · trans. Anonymous (*Pirqei Abuqraṭ*), 7.51 (403): אמר אבוקרט: העטוש ⟨ש⟩יהיה בראש כשנתחמם המוח ונרטב המקום החלל אשר בראש ונלכד שמה הרוח ונשמע לו קול רעם כי התפלשותו ויציאתו יהיה במקום צר. → NM 3:139.

• **מקום המעשה** · **scar**: Arab. موضع الأثر · Maimonides, *Šarḥ fuṣūl Abūqrāṭ* · trans. Zeraḥyah Ḥen (*Pirqei Abuqraṭ*), 6.45 (337): אמר בקראט: כשיעבור על החבלה זמן והיא נגרת מוגלא ראוי בהכרח שזה התאחז בעצם ושיהיה מקום המעשה עמוק אחר היותה מתחילה להתרפאות. → NM 3:139.

• **מקום הנגע** · **scar**: Arab. موضع الأثر · Maimonides, *Šarḥ fuṣūl Abūqrāṭ* · trans. Moses ibn Tibbon (*Pirqei Abuqraṭ*), 6.45 (337): אמר אבקראט: כאשר עבר על הנגע שנה או זמן יותר גדול מזה יתחייב בהכרח שיצאו ממנו עצמות ושיהיה מקום הנגע אחר החתמו עמו. → NM 3:139.

• **נקב אותו מקום של אשה** → **נֶקֶב**.

• **עצם מקום שער הרגלים** → **עֶצֶם**.

• **מקום הערוה** · **lower abdomen**: Hippocrates, *Aphorisms* · trans. Do'eg ha-Edomi (*Sefer Agur*), 2.35 (87) (fol. 43[a]): אמר אפוקרט: עור בטן החולה בהיותו למטה מן הטבור עד מקום הערוה והוא דק ורזה במשוש אריכות חולי ורעה יגיד. → NM 3:139.

• **המקום הפנוי** · **cavity**: a) Arab. فضاء · Maimonides, *Šarḥ fuṣūl Abūqrāṭ* · trans. Moses ibn Tibbon (*Pirqei Abuqraṭ*), 6.27 (319): אמר המפרש: הנפוחים יקרא כל מי שהיה בו מוגלא במקום הפנוי אשר בין החזה והריאה ויצטרך אל הכויה בעל החולי הזה כדי שיתנגב הלחות ההוא כאשר יגע מיציאתו ברקיקה. → NM 3:140.

b) Arab. الموضع الخالي / Gr. κενόν · Maimonides, *Šarḥ fuṣūl Abūqrāṭ* · trans. Moses ibn Tibbon (*Pirqei Abuqraṭ*), 7.5 (403): אמר אבקראט: העיטוש יהיה בראש כאשר נתחמם המוח ונרטב המקום הפנוי בראש וירד האויר אשר בו ונשמע לו קול כי עברו ותנועתו יהיה במקום צר. → NM 3:140.

• **קיים במקומו** → [קום].

• **מקום הרושם** · **scar**: Arab. موضع الأثر · Hippocrates, *Aphorisms* · trans. Nathan ha-

Me'ati, 6.45 (337) (fol. 121[a]): אמר אבוקרט: כשיעבור בשחין שנה או זמן יותר ארוך מזה ראוי בהכרח שיתבאר ממנו עצם ושיהיה מקום הרושם אחר שיבריא שוקע. → NM 3:140.

• **מקום רחב** · **convex part of a vertebra; epiphysis**: Arab. قمة · Ibn Sīnā, *K. al-Qānūn fī al-ṭibb* · trans. Zeraḥyah Ḥen (*Sefer ha-Qanun*), bk. 1 (fol. 20[a]): והיו שתי קצוות הגב יטו אל הפגישה לא נוצר להם מקום רחב. → NM 4:103–4.

• **המקום הריק** · **cavity**: Arab. الموضع الخالي · Hippocrates, *Aphorisms* · trans. Nathan ha-Me'ati, 7.51 (403) (fol. 137[b]): אמר אבוקרט: העיטוש שיהיה מן הראש כשיתחמם המוח ויתרטב המקום הריק אשר בראש אז ירד האויר אשר בו וישמע לו קולו כי עבר ותנועתו במקום צר. → NM 3:140–1.

• **מקום השמיעה** · **the external acoustic meatus; the inner cavity of the ear; the middle ear; the tympanic cavity**: Arab. صماخ · Ibn Sīnā, *K. al-Qānūn fī al-ṭibb* · trans. Zeraḥyah Ḥen (*Sefer ha-Qanun*), bk. 1 (fol. 30[b]): והחלק הראשון מכל זוג ממנו ילך אל הקרום הפנימי שהוא מקום השמיעה. → NM 4:104.

• **מקום השתן** · **urinary bladder**: Hippocrates, *Aphorisms* · trans. Do'eg ha-Edomi (*Sefer Agur*), 7.54 (406) (fol. 120[b]): אמר אפוקרט: שפעת ליחה בהתגברה בין הקרב והריאה יחול כאב אם לא תמצא מקום לעבור דרך המקורות אל מקום השתן. → NM 3:141.

מְקוֹמִי · **conventional**: Arab. وضعي · Maimonides, *K. al-fuṣūl fī al-ṭibb* · trans. Zeraḥyah Ḥen (*Sefer ha-Peraqim*), 25.59: מבעלי זה החולי הכולל נמצא מינים מבני אדם בעלי זריזות והבנה שידעו אחת מהחכמות הפילוסופיות או העיוניות או שידעו אחת מהחכמות המקומיות. → NM 1:166.

מקוצף → **מְקֻצָּף**.

מָקוֹר • **הזלת מקור** → **הַזָּלָה**.

• *Plur.*[1] **מקורים** · **minerals**: Arab. معادن · Maimonides, *K. al-fuṣūl fī al-ṭibb* · trans. Zeraḥyah Ḥen (*Sefer ha-Peraqim*), 7.72: אמר משה זה אמת כי השחוק מסגולות האדם. וידוע כי כל סגולה היא נמשכת אחר הצורות המיניות בין שיהיו אותם הסגולות לאי זו מין ממיני בעל חיים או הצמחים או המקורים. → NM 1:166.

• *Plur.*[2] **מקורות** · I. **arteries; veins; vessels**: Hippocrates, *Aphorisms* · trans. Do'eg ha-Edomi (*Sefer Agur*), 1.2 (29) (fol. 21[b]): ברצותך לחסר דם המקורות שמור כח הסובל. → NM 3:141.

· II. **fontanels**: Lat. fontinellae · Arnau de Vilanova, *Medicationis Parabole* · trans. Abraham Avigdor (*Pirqei Arnauṭ de Vilanova*), 5.26 (90): הכויות המריקות ראוי שיעשו לעולם במקורות, והוא המקום אשר יפרדו שם העצלים זה מזה הפרד מבואר או המקום אשר אין שם מונע שלא יתחבר חבור נאות. → NM 4:104.

מַקּוֹר · **forceps**: Arab. منقاش · Al-Zahrāwī, *K. al-taṣrīf li-man ʿağiza ʿan at-taʾlīf* · trans. Shem Tov ben Isaac (*Sefer ha-Shimmush*), bk. 30, 2.50 (fol. 217[a]): ואם יהיה הצמח קטון ראוי לחפשו במקור ולחתכו מן השרש. → NM 1:104–5.

מְקוֹרִי · **mineral**: Arab. معدني · Maimonides, *K. al-fuṣūl fī al-ṭibb* · trans. Zeraḥyah Ḥen (*Sefer ha-Peraqim*), 9.97: והרפואה המקררת המייבשת ברוב היא עוצרת והעוצר יהיה נושך והוא לא יסבול הנשיכה ועל כן הטוב שברפואותיה הוא המקוריות שאינם חמות כשיגיעו. → NM 1:166–7.

מַקֵּל • **מקל הרועה** • knotgrass [*Polygonum aviculare*]: Arab. عصا الراعي • Al-Rāzī, *K. al-Manṣūrī* • trans. Shem Tov ben Isaac (*Sefer Almansur*), Ayin 1: עצה אלראעי ובלעז וירגא פשטורא וב״מ מקל הרועה וב״ח חוטרא רעיא: קר טוב למורסות החמות ולהבת האצטומכה כשיחובש בו. → NM 2:15.

מְקַלֵּחַ (*Part. Pi'el*) → [קלח].

מֻקְצָץ (*Part. Hof'al*) → [קיץ].

מְקֻצָּף (*Part. Pu'al*) → [קצף].

מְקָרֵב (*Part Pi'el*) → [קרב].

מִקְרֶה • *Plur.* **מקרים** • symptoms: Arab. أعراض • Maimonides, *Šarḥ fuṣūl Abūqrāṭ* • trans. Moses ibn Tibbon (*Pirqei Abuqraṭ*), 7.4 (356): אמר המפרש: כבר אמר אבקראט כי מקרי הנקיון כשלא יתחדש מהם נקיון יורה על מות או קשי נקיון כי הטבע נבוך. → NM 3:141.

מְקַרְקֵר (*Part. Pi'el*) → [קרקר].

מְקָרֵר (*Part. Pi'el*) → [קרר].

מִקְשִׁי • dense: Arab. متكاثف • Maimonides, *Šarḥ fuṣūl Abūqrāṭ* • trans. Anonymous (*Pirqei Abuqraṭ*), 5.62 (282): אמר אבוקרט: כשתהיה פי הרחם מן האשה קר ומקשיי לא תתעבר. → NM 3:141–2.

מקשיי → מִקְשִׁי.

מְקַשֵּׁר (*Part. Pi'el*) → [קשר].

מַר • **קשואים מרים** → קִשּׁוּא.

מַרְאֶה • color: Arab. لون • a) Ibn al-Jazzār, *Zād al-musāfir wa-qūt al-ḥādir* • trans. Moses ibn Tibbon (*Sefer Ṣedat ha-Derakhim*), bk. 7, 7.1: והשתנותה באיכותה יהיה לפי המותר המורק ותהיה משתנה אם במראה כמו שיקרה כשתהיה אדומה או כרכומית או ירוקה או לבנה. → NM 1:61.

b) Maimonides, *K. al-fuṣūl fī al-ṭibb* • trans. Zeraḥyah Ḥen (*Sefer ha-Peraqim*), 9.8: הכתמים אשר יראה האדם לפני עיניו הם מן הליחות עצמותם ומראיהם מנגד ללחות הביציי ויתקבצו בין הכפורית והקרנית. → NM 1:167.

• **אפיסת המראה** → אֲפִיסָה.

• **חשוך המראה** → חָשׁוּךְ.

• *Plur.*[1] **מראים** • kinds: Arab. ألوان / Gr. μεταβολαί • Maimonides, *Šarḥ fuṣūl Abūqrāṭ* • trans. Zeraḥyah Ḥen (*Pirqei Abuqraṭ*), 2.14 (66): אמר בקראט: בהגרת הבטן יועיל בשינוי המראים שיתראו בצואה כל זמן שזה השינוי לא יהיה נוטה אל מינים רעים. → NM 3:142.

• *Plur.*[2] **מראות** • kinds: Hippocrates, *Aphorisms* • trans. Do'eg ha-Edomi (*Sefer Agur*), 2.14 (66) (fol. 36[b]): אמר אפוקרט: הזלת הבטן בבאה במראה הדבר הראוי להזיל אות מרפא הוא. התהפך החולה למראות אחרות אות רע הוא. → NM 3:142; corr. 4:230.

מְרֻבָּע (*Part. Pu'al*) → [רבע].

מַרְדִּים (*Part. Hif'il*) → [רדם].

מָרָה • **כיס המרה** → כִּיס.

מרובע → מְרֻבָּע.

מְרוּצָה • channel: Arab. مجرى • Maimonides, *K. al-fuṣūl fī al-ṭibb* • trans. Zeraḥyah Ḥen (*Sefer ha-Peraqim*), 1.67: וזה העצב החלול ... כלומר ראש האמה מרוצתו רחוק מהגיד ומרוצת הזרע בו ממה שסמוך הצד השפל משוך בארך באמצעיתו. → NM 1:167.

מַרְחִיק (*Part. Hifʿil*) → [רחק].
מֶרְחָץ • **הרגיל במרחץ** → [רגל].
• **זוהמת המרחץ** → זֻהֲמָה.
מריכות • **מריכות נפש** · **fainting**: Arab. ذبول نفس · Maimonides, *Šarḥ fuṣūl Abūqrāṭ* · trans. Anonymous (*Pirqei Abuqraṭ*), 7.8 (360): אמר אבוקרט: כשנתפתח הצמח ונשפך לצד פנימי הגוף יבא מזה נפילת הכח וקיא ומריכות נפש. → NM 3:142.
מְרָיִם • אִילָן→אילן מרים.
מֹרֶךְ · **emaciation**: Arab. سخافة · Maimonides, *K. al-fuṣūl fī al-ṭibb* · trans. Zeraḥyah Ḥen (*Sefer ha-Peraqim*), 9.116: אשר יקרה להם העילוף בעבור מורך גופם ורוב התרת הרוח תפרנס במזון שאינה ממהרת ההתרה. → NM 1:167.
• **מורך הגוף** · **limpness of the body**: Arab. رخاوة من البدن · Maimonides, *Šarḥ fuṣūl Abūqrāṭ* · trans. Zeraḥyah Ḥen (*Pirqei Abuqraṭ*), 1.20 (47): תשובה על זה שאפשר זה כשההרקה תהיה מרובה ושתהיה מן המין הראוי להוציא עם שאר התנאים כי כשיתרבה ולא יבוא בסופו מנוחה אבל חולשה ומורך הגוף ואיפשר שיתעלפה עילוף חזק. ודע זה. → NM 3:142–3.
מרכב · **thickened juice**: Arab. عقيد · Maimonides, *K. al-fuṣūl fī al-ṭibb* · trans. Zeraḥyah Ḥen (*Sefer ha-Peraqim*), 21.61: רפואה שתטהר ותנקה מבלתי נשיכה כמו השורבו העשוי מן הפולים ומים שלפארי מהשעורים וזרע הפשתן הקלוי והמירכב העשוי מן התאנים היבישים. אבל מירכב הענבים כחו שיטהר וידבק והוא רחוק מהנשיכה יותר מכל דבר. → NM 1:167–8.
מֶרְסָא (*Aram.*) • **מורסת הבשר הרך** · **bubo**: Arab. ورم اللحم الرخو · Maimonides, *Šarḥ fuṣūl Abūqrāṭ* · trans. Zeraḥyah Ḥen (*Pirqei Abuqraṭ*), 4.55 (192): אמר בקראט: כל קדחת שתהיה עם מורסת הבשר הרך אשר באינגוינלי ודומיהם היא רעה אלא אם תהיה קדחת יום. → NM 3:143.
• **מורסת הבשר הרפה** · **bubo**: Arab. ورم اللحم الرخو · Maimonides, *Šarḥ fuṣūl Abūqrāṭ* · trans. Moses ibn Tibbon (*Pirqei Abuqraṭ*), 4.55 (192): אמר אבקראט: כל קדחת תהיה עם מורסת הבשר הרפה אשר ראינג׳ש וזולתו ממה שדומה לו הנה היא רעה אם לא שתהיה קדחת יום. → NM 3:143.
• **יציאת מורסא** → יְצִיאָה.
• **מורסא לחיית** · **a phlegmatic aposteme**: Lat. apostema flegmaticum / Arab. الورم البلغمي · Galen, *De inaequali intemperie* · trans. David Caslari (*Sefer Roʿa Mezeg Mitḥallef*), 1.2: ורוע מזג מתחלף יהיה בכל אחד ואחד מן האיברים, אי זה שיהיה כמו שיהיה לו רכות שהוא מורסא לחיית. → NM 2:167.
• **מורסת המוח** · **an inflammation of the brain (phrenitis)**: Arab. ورم الدماغ · Maimonides, *Šarḥ fuṣūl Abūqrāṭ* · trans. Moses ibn Tibbon (*Pirqei Abuqraṭ*), 4.72 (209): אמר אבקראט: כשיהיה השתן ספירי לבן הנה הוא רע וכל שכן בבעלי הקדחת אשר עם מורסת המוח. → NM 3:143.
• **מורסת המסך** · **pleurisy**: Arab. شوصة · Ibn al-Jazzār, *Zād al-musāfir wa-qūt al-ḥādir* · trans. Moses ibn Tibbon (*Sefer Ṣedat ha-Derakhim*), introduction (fol. 3[a]): השער הי״ב במורסת המסך הנקרא שוצה ומדוה הצד. → NM 4:105.

• **המורסא המתרחבת** › **shingles**: Arab. الورم الساعي · Maimonides, *K. al-fuṣūl fī al-ṭibb* · trans. Nathan ha-Me'ati (*Sefer ha-Peraqim*), 2.25: בהיות המאכלים הרעים הכימוס שני מינים דקים וגסים והנה מה שיהיה מן הכימוס הרע דק מחדש חלאים רעים וחדים וקדחות מגונות וכשיגיע אל אבר יחדש מורסא הנקראת חמרא והמורסא המתרחבת וכאבים זולתם. → NM 2:62.

• **מורסת העין** › **ophthalmia**: Arab. رمد · Maimonides, *Šarḥ fuṣūl Abūqrāṭ* · trans. Anonymous (*Pirqei Abuqraṭ*), 3.21 (127): אמר אבוקרט: ואמנם בקיץ יקרה להם קצת אלו התחלואים וקדחת תמידית ושורפת ושלישית הרבה וקיא ודפיקה ומורסת העין וכאב האזן ונגעים בפה ועפוש בנגעים ובשר מת. → NM 3:144.

• **מורסת הראש** › **phrenitis**: a) Pers. سرسام · Ibn al-Jazzār, *Zād al-musāfir wa-qūt al-ḥādir* · trans. Moses ibn Tibbon (*Sefer Ṣedat ha-Derakhim*), bk. 1, ch. 18 (fol. 26[a]): מורסת הראש במאמר מוחלט היא מורסא חמה תקרה בקצת קרומות המוח ישיגהו תמיד צער ושגעון וערבוב השכל. → NM 4:105.

b) Arab. برسام / Gr. φρενῖτις · Maimonides, *Šarḥ fuṣūl Abūqrāṭ* · trans. Moses ibn Tibbon (*Pirqei Abuqraṭ*), 7.12 (364): אמר אבקראט: ומחולי הריאה מורסת הראש. → NM 3:144.

• **מורסת הריאה** › **pneumonia**: Hippocrates, *Aphorisms* · trans. Judah Shalom, 3.23 (129) (fol. 46[b]): ובסתו פלברשין ומורסת הריאה וזכאם ונזילה ושעול וכאבי הצד והחזה והכסלים וכאב הראש וסבוב ושתוק. → NM 3:144.

• **המורסא השורצת** › **shingles**: Arab. الورم الساعي · Maimonides, *K. al-fuṣūl fī al-ṭibb* · trans. Zeraḥyah Ḥen (*Sefer ha-Peraqim*), 2.25: מפני היות המזונות שהם רעים בכימוס שתי מינים דקים ועבים כי מה שהוא מן הכימוס הרע דק יחדש חליים חדים וקדחות פוראלינטי ואם יבוא אל אבר יחדש מורסת הריזיפילה בער׳ חמרה והמורסא השורצת כלומר המתפשטת הנה והנה וכאבים וחליים אחרים. → NM 1:191.

• *Plur.* **מורסות** › **wounds**: Lat. vulnera · Hippocrates, *Aphorisms* · trans. Hillel ben Samuel, 5.66 (286) (fol. 37[b]): א״א: המורסות שהן גדולות ורעות אם לא יראה בהם נפח הרעה גדולה מאד. → NM 3:143.

• **מורסות קרומי המוח** › **phrenitis**: Gr. φρενίτιδες · Hippocrates, *Aphorisms* · trans. Joseph Delmedigo, 3.30 (136): וליוצאים מאלו השנים יקרם קוצר הנשימה וחולי הצד ומורסת הריאה ותנומות ומורסות קרומי המוח וקדחות בוערות ושלשולי הבטן ארוכים והרקת הירוקה מלמעלה ומלמטה ושלשול הדם וחלקות הבטן והטחורים. → NM 3:144–5.

[מרסם] • *Part. Puʿal* **מְמֹרְסָם** › **tumorous**: Arab. وارم · Maimonides, *K. al-fuṣūl fī al-ṭibb* · trans. Zeraḥyah Ḥen (*Sefer ha-Peraqim*), 3.109: ברופאים כת שחושבים כי כל אשר יהיה יותר קובץ בחוזק יהיה יותר טוב במה שירצו בו לעשות דברים מקבצים וכן מה שהיה מן הרפואות יותר מתיר שהוא יותר טוב ומועיל יותר במה שירצו להתירו. ולא יבינו כי כל אחד משתי אילו הכחות כל אשר הוא יותר חזק יהיה מה שיתחדש באבר הממורסם מן הכאב יותר חזק. → NM 1:163.

• *Nitpaʿel* **נִתְמַרְסֵם** › 1. **to have a tumor**: Arab. تورّم · Maimonides, *K. al-fuṣūl fī al-ṭibb* · trans. Zeraḥyah Ḥen (*Sefer ha-Peraqim*), 3.61: בהאריך לעמוד הלחויות המורקות אל המקום הפנוי באברים אשר נתמרסמו יתחדש בהם שינויים משונים מאד. → NM 1:168.

‣ II. to swell: Arab. ورم · Maimonides, *Šarḥ fuṣūl Abūqrāṭ* · trans. Zeraḥyah Ḥen (*Pirqei Abuqraṭ*), 3.26 (132): וכל זאת ההנהגה מפסידה המזון ומרבה הליחות וגופותם עם זה לח ואיבריהם רפים והוא ראוי להיות כל מה שזכר כי כשיתמרסם המושקולי של הגרון ימשוך החוליה מן העורף בעבור חלקות הקישורים. → NM 3:145.

מַרְפֶּה (*Part. Hif'il*) → [רפה].

מַרְפֵּק • **כפיפת המרפק** → **כְּפִיפָה**.

• **פרק המרפק** → **פֶּרֶק**.

[מרק] • *Part. Pi'el* **מְמָרֵק** • **הסם הממורק** → **סַם**.

מָרָק • **מרק תרנגולים קטנים** ‣ a kind of broth: Arab. زيرباج / Lat. species cibi iusculenti · Ibn al-Jazzār, *Zād al-musāfir wa-qūt al-ḥādir* · trans. Moses ibn Tibbon (*Sefer Ṣedat ha-Derakhim*), bk. 1, ch. 10 (fol. 16[b]): מזה תאר גירא וחבר אותה בן מאסויה יועיל מהסבוב הנקרא סדר בערבי ומכאב הראש שיקרה מליחה לבנה ומרה שחורה יטהר האצטומכא ויתחזק הכבד והוא עומד במעמד הגיראש הגדולות והלקיחה ממנו מדרהם עד שקל ויקחנו במים חמים ויאכל אחריו מרק תרנגולים קטנים או פיישאן. → NM 4:105–6.

מֶרְקָח • *Plur.* **מרקחים** ‣ stomachic: Arab. جوارشن; جوارش, *Plur.* جوارشنات / Pers. گوارش · Al-Zahrāwī, *K. al-taṣrīf li-man ʿağiza ʿan at-taʾlīf* · trans. Shem Tov ben Isaac (*Sefer ha-Shimmush*), bk. 27, fol. 124[b], col. a: ודחיית נזקו לבשלו היטב עם יועזר הרבה מבלי שתיית מים אחריו כלל עד שיתעכל וירד מן האסטומ׳ ואחר כך להרגיל אחריו מה שידקדק ויגיר השתן מן המרקחים. → NM 4:106.

• **מרקחים חמים** ‣ stomachics: Arab. جوارشنات · Al-Zahrāwī, *K. al-taṣrīf li-man ʿağiza ʿan at-taʾlīf* · trans. Shem Tov ben Isaac (*Sefer ha-Shimmush*), bk. 27, fol. 123[b], cols. a–b: ואמר אסחק בן סלימאן בלחם מצות כי הוא לא יאות לשום אדם אע״פ שרבים מן הקוצרים והאכרים אוכלים אותו ויתעכל באצטומכתם מרוב יגיעתם ועמלם והנהגתם עליו ונזקו גדול לבעלי המנוחה ומי שהוא חלוש העכול. ותקונו ודחיית נזקו יהיה במה שזכרתי מתקון לחם הסלת בדברים המדקדקים והמגירים השתן מן המרקחים החמים ודומיהם. → NM 4:106–7.

מִרְקַחַת ‣ I. electuary: Arab. معجون · a) Ibn al-Jazzār, *Zād al-musāfir wa-qūt al-ḥādir* · trans. Moses ibn Tibbon (*Sefer Ṣedat ha-Derakhim*), bk. 1, ch. 23 (fol. 36[a]): תאר מרקחת יועיל בע״ה מן הרוחות העבות ומן הפלג ועקום הפה והרפיון והרעש והגלגול ותרדמת האיברים ורוח הגבנות וקווץ העצבים וכל חולי שיולד מליחה לבנה דבקה. → NM 4:107.

b) Maimonides, *K. al-fuṣūl fī al-ṭibb* · trans. Nathan ha-Me'ati (*Sefer ha-Peraqim*), 10.56: הנה רפאתי אנשים רבים מקדחת רביעית בשתית התריאק אלא שהייתי מריק גופם תחלה ואחר הייתי משקה אותם סחיטת אפסנתין ואחריהם הייתי משקה אותם זה המרקחת קודם עת הקדחת בשתי שעות והיה המוקדח מתרפא בשתי שתיות או שלש. → NM 2:62–3.

‣ II. stomachic: Arab. جوارشن · Al-Zahrāwī, *K. al-taṣrīf li-man ʿağiza ʿan at-taʾlīf* · trans. Shem Tov ben Isaac (*Sefer ha-Shimmush*), bk. 27, fol. 138[b], col. a: וראוי להנזר ממנו מי שירבו בו הרוחות וימהר אליו הגעש החמוץ ואם יגבר עליו יצרו ויאכל ממנו ראוי לשתות אחריו מיד מן היין החי או לאכול ממרקחת הכמון הלבן או מרקחת הלבוניי. → NM 4:107.

• **מרקחת החבושים** ‣ the quince stomachic: Arab. جوارشن السفرجل · a) Al-Zahrāwī, *K.*

al-taṣrīf li-man ʿağiza ʿan at-taʾlīf · trans. Shem Tov ben Isaac (*Sefer ha-Shimmush*), bk. 27, fol. 141b, col. b: והמרבה מאכילת השקדים הרטובים החדשים ראוי לקחת עליהם ממרקחת התמרי או ממרקחת החבושים המשלשל. → NM 4:107.

b) Maimonides, *K. al-fuṣūl fī al-ṭibb* · trans. Zeraḥyah Ḥen (*Sefer ha-Peraqim*), 9.47: המילוי אשר ישתלשל עמו הטבע עד שיתרבה ויחטוף הכח תפרנסנו בדברים עוצרים בסדר והרבה פעמים תפול תאות המזון עם אחד ממיני השלשול הנק׳ דרב וצריך שיקח החולה מרקחת החבושים ודומיהו. → NM 1:168.

c) Maimonides, *K. al-fuṣūl fī al-ṭibb* · trans. Nathan ha-Meʾati (*Sefer ha-Peraqim*), 9.47: הקבסא שיותר עמה הטבע עד שיפליג ויתיש הכח יונהג בה בדברים הקובצים בהדרגה ורבים יפול עם השלשול תאות המאכל ואז יקח העלול מרקחת החבושים וכיוצא בו. → NM 2:62.

• **מרקחת התמרי** · **the date stomachic**: Arab. جوارشن التمري · Al-Zahrāwī, *K. al-taṣrīf li-man ʿağiza ʿan at-taʾlīf* · trans. Shem Tov ben Isaac (*Sefer ha-Shimmush*), bk. 27, fol. 141b, col. b: והמרבה מאכילת השקדים הרטובים החדשים ראוי לקחת עליהם ממרקחת התמרי או ממרקחת החבושים המשלשל. → NM 4:108.

מְרֵרָה • **מררת הפיל** · **(lit., elephant's bile); lycium**: Arab. فيل زهرج · Al-Rāzī, *K. al-Manṣūrī* · trans. Shem Tov ben Isaac (*Sefer Almansur*), Pe 4 (64): פילזהרג הוא לשון פרס וב״מ מררת הפיל ובלעז ליסיאום: יחזק השער כשינתן על הראש. → NM 2:15.

מַרְתִּיעַ (*Part. Hifʿil*) → [רתע].

מְשַׁבֵּר (*Part. Piʿel*) → שָׁבַר.

מְשֻׁבָּשׁ (*Part. Puʿal*) → [שבש].

משובש → מְשֻׁבָּשׁ.

משוחף → מְשֻׁחָף.

משוכר → מְשֻׁכָּר.

משוכשך → מְשֻׁכְשָׁךְ.

משונה → מְשֻׁנֶּה.

משועמם → מְשֻׁעֲמָם.

משוקה → מְשֻׁקֶּה.

משורי • דפק משורי → דֹּפֶק.

מְשׁוּשׁ · **fomentation; fomenting**: Arab. تكميد · Maimonides, *Šarḥ fuṣūl Abūqrāṭ* · trans. Zeraḥyah Ḥen (*Pirqei Abuqraṭ*), 6.31 (323): אמר בקראט: כאבי העינים יתיר אותם שתות היין שאינו מזוג או המרחץ או המישוש הנק׳ תכמיד בערבי או הקזת הגיד או שתיית הרפואה. → NM 3:145–6.

משותק → מְשֻׁתָּק.

מָשַׁח • **משח הנחירים** · **to apply an errhine**: Arab. سَعَّطَ · Ibn al-Jazzār, *Zād al-musāfir wa-qūt al-ḥādir* · trans. Moses ibn Tibbon (*Sefer Ṣedat ha-Derakhim*), bk. 1, ch. 10 (fol. 15a): וימשח נחיריו אחרי הרקת הגוף בשחיטת כרוב או בשחיטת בלידש או בשמן קמוילא או בקצת השמנים החמים אשר זכרנו. → NM 4:108.

מַשְׁחֶזֶת · **whetstone**: Arab. مسن · Ibn al-Jazzār, *Zād al-musāfir wa-qūt al-ḥādir* · trans. Moses ibn Tibbon (*Sefer Ṣedat ha-Derakhim*), bk. 2, ch. 4 (fol. 45a): ויעשה ממנו גרגרים

קטנים ויקח ממנו אחת וישרה אותה במי מטר ויטיף ממנו בעין או תחכך אותה על המשחזת ויכחול בו. → NM 4:108.

מַשְׁחִין (*Part. Hifʿil*) → [שחן].

מְשֻׁחָף (*Part. Puʿal*) → [שחף].

מֻשְׁחָת (*Part. Hofʿal*) → [שחת].

מְשִׁיחָה · **fomentation; fomenting**: Arab. تكميد · Maimonides, *Šarḥ fuṣūl Abūqrāṭ* · trans. Zeraḥyah Ḥen (*Pirqei Abuqraṭ*), 5.28 (248): אמר בקראט: המשיחה עם התבלין ימשוך הדם הבא מן הנשים ויועיל במקומות אחרים הרבה אלא שהוא יחדש בראש כובד. → NM 3:146.

• **משיחת הנחירים** · **errhine; snuff medicine**: Arab. سعوط · Ibn al-Jazzār, *Zād al-musāfir wa-qūt al-ḥāḍir* · trans. Moses ibn Tibbon (*Sefer Ṣedat ha-Derakhim*), bk. 1, ch. 10 (Ms. Oxford, Bodleian Library, Poc. 353, Uri Heb. 314, fol. 4[b]): ויזהר החולה שלא יעשה שפיכת המים על הראש ומשיחת הנחירים רק אחר הרקת הגוף. → NM 4:108–9.

מְשִׁיחוּת · **greasy quality**: Lat. unctuositas · Bruno Longobucco, *Cyrurgia Magna* · trans. Hillel ben Samuel (*Sefer Keritut*), 30[b]: משיחות שמרכבות ומחליקות האבר בלחותם ומשיחותם. → NM 1:31.

מְשִׁיכָה · **tetanus**: Arab. تمدّد / Gr. τέτανος · Maimonides, *Šarḥ fuṣūl Abūqrāṭ* · trans. Moses ibn Tibbon (*Pirqei Abuqraṭ*), 4.57 (194): אמר אבקראט: מי שקרהו קווץ או משיכה ואחר כן תמצאהו קדחת יותך בה חליו. → NM 3:146.

מָשַׁךְ · **to supply with [food]**: Arab. مدّ · Ibn al-Jazzār, *Zād al-musāfir wa-qūt al-ḥāḍir* · trans. Moses ibn Tibbon (*Sefer Ṣedat ha-Derakhim*), bk. 1, ch. 1 (fol. 5[a]): השער מתילד מאיד עשני עב מתחדש מן החום האשי בגוף ויצמח השער ויתוסף במה שימשך מן האיד הזה. → NM 4:109.

• *Part.* **מוֹשֵׁךְ** • **הסם המושך** → סַם.

• *Part. Nifʿal* **נִמְשָׁךְ** • **נמשך זה אחר זה** · **synonymous**: Arab. مترادف · Maimonides, *K. al-fuṣūl fī al-ṭibb* · trans. Zeraḥyah Ḥen (*Sefer ha-Peraqim*), 23.21: אמר משה בהיותך משתכל מה שזכר גליאנוס בספרו הוקרא הרעד והרפפות והריגור והכיווץ ובאר זה כי שם הרעד והרעש שתי שמות נמשכות זו אחר זו. → NM 1:168; corr. 4:229.

מְשַׁכֵּךְ (*Part. Piʿel*) → [שכך].

מְשֻׁכָּר (*Part. Puʿal*) → [שכר].

מְשֻׁכְשָׁךְ (*Part. Puʿal*) → [שכשך].

מָשַׁל · **to mould**: Arab. مثّل · Maimonides, *K. al-fuṣūl fī al-ṭibb* · trans. Nathan ha-Me'ati (*Sefer ha-Peraqim*), 7.73: ולפעמים ימשל הראות ויחקקהו חק נסתר ולפעמים יציירהו ולא ישלם כחו. → NM 2:63.

• *Part.* **מוֹשֵׁל** • **האבר המושל** → אֵבֶר.

מִשְׁלַחַת · **flowing; pouring**: Lat. effusio · Bruno Longobucco, *Cyrurgia Magna* · trans. Hillel ben Samuel (*Sefer Keritut*), fol. 96[a]: הבשרית האות עליה הכובד והקושי והעובי עם כאב גדול וסבתה משלחת החומר מן המעים אל הבצים או הכאה. → NM 1:31.

מַשְׁלִיךְ (*Part. Hifʿil*) → [שלך].

מְשַׁלְשֵׁל (*Part. Piʿel*) → [שלשל].

מִשְׁמוּשׁ • **המישמוש בידים** · a warm compress: Arab. التكميد · Maimonides, *K. al-fuṣūl fī al-ṭibb* · trans. Zeraḥyah Ḥen (*Sefer ha-Peraqim*), 23.33: המישמוש בידים או בדבר אחר ונקרא בערבי תכמיד והוא נופל על מה שיחמם הגוף מחוצה ומיניו חמשה. → NM 1:168.

[משמש] • *Pi'el* **מִשְׁמֵשׁ** · to apply a hot compress: Arab. كمّد · Maimonides, *K. al-fuṣūl fī al-ṭibb* · trans. Zeraḥyah Ḥen (*Sefer ha-Peraqim*), 23.33: והממוצע הוא שיוקח שעורים וכרסנה תשחקם ותבשלם בחומץ חזק ומזוג יותר חזק יהיה מאותו ששותים בני אדם ותשימנו בכיס ותמשמש בו האברים וכן תעשה בסובין. → NM 1:169.

מְשֻׁנֶּה (*Part. Pu'al*) → [שנה].

מְשֻׁעְמָם (*Part. Pu'al*) → [שעמם].

מִשְׁפָּט • **החקדמה במשפט** → הַקְדָּמָה.

• *Plur.* **משפטים** · effects; virtues: Arab. أحكام · Ibn Sīnā, *K. al-adwiya al-qalbiya* · trans. Anonymous (*Sammim Libbiyim*), fol. 130ª: סוסן אראה אותו קרוב הטבע מן הזעפראן קרוב המשפט ממשפטיו. → NM 4:109.

מַשְׁקֶה · wine: Arab. شراب / Gr. θώρηξις · Maimonides, *Šarḥ fuṣūl Abūqrāṭ* · trans. Moses ibn Tibbon (*Pirqei Abuqraṭ*), 2.21 (73): אמר אבקראט: שתיית המשקה יסיר הרעב. → NM 3:146–7.

• **משקה הדבש** · honey drink (h.l., hydromel): *Anonymous Glossary*, Ms. Oxford, Bodleian Library, Mich. Add. 22, fol. 6ª: אדרומיל משקה הדבש. → NM 4:109.

• **משקה סוכרי** · julep (i.e., a syrup made with rose water and sugar or honey): Arab. جلّاب · Ibn al-Jazzār, *Zād al-musāfir wa-qūt al-ḥādir* · trans. Moses ibn Tibbon (*Sefer Ṣedat ha-Derakhim*), bk. 1, ch. 18 (fol. 27ᵇ): וישקוהו בערב מי רמונים עם משקה סוכרי. → NM 4:109–10.

מְשֻׁקֶּה (*Part. Pu'al*) → [שקה].

מִשְׁקָל • *Plur.* **משקלים** · *mithqāl* (i.e., 4.46 grams), *Plur. mithqāls*: Arab. مثاقيل · Maimonides, *K. al-fuṣūl fī al-ṭibb* · trans. Nathan ha-Me'ati (*Sefer ha-Peraqim*), 9.46: ותואר הגירא: יוקח דארציני הוא סינאמומי ושבלת נרד וזעפרן ואשארי ומצטכי ועץ בלשמו מכל אחד ששה משקלים אלואן מאה השקלים. → NM 2:63–4.

מִשְׁקָע · base; insertion; origin; the place of growth; root: Arab. مغرز · Ibn Sīnā, *K. al-Qānūn fī al-ṭibb* · trans. Nathan ha-Me'ati (*Sefer ha-Qanun*), bk. 1 (fol. 44ª): ולפעמים יקרבו מאד משקע האוזן בקצת האנשים ומתחברים בו ויניע(ו) אזניו. → NM 4:110.

מַשְׂרֵט • *Plur.* **משרטים** · scarifying scalpels: Arab. مشارط · Al-Zahrāwī, *K. al-taṣrīf li-man 'ağiza 'an at-ta'līf* · trans. Shem Tov ben Isaac (*Sefer ha-Shimmush*), bk. 30, 2.46 (fol. 216ᵇ): ואלה הם המשרטים אשר יבוקעו ויופשטו בהם האגודות והצמחים והם שלשה מינים גדולים ואמצעים וקטנים. → NM 1:105.

[משש] • *Part. Pi'el* **מְמַשֵּׁשׁ** • **כלי הממשש** → כְּלִי.

מִשְׁתַּדֵּף (*Part. Hitpa'el*) → שָׁדַף.

מִשְׁתַּנֶּה (*Part. Hitpa'el*) → [שנה].

מְשֻׁתָּק (*Part. Pu'al*) → שָׁתַק.

מַתְאִים (*Part. Hif'il*) → [תאם].

מִתְאַכֵּל (*Part. Hitpa'el*) → [אכל].

מְתֻבָּל (*Part. Pu'al*) → [**תבל**].
מִתְהַפֵּךְ (*Part. Hitpa'el*) → **הָפַךְ**.
מתובל → **מְתֻבָּל**.
מִתּוּחַ · **tetanus:** Arab. تمدّد · Maimonides, *Šarḥ fuṣūl Abūqrāṭ* · trans. Anonymous (*Pirqei Abuqraṭ*), 4.57 (194): אמר אבוקרט: מי שארעו חולי הקווץ או המתוח ואחר כך אירע לו קדחת הותר בו החולי. → NM 3:148.
מִתּוּן • **המתון מן האכילה** · **abstention from food (i.e., fasting):** Arab. الصبر عن الطعام · Maimonides, *Šarḥ fuṣūl Abūqrāṭ* · trans. Moses ibn Tibbon (*Pirqei Abuqraṭ*), 1.13 (40): אבל הישישים אשר בתכלית הישישות הנה לא יסבלו המתון מן האכילה אבל יצטרכו שיקחו אותו מעט מעט פעם אחר פעם לקרבת חמימותם מן הכבוי ויצטרכו אל התמדת מה שימשכה מעט אחר מעט. → NM 3:148.
מתוקן → **מְתֻקָּן**.
[**מתח**] • *Part. Nif'al* **נִמְתָּח** · **spasmodic:** Arab. متواتر · Maimonides, *K. al-fuṣūl fī al-ṭibb* · trans. Nathan ha-Me'ati (*Sefer ha-Peraqim*), 4.12: הדפק החזק יהלום לעולם הלימה כבדה וכן מין הדפק הקשה יהלום הלימה כבדה כמו דפק הנרעד והדפק הנמתח. → NM 2:68.
• *Hif'il* **הִמְתִּיחַ** • **המתיח הרוח** · **to dilate the pneuma:** Lat. dilato spiritum · Ibn Sīnā, *K. al-adwiya al-qalbiya* · trans. Anonymous (*Sefer ha-Refu'ot ha-Libbiyot*), fol. 250[b]: ובו סגולה לחזק הלב ולשמח והיא מתחדשת ממה שקדמנו בו ובזה הוא ממתיח הרוח ומחזקו וממרקו ומזהירו. → NM 4:110.
מִתְחַלֵּף (*Part. Hitpa'el*) → [**חלף**].
מְתִיחָה · **tetanus:** Arab. تمدّد · Hippocrates, *Aphorisms* · trans. Nathan ha-Me'ati, 4.57 (194) (fol. 45[b]): אמר אבוקרט: מי שיקרהו כויצה הוא אישפשמי או מתיחה ואחר ימצאהו קדחת נתך בה חליו. → NM 3:148.
מַתִּיךְ (*Part. Hif'il*) → [**נתך**].
מְתִיקָה → **מתקה**.
מִתְלַבֵּד (*Part. Hitpa'el*) → [**לבד**].
מִתְלַהֵב (*Part. Hitpa'el*) → [**לחב**].
מִתְלַחֵם (*Part. Hitpa'el*) → [**לחם**].
מתלעת · **jaw (bone):** Lat. mandibula · Bruno Longobucco, *Cyrurgia Magna* · trans. Hillel ben Samuel (*Sefer Keritut*), fol. 59[b]: ההשמטה מעצם המתלעת תבוא לעתים רחוקות וההוראה על זה היא בהיות שורת השנים התחתונים בלתי שוה בעליונה. → NM 1:31.
[**מתן**] • *Hif'il* **הִמְתִּין** • **המתין על** · **to bear:** Arab. صبر على · Maimonides, *K. al-fuṣūl fī al-ṭibb* · trans. Zeraḥyah Ḥen (*Sefer ha-Peraqim*), 20.65: הדברים אשר להם שמנונית ודבקות כמו החלבים מיד שיגיעו אל האסטומכא בתחלת אכלם הם שובעים וימלאו גוף האוכל אותם ואחרי כן ישובו וימעטו התאוה למזון והאדם לא ימתין על התמדתם. → NM 1:169.
מִתְנַגֵּעַ (*Part. Hitpa'el*) → **נָגַע**.
מִתְנַכֵּר (*Part. Hitpa'el*) → [**נכר**].
מִתְפַּרְנֵס (*Part. Hitpa'el*) → [**פרנס**].
מִתְפַּשֵּׁט (*Part. Hitpa'el*) → **פָּשַׁט**.
מתקה · **sweetness:** Arab. حلاوة · Al-Zahrāwī, *K. al-taṣrīf li-man 'ağiza 'an at-ta'līf* · trans.

Shem Tov ben Isaac (*Sefer ha-Shimmush*), bk. 27, fol. 133[a], col. b: ודחיית נזקו תהיה באכילת מיני מתקה. → NM 4:110.

מְתֻקָּן (*Part. Pu'al*) → [תקן].

מִתְרַגֵּשׁ (*Part. Hitpa'el*) → [רגש].

מִתְרַחֵב (*Part. Hitpa'el*) → [רחב].

נ

נאד • החדרוקן אשר בו חמים כמי הנאד → הִידְרוֹקָן.

נאדי • השקוי הנאדי → שִׁקּוּי.

נָאוּת · crudeness: Arab. فجاجة · Maimonides, *Šarḥ fuṣūl Abūqrāṭ* · trans. Moses ibn Tibbon (*Pirqei Abuqraṭ*), 4.37 (174): אמר המפרש: חוזק הקדחת יכבה החום הטבעי ולא יתבשלו הליחות הקרות מאד אשר בנראה מן הגוף אשר מהם תצא הזיעה הקרה ותורה על נאות הליחות האלה וחוזק קרירותם היות חום הקדחת החזקה לא יוכל לחמם מה שיצא מהם. → NM 3:149.

נְאוֹתוּת • יש ביניהם נאותות · **they are mutually appropriate:** Lat. ad invicem convenientes sunt / Arab. وافق بعضه بعضا · Galen, *De inaequali intemperie* · trans. David Caslari (*Sefer Ro'a Mezeg Mithallef*), 6.3: ומפני זה היה שהליחות שהם בקצת בעלי חיים יש ביניהם נאותות. → NM 2:167.

נֶאֱכָל (*Part. Nif'al*) → [אכל].

נֶאֱמָן (*Part. Nif'al*) → [אמן].

נָבוּב • הנבוב · **vena cava:** Arab. الأجوف · Ibn Sīnā, *K. al-Qānūn fī al-ṭibb* · trans. Nathan ha-Me'ati (*Sefer ha-Qanun*), bk. 1 (fol. 66[a]): הפרק החמישי בנתוח הנבוב היורד הנה חתמנו הדבור בחלק העולה מן הנבוב והוא הקטון שבחלקיו. → NM 4:110–1.

• הוריד הנבוב → וְרִיד.

• הנבוב היורד · **the inferior vena cava:** Arab. الأجوف النازل · Ibn Sīnā, *K. al-Qānūn fī al-ṭibb* · trans. Nathan ha-Me'ati (*Sefer ha-Qanun*), bk. 1 (fol. 66[a]): הפרק החמישי בנתוח הנבוב היורד הנה חתמנו הדבור בחלק העולה מן הנבוב והוא הקטון שבחלקיו. → NM 4:111.

נָבוֹךְ • קדחות נבוכות → קַדַּחַת.

נְבוֹכוּת · **confusion:** Arab. تحيّر · Ibn al-Jazzār, *Zād al-musāfir wa-qūt al-ḥāḍir* · trans. Moses ibn Tibbon (*Sefer Ṣedat ha-Derakhim*), bk. 2, ch. 6 (fol. 45[b]): ואם סר חליו יורה זה כי החולי היה מפני שתוף האצטמ׳ ואם עמד הדמיון והנבוכות והאופל יורה כי החולי ההוא בעין לבד. → NM 4:111.

[נבט] • *Hif'il* **הִבִּיט** · **to indicate:** Arab. أنذر · Maimonides, *Šarḥ fuṣūl Abūqrāṭ* · trans. Anonymous (*Pirqei Abuqraṭ*), 2.28 (80): אמר אבוקרט: מי שהיה בו הקדחת בלתי חלושה מאד אם ישאר גופו על ענינו לא יחסר ממנו כלום או יותך ביותר מן הראוי הוא רע כי הראשון יביט באורך חולי והשני יורה על חלישות הכח. → NM 3:149.

• הביט בעיקום · **to squint:** Lat. obliquitas aspectus · Al-Rāzī, attr., *On the Treatment of Small Children* · trans. Anonymous, ch. 12: כשהילד הוא מביט בעיקום. → NM 2:179.

נִגְלֶה (*Part. Nif'al*) → [גלה].

נָגַע · **to inflame:** Arab. قرّح · Maimonides, *Šarḥ fuṣūl Abūqrāṭ* · trans. Zeraḥyah Ḥen (*Pirqei Abuqraṭ*), 4.24 (161): אבל אם תהיה זאת הליחה המלנקוניאה היא אשר עשתה הפונטי וגם נגעה המעיים ואחר כן באה הדם על כל פנים יחדש במעיים דמיון הסרטן המתחדש בשטח העור. → NM 3:149–50.

• *Nif'al* **נִגַּע** · **to cause ulceration:** Arab. أقرح · Maimonides, *Šarḥ fuṣūl Abūqrāṭ* · trans. Moses ibn Tibbon (*Pirqei Abuqraṭ*), 5.15 (235): אמר המפרש: כאשר לא יצא החומר אשר נבקע והגיע בריקות החזה הנה יתעפש ויקפא וינגע הריאה. → NM 3:150.

• *Part. Pi'el* **מְנַגֵּעַ** • **הסם המנגע** → **סַם**.

• **סמים מנגעים** → **סַם**.

• *Part. Pu'al* **מְנֻגָּע** ‣ **ulcerous:** Lat. vulneratus / Gr. ἑλκούμενος · Hippocrates, *Aphorisms* · trans. Hillel ben Samuel, 5.23 (243) (fol. 32[b]): וגם באיריסיפילה הבלתי מנוגעת. → NM 3:132.

• *Hitpa'el* **הִתְנַגֵּעַ** ‣ **to develop an ulcer:** a) Arab. تقرّح · Maimonides, *Šarḥ fuṣūl Abūqrāṭ* · trans. Moses ibn Tibbon (*Pirqei Abuqraṭ*), 3.20 (126): וחליים ממרה אדומה כמו השחין אשר יתנגע בהם העור והמורסות. → NM 3:150.

b) Arab. قرح · Maimonides, *K. al-fuṣūl fī al-ṭibb* · trans. Nathan ha-Me'ati (*Sefer ha-Peraqim*), 6.72: כשיתנגע מעי מן המעים מן המרה השחורה לא יהיה לו רפואה. → NM 2:65.

• *Part. Hitpa'el* **מִתְנַגֵּעַ** ‣ **ulcerous:** Arab. متقرّح · Ibn al-Jazzār, *Zād al-musāfir wa-qūt al-ḥādir* · trans. Moses ibn Tibbon (*Sefer Ṣedat ha-Derakhim*), bk. 7, 20.3: וזכר שהוא כשיעורב גפרית עם גומא טרבנטינה יסיר הגרב המתנגע והקובא והרשמים הלבנים אשר יקרו בצפרנים. → NM 1:62.

נֶגַע ‣ I. **fistula:** Lat. fistula · Bruno Longobucco, *Cyrurgia Magna* · trans. Hillel ben Samuel (*Sefer Keritut*), fol. 36[b]: הנגע היא חבלה עמוקה וצרה מעוקלת כלומר במקום אחד רחבה ובמקום אחר צרה עם קושי הבשר שסביבה והיא כמו קנה נוצת אווז בענין הכנסה. → NM 1:31–2.

‣ II. **ulcer:** Arab. قرحة · Ibn al-Jazzār, *Zād al-musāfir wa-qūt al-ḥādir* · trans. Moses ibn Tibbon (*Sefer Ṣedat ha-Derakhim*), bk. 7, 14.2: ואם הרתיחה ולא תתעפש תחדש המין אשר יתחדש עמו דומה בכאב הנגע בכל שטח הגוף ותהיה עמו עקיצה דומה לעקיצת המחטים. → NM 1:62.

‣ III. **wound:** Arab. جراحة · Ibn al-Jazzār, *Zād al-musāfir wa-qūt al-ḥādir* · trans. Moses ibn Tibbon (*Sefer Ṣedat ha-Derakhim*), bk. 7, 15.1: הנה כל מורסא תתחדש מהגרת ליחה אל אבר מהאברים וסבות ההגרה מהם מתחילות באות מחוץ ומהם קודמות פנימיות והמתחילות כמו הכאה או נגע או ריצוץ או הקעה או שבר או סדק. → NM 1:62.

• **מקום הנגע** → **מָקוֹם**.

• **עשה הנגע** → **עָשָׂה**.

• *Plur.* **נגעים** ‣ **ulcers:** Arab. قروح · Maimonides, *K. al-fuṣūl fī al-ṭibb* · trans. Nathan ha-Me'ati (*Sefer ha-Peraqim*), 6.83: הדם אשר יצא מן הכבד עם הציאה זה לפעמים יעצר ביום או ביומים או שלשה ויבא יותר רע ממה שהיה בפעם הראשון ולא יבאו עמו גרידות. ואלו הם שני אותות שאינן כלום מנגעי המעים. → NM 2:65.

• **נגעים אשר יתרחבו** ‣ **herpes:** Arab. القروح التي تسعى · Maimonides, *Šarḥ fuṣūl Abūqrāṭ* · trans. Moses ibn Tibbon (*Pirqei Abuqraṭ*), 5.22 (242): והוא היותר טוב מכל הדברים לשבר העצמות וכל שכן המופשטים מן העור ומן העצמות בפרט לעצמות הראש וכל מה שהמיתו הקור או נגעו ולנגעים אשר יתרחבו. → NM 3:150.

• **הנגעים המתרחבים** ‣ **herpes:** Arab. القروح التي تسعى · Maimonides, *Šarḥ fuṣūl Abūqrāṭ* · trans. Anonymous (*Pirqei Abuqraṭ*), 5.22 (242): והוא מן הנאותים שבענינים לשברון העצמות וכ״ש לערומים מהם מן הבשר וכ״ש לעצמות הראש ולכל מי שאחזו הקור וניגעתהו והנגעים המתרחבים והמתאכלים. → NM 3:150–1.

• **הנגעים הנוקבים** ‧ **penetrating fistulas:** Lat. fistule penetrantes · Bruno Longobucco, *Cyrurgia Magna* · trans. Hillel ben Samuel (*Sefer Keritut*), fol. 100[a]: ואל תחשוב שיש דרך אחרת בנגעים הנוקבים. → NM 1:32.

• **נגעי הפה** ‧ **aphthae:** Arab. قلاع · Hippocrates, *Aphorisms* · trans. Nathan ha-Me'ati, 3.24 (130) (fol. 53[b]): אמר אבוקרט: ואמנם בשנים הנה יקרו אלו החליים: הנערים הקטנים בעת הולדם יקרה להם נגעי הפה הנקראים אלקלעא. → NM 3:151.

[נגר] • *Part. Hif'il* **מַגִּיר** • **הסם המגיר הדם** → **סַם**.

• **הסם המגיר לזיעה** → **סַם**.

• **הסם המגיר השתן** → **סַם**.

נִדְבָּק (*Part. Nif'al*) → **[דבק]**.

נָהַג ‧ I. **to administer (a remedy):** Lat. administrare · Bruno Longobucco, *Cyrurgia Magna* · trans. Hillel ben Samuel (*Sefer Keritut*), fol. 16[b]: ואפילו בגופים הקשים והיבשים מאד הסרפינו עם טירבינטינה תנהוג. → NM 1:32.

‧ II. **to apply:** Lat. uti · Al-Rāzī, attr., *On the Treatment of Small Children* · trans. Anonymous, ch. 24: וינהג זה השמן תמיד. → NM 2:179.

• *Hitpa'el* **הִתְנַהֵג** ‧ **to be treated:** Arab. تدبّر · Maimonides, *Šarḥ fuṣūl Abūqrāṭ* · trans. Moses ibn Tibbon (*Pirqei Abuqraṭ*), 1.1 (19): אמר המחבר: ועם השתמשו בה ידע כי כל מי שהוא בלתי שלם בה הנה יזיק יותר ממה שיועיל כי היות האיש בריא או חולה יותר טוב שלא יתנהג בעצת רופא כלל משיתנהג בעצת רופא יטעה בו. → NM 3:151.

נוֹדָע (*Part. Nif'al*) → **יָדַע**.

[נוח] • *Part.* **נָח** • **הגידים הנחים** → **גִּיד**.

• **העורקים הנחים** → **עוֹרֶק**.

• *Hif'il* **הֵנִיחַ** ‧ I. **to compose:** Arab. وضع · Galen, attr., *Prohibition of Burial* · trans. Judah al-Ḥarizi (*Sefer Issur ha-Qevurah le-Galienus*), par. 1: אמר גליינוס: אני הנחתי ספר בד' מאמרים. → NM 4:111.

‧ II. **to put an end to:** Arab. سكّن / Gr. παύω · Maimonides, *Šarḥ fuṣūl Abūqrāṭ* · trans. Moses ibn Tibbon (*Pirqei Abuqraṭ*), 2.2 (54): אמר אבקראט: כאשר הניחה השינה ערבוב השכל הנה הוא סימן טוב. → NM 3:151.

• **הניח מן** ‧ **to refrain from:** Arab. اجتنب عن · Maimonides, *K. al-fuṣūl fī al-ṭibb* · trans. Zeraḥyah Ḥen (*Sefer ha-Peraqim*), 8.22: הייתי מקדים על הרבה בני אדם וקצתם השקיתים המים הקרים בהבטחה ונאמנות בכל זמן שהם חולים ומהם בזמן בלתי זמן עם שזולתי מן הרופאים היו מניחים מהשקותם אילו. → NM 1:169.

• **הניח למטה** ‧ **to use as a suppository:** Arab. احتمل · Maimonides, *K. al-fuṣūl fī al-ṭibb* · trans. Nathan ha-Me'ati (*Sefer ha-Peraqim*), 13.34: קצת הקדמונים היו מצויים למי שמצאו קולנג' שיהיה לוקח אבן קטן מן המלח ומניחים למטה ויהיה הפרש יוצא יציאה נקלה מהרה. → NM 2:65–6.

• *Part. Hof'al* **מֻנָּח** ‧ I. **composed:** Arab. موضوع · Maimonides, *Šarḥ fuṣūl Abūqrāṭ* · trans. Moses ibn Tibbon (*Pirqei Abuqraṭ*), 1.1 (17): וידוע כי ידיעת אלו החלקים השבעה כלם ולדעת אותם על פה הוא מן הספרים המונחים לכל חלק מהם לא יגיע בו תכלית פעולת הרופא ולא יגיע בעבור החכמות ההם שלמות המלאכה עד שיהיה מוחזק שיראה האישים בענין בריאותם וענין חלייהם. → NM 3:132–3.

‣ II. **established**: Arab. مستقرّ · Maimonides, *K. al-fuṣūl fī al-ṭibb* · trans. Nathan ha-Me'ati (*Sefer ha-Peraqim*), 25.65: ומבואר הוא אצל מי שיבין מה שיתחייב מן הסברא שהאומר בקדמות העולם על זה הענין אין לשם רצון מתחדש ולא חפץ חדש ואין במציאות אפשר נתלה בו יכלתו ורצונו עד שהוא על דרך משל שלא יוכל שיב⟨י⟩א לנו מטר יום מה או ימנעהו יום מה כפי רצונו כי ירידת המטר בזה הטבע המונח נמשך אחר הכנת האידים הממציאים אותו או המונעים אותו. → NM 2:60.

נוֹטֶה (*Part.*) → **נָטָה**.

נוֹפֵחַ (*Part.*) → **נָפַח**.

נוֹפֵל (*Part.*) → **נָפַל**.

נוֹפֶת → **נֹפֶת**.

נוֹסֵחַ (*Part.*) → **נָסַח**.

נוֹסָף (*Part. Nif'al*) → [**יסף**].

[נוע] • *Hif'il* **הֵנִיעַ** ‣ **to move (i.e., to administer an emetic, an enema, a purge)**: Arab. حرك / Gr. κινέω · Maimonides, *Šarḥ fuṣūl Abūqrāṭ* · trans. Moses ibn Tibbon (*Pirqei Abuqraṭ*), 2.29 (81): כל זמן שיהיה החולי בהתחלתו אם תראה בדעתך להניע שום דבר תניעהו כי הוא בהגיע החולי אל עמידתו ראוי שינוח החולה ויעמוד. → NM 3:152.

נוֹקֵב (*Part.*) → **נָקַב**.

נוֹשֵׁךְ (*Part.*) → **נָשַׁךְ**.

נְזִילָה • **נזילה על הריאה** ‣ **asthma**: Arab. ربو / Gr. ἄσθμα · Maimonides, *Šarḥ fuṣūl Abūqrāṭ* · trans. Anonymous (*Pirqei Abuqraṭ*), 3.26 (132): אמר אבוקרט: כשיעבור הנער אלו השנים יקרה לו מורסת הגרון וכניסת חוליא שבעורף ונזילה על הריאה והאבן והרימה ותולעים שבגוף והשומות התלויים והחזירים ושאר האבעבועות. → NM 3:153.

• *Plur.* **נזילות** ‣ **catarrhs**: Arab. نزلات / Gr. κατάρροοι · Maimonides, *Šarḥ fuṣūl Abūqrāṭ* · trans. Zeraḥyah Ḥen (*Pirqei Abuqraṭ*), 7.38 (390): אמר בקראט: הנזילות היורדות אל התוך העליון יבואו לידי מגל בעשרים יום. → NM 3:152–3.

[נזל] • *Hif'il* **הִזִּיל** ‣ **to purge**: Hippocrates, *Aphorisms* · trans. Do'eg ha-Edomi (*Sefer Agur*), 4.4 (143) (fol. 60[a]): בהיות הגוף בריא ושלם אם יקרהו ⟨הקיא⟩ יאות להזילו למעלה אך לא בימי הקור. → NM 3:153.

נַזֶּלֶת • **נזלת האף** ‣ **rheum**: Hippocrates, *Aphorisms* · trans. Do'eg ha-Edomi (*Sefer Agur*), 3.14 (120) (fol. 53[a]): אמר אפוקרט: טוב הרוח צפונית לנשים ולבעלי מזג לח טורפת(?) שאר אישים בחולי יבש בעיניהם טנפה(?) אחרים בנזלת האף ובמדוה מחודד גם בהגרת השחורה. → NM 3:154.

• **נזלת דם** ‣ **dysentery**: Hippocrates, *Aphorisms* · trans. Do'eg ha-Edomi (*Sefer Agur*), 3.16 (122) (fol. 53[b]): אמר אפוקרט: כח יבשות האויר בהמנע הגשם יוליד תחלואי העיניים כאב קשרי הדבקים כובד הזלת השתן ונזלת דם. → NM 3:154.

נֵזֶר ‣ **rim around the cornea**: Arab. إكليل · Maimonides, *K. al-fuṣūl fī al-ṭibb* · trans. Nathan ha-Me'ati (*Sefer ha-Peraqim*), 15.25: הברד אשר בעין יצטרך לחתך וכן המוגלא המקובצת בעין בעלה הנקראת אלכמנה ורוב מה שתרפא ברפואות מתיכות לא במה שינגב נגוב חזק כי יריק היותר גדול שבו ויקפיא הנשאר. והנה אנחנו הריקונו המוגלא הזאת ששטחנו הכתונת הקרניית במקום הנזר. → NM 2:66.

נָח (*Part.*) → [נוח].
נֶחְבָּא (*Part. Nif'al*) → [חבא].
נִחוּר • **ניחור הגרון** • **hoarseness:** Hippocrates, *Aphorisms* · trans. Do'eg ha-Edomi (*Sefer Agur*), 2.40 (92) (fol. 45[a]): צרת ניחור הגרון וזוב הנחירים קשה להתבשל בזקנים. → NM 3:154–5.
• **ניחור הקול** • **roughness of the voice:** Arab. خشونة الصوت · Ibn al-Jazzār, *Zād al-musāfir wa-qūt al-ḥādir* · trans. Moses ibn Tibbon (*Sefer Ṣedat ha-Derakhim*), introduction (fol. 3[a]): השער הה' בניחור הקול. → NM 4:111.
נְחִיר • *Dual* **נְחִירַיִם** • **הגרת דם מהנחירים** → הֲגָּרָה.
• **הושם בנחיריו** → [שים].
• **חולת דם הנחירים** → חֲזָלָה.
• **הטפת דם מהנחירים** → הַטָּפָה.
• **זוב דם הנחירים** → זוֹב.
• **זוב הנחירים** → זוֹב.
• **יציאת דם הנחירים** → יְצִיאָה.
• **משח הנחירים** → מָשַׁח.
• **משיחת הנחירים** → מְשִׁיחָה.
• **עריפת דם הנחירים** → עֲרִיפָה.
• **צאת דם הנחירים** → יָצָא.
• **רעיפת דם מן הנחירים** → רְעִיפָה.
נְחִירָה • *Plur.* **נחירות** • **errhines; snuff medicines:** Arab. سعوط, *Plur.* سعوطات · Ibn al-Jazzār, *Zād al-musāfir wa-qūt al-ḥādir* · trans. Moses ibn Tibbon (*Sefer Ṣedat ha-Derakhim*), bk. 1, ch. 23 (Ms. Oxford, Bodleian Library, Poc. 353, Uri Heb. 314, fol. 10[a]): וישים בנחירי החולה הנחירות אשר נזכור אחר זה. → NM 4:111.
[נחר] • *Part. Hif'il* **מַנְחִיר** • **הסם המנחיר** → סַם.
נַחֲרָה • **roughness:** Arab. خشونة / Gr. τράχυτης · Al-Zahrāwī, *K. al-taṣrīf li-man ʿağiza ʿan at-taʾlīf* · trans. Shem Tov ben Isaac (*Sefer ha-Shimmush*), bk. 27, fol. 133, col. a: וכחו לרפות המעים ואיננו לנפח כלל ולא מעורר הקיא ועובר בגוף מהרה ומרכך נחרת החזה ומגיר השתן. → NM 4:112.
• **נחרת הגרון** • **hoarseness:** Arab. بحوحة الصوت · Al-Zahrāwī, *K. al-taṣrīf li-man ʿağiza ʿan at-taʾlīf* · trans. Shem Tov ben Isaac (*Sefer ha-Shimmush*), bk. 30, 1.23 (fol. 202[a]): שער כג' בכויה מנחרת הגרון וצרות הנשימה. → NM 1:105.
נָחָשׁ • **חולי הנחש** → חֳלִי.
• *Plur.* **נחשים** • I. **[intestinal] worms:** Arab. حيات · Maimonides, *K. al-fuṣūl fī al-ṭibb* · trans. Nathan ha-Me'ati (*Sefer ha-Peraqim*), 6.21: והקבסא התכופה זו אחר זו ואכילת הדברים אשר כבר התחילו להתעפש והלחם הגס מוליד הנחשים בבטן. → NM 2:66.
• II. **round worms:** Arab. حيّات / Gr. ἕλμινθες · a) Ibn al-Jazzār, *Zād al-musāfir wa-qūt al-ḥādir* · trans. Moses ibn Tibbon (*Sefer Ṣedat ha-Derakhim*), introduction (fol. 3[b]): השער הי"ח בתולעים והנחשים המתילדים במעים. → NM 4:112.
b) Hippocrates, *Aphorisms* · trans. Nathan ha-Me'ati, 3.26 (132) (fol. 54[a]): אמר

אבוקרט: ואם יעבור הנער אלו השנים יקרה לו מורסת הגרון והכנסת חוליות העורף והגניחה הנקרא רבו והחצץ והנחשים והתולעים הקטנים והיבלות התלויות והחזירים ושאר היציאות.
→ NM 3:155.

נְחֹשֶׁת • **פרח הנחשת** → **פֶּרַח**.
• **קלפת נחשת** → **קְלִפָּה**.

נָטָה • *Part.* **נוֹטֶה** • **נוטה ל-** · **similar to**: Arab. -شبيه ب · Ibn Sīnā, *K. al-Qānūn fī al-ṭibb* · trans. Nathan ha-Me'ati (*Sefer ha-Qanun*), bk. 1 (fol. 35b): ועצמות העגז נוטים לעצמות הקטן. → NM 4:111.

נְטִיָּה • **נטית הפה** · **twisted mouth (crooked mouth; facial paresis; paralysis of the facial nerve)**: Arab. لقوة · a) Al-Zahrāwī, *K. al-taṣrīf li-man 'ağiza 'an at-ta'līf* · trans. Shem Tov ben Isaac (*Sefer ha-Shimmush*), bk. 27, fol. 134b, col. b: ואם יושם ממנה בנחירים מעורבים במרירת עגור תועיל מנטית הפה. → NM 4:112.
b) Al-Zahrāwī, *K. al-taṣrīf li-man 'ağiza 'an at-ta'līf* · trans. Shem Tov ben Isaac (*Sefer ha-Shimmush*), bk. 30, 1.6 (fol. 203b): השער הששי בכוית נטיית הפה הנטייה הראויה לרפאתה בכויה היא המתחדשת מן הלחה הלבנה על מה שזכרתי בחלוקות החליים.
→ NM 1:105–6.

נטייה → **נְטִיָּה**.

נְטִילָה · **applying fomentations**: Arab. تنطيل · Maimonides, *Šarḥ fuṣūl Abūqrāṭ* · trans. Anonymous (*Pirqei Abuqraṭ*), 1.1 (16): החלק השביעי: ידיעת הכלים אשר בהם יעשה הרופא עד שתתמיד הבריאות שנמצאת או תושב הבריאות הנחסרה כמו מזונות האדם ורפואת סממניו לפי חלוף מיניהם ופשוטיהם ומורכביהם והדחיקה והקשירה והנטילה מזה המין. → NM 3:155.

נִיּוּת · **crude (matter)**: Arab. خام · Maimonides, *K. al-fuṣūl fī al-ṭibb* · trans. Zeraḥyah Ḥen (*Sefer ha-Peraqim*), 5.19: והשתן הדשן יורה על התכת השומן והדומה לשתן הבהמות יורה על ריבוי הניות. → NM 1:170.

ניחור → **נִחוּר**.

ניעול → **נִעוּל**.

ניפוש → **נִפּוּשׁ**.

ניצול → **נִצּוּל**.

ניצוציות · **radiance**: Arab. شعاعيّة · Ibn Sīnā, *K. al-adwiya al-qalbiya* · trans. Anonymous (*Sammim Libbiyim*), fol. 129a: כהרבא חם בראשונה יבש בשנית וכבר חשבו שהוא קר ויש לו בושמיות כמפוריית ויש לו מעט ניצוציות. → NM 4:112.

ניקודים → **נִקּוּדִים**.

נִכְאָה (*Part. Nif'al*) → [**כאה**].

נִכְאוּת · **sadness**: Arab. كآبة · Maimonides, *K. al-fuṣūl fī al-ṭibb* · trans. Zeraḥyah Ḥen (*Sefer ha-Peraqim*), 6.52: סימני המראקיא שיהיה לו אחר אכלו רוטו חמוץ ורקיקה לחה בשיעור ושריפה מתחת החלצים וקולות לא תתחדש אלא אחר האכילה בשעה אחת ויתחדש ריעות נפש ונכאות ויקרה לשכלו כמו מקרה השעמום המלינקוניקו. → NM 1:170.

[**נכה**] • *Hif'il* **הִכָּה** · **to proceed randomly**: Arab. خبط · Maimonides, *K. al-fuṣūl fī al-ṭibb* · trans. Zeraḥyah Ḥen (*Sefer ha-Peraqim*), 25.64: גליאנוס לא יאבה בשום דבר מזה ולא ידענו אבל הוא מכה לבד. → NM 1:170.

נְכוּת · **disability**: Arab. زمانة · Al-Zahrāwī, *K. al-taṣrīf li-man ʿağiza ʿan at-taʾlīf* · trans. Shem Tov ben Isaac (*Sefer ha-Shimmush*), bk. 27, fol. 130[a], col. b: ומנזק היין אל הגוף בכלל למי שיתמידו וישתהו על בלי סדר ויבקש בו השכרות כי הוא יוליד חליים ישנים ... ויחדש הרטט הארוך והפדגרא והנכות. → NM 4:112–3.

נִכְנָס (*Part. Nifʿal*) → [כנס].

נִכְפָּל (*Part. Nifʿal*) → כָּפַל.

[נכר] • *Hifʿil* הִכִּיר • הכיר על · **to conclude from**: Arab. استدلّ على · Maimonides, *K. al-fuṣūl fī al-ṭibb* · trans. Zeraḥyah Ḥen (*Sefer ha-Peraqim*), 11.30: משׁשה דברים תכיר על הבחראן השלם. → NM 1:170.

• *Part. Hitpaʿel* מִתְנַכֵּר · **foul**: Arab. منكر / Gr. βαρύς · Hippocrates, *Aphorisms* · trans. Nathan ha-Me'ati, 4.81 (218) (fol. 84[b]): אמר אבוקרט: מי ישתין דם ומוגלא ויהיה לשתנו ריח מתנכר הנה זה יורה על שחין במקותו. → NM 3:156.

נָכְרִי · I. **extraordinary; strange; unnatural; unusual**: Arab. غريب · Al-Zahrāwī, *K. al-taṣrīf li-man ʿağiza ʿan at-taʾlīf* · trans. Shem Tov ben Isaac (*Sefer ha-Shimmush*), bk. 27, fol. 147[b]. col. a: כל הקיבות יש בהן חמימות נכרית וחריפות מקרית. → NM 4:113.

· II. **savage; wild**: Arab. وحش · Ibn al-Jazzār, *Zād al-musāfir wa-qūt al-ḥādir* · trans. Moses ibn Tibbon (*Sefer Ṣedat ha-Derakhim*), bk. 7, ch. 19.1: הקובא שני מינים: ממנו מין שהוא שוה עם שטח הגוף והויתו ממרה שחורה מתילדת מעבירות הדם ופעמים שיהיה עמו חכוך כשיהיה החומר חזק התנועה ואמנם תתחזק כשיהיה החומר מעופש מאד או נלהב מאד ואולם המין האחר יקרא הנכרי. → NM 4:113.

• חום נכרי → חֹם.

נִלְהָב (*Part. Nifʿal*) → [להב].

נִלְחָם (*Part. Nifʿal*) → [לחם].

נְמִיכוּת • נמיכות הקול · **hoarseness**: Arab. بحوحة / Gr. βράγχος · Maimonides, *Šarḥ fuṣūl Abūqrāṭ* · trans. Anonymous (*Pirqei Abuqraṭ*), 3.20 (126): אמר אבוקרט: כבר יקרה באביב הדאגה השחורי והשטות וחולי הנופל והשתוק ונביעת הדם והאסכרה וסתום הנחירים ונמיכות הקול והשעול והחולי אשר יופשט בעבורו הגלד והילפת והבהק והכתמים גדולים אשר יתנגעו והאבעבעות וכאב הפרקים. → NM 3:157 (corr.).

נְמָלָה · **shingles**: a) Lat. formica · Bruno Longobucco, *Cyrurgia Magna* · trans. Hillel ben Samuel (*Sefer Keritut*), fol. 81[a]: הנמלה היא מורסא קטנה המתילדת מחומר מרירי. → NM 1:32.

b) Arab. نملة · i. Maimonides, *K. al-fuṣūl fī al-ṭibb* · trans. Zeraḥyah Ḥen (*Sefer ha-Peraqim*), 9.105: מה שתהיה מן הנמלה עמה איכול תהיה רפואתה רפואה מקררת לא מלחלחת כשאר מיני הנמלה. → NM 1:170–1.

· ii. Maimonides, *K. al-fuṣūl fī al-ṭibb* · trans. Nathan ha-Me'ati (*Sefer ha-Peraqim*), 9.105: מה שיהיה מן הנמלה שיהיה עמה אכול אז יהיו רפואותיה מקרירות ולא מרטיבות כשאר מיני הנמלה אבל יהיה בהם עם קרורם נגוב. → NM 2:67.

נִמְלָט (*Part. Nifʿal*) → [מלט].

נִמְשָׁךְ (*Part. Nifʿal*) → מָשַׁךְ.

נִמְתָּח (*Part. Nifʿal*) → [מתח].

נָסַח • *Part.* נוֹסֵחַ · **copyist**: Arab. ناسخ · Maimonides, *K. al-fuṣūl fī al-ṭibb* · trans. Nathan ha-Me'ati (*Sefer ha-Peraqim*), 25.45: והיותר קרוב אצלי שזאת הכפיאה האמור בבחארן הוא טעות הנוסח משרש. → NM 2:66.

נִסְתָּר (*Part. Nif'al*) → [סתר].

נִעוּל • ניעול המאכלים · **want of appetite**: Hippocrates, *Aphorisms* · trans. Judah Shalom, 4.17 (154) (fol. 56[b]): בלא מוקדח בהיות ניעול המאכלים ונשיכת הלב וחשיכות והפה מר יורה שיצטרך הרקה מלמעלה. → NM 3:157.

נעיי · **mucous**: Arab. مخاطي · Al-Zahrāwī, *K. al-taṣrīf li-man ʿağiza ʿan at-taʾlīf* · trans. Shem Tov ben Isaac (*Sefer ha-Shimmush*), bk. 27, fol. 143[b], cols. a–b: בשר הדוב נעיי חלוק קשה להתעכל ממהר לרדת מן האסטומ' מגונה המזון מאד. → NM 4:113.

[נעם] • *Hifʿil* **הִנְעִים** · **to fatten**: Arab. خصب · Al-Zahrāwī, *K. al-taṣrīf li-man ʿağiza ʿan at-taʾlīf* · trans. Shem Tov ben Isaac (*Sefer ha-Shimmush*), bk. 27, fol. 124[b], col. a: וינעים הגופים הבריאים וכל שכן כשיהיה מן החטה האדומה הכבדה. → NM 4:114.

נֶעֱסָק (*Part. Nif'al*) → [עסק].

נַעַר · **pupil (of the eye)**: Arab. صبيّ · Al-Zahrāwī, *K. al-taṣrīf li-man ʿağiza ʿan at-taʾlīf* · trans. Shem Tov ben Isaac (*Sefer ha-Shimmush*), bk. 30, 2.23 (fol. 212[a]): וראוי לתת שעור הכנסת המקדיח כעין שעור הרוחק אשר יהיה מן הנער אל סוף השחרות והוא עגול העין. → NM 1:106.

• *Plur.* **נערים • אם הנערים** → **אֵם**.

נֶעֱתָק (*Part. Nif'al*) → **עָתַק**.

נָפוּחַ (*Pass. Part.*) → **נָפַח**.

נפוס • תבשיל הנפוס → **תַּבְשִׁיל**.

נִפּוּשׁ · **respiration**: Arab. تنفّس · Maimonides, *K. al-fuṣūl fī al-ṭibb* · trans. Zeraḥyah Ḥen (*Sefer ha-Peraqim*), 24.38: פגשתי יום אחד רופא אחד מפורסם במלאכת הרפואות ומששתי לו הדפק ומצאתי בו כל מין ממיני השינוי בלא קדחת ולא היה מרגיש בניפושו שום דבר כלל ואמרתי לו אני רואה שזה השינוי יהיה מדוחק וצרות שיהיה בגידים אשר בריאה או בעבור סתימה מליחות עבות דבקות או מתולדת צמח שלא נתבשל ואמר לי אם כן היה ראוי שהיה לי בניפוש מצב מרימפלי ואמרתי לו כי המצב יהיה בהתקבץ הליחה הדבקה בחלקי קנה הריאה לא בהתקבצו בגידים הדופקים. → NM 1:171.

• **עוצר הניפוש** → **עֹצֶר**.

• **צרות הניפוש** → **צָרוּת**.

• **רוע הניפוש** → **רֹעַ**.

נָפַח • *Part.* **נוֹפֵחַ • הסם הנופח** → **סַם**.

• *Pass. Part.* **נָפוּחַ** • *Plur.* **הנפוחים** · **those suffering from an empyema**: Arab. المتقيّحون · Maimonides, *Šarḥ fuṣūl Abūqrāṭ* · trans. Moses ibn Tibbon (*Pirqei Abuqraṭ*), 6.27 (319): אמר אבקראט: מי שנכוה או נבקע מן הנפוחים או המשוקים ויגר ממנו מן החומר או מן המים שעור רב פתאום הנה הוא ימות בלא ספק. → NM 3:157–8.

• *Part. Piʿel* **מְנַפֵּחַ • הסם המנפח** → **סַם**.

• *Inf. Hitpaʿel* **הִתְנַפֵּחַ** · **being inflamed**: Arab. تورّم · Maimonides, *Šarḥ fuṣūl Abūqrāṭ* · trans. Moses ibn Tibbon (*Pirqei Abuqraṭ*), 5.2 (222): אמר המפרש: זה יהיה להתנפח העצבים ויעלה הכאב אל המוח. → NM 3:158.

נֶפַח ‧ I. **flatulence; gas**: Arab. نفخ · Ibn Sīnā, *K. al-Qānūn fī al-ṭibb* · trans. Nathan ha-Me'ati (*Sefer ha-Qanun*), bk. 1 (fol. 36[a]): וימלאו הקרבים מן המזון והנפח ויצטרך אל מקום רחב לאויר הנמשך. → NM 4:114.

‧ II. **inflammation**: Hippocrates, *Aphorisms* · trans. Judah Shalom, 3.24 (130) (fol. 47[a]): ובשנים אלו ⟨יקרו⟩ לקטנים הילדים הנולדים מחדש שחיני הפה וקיא ושעול ויקיצה ופּחד ונפח הטבור ולחות האזנים. → NM 3:158.

‧ III. **suppuration**: Arab. تقيح · Maimonides, *Šarḥ fuṣūl Abūqrāṭ* · trans. Moses ibn Tibbon (*Pirqei Abuqraṭ*), 7.20 (372): אמר אבקראט: ומהמורסא אשר יקרא אלחומרא העפוש והנפח. → NM 3:158.

‧ IV. **watery vesicle**: Arab. نفّاخة · Maimonides, *Šarḥ fuṣūl Abūqrāṭ* · trans. Moses ibn Tibbon (*Pirqei Abuqraṭ*), 7.55 (407): פעמים יתחדשו נפחים רבים ואמרו כי מי שנמלא בטנו ממים ימות זה על הרוב. → NM 3:158.

• **נפח הגידים השפלים** ‧ **hemorrhoids**: Hippocrates, *Aphorisms* · trans. Do'eg ha-Edomi (*Sefer Agur*), 3.30 (136) (fol. 58[a]): תגיע אליהם בהגיעם לארבעים צרת כאב הצדדים ולמטה מן הצלעות גם כאב הריאה וקדחות עם תעורה ואפיסת הדעת ההזלה הארוכה וקיא ונפח הגידים השפלים. → NM 3:158–9.

נְפִיחָה ‧ I. **flatulence**: Arab. نفخة · Ibn Sīnā, *K. al-adwiya al-qalbiya* · trans. Anonymous (*Sammim Libbiyim*), fol. 126[b]: והעצם המזוני אשר בו יתילד ממנו דם עכור שחוריי והלחות המותרי אשר בו יתחדש ממנו הנפיחה בעורקים וכבר ידעת הזק שני אלו הענינים. → NM 4:114.

‧ II. **inflammation**: Gr. φλεγμονή · Hippocrates, *Aphorisms* · trans. Joseph Delmedigo, 3.24 (130): אמנם לפי השנים יקרו אלו החולאים לקטנים ושנולדו מחדש יבואו שחינים בפה וקיא ושעול ויקיצה או תעורה ופחד ונפיחת הטבור וליחות האזנים. → NM 3:159.

• **נפיחת פיות העורקים מלמטה** ‧ **hemorrhoids**: Arab. انتفاخ أفواه العروق من أسفل · Hippocrates, *Aphorisms* · trans. Nathan ha-Me'ati, 3.30 (136) (fol. 56[b]): אמר אבוקרט: ואמנם מי שיעבור אלו השנים יקרה להם הגניחה הוא רבו ובעלת הצד ובעלת הריאה וקדחת שיהיה עמה התעורה והקדחת שיהיה עמה בלבול השכל והדלקת והיצא הוא שלשול וקיא יחדיו ושלשול ארוך והפשט המעים וחלקלקות המעים ונפיחת פיות העורקים מלמטה. → NM 3:159.

נְפִיחוּת ‧ **distension; inflation (h.l., bubbling)**: Arab. انتفاخ · Maimonides, *K. al-fuṣūl fī al-ṭibb* · trans. Nathan ha-Me'ati (*Sefer ha-Peraqim*), 2.30: הליחה השחורית מה שלא יתחדש ממנה כשתשפך על הארץ אבעבועות ונפיחות הנה היא טבעית. → NM 2:68.

נְפִילָה ‧ **miscarriage**: Arab. إسقاط / Gr. τρωσμός · Maimonides, *Šarḥ fuṣūl Abūqrāṭ* · trans. Moses ibn Tibbon (*Pirqei Abuqraṭ*), 4.23 (160): אמר אבקראט: מי שכבר החלישו חולי חד או נושן או נפילה או זולת זה ואחר כן יצא ממנו מרה שחורה או כמו דם שחור הנה הוא ימות ממחרת היום ההוא. → NM 3:160.

• **חלי הנפילה** → חֳלִי.

• **נפילת כח** ‧ **collapse of strength**: Arab. سقوط قوّة / Gr. ἔκλυσις · Maimonides, *Šarḥ fuṣūl Abūqrāṭ* · trans. Moses ibn Tibbon (*Pirqei Abuqraṭ*), 7.8 (360): אמר אבקראט: כאשר נפתחה היציאה לפנים יתחדש מזה נפילת כח וקיא והתכת נפש. → NM 3:160.

• **מחלת הנפילה** → מַחֲלָה.

• **נפילת התאוה** · **loss of appetite**: Arab. سقوط الشهوة · Maimonides, *K. al-fuṣūl fī al-ṭibb* · trans. Nathan ha-Me'ati (*Sefer ha-Peraqim*), 6.90: ואמנם אם תארך העלה אז יתחדש נפילת התאוה ואז היא אות רע כי זה יורה על מיתת הכחות. → NM 2:68.

נָפַל · **to expect**: Arab. توقّع · Hippocrates, *Aphorisms* · trans. Nathan ha-Me'ati, 3.6 (112) (fol. 42[b]): אמר אבקראט: כשיהיה הקייץ דומה לאביב יפול בקדחת זיעה רבה. → NM 3:160–1.

• *Part.* **נוֹפֵל** • **החולי הנופל** → חֹלִי.

• *Part. Hif'il* **מַפִּיל** • **החולי המפיל** → חֹלִי.

נִפְסָק (*Part. Nif'al*) → פָּסַק.

נֶפֶשׁ • **הפוך נפש** → הִפּוּךְ.

• **הרחיב הנפש** → [רחב].

• **התכת נפש** → הַתָּכָה.

• **חלשת הנפש** → חֻלְשָׁה.

• **מריכות נפש** → מריכות.

• **רוע נפש** → רֹעַ.

• **בריקות נפש** → רֵיקוּת.

נַפְשִׁי • **האיברים הנפשיים** → אֵבֶר.

• **ההאצלות הנפשיות** → הַאֲצָלָה.

נֹפֶת · **honeycomb**: Arab. شهدة / Gr. κηρός · Ibn al-Jazzār, *Zād al-musāfir wa-qūt al-ḥādir* · trans. Moses ibn Tibbon (*Sefer Ṣedat ha-Derakhim*), bk. 1, ch. 7 (fol. 11[b]): השער הז' בחולי הנקרא הנופת ובלעז' ברשקש ובערבי אלשהדה פעמים יקרה גם כן בעור הראש נגעים שיהיו בהם נקבים קטנים יצא מהם לחות עב דבק דומה בדבש ולכן נקרא החולי הזה נופת והתילדו מלחה לבנה מלוחה. → NM 4:115.

נִצּוֹל • **הניצול מן החולי** · **the convalescent**: Arab. الناقه · Maimonides, *Šarḥ fuṣūl Abūqrāṭ* · trans. Anonymous (*Pirqei Abuqraṭ*), 2.8 (60): אמר אבוקרט: הניצול מן החולי כשיקח מן המזון ולא יתחזק בו זה יורה על שעמס על גופו מן המזון יותר ממה שיסבול וכאשר היה זה והוא לא יקח ממנו יורה על שגופו צריך אל ההרקה. → NM 3:161.

נָצוֹר • **הנצור אשר יהיה בדמע העין** · **lacrimal fistula**: Lat. fistula lacrimalis · Arnau de Vilanova, *Medicationis Parabole* · trans. Abraham Avigdor (*Pirqei Arnauṭ de Vilanova*), 5.88 (88): ההגרה הבלתי טבעית יאות להטותה אל מעבר טבעי, כמו הזלת הנצור אשר יהיה בדמע העין נטה אותו אל מסננת האף אם העצם כבר נתעפש. → NM 4:115.

[נצל] • *Part. Nif'al* **נִצָּל** • **נצל מן** · **free from**: a) Arab. معرّا من · Al-Zahrāwī, *K. al-taṣrīf li-man 'ağiza 'an at-ta'līf* · trans. Shem Tov ben Isaac (*Sefer ha-Shimmush*), bk. 27, fol. 128[b], col. a: מצד ריחם להיותם נצלים מן הסרחון. → NM 4:115–6.

b) Arab. سليم من · Al-Zahrāwī, *K. al-taṣrīf li-man 'ağiza 'an at-ta'līf* · trans. Shem Tov ben Isaac (*Sefer ha-Shimmush*), bk. 27, fol. 146[a], col. b: החלב החשוב הוא ההולך על מהלך טבע הבעל חיים אשר הוא ממנו כשיהיה הבעל חיים בריא הגוף יפה המראה ממוצע השומן נצל מן הרזון והמחלות ויתר ההוות.

• *Part. Hif'il* **מַצִּיל** · **antidote**: Arab. مخلّص · Maimonides, *Šarḥ fuṣūl Abūqrāṭ* · trans. Moses ibn Tibbon (*Pirqei Abuqraṭ*), 1.1 (27): ויש סמנים תהיה פעולתם בגופותינו הנמשכת אחר צורתם נגלית גדולה כסמנים המשלשלים והסמים הממיתים והמצילים. → NM 3:137.

נִצָּל (*Part. Nif'al*) → [**נצל**].

נָקַב • *Part.* **נוֹקֵב** • **כלי נוקב** → **כְּלִי**.

• **הנגעים הנוקבים** → **נֶגַע**.

נֶקֶב • **נקב האזן** • I. **ear canal**: Arab. (الأذن) ثقب • Ibn al-Jazzār, *Zād al-musāfir wa-qūt al-ḥāḍir* • trans. Moses ibn Tibbon (*Sefer Ṣedat ha-Derakhim*), bk. 2, ch. 7 (fol. 47[b]): ואם לא נראה דבר מזה וראינו נקב האזן בריא אין בו נזק ידענו כי העצב אשר בו ילך השמע כואב ואם היה כאב העצב השומע מפני מותר עב קר דבק או מפני רוח עבה או מורסא קרה ... אז ראוי לשלשל המותרות ההם. → NM 4:116.

• II. **the external acoustic meatus; the inner cavity of the ear; inner earhole; the middle ear; the tympanic cavity**: a) Arab. السماخ • Maimonides, *K. al-fuṣūl fī al-ṭibb* • trans. Nathan ha-Me'ati (*Sefer ha-Peraqim*), 6.94: כי אתה ידעת שרבים מהשוטים ובעלי המלאנכוניא יחיו זמן ארוך והם חזקי הגשמים כי הפסד שכלם הוא מפני פגע במוח לבדו לא מפני חולשת הכח המנהיג כמו מה שיקרה לחולים בעת הגוססות כמו שחולשת הראות ההוה מפני פגע בעין או חולשת השמע ההוה מפני פגע בנקב האוזן אינו כמו חולשת הראות או השמע ההוה בעת המות מפני נפילת הכח הכולל המנהיג. → NM 2:68.

b) Arab. صماخ • Ibn Sīnā, *K. al-Qānūn fī al-ṭibb* • trans. Nathan ha-Me'ati (*Sefer ha-Qanun*), bk. 1 (fol. 57[a]): והחלק הראשון מכל זוג ממנו יכוון אל הקרום המחפה בתוך אלסמך הוא נקב האוזן. → NM 4:116.

• **נקב אותו מקום של אשה** • **vulva**: Lat. vulva mulieris • Bruno Longobucco, *Cyrurgia Magna* • trans. Hillel ben Samuel (*Sefer Keritut*), fol. 97[a]: הראשון שבאנשים שנראה בעור הבצים באותו שהוא באמצע שניהן תבנית נקב אותו מקום של אשה ויש שם שערות. → NM 1:33.

• **הנקב התחתון** • **anus**: Lat. anus • Bruno Longobucco, *Cyrurgia Magna* • trans. Hillel ben Samuel (*Sefer Keritut*), fol. 65[a]: שער הי"ו מן הנגעים הבאים בנקב התחתון. → NM 1:33.

• *Plur.* **נקבים** • **pores**: Arab. مسامّ • Ibn Sīnā, *K. al-adwiya al-qalbiya* • trans. Anonymous (*Sammim Libbiyim*), fol. 120[b]: והממרק הוא הסם אשר יכלה מן הליחה הנקפאת והדבקה מה שהיה על ישטח האבר ופיות הנקבים. → NM 4:116.

• **רפה הנקבים** → **רָפֶה**.

נקביות • **נקביות הבשר** • **softening of the flesh**: Lat. carnium effeminatio • Hippocrates, *Aphorisms* • trans. Judah Shalom, 5.16 (236) (fols. 78[a–b]): החום מזיק למרגילים אותו תמיד אלו ההזקים: נקביות הבשר ובלתי קיום העצבים והרדמת השכל והגרת דם וחסרון הרוח אשר מאלו תמשך המות. → NM 3:161.

נִקְבָּס (*Part. Nif'al*) → [**קבס**].

נִקְבָּע (*Part. Nif'al*) → [**קבע**].

[נקה] • *Inf. Nif'al* **הִנָּקוֹת** • **to heal**: Lat. ad curandum • Bruno Longobucco, *Cyrurgia Magna* • trans. Hillel ben Samuel (*Sefer Keritut*), fol. 5[b]: שער שמני יבקש למה המכות מתאחרות להנקות ומתחבולות הנקיות מאותן המכות. → NM 1:33.

• *Pu'al* **נֻקָּה** • **to heal**: Lat. curatus esse • Bruno Longobucco, *Cyrurgia Magna* • trans. Hillel ben Samuel (*Sefer Keritut*), fol. 36[b]: וסבותיה שתים אחת פנימית ואחת חיצונית הפנימית היא מלחות נפסדות והחיצונית היא ממכות או מחבלות מבלתי נוקו כהוגן. → NM 1:33.

נָקוּב · **cavity**: Arab. نقب · Ibn al-Jazzār, *Zād al-musāfir wa-qūt al-ḥādir* · trans. Moses ibn Tibbon (*Sefer Ṣedat ha-Derakhim*), bk. 2, ch. 18 (fol. 59[a]): כאשר יכאבו ויפסדו יחסר פעולתם ויראו בהם חליים מתחלפים ומהם חליים נראה אותם לעין כמו אכול השנים ונקובם ועפושם ותנועתם ולכלוכם אשר יהיה עליהם ומה שדומה לזה. → NM 4:116.

נִקּוּדִים • **לחם ניקודים** → **לֶחֶם**.

נָקִי • **הנקי** · **the convalescent**: Arab. الناقه · Maimonides, *Šarḥ fuṣūl Abūqrāṭ* · trans. Zeraḥyah Ḥen (*Pirqei Abuqraṭ*), 2.32 (84): המאמר במקום זה הוא בנקי. → NM 3:161.

• **הנקי מן החולי** · **the convalescent**: Arab. الناقه · Maimonides, *Šarḥ fuṣūl Abūqrāṭ* · trans. Zeraḥyah Ḥen (*Pirqei Abuqraṭ*), 2.8 (60): הנקי מן החולי בקחתו מן המזון ולא יתחזק זה יורה על שהוא יסבול מן המזון יותר ממה שהוא סובל ובהיות זה שהוא לא יבואנו ממנו זה יורה על שגופו צריך אל ההרקה. → NM 3:162.

נִקָּיוֹן · I. **crisis**: Arab. بحران · a) Ibn al-Jazzār, *Zād al-musāfir wa-qūt al-ḥādir* · trans. Moses ibn Tibbon (*Sefer Ṣedat ha-Derakhim*), bk. 7, 7.1: והזיעה הטבעית היא כמו הזיעה אשר תהיה מן הנקיון הטוב. → NM 1:62–3.

b) Maimonides, *Šarḥ fuṣūl Abūqrāṭ* · trans. Moses ibn Tibbon (*Pirqei Abuqraṭ*), 2.12 (64): אמר אבקראט: השאריות אשר ישארו מן החליים אחר הנקיון ממנהגם שיסבבו חזרת החולי. → NM 3:162.

· II. **cure; therapy**: Lat. curatio · Bruno Longobucco, *Cyrurgia Magna* · trans. Hillel ben Samuel (*Sefer Keritut*), fol. 5[b]: שער חמישי מן סוג הכולל הנקיון מן החבלות שבגידין. → NM 1:34.

· III. **purgation**: Lat. purgatio · Hippocrates, *Aphorisms* · trans. Hillel ben Samuel, 2.35 (87) (fol. 13[a]): א״א: בכל החלאים שיהיה מה שסמוך לטבור ולעצם הערוה עבים הוא טוב ובהיותם דקים ורזים הוא רע מפני שזה מזיק בנקיון של מטה. → NM 3:162.

נְקִיּוּת · **cure; therapy**: Lat. curatio · Bruno Longobucco, *Cyrurgia Magna* · trans. Hillel ben Samuel (*Sefer Keritut*), fol. 5[b]: שער שמיני יבקש למה המכות מתאחרות להנקות ומתחבולות הנקיות מאותן המכות. → NM 1:34.

נְקִירָה · **caries**: Arab. نخر · Maimonides, *K. al-fuṣūl fī al-ṭibb* · trans. Zeraḥyah Ḥen (*Sefer ha-Peraqim*), 7.25: הליחות החדות או הרפואה המחודדת אשר יעבה האברים כשיהיה עמם מותר כח מרובה שיחום(?) באברים הבשריים חבלות ובעצמות נקירה. → NM 1:171.

נִקְנָה (*Part. Nif'al*) → [קנה].

נָקַע · **to become dislocated**: Arab. انخلع / Gr. ἐξίσταμαι · Maimonides, *Šarḥ fuṣūl Abūqrāṭ* · trans. Moses ibn Tibbon (*Pirqei Abuqraṭ*), 6.60 (352): אמר אבקראט: מי שקרהו כאב הירך זמן גדול והיתה ירכו נוקעת הנה כל רגלו תצמוק וישוב חגר אם לא יכוה. → NM 3:162–3.

• *Part. Nif'al* **נִקָּע** · **macerated; steeped**: Arab. نقيع · Al-Zahrāwī, *K. al-taṣrīf li-man 'ağiza 'an at-ta'līf* · trans. Shem Tov ben Isaac (*Sefer ha-Shimmush*), bk. 27, fol. 131[b], col. a: שכר התאנים: זה השכר יעשה נקע ויעשה מבושל והנקע יותר לח מן המבושל הרבה והוא מוליד רוחות רבות ונפח. → NM 4:117.

נִקָּע (*Part. Nif'al*) → **נָקַע**.

נִקְפָּא (*Part. Nif'al*) → **קָפָא**.

נְקָרָה · **cavity**: Arab. نقرة · Ibn Sīnā, *K. al-Qānūn fī al-ṭibb* · trans. Nathan ha-Me'ati (*Sefer *ha-Qanun*), bk. 1 (fol. 32ᵇ): ולכל כנף מהם יש שתי נקרות ולכל צלע שתי תוספות מגובנים. → NM 4:117.

[נקרס] • *Puʿal* **נֻקְרַס** · **to suffer from gout**: Hippocrates, *Aphorisms* · trans. Judah Shalom, 6.28 (320) (fol. 102ᵇ): הסריסים לא ינוקרסו ולא יעשו קרחים. → NM 3:163.

נִרְאֶה (*Part. Nifʿal*) → **רָאָה**.

נרדי (here: **תרדי**) • **עצם תרדי** → **עֶצֶם**.

נִרְדָּם (*Part. Nifʿal*) → [**רדם**].

נִרְחָב (*Part. Nifʿal*) → [**רחב**].

נִרְעָד (*Part. Nifʿal*) → [**רעד**].

נָשָׂא · **to apply as a suppository**: Arab. احتمل · Al-Rāzī, *K. al-Manṣūrī* · trans. Shem Tov ben Isaac (*Sefer Almansur*), Alef 16 (16): אתמד: קר יבש מחזק העין שומר בריאותה ויועיל עוד מהגרת דם הנדות כשתשא ממנו האשה. → NM 2:15.

• **נשא ונתן** · **to attend to**: Arab. باشر · Maimonides, *Šarḥ fuṣūl Abūqrāṭ* · trans. Zeraḥyah Ḥen (*Pirqei Abuqraṭ*), 1.1 (17): וידוע כי ידיעת אילו החלקים השבעה כולם ושמירתם הוא מן הספרים המונחים לכל חלק מהם לא יגיעו בו תכלית פעולת הרופא ולא יגיע לאותו היודע שלימות המלאכה עד שישא ויתן עם האנשים בזמן בריאותם ועניין חליים. → NM 3:163–4.

[נשג] • *Hifʿil* **הִשִּׂיג** · I. **to correct**: Arab. استدرك · Maimonides, *K. al-fuṣūl fī al-ṭibb* · trans. Zeraḥyah Ḥen (*Sefer ha-Peraqim*), 25.43: ואמר בזה המאמר בדברו על עניין זה האיש בעצמו זה המאמר אמר: אין ראוי שיהיה היובש נשאר כמו שהוא לבדו ויהיה החמימות והקרירות משתוים לא יחסר דבר כי האברים כשאינם מתפרנסים יתקררו בזמן קצר. זה לשונו כמו כן שם וזהו האמת. ובזוכרו מה שקדם לו ממאמרו בזה האיש שהוא היה בין החמימות והקרירות בריא לקח להשיג זה בזה הלשון. → NM 1:171.

· II. **to take**: Arab. نال / Gr. λάμβανω · Hippocrates, *Aphorisms* · trans. Nathan ha-Me'ati, 2.8 (60) (fol. 21ᵇ): אמר אבוקרט: הנמלט מחולי כשיקח מן המזון ולא יתחזק הנה זה יורה שהוא לוקח יותר מן המזון ממה שיסבול וכשיהיה זה והוא לא ישיג ממנו מורה שגופו יצטרך אל הרקה. → NM 3:164.

נְשִׁיכָה • **נשיכת חלב** · **cardialgia**: Hippocrates, *Aphorisms* · trans. Judah Shalom, 4.17 (154): בלא מוקדח בהיות ניעול המאכלים ונשיכת הלב וחשיכות והפה מר יורה שיצטרך הרקה מלמעלה. → NM 3:165.

• **נשיכה בלב** · **cardialgia**: Lat. cordis morsus · Hippocrates, *Aphorisms* · trans. Hillel ben Samuel, 4.65 (202) (fol. 27ᵇ): א״א: בקדחת בערה רבה קרוב לבטן ונשיכה בלב רע. → NM 3:164.

• **נשיכה במוראה** · **cardialgia**: Arab. نخس في الفؤاد · Maimonides, *Šarḥ fuṣūl Abūqrāṭ* · trans. Moses ibn Tibbon (*Pirqei Abuqraṭ*), 4.17 (154): אמר אבקראט: מי שלא תהיה בו קדחת והיה בו מניעה מן המאכל ונשיכה במוראה וסבוב ומרירות בפה הנה זה יורה על שהרקתו ברפואה מלמעלה. → NM 3:164–5.

• **נשיכה בפי האצטומכה** · **cardialgia**: Arab. نخس في الفؤاد · Maimonides, *Šarḥ fuṣūl Abūqrāṭ* · trans. Anonymous (*Pirqei Abuqraṭ*), 4.17 (154): אמר אבוקרט: מי שאין לו קדחת ויש לו מניעה מהמאכל ונשיכה בפי האצטומכא וסבוב ראש ומרירה בפה כל זה ראיה על צורך ההרקה בסם מלמעלה. → NM 3:165.

נְשִׁימָה • חסרון נשימה → חֶסְרוֹן.

• צרות הנשימה → צָרוּת.

• רוע הנשימה → רֹעַ.

נְשִׁירוּת • נשירות שער הראש · **loss of hair**: Arab. ذهاب شعر الرأس · Maimonides, *Šarḥ fuṣūl Abūqrāṭ* · trans. Moses ibn Tibbon (*Pirqei Abuqraṭ*), 5.11 (231): אמר המפרש: סרחון הריח ראיה על הפסד הליחות וחוזק עפושם ונשירות שער הראש ממה שיחזק ראית הפסד הליחות וגם כן יורה על העדר המזון מן האברים. → NM 3:165.

נָשַׁךְ · **to prick**: Arab. نخس · Maimonides, *K. al-fuṣūl fī al-ṭibb* · trans. Zeraḥyah Ḥen (*Sefer ha-Peraqim*), 15.10: האבר כשהוא מת ולא ירגיש כשאתה תנשכנו או תחתכנו או תשרפנו באש בלא ספק כי זה האבר ישתחר ועל כן ראוי שתמהר לחתכו כדי שלא יפסיד המקום הבריא אשר לצדו. → NM 1:172.

• *Part.* **נוֹשֵׁךְ • הסם הנושך** → סַם.

[נתך] **•** *Part. Nif'al* **נִתָּךְ** · **reaching its crisis**: Arab. انقضى · Maimonides, *Šarḥ fuṣūl Abūqrāṭ* · trans. Zeraḥyah Ḥen (*Pirqei Abuqraṭ*), 4.59 (196): אמר בקראט: הקדחת השלישית ברוב תהיה נתכת בשבעה עונות. → NM 3:165.

• *Part. Hif'il* **מַתִּיךְ • הסם המתיך** → סַם.

נִתָּךְ (*Part. Nif'al*) → [**נתך**].

נִתְלֶה (*Part. Nif'al*) → [**תלה**].

נָתַן • נשא ונתן → נָשָׂא.

• נתן הרפואה · **to administer purgative drugs**: Arab. سقى الدواء / Gr. φαρμακεύω · Maimonides, *Šarḥ fuṣūl Abūqrāṭ* · trans. Moses ibn Tibbon (*Pirqei Abuqraṭ*), 4.1 (138): אמר אבקראט: ראוי שתנתן הרפואה למעוברת כאשר יהיו הליחות מתעוררות אחר שיעבור על הולד ארבעה חדשים עד שיעברו עליו שבעה חדשים ויכניס עצמו בזה מעט ואולם המעט מזה והיותר הנה ראוי שישמור ממנו. → NM 3:165–6; corr. 4:230.

נֶתֶק · I. **cradle cap**: Arab. سعفة · Maimonides, *K. al-fuṣūl fī al-ṭibb* · trans. Nathan ha-Me'ati (*Sefer ha-Peraqim*), 23.54: יתחדש בעור הראש עלה ממין המורסא יהיה בה נקבים קטנים דקים מלאים לחות דקה דבקה נקרא סעפה והוא הנתק. → NM 2:69.

· II. **freckles**: Arab. كلف · Al-Rāzī, *K. al-Manṣūrī* · trans. Shem Tov ben Isaac (*Sefer Almansur*), Bet 7 (18): בלבוס הוא בצל נאכל: יסכסך תאות המשגל וכשיוטח בו הפנים יסיר בו הנתק. → NM 2:15.

[נתר] **•** *Nif'al* **נִתַּר** · **to dissolve**: Arab. تحلّل · Maimonides, *K. al-fuṣūl fī al-ṭibb* · trans. Zeraḥyah Ḥen (*Sefer ha-Peraqim*), 15.20: הצמחים אשר ברוב יתחדשו בשטח הגוף הכוונות הכוללות ברפואתם הם שלושה: ההתרה או העיפוש או לחתוך בברזל והדבשית מהם תצטרך אל אחת מאילו לבד אבל אשר תהיה בתוכה כדמות קמח מבושל במים ראוי לך שתחתכנה והוא עובר שתעפשנה והדומה לחלב או לשומן תרפאנה בברזל לבדו אחר שאי אפשר בה שתתעפש ולא שתהיה ניתרת. → NM 1:173.

• *Hif'il* **הִתִּיר** · I. **to cure**: Lat. solvo · Hippocrates, *Aphorisms* · trans. Hillel ben Samuel, 2.42 (94) (fol. 14[a]): א"א: להתיר האפופלוסיה החזקה אי אפשר והחלושה לא תהיה נתרת בקלות. → NM 3:166.

· II. **to state definitely**: Arab. أطلق (القضية) · Maimonides, *K. al-fuṣūl fī al-ṭibb* · trans.

Zeraḥyah Ḥen (*Sefer ha-Peraqim*), 25.36: ומקום הספק מבואר מאד והוא היותו מתיר הגזרה בתועלת האברים בעצבי העור אמנם הוא מן המושקלי אשר יבוא למושקולי הפנימי ובשלישי מההכרות יאמר כי עצב יבוא לעור מן היד זולתי העצבים אשר יבואו למושקלי המניע היד וזה פלא אם יהיה מיוחד ליד מבין שאר האברים איך לא זכר זה. → NM 1:172.

• **התיר הפסק דין** · **to make a definite statement:** Arab. أطلق القضيّة · Maimonides, *Šarḥ fuṣūl Abūqrāṭ* · trans. Zeraḥyah Ḥen (*Pirqei Abuqraṭ*), 5.40 (260): אמר המפרש: היותר קרוב אצלי שאבקראט ראה זה העניין פעם או פעמיים והתיר הפסק דין כמנהגו בספרו ספר איפידימיאה. → NM 3:166.

• *Part. Hif'il* **מַתִּיר** • **הסם המתיר הזיעה** → **סַם**.

• **הסם המתיר השתן** → **סַם**.

• **רפואה מתירה** → **רְפוּאָה**.

• *Hof'al* **הֻתַּר** • **הותר בטנו** · **to suffer from diarrhea:** Arab. استطلق بطنه / Gr. κοιλίη ἐκταραχθεῖσα · Hippocrates, *Aphorisms* · trans. Nathan ha-Me'ati, 4.60 (197) (fol. 76[b]): אמר אבוקרט: מי שימצאהו בקדחת החדה באזניו חרשות ויזול מנחיריו דם או שיותר בטנו יותך בזה חליו. → NM 3:166–7.

ס

[סבב] • *Part. Piʿel* **מְסַבֵּב** • **חעצל המסבב** → **עָצֵל**.

סִבָּה • **באין סבה ידועה אליו** · **spontaneous:** Hippocrates, *Aphorisms* · trans. Do'eg ha-Edomi (*Sefer Agur*), 2.5 (57) (fol. 34[a]): אנוש עיף ויגע באין סבה ידועה אליו אות מחלה הוא. → NM 3:167.

• **לא נודע אליה סבה** → **יָדַע**.

• *Plur.* **סבות** • **מסבות נסתרות** · **spontaneous:** Hippocrates, *Aphorisms* · trans. Judah Shalom, 2.5 (57) (fol. 16[b]): היגיעות מסבות נסתרות מורות חליים. → NM 3:167.

סִבּוּב · **dizziness; vertigo:** a) Arab. دوار · Ibn al-Jazzār, *Zād al-musāfir wa-qūt al-ḥādir* · trans. Moses ibn Tibbon (*Sefer Ṣedat ha-Derakhim*), introduction (Ms. Oxford, Bodleian Library, Poc. 353, Uri Heb. 314, fol. 1[b]): השער הי״ג בגלגול והסבוב. → NM 4:117–8.

b) Arab. سدر · Ibn al-Jazzār, *Zād al-musāfir wa-qūt al-ḥādir* · trans. Moses ibn Tibbon (*Sefer Ṣedat ha-Derakhim*), bk. 7, 10.1: ויקרה לו עלוף רב וסבוב וזיעה קרה ועוצר השתן ועצור ויקיא מרה כרכומית. → NM 1:63.

• **סבוב חשוכי** · **dizziness:** Gr. σκοτόδινος · Hippocrates, *Aphorisms* · trans. Joseph Delmedigo, 4.17 (154): מי שהוא נעדר הקדחת ויש לו תיעוב המאכל ונשיכת פי האצטומכה וסבוב חשוכי ומרירות הפה מורה שצריך שיורק דרך מעלה. → NM 3:167–8.

סָבִיב • **צמיחת השער סביב הערוה** → **צְמִיחָה**.

סְדִיקָה • *Plur.* **סדיקות** · **fissures:** Arab. شقاق · Ibn al-Jazzār, *Zād al-musāfir wa-qūt al-ḥādir* · trans. Moses ibn Tibbon (*Sefer Ṣedat ha-Derakhim*), bk. 7, ch. 30.1: הנה כשיעורב עם דם המזון מרה שחורה עבה או כרכומית מחודדת יוליד ברגלים ובידים סדיקות מפני תגבורת היובש על דם המזון אבל כי המרה השחורה לכבדותה ועביה תצלול ואמנם תוליד הסדיקות בשפל הרגלים והמרה הכרכומית לקלותה רוב מה שתוליד הסדיקות בידים. → NM 4:118 (corr.).

[סדר] • *Piʿel* **סִדֵּר** · **to write (h.l., to formulate):** Arab. حرّر · Maimonides, *Šarḥ fuṣūl Abūqrāṭ* · trans. Moses ibn Tibbon (*Pirqei Abuqraṭ*), 5.49 (268): זה מבואר כי הצד הימני יותר חם וזכר גאלינוס כי הזרע אשר יבא מן האשה מן הצד הימני מן אחד מביציה בו עובי וחום ואשר יבוא מן הצד השמאלי דק מימי ויותר קר מן האחר ואיני יודע אם הגיע לו זה בנבואה או שהגיע אליו בהקש ואם היה שגדר וסדר זה הסדר זה בהקש הנה הוא הקש נפלא. → NM 3:168.

סֵדֶר · I. **(piece of) writing (h.l., argument):** Arab. تحرير · Maimonides, *Šarḥ fuṣūl Abūqrāṭ* · trans. Moses ibn Tibbon (*Pirqei Abuqraṭ*), 5.49 (268): זה מבואר כי הצד הימני יותר חם וזכר גאלינוס כי הזרע אשר יבא מן האשה מן הצד הימני מן אחד מביציה בו עובי וחום ואשר יבוא מן הצד השמאלי דק מימי ויותר קר מן האחר ואיני יודע אם הגיע לו זה בנבואה או שהגיע אליו בהקש ואם היה שגדר וסדר זה הסדר זה בהקש הנה הוא הקש נפלא. → NM 3:168.

· II. **rule:** Arab. قانون · Ibn al-Jazzār, *Zād al-musāfir wa-qūt al-ḥādir* · trans. Moses ibn Tibbon (*Sefer Ṣedat ha-Derakhim*), bk. 1, ch. 10 (fol. 16[b]): ובמה שזכרנו מרפואת כאב הראש על דרך הסדר הלמודי מחכמת הרפואה די ספוק. → NM 4:118.

• *Plur.* **סדרים** · **rules:** Arab. قانون, *Plur.* قوانين · Maimonides, *Šarḥ fuṣūl Abūqrāṭ* · trans. Zeraḥyah Ḥen (*Pirqei Abuqraṭ*), 1.1 (16): והחלק הרביעי לדעת סדרי הראיות והם איך יוקחו

מאותם המקרים המשיגים לגוף סימנים מורים על מין ומין ממיני הבריאות ועל כל מין ומין ממיני החולי. → NM 3:168.

סוכר → סֻכָּר.

סוכרי • משקה סוכרי → מַשְׁקֶה.

סוּס • סוס חים › hippopotamus: Arab. فرس البحر · Maimonides, *K. al-fuṣūl fī al-ṭibb* · trans. Nathan ha-Me'ati (*Sefer ha-Peraqim*), 22.15: עור סוס הים שרוף מועיל מן המורסות הקשות. → NM 2:69.

סוּסִי • צפורן סוסית → צִפֹּרֶן.

סוֹף • סוף הפרשות › coccyx: Arab. عجز الذنب · Al-Zahrāwī, *K. al-taṣrīf li-man ʿağiza ʿan at-ta'līf* · trans. Shem Tov ben Isaac (*Sefer ha-Shimmush*), bk. 30, 2.80 (fol. 222[b]). → NM 1:106.

[סור] • *Inf.* סור › **to be on one's guard; to guard against; to take care:** Lat. cavere · Bruno Longobucco, *Cyrurgia Magna* · trans. Hillel ben Samuel (*Sefer Keritut*), fol. 84[b]: וסור מאד שלא יבוא שמן או מים או שום דבר שמן אחרי שנפתחה. → NM 1:34.

סוֹתֵם (*Part.*) → סָתַם.

סְחוּסִי › cartilaginous: Arab. غضروفي · Al-Zahrāwī, *K. al-taṣrīf li-man ʿağiza ʿan at-ta'līf* · trans. Shem Tov ben Isaac (*Sefer ha-Shimmush*), bk. 27, fol. 144[a], col. a: האף קר יבש סחוסי קשה להתעכל מעט המזון. → NM 4:118.

• הבשר הסחוסי → בָּשָׂר.

סטני › quince: Lat. citonia · Al-Zahrāwī, *K. al-taṣrīf li-man ʿağiza ʿan at-ta'līf* · trans. Shem Tov ben Isaac (*Sefer ha-Shimmush*), bk. 27, fol. 138[b], col. a: והוא מנוגב מעט המימות יקרא המתפלח ובלשון רבותינו הסיטני. → NM 4:118–9.

סִיבִי › fibrous: Arab. ليفي · Al-Zahrāwī, *K. al-taṣrīf li-man ʿağiza ʿan at-ta'līf* · trans. Shem Tov ben Isaac (*Sefer ha-Shimmush*), bk. 27, fol. 143[a], col. b: בשר הבקר המוכלח איננו טוב כלל מפני התחברות הנגוב והכחשות וחולשת החמימות בו ולפיכך יהיה בשרו סיבי. → NM 4:120.

סִיג • סיג הזהב › gold calamine: Arab. إقليميا الذهب · Ibn al Jazzār, *Zād al musāfir wa-qūt al-ḥādir* · trans. Moses ibn Tibbon (*Sefer Ṣedat ha-Derakhim*), bk. 2, ch. 6 (fol. 47[a]): ואם לא ימצא הפלפל הלבן יושם תמורתו סיג הזהב. → NM 4:119.

• סיג הכסף › silver cadmia; silver calamine: Arab. إقليميا الفضّة · Ibn al-Jazzār, *Zād al-musāfir wa-qūt al-ḥādir* · trans. Moses ibn Tibbon (*Sefer Ṣedat ha-Derakhim*), bk. 1, ch. 7 (fol. 12[a]): או יקח סיג הכסף ובלנקט ויודקו בחומץ ושמן ורדים ויטוח בו. → NM 4:119.

• סיג הצפרנים › nail cuttings: Arab. قلامة الأظفار · Galen, attr., *Prohibition of Burial* · trans. Judah al-Ḥarizi (*Sefer Issur ha-Qevurah le-Galienus*), par. 117 (Ms. Leeuwarden, Tresoar Fr. 23, no foliation): ורפואת עלות המאמר הג' שיתעשנו בדאם ושישון וקלי החטה המשורפ' וסיג הצפרנים והם יקומו לשעתם. → NM 4:119–20.

סִיד • הסיד החי › quicklime: Lat. calx viva · Bruno Longobucco, *Cyrurgia Magna* · trans. Hillel ben Samuel (*Sefer Keritut*), fol. 16[a]. → NM 1:34.

סיטני → סטני.

סִימְפּוֹנָא → סמפונא.

סינון → סִנּוּן.

סַכִּינִי • מכוה סכיני → מִכְוָה.

סִכְלוּת · **delirium; mental confusion:** Hippocrates, *Aphorisms* · trans. Judah Shalom, 4.50 (187) (fol. 65^b): בכל מי אשר בקדחת בלתי נפסקת יהיה דישמא וסכלות הוא ממית. → NM 3:168–9.

סִכְסוּךְ • סכסוך הרוחות · **arousing winds; flatulences:** Arab. تهييج الرياح · Al-Zahrāwī, *K. al-taṣrīf li-man ʿağiza ʿan at-taʾlīf* · trans. Shem Tov ben Isaac (*Sefer ha-Shimmush*), bk. 27, fol. 125^b, col. a: והמצה ממנו עבה וחלוקה ומתאחרת להתעכל וכבדה על האצטומ׳ ומוסיפה בסכסוך הרוחות רבת הנזק לבעלי החליים הקרים. → NM 4:120.

[סכסך] • *Piʿel* **סִכְסֵךְ** · **to move; to stimulate:** Arab. حرّك · Al-Rāzī, *K. al-Manṣūrī* · trans. Shem Tov ben Isaac (*Sefer Almansur*), Alef 12 (16): אניסון: חם יגרש הרוחות ויפתח סתומי הכבד ויסכסך תאות המשגל. → NM 2:16.

סֻכָּר • סוכר ויאולש · **violet preserve:** Arab. بنفسج مربّا · Ibn al-Jazzār, *Zād al-musāfir wa-qūt al-ḥādir* · trans. Moses ibn Tibbon (*Sefer Ṣedat ha-Derakhim*), bk. 1, ch. 18 (fol. 27^b): ויורק אחר כן בבשול תמראינדיש ופרונש וגוגובש ופרחי ויאולש עם קשיא פישטולא ומאנא ומה שדומה להם וישתה בכל יום מה שירכך הטבע ויכבה חום מרה כרכומית כמו שיקח מנא וסוכר ויאולש מ״א עשרה דרהם וקשיא פשטולא מנוקה ה׳ דרהם וימרסהו במי קרא צלויה או במי קשואים וישתה אותו בהיותו צם. → NM 4:120.

• **סוכר כנדי** (also: **סוכרי קנדי**) · I. **concentrated juice of the sugar cane:** Arab. سكّر الفانيد · Ibn al-Jazzār, *Zād al-musāfir wa-qūt al-ḥādir* · trans. Moses ibn Tibbon (*Sefer Ṣedat ha-Derakhim*), bk, 2, ch. 2 (Ms. Oxford, Bodleian Library, Poc. 353, Uri Heb. 314, fol. 12^a): ויועיל מן הלובן שיקח סוכר טוב ב׳ חלקים וקצף הים חלק יודק וינופה וירפא בו או יקח אמידום וסוכר כנדי מכל אחד חלק ויודקו ויתרפא בהם. → NM 4:121.

· II. **ṭabarzad sugar (i.e., fine-quality white and refined cane sugar *qand*):** Arab. سكّر طبرزد · Ibn al-Jazzār, *Zād al-musāfir wa-qūt al-ḥādir* · trans. Moses ibn Tibbon (*Sefer Ṣedat ha-Derakhim*), bk. 2, ch. 2 (fol. 43^b): ולו ג״כ תאר עגולים מועילים ללובן ולשחין המתהוה בעין והוא נפלא יקח בלנקט ב׳ שקלים סרקאקולא מתוקנת ב׳ דר׳ דרגגאן וגומא ארביקא וסוכרי קנדי וכאנפר מ״א חצי דרהם. → NM 4:121–2.

• **קני הסוכר** → קָנֶה.

• **סוכר קשה** · **ṭabarzad sugar (i.e., fine-quality white and refined cane sugar *qand*):** Arab. سكّر طبرزد · Ibn al-Jazzār, *Zād al-musāfir wa-qūt al-ḥādir* · trans. Moses ibn Tibbon (*Sefer Ṣedat ha-Derakhim*), bk. 7, ch. 8.3: ומזה גם כן רפואה נסינו אותה ושבחנוה ישתה אותה בתחלת השנפיו והויירולא ותמהר ראותם: יקח ורדים ועדשים קלופים מ״א ארבעה דרהם לאכא מנוקה מעיציה שני דרהם זרע שומר רחב וזרע חבושים ודרגאגאן לבן מכל אחד שקל משתיק דרהם יבושל זה בליטר׳ מים באש רכה עד שיסור החצי וימרסהו ויסננהו וישתה ממנו רביע ליטר׳ עם שבעה דרהם סוכר קשה. → NM 4:122.

• **סכר הרטוב** · ***Sulaimānī* sugar:** Arab. السكّر السليماني · Ibn al-Jazzār, *Zād al-musāfir wa-qūt al-ḥādir* · trans. Moses ibn Tibbon (*Sefer Ṣedat ha-Derakhim*), bk. 1, ch. 10 (Ms. Oxford, Bodleian Library, Poc. 353, Uri Heb. 314, fol. 4^b): או ישתה מיץ שני הרמונים עם סוכר הרטוב. → NM 4:122.

סַם • הסם הדק › **the attenuant (refining) remedy**: Lat. subtiliativa medicina · Ibn Sīnā, *K. al-adwiya al-qalbiya* · trans. Anonymous (*Sefer ha-Refu'ot ha-Libbiyot*), fol. 244[a]: הסם הדק נאמר אותו שמדקדק עצם הליחה מתיך בקלות בחום מזוג. → NM 4:122–3.

• **הסם החותך** › **the incisive remedy**: Lat. incisiva medicina · Ibn Sīnā, *K. al-adwiya al-qalbiya* · trans. Anonymous (*Sefer ha-Refu'ot ha-Libbiyot*), fol. 120[b]: החותך הוא סם דק נוקב בין שטח האבר ושטח הליחה הדבקה עד שיפרידנו ממנו. → NM 4:123.

• **הסם הטריאקי** › **theriac**: Arab. ترياق · Ibn Sīnā, *K. al-adwiya al-qalbiya* · trans. Anonymous (*Sammim Libbiyim*), fol. 122[b]: והטריאקי והבאדזהר הוא הסם אשר ישנה מזג הרוח הקורה מסם ארסיי אל מזגו הטבעי וישמרהו עליו בסגולה שבו. → NM 4:123.

• **הסם הכווה** › **the caustic remedy**: Arab. الدواء الكاوي · Ibn Sīnā, *K. al-adwiya al-qalbiya* · trans. Anonymous (*Sammim Libbiyim*), fol. 121[b]: והכווה הוא הסם אשר ישרוף העור שריפה יכלה לחותו עד שיתקבצו חלקיו ויקשהו וישוב עצם זה העור סתום המעברים ⟨מ⟩ליחה נוזלת. → NM 4:123.

• **הסם המאדם** › **the reddening (rubefacient) remedy**: Arab. الدواء المحمّر · Ibn Sīnā, *K. al-adwiya al-qalbiya* · trans. Anonymous (*Sammim Libbiyim*), fol. 121[a]: והמאדם הוא הסם אשר יחמם האבר אשר ימשכהו חמום חזק עד שימשוך אליו הדם הרקיק משיכה חזק יגיע לנראה ממנו ויאדמהו. → NM 4:123–4.

• **הסם המאכל** › **the erosive (corroding) remedy**: Arab. الدواء الأكّال · Ibn Sīnā, *K. al-adwiya al-qalbiya* · trans. Anonymous (*Sammim Libbiyim*), fol. 121[a]: והמאכל הוא הסם אשר יגיע מהתכתו והתבערותו שיחסר מעצם הבשר. → NM 4:124.

• **הסם המביא הדם** › **the hemorrhagic remedy**: Lat. medicina sanguinis eductiva · Ibn Sīnā, *K. al-adwiya al-qalbiya* · trans. Anonymous (*Sefer ha-Refu'ot ha-Libbiyot*), fol. 245[b]: הסם המתיר השתן וזיעה וסם משלשל ומביא הדם או העוצר אותו ודומים יש להם ידיעה נגלית ולכן אינן צריכין ביאור. → NM 4:124.

• **הסם המבשל** › **the ripening (coctive) remedy**: Arab. الدواء المنضج · Ibn Sīnā, *K. al-adwiya al-qalbiya* · trans. Anonymous (*Sammim Libbiyim*), fol. 121[b]: והמבשל הוא הסם אשר יתקן ממשות הליחה אם היה עבה ידקדקהו בשווי ואם היה דק יעבחו עד שיתוקן לדחותו. → NM 4:124.

• **הסם המגיר הדם** › **the hemorrhagic remedy**: Arab. الدواء مسيّل الدم · Ibn Sīnā, *K. al-adwiya al-qalbiya* · trans. Anonymous (*Sammim Libbiyim*), fol. 122[b]: הסם המגיר השתן ולזיעה והמשלשל ומגיר הדם ועוצר אותו ומה שנשאר מאלו ענינם ידוע לא נצטרך להגדרתם. → NM 4:124–5.

• **הסם המגיר לזיעה** › **the diaphoretic remedy**: Arab. الدواء المدرّ للعرق · Ibn Sīnā, *K. al-adwiya al-qalbiya* · trans. Anonymous (*Sammim Libbiyim*), fol. 122[b]: הסם המגיר השתן ולזיעה והמשלשל ומגיר הדם ועוצר אותו ומה שנשאר מאלו ענינם ידוע לא נצטרך להגדרתם. → NM 4:125.

• **הסם המגיר השתן** › **the diuretic remedy**: Arab. الدواء المدرّ للبول · Ibn Sīnā, *K. al-adwiya al-qalbiya* · trans. Anonymous (*Sammim Libbiyim*), fol. 122[b]: הסם המגיר השתן ולזיעה והמשלשל ומגיר הדם ועוצר אותו ומה שנשאר מאלו ענינם ידוע לא נצטרך להגדרתם. → NM 4:125.

• **הסם המדביק או המחליק** · **the agglutinant or mollifacient remedy**: Lat. inviscativa seu lenificativa medicina · Ibn Sīnā, *K. al-adwiya al-qalbiya* · trans. Anonymous (*Sefer ha-Refu'ot ha-Libbiyot*), fol. 245[a]: המדביק או המחליק הוא אותו שהוא בדבקות ימתח על שטח האבר מתחלף החלקים כמו האצטומ׳ או הרחם או הקנה הישר ולזה יתחדש ויסבב בהם שטח זר וחלק. → NM 4:125.

• **הסם המדקדק** · **the attenuant (refining) remedy**: Arab. الدواء الملطّف · Ibn Sīnā, *K. al-adwiya al-qalbiya* · trans. Anonymous (*Sammim Libbiyim*), fol. 120[a]: המדקדק הוא הסם אשר מדרכו שישים ממשות הליחות יותר רקיק בהתכה חסרה בחום שוה. → NM 4:125.

• **הסם המושך** · **the attracting remedy**: Arab. الدواء الجاذب · Ibn Sīnā, *K. al-adwiya al-qalbiya* · trans. Anonymous (*Sammim Libbiyim*), fol. 121[a]: והמושך הוא הסם אשר לו איכות עוברת מאד יגיע הליחה לצד השטח אשר ימששהו אם בסגולה אם בחמום. → NM 4:125–6.

• **הסם המחזק** · **the tonic (strengthening) remedy**: Arab. الدواء المقوّي · Ibn Sīnā, *K. al-adwiya al-qalbiya* · trans. Anonymous (*Sammim Libbiyim*), fol. 122[b]: והמחזק הוא הסם אשר ישוה מזג האבר עד שימנעהו מקבלת הפגעים אם לסגולה שבו ואם לשווי מזגו ויקרר מה שהוא יותר חם ויחמם מה שהוא יותר קר לפי מה שזכרו גאלינוס בשמן הוורד. → NM 4:126.

• **הסם המחכך** · **the pruritic remedy**: Arab. الدواء المحكّك · Ibn Sīnā, *K. al-adwiya al-qalbiya* · trans. Anonymous (*Sammim Libbiyim*), fol. 121[a]: והמחכך הוא הסם אשר יגיע מחדותו שימשוך אל הנקבים ליחות עוקצות ולא יגיע אל שישחין כמו האלסכבינג. → NM 4:126.

• **הסם המחתך** · **the incisive (biting, cutting, pungent) remedy**: Arab. الدواء المقطّع · Ibn Sīnā, *K. al-adwiya al-qalbiya* · trans. Anonymous (*Sammim Libbiyim*), fol. 120[b]: והמחתך הנה הוא הסם הדק אשר אפשר לו שיעבור במה שבין שטח האבר ושטח הליחה הדבקה המדובקת בו עד שינקה אותה ממנו. → NM 4:126–7.

• **הסם המטיח** · **the smoothing remedy**: Arab. الدواء المملّس · Ibn Sīnā, *K. al-adwiya al-qalbiya* · trans. Anonymous (*Sammim Libbiyim*), fol. 122[a]: והמטיח הוא המתדבק אשר יתפשט על פני האבר המתחלף החלקים בהנחה ר״ל כל הנחורים כמו האצטומכא והרחם וקנה הריאה ויתדבק בהם ויתחדש עליהם שטח זר חלק. → NM 4:127.

• **הסם הממית** · **the lethal remedy**: Arab. الدواء القاتل · Ibn Sīnā, *K. al-adwiya al-qalbiya* · trans. Anonymous (*Sammim Libbiyim*), fol. 122[b]: והסם הממית הוא הסם אשר יפסיד עצם מזג הרוח והגוף אם מעצמיותו וצורתו אשר הוא מינו כמו הארסים ואם לתגבורת האיכות הפועלת בו כמו האפיון בקרירותו והאפריביון בחמימותו. → NM 4:127.

• **הסם הממעיד** · **the lubricant remedy**: Arab. الدواء المزلّق · Ibn Sīnā, *K. al-adwiya al-qalbiya* · trans. Anonymous (*Sammim Libbiyim*), fol. 122[a]: והממעיד הוא הסם אשר יטפיח שטח גשם נעצר במעברים ויפרידהו ממה שנעצר בו ואחר יתנועע זה הגשם בכבדותו הטבעי ויהיה מניע אותו במקרה והוא כמו אל⟨אגא⟩ש ואללעאבאת. → NM 4:127–8.

• **הסם הממרק** · **the detergent (cleansing, clearing) remedy**: Arab. الدواء الجالي · Ibn Sīnā, *K. al-adwiya al-qalbiya* · trans. Anonymous (*Sammim Libbiyim*), fol. 120[b]: והממרק הוא הסם אשר יכלה מן הליחה הנקפאת והדבקה מה שהיה על שטח האבר ופיות הנקבים. → NM 4:128.

• **הסם המנגע** · **ulcerative [remedy]**: Lat. ulcerativa · Ibn Sīnā, *K. al-adwiya al-qalbiya* · trans. Anonymous (*Sefer ha-Refu'ot ha-Libbiyot*), fol. 244[b]: והמנגע הוא אותו שיש לו

כח חזק לאדם עד שתתך הליחות הנדבקות מהחלקים שיגע בהם ומסבב החבורות ומושך להם המותרות שמהם הוות היציאות כמו סם האנקרדי. → NM 4:128.

• **הסם המנחיר** · **the roughening remedy**: Arab. الدواء المخشّن · Ibn Sīnā, *K. al-adwiya al-qalbiya* · trans. Anonymous (*Sammim Libbiyim*), fol. 120[b]: והמנחיר הוא הסם אשר ימרק מאבר קשה העצם כמו העצמות והשחוסים והעצבים כאשר יהיה הנחת חלקי האבר מתחלפים וכבר עבר עליו לחות החליק אותו ישיבהו אל נחירותו. → NM 4:128–9.

• **הסם המנפח** · **the flatulent remedy**: Lat. inflativa medicina · Ibn Sīnā, *K. al-adwiya al-qalbiya* · trans. Anonymous (*Sefer ha-Refu'ot ha-Libbiyot*), fol. 245[a]: המנפח הוא אותו אשר בעצמו לחות גסה זרה מתגברת מעורבת אל היושר וכשיפעל בה החום הטבעי יוליד רוח שאינו נתך כמו הפישולש. → NM 4:129.

• **הסם המעבה** · **the thickening remedy**: Arab. الدواء المغلّظ · Ibn Sīnā, *K. al-adwiya al-qalbiya* · trans. Anonymous (*Sammim Libbiyim*), fol. 122[a]: הסם המעבה הפך המדקדק. → NM 4:129.

• **הסם המעכל** · **the digestive remedy**: Arab. الدواء الهاضم · Ibn Sīnā, *K. al-adwiya al-qalbiya* · trans. Anonymous (*Sammim Libbiyim*), fol. 120[b]: והמעכל הוא הסם אשר ישנה המזון אל הדמות הליחות המשובחות אשר יזונו הגוף והליחות אל הדמות הגוף. → NM 4:129.

• **הסם המעפש** · **the putrefying remedy**: Arab. الدواء المعفّن · Ibn Sīnā, *K. al-adwiya al-qalbiya* · trans. Anonymous (*Sammim Libbiyim*), fol. 121[b]: והמעפש הוא הסם אשר יפסיד התדבקות האבר בהתכתו מה שבו מן הרוח הטבעי והתכת חומו הטבעי ולא יגיע אל שיאכלהו או יצ⟩י⟨להו או ישרפהו אבל ישאר בו לחות יתעצם בו חום בלתי טבעי. → NM 4:129.

• **הסם המפיג** · **the remedy that makes crude (unripe)**: Arab. الدواء المفجّج · Ibn Sīnā, *K. al-adwiya al-qalbiya* · trans. Anonymous (*Sammim Libbiyim*), fol. 122[b]: והמפיג הוא הסם המונע מהבשול והעכול לקרירותו כמו המים הקרים כאשר ישתו במורסות האצטומכא. → NM 4:130.

• **הסם המרדים** · **the benumbing (narcotic, soporific, stupefying) remedy**: Arab. الدواء المخدّر · Ibn Sīnā, *K. al-adwiya al-qalbiya* · trans. Anonymous (*Sammim Libbiyim*), fol. 122[b]: והמרדים הוא הסם הקר אשר יגיע מקרירותו לאבר אל שישנה עצם מח שיעבור בו מן הרוח אל מזג קר יבש יוצא ממזגו אשר בו יקבל הכוחות המרגישות והמניעות וישנה מזג האבר ככה ויבטל החוש. → NM 4:130.

• **הסם המרפה** · **the relaxant (slackening) remedy**: Arab. الدواء المرخي · Ibn Sīnā, *K. al-adwiya al-qalbiya* · trans. Anonymous (*Sammim Libbiyim*), fol. 120[b]: והמרפה הוא אשר ישים ממשות האברים קצרי הנקבים יותר רך ללחותו וחומו ויקרה מזה שישים הנקבים רחבים וידחה מה שבהם מן המותרים יותר נקל. → NM 4:130.

• **הסם המרתיע** · **the repellent remedy**: Arab. الدواء الرادع · Ibn Sīnā, *K. al-adwiya al-qalbiya* · trans. Anonymous (*Sammim Libbiyim*), fol. 122[b]: והמרתיע הוא הסם הקר אשר יחדש באבר קור יעבה אותו וייצר נקביו ויקפיא הנוזל אליו ויעבהו בכבוי חומו וימנעהו ובפרט כאשר היה עב הממשות כמו שמן הורד המקורר וה⟩ד⟨בסרקאטונא וזולתה. → NM 4:131.

• **הסם המשבר הרוח** · **the carminative remedy**: Arab. الدواء الكاسر الرياح · Ibn Sīnā, *K. al-adwiya al-qalbiya* · trans. Anonymous (*Sammim Libbiyim*), fol. 122[a]: הסם המשבר הרוח הוא הסם אשר ישיג בחומו הדק העובר מה שיקצר בו ⟨החום⟩ החלוש אם ישתנה הלחות אל רוח

ולא יותך ולפעמים יהיה מגיע התכתו להתיך מה שבעורקים מנפח המזונות והסמים כמו זרע רודא ואנג׳ילקשטי. → NM 4:131.

• **הסם המשחין** · **the ulcerative remedy**: Arab. الدواء المقرّح · Ibn Sīnā, *K. al-adwiya al-qalbiya* · trans. Anonymous (*Sammim Libbiyim*), fol. 121[a]: והמשחין הוא הסם אשר יפליג התאדמותו עד שיתיך הליחות המגיעות בין חלקי מה שיפגשהו ויחדש אליהם חבורות וימשוך אליהם מותרים וישוב כמו נגע וזה כמו הבלאדור. → NM 4:131–2.

• **הסם המשלשל** · **the purgative remedy**: Arab. الدواء المسهل · Ibn Sīnā, *K. al-adwiya al-qalbiya* · trans. Anonymous (*Sammim Libbiyim*), fol. 122[b]: הסם המגיר השתן ולזיעה והמשלשל ומגיר הדם ועוצר אותו ומה שנשאר מאלו ענינם ידוע לא נצטרך להגדרתם. → NM 4:132.

• **הסם המתיך** · **the resolvent (melting, reducing) remedy**: Arab. الدواء المحلّل · Ibn Sīnā, *K. al-adwiya al-qalbiya* · trans. Anonymous (*Sammim Libbiyim*), fol. 120[a–b]: המתיך הוא הסם אשר יתיך הליחה בהפרידו אותה והוציאו אותה מן המקום אשר נסתבכה בו חלק אחר חלק עד יכלה אותו להפלגת חומו. → NM 4:132.

• **הסם המתיר הזיעה** · **the diaphoretic remedy**: Lat. medicina provocativa sudoris · Ibn Sīnā, *K. al-adwiya al-qalbiya* · trans. Anonymous (*Sefer ha-Refu'ot ha-Libbiyot*), fol. 245[b]: הסם המתיר השתן וזיעה וסם משלשל ומביא דם או העוצר אותו ודומים יש להם ידיעה נגלית ולכן אינן צריכין ביאור. → NM 4:132.

• **הסם המתיר השתן** · **the diuretic remedy**: Lat. medicina provocativa urine · Ibn Sīnā, *K. al-adwiya al-qalbiya* · trans. Anonymous (*Sefer ha-Refu'ot ha-Libbiyot*), fol. 245[b]: הסם המתיר השתן וזיעה וסם משלשל ומביא דם או העוצר אותו ודומים יש להם ידיעה נגלית ולכן אינן צריכין ביאור. → NM 4:132–3.

• **הסם הנופח** · **the flatulent remedy**: Arab. الدواء المنفخ · Ibn Sīnā, *K. al-adwiya al-qalbiya* · trans. Anonymous (*Sammim Libbiyim*), fol. 121[b]: והנופח הוא הסם בעצמיותו ליחות עבה זרה וכאשר יפעל בו החום הטבעי השוה ישתנה רוח ולא יותך כמו הלוביא. → NM 4:133.

• **הסם הנושך** · **the irritant remedy**: Lat. mordicativa medicina · Ibn Sīnā, *K. al-adwiya al-qalbiya* · trans. Anonymous (*Sefer ha-Refu'ot ha-Libbiyot*), fol. 244[b]: הנושך הוא אותו שיש בו איכות דק נושך עושה בפרוק חבור מרבה המספר מהחלקים הקטנים ומקרובי ההנחה. → NM 4:133.

• **הסם הסותם** · **the obstruent (clogging, stopping the pores) remedy**: Arab. الدواء المسدّد · Ibn Sīnā, *K. al-adwiya al-qalbiya* · trans. Anonymous (*Sammim Libbiyim*), fol. 122[a]: והסותם הוא הסם אשר כאשר עבר במעברים התגבר על הכח המניע לדחותו ועמד נגד כל מציק ומלא את החלל כמו הטיט הנאכל. → NM 4:133.

• **הסם העוצר** · I. **the astringent remedy**: Lat. compressiva medicina · Ibn Sīnā, *K. al-adwiya al-qalbiya* · trans. Anonymous (*Sefer ha-Refu'ot ha-Libbiyot*), fol. 245[a]: העוצר הוא אותו שהוא יבש מסבב לאבר יובש ומקבץ אותו לעצמו ולזה סותם המעברים. → NM 4:133–4.

· II. **the constrictive remedy**: Arab. الدواء العاصر · Ibn Sīnā, *K. al-adwiya al-qalbiya* · trans. Anonymous (*Sammim Libbiyim*), fol. 125[a]: והעוצר הוא הסם אשר יגיע מקביצותו וחברו חלקי האבר קצתם אל קצת אל שיוכרחו הלחויות הרקיקים אשר יעמדו בפנימיותו אל שיתלחצו ושיתנועעו התנועה הנבדלת ממנו. → NM 4:134.

• **הסם העוצר הדם** · **the styptic remedy**: Arab. الدواء الحابس الدم · Ibn Sīnā, *K. al-adwiya* *al-qalbiya* · trans. Anonymous (*Sammim Libbiyim*), fol. 122[b]: הסם המגיר השתן ולזיעה והמשלשל ומגיר הדם ועוצר אותו ומהשנשאר מאלו ענינם ידוע לא נצטרך להגדרתם. → NM 4:134.

• **הסם העוקץ** · **the irritant (corrosive) remedy:** Arab. الدواء اللاذع · Ibn Sīnā, *K. al-adwiya al-qalbiya*· trans. Anonymous (*Sammim Libbiyim*), fol. 121[a]: והעוקץ הוא הסם אשר לו איכות דקה עוברת תחדש פרוק במחובר רב המספר מתקרב ההנחה קטון השעור. → NM 4:134.

• **עשיית הסם** → עֲשִׂיָּה.

• **הסם הפותח** · **the deobstruent remedy:** Arab. الدواء المفتّح · Ibn Sīnā, *K. al-adwiya al-qalbiya* · trans. Anonymous (*Sammim Libbiyim*), fol. 120[b]: והפותח הוא אשר יגיע החומר הנופל בחללות המעברים ויוציאהו לא בפיותיהם לבד. → NM 4:134–5.

• **הסם הקובץ** · **the astringent remedy:** Arab. الدواء المقبّض · Ibn Sīnā, *K. al-adwiya al-qalbiya* · trans. Anonymous (*Sammim Libbiyim*), fol. 122[a]: והקובץ הוא הסם היבש אשר יחדש באבר יובש והתקבצות אל עצמו ויסתים לזה המעברים. → NM 4:135.

• **הסם הרוחץ** · **the abluent remedy:** Arab. الدواء الغسّال · Ibn Sīnā, *K. al-adwiya al-qalbiya* · trans. Anonymous (*Sammim Libbiyim*), fol. 120[b]: והרוחץ הוא הסם אשר ימרק לא בכח פועלת בו אבל בכח מתפעלת והוא הלחות כשילך על פיות הנקבים וירכך מה שיש עליהם מן הליחות הדבקות והנקפאות בלחותו והזלתו והתערבו בהם. → NM 4:135.

• **הסם השובר רוח** · **the carminative remedy:** Lat. frangitiva ventositatis medicina · Ibn Sīnā, *K. al-adwiya al-qalbiya* · trans. Anonymous (*Sefer ha-Refu'ot ha-Libbiyot*), fol. 245[a]: השובר רוח הוא הסם ממלא בחומו הדק העובר חסרון החום החלוש אשר הוא בלתי יכול להתיך הלחות המנפח כשפועל בה והתרת זאת הרפואה הגיע לפעמים להתיך הנפח ההווה בגידים מהמזונות ומהסמים כמו זרע רודא ואנגילקושט. → NM 4:135–6.

• **הסם השורף** · **the corrosive remedy:** Arab. الدواء المحرق · Ibn Sīnā, *K. al-adwiya al-qalbiya* · trans. Anonymous (*Sammim Libbiyim*), fol. 120[b]: והשורף הוא הסם אשר ישרוף לחות הליחות וישאיר אפריותם כמו אלפרביון ואלחלתית. → NM 4:136.

• *Plur.* **סמים** • **סמים מנגעים** · **ulcerating drugs:** Arab. الأدوية التي تقرّح · Ibn al-Jazzār, *Zād al-musāfir wa-qūt al-ḥāḍir* · trans. Moses ibn Tibbon (*Sefer Ṣedat ha-Derakhim*), bk. 7, 13.3: וראוי שנתחיל ברפואתו קודם שיראו בו האותות הרעות שנשתדל לשרוף המקום הנשוך בכויה עמוקה מרחבת הנשיכה או בסמים מנגעים ומרחיבים אותה ולא יושם עליה רפואה שתנגבה ויסתמה ויעשה הארס לפנים. → NM 1:60.

• **סמים מרפים ומחלחלים** · **thinning and rarefying medicines:** Arab. أدوية مسخّفة ومخلخلة · Maimonides, *K. al-fuṣūl fī al-ṭibb* · trans. Nathan ha-Me'ati (*Sefer ha-Peraqim*), 23.99: ולכן נקראים סמים מרפים ומחלחלים. → NM 2:58.

• **הסמים הצריים** · **theriacs:** Lat. medicina tyriacalis · Ibn Sīnā, *K. al-adwiya al-qalbiya* · trans. Anonymous (*Sefer ha-Refu'ot ha-Libbiyot*), fol. 251[a]: פוסתיק: יש לו ריחניות ועפיצות עם דביקות ומפני זה הוא משמח הלב ולזה הוא נמנה בכל הסמים הצריים. → NM 4:135.

סָמוּךְ (*Pass. Part.*) → סָמַךְ.

סַמּוּר · **sable** [*Martes zibellina*]: Arab. سمّور · Al-Zahrāwī, *K. al-taṣrīf li-man ʿağiza ʿan at-taʾlīf* · trans. Shem Tov ben Isaac (*Sefer ha-Shimmush*), bk. 27, fol. 150[b], col. a: הסמור חשוב וטוב אל החזה והכליות והכבד. → NM 4:136.

סִמּוּר · **tremor**: Lat. tremor / Arab. نافض · Galen, *De inaequali intemperie* · trans. David Caslari (*Sefer Ro'a Mezeg Mitḥallef*), 6.4: ומהם עדיין יש בקצתם שיחדשו סמור. → NM 2:167.

סַמּוּת · **poisonous effect**: Arab. سمّية · Maimonides, *K. al-fuṣūl fī al-ṭibb* · trans. Zeraḥyah Ḥen (*Sefer ha-Peraqim*), 13.50: אמר משה זה אמת כל זמן שיהיה השלשול ברפואה בעלת סם או חזקה כמו הקולוקוינטידא והתורפד מפני סמותם או הקטפוץ מרוב כחו. → NM 1:173.

סָמַךְ • *Pass. Part.* סָמוּךְ • פרק קנה הזרוע הסמוך ליד → פֶּרֶק.

סִמָּן • סמן התחתון · **puberty**: Hippocrates, *Aphorisms* · trans. Judah Shalom, 5.7 (227) (fol. 76[b]): הכפיה אשר תהיה קודם סמן התחתון יש לה העתק. → NM 3:169.

סִמְפּוֹן • *Plur.* סמפונות · **[nasal] arteries**: Arab. خيشوم, *Plur.* خياشيم / Lat. venae in interiore naso · Ibn al-Jazzār, *Zād al-musāfir wa-qūt al-ḥādir* · trans. Moses ibn Tibbon (*Sefer Ṣedat ha-Derakhim*), bk. 2, ch. 14 (fol. 54[a]): ואם יקרה הרבמס מפני ליחה חמה חדה נגרת מן המוח אל הנחירים ימצא החולה מזה תגבורת שרפה בחוטם וחום ולהבה ושעירות בגרונו ובשני בסמפונות אשר מן החוטם אל הפה הנקראים כיאשם דומה לעשן. → NM 4:136.

סמפונא (*Aram.*) • *Plur.* סמפונין · **passages (i.e., blood vessels)**: Arab. مجار · Al-Zahrāwī, *K. al-taṣrīf li-man ʿağiza ʿan at-taʾlīf* · trans. Shem Tov ben Isaac (*Sefer ha-Shimmush*), bk. 27 (Ms. Oxford, Bodleian Library, Hunt. Donat 2, fol. 211[a], col. a): ומי שלא יוכל למצוא דרך לסננם מרוב טרדתו אם יהיה בדרך או בים צריך לקחת אחריהם דברים פותחים הסתומים ומנקים סמפוני הכבד והכליות וכיס מקוה המים. → NM 4:136–7.

סמרות · **shivering**: Arab. اقشعرار · Maimonides, *K. al-fuṣūl fī al-ṭibb* · trans. Zeraḥyah Ḥen (*Sefer ha-Peraqim*), 19.37: התרחץ במרחץ בקדחות כולם ראוי שתכווין בו שלשה כוונות: האחד שלא יחדש פלצות ולא סמרות בהכנסתו והשני שלא יהיה אבר שפריטואלי חלוש והשלישי שלא יהיה בגידים הראשונים מהליחות הניות שיעור מרובה מקובץ וכלוא. → NM 1:173.

סִנּוּן • *Plur.* סינונים · **dentifrices**: Arab. سنونات · Ibn al-Jazzār, *Zād al-musāfir wa-qūt al-ḥādir* · trans. Moses ibn Tibbon (*Sefer Ṣedat ha-Derakhim*), introduction (fol. 2[b]): השער הכ״א בסינונים אשר ינקו השנים. → NM 4:137.

[סנן] • *Puʿal* סֻנַּן · **to be dripped; to be poured in by drops**: Lat. instillare · Bruno Longobucco, *Cyrurgia Magna* · trans. Hillel ben Samuel (*Sefer Keritut*), fol. 48[b]: וגם יסונן שמן רוסטו באזנים. → NM 1:34.

סַנְסַן • *Plur.* סנסנים · **spinous processes**: Arab. سنسنة, *Plur.* سناسن / Gr. ἄκανθα · Ibn Sīnā, *K. al-Qānūn fī al-ṭibb* · trans. Nathan ha-Me'ati (*Sefer ha-Qanun*), bk. 1 (fol. 32[a]): ובעד השנית שהשדרה מחסה ומגן לאיברים הנכבדים המונחים לפניה ולכן ברא לה קוצים וסנסנים. → NM 4:137.

סְנַפִּיר • *Plur.* סנפירות · I. **dandruff; scurf**: Arab. إبرية / Lat. furfuratio capitis / Gr. πιτυρίασις · Ibn al-Jazzār, *Zād al-musāfir wa-qūt al-ḥādir* · trans. Moses ibn Tibbon (*Sefer Ṣedat ha-Derakhim*), introduction (Ms. Oxford, Bodleian Library, Poc. 353, Uri Heb. 314, fol. 1[b]): השער הה׳ בסנפירות המתילדות בעור הראש. → NM 4:137.

· II. **eschars**: Arab. خشكريشة · Ibn al-Jazzār, *Zād al-musāfir wa-qūt al-ḥādir* · trans. Moses ibn Tibbon (*Sefer Ṣedat ha-Derakhim*), bk. 7, 22.1: הנגעים אמנם יתילדו ממשיכת הדם וכל שכן הנגעים האדומים והם נגעים רעים שיש עמהם קדחת ועליהם סנפירות ומראיהם אדום ואדמימותם נוטה למראה אפר. → NM 1:63; 4:138.

› III. **scales:** Arab. نخالة · Ibn al-Jazzār, *Zād al-musāfir wa-qūt al-ḥādir* · trans. Moses ibn Tibbon (*Sefer Ṣedat ha-Derakhim*), bk. 7, ch. 19.1: הקובא שני מינים: ממנו מין שהוא שוה עם שטח הגוף והויתו ממרה שחורה מתילדת מעכירות הדם ופעמים שיהיה עמו חכוך כשיהיה החומר חזק התנועה ואמנם תתחזק כשיהיה החומר מעופש מאד או נלהב מאד. ואולם המין האחר יקרא הנכרי ובו שריפה והוא בולט יוצא משטח הגוף והוא נוטה למראה תכלת והקודם נוטה אל האדמימות ובמין הזה השני סנפירות רב כעין מורסן ונגוב ופעמים סדיקות וחכוך. → NM 4:137–8.

ססי › I. **hard; rough:** أخرش · Al-Zahrāwī, *K. al-taṣrīf li-man ʿağiza ʿan at-taʾlīf* · trans. Shem Tov ben Isaac (*Sefer ha-Shimmush*), bk. 27, fol. 149[a]: הדגים הימיים על שני מינים: המין האחד האדום הנקרא רויל הנצוד בסלעי הים והדגים הססיים. → NM 4:138.

› II. **that which is harsh, rough:** Arab. ما كان به خشونة / Gr. αὐστηρός · Al-Zahrāwī, *K. al-taṣrīf li-man ʿağiza ʿan at-taʾlīf* · trans. Shem Tov ben Isaac (*Sefer ha-Shimmush*), bk. 27, fol. 137[a], cols. a–b: והצמוקים הקובצים והססיים מורכבים משתי כחות כח מבשל ומתיך התכה בינוני וכח קובץ ומחזק. → NM 4:138.

• **חירק חססי** → יָרֵק.

[סער] • *Inf. Hitpaʿel* **הִסְתַּעֵר** • **הסתער הבטן** › **diarrhea:** Lat. perturbationes ventris · Hippocrates, *Aphorisms* · trans. Hillel ben Samuel, 1.2 (29): א״א: בהסתער הבטן והקיא כשבאים מהטבע אם מה שצריך להתנקות יתנקה יועילהו זה ויקל שאתו ואם לאו יהיה בהפך. → NM 3:169.

• *Part. Hitpaʿel* **מִסְתַּעֵר** › **stirred up:** Arab. مهتاج / Gr. ὀργάω · Maimonides, *Šarḥ fuṣūl Abūqrāṭ* · trans. Moses ibn Tibbon (*Pirqei Abuqraṭ*), 1.22 (49): אמר אבקראט: אמנם ראוי לך שתעשה הרפואה וההנעה אחר שיתבשל החולי אבל כל זמן שהוא נא ובתחלת החולי אין ראוי זה אם לא שיהיה החולי מסתער ואי אפשר ברוב הענין שיהיה החולי מסתער. → NM 3:133–4.

סַעַר › I. **anxiety:** Arab. قَلَق / Gr. ἀλύκη · Maimonides, *Šarḥ fuṣūl Abūqrāṭ* · trans. Moses ibn Tibbon (*Pirqei Abuqraṭ*), 7.56 (408): אמר אבקראט: הסער והאשתרילאר והפלצות ירפאהו היין כאשר נמזג אחד שוה באחד שוה. → NM 3:169.

› II. **distress:** Arab. كرب · a) Ibn al-Jazzār, *Zād al-musāfir wa-qūt al-ḥādir* · trans. Moses ibn Tibbon (*Sefer Ṣedat ha-Derakhim*), bk. 1, ch. 18 (fol. 26[a]): ויקרה לחולה עם עלות החולי וקרוב חזקתו מקרים מפחידים כמו צמא חזק ונגוב פה ושעירות לשון ושחרותה וסער ודפיקת לב. → NM 4:139.

b) Maimonides, *K. al-fuṣūl fī al-ṭibb* · trans. Zeraḥyah Ḥen (*Sefer ha-Peraqim*), 13.47: ותעלה בדעתך כי מי ששוקה רפואה משלשלת וליחותיו גסות והאויר קר כי יחדש לו סער והמיה וכאב באסטומכא ובמיעים ולא ישלשלנו. → NM 1:173–4.

› III. **sleeplessness; wakefulness, engendered by anxiety and grief:** Arab. أرق · Ibn al-Jazzār, *Zād al-musāfir wa-qūt al-ḥādir* · trans. Moses ibn Tibbon (*Sefer Ṣedat ha-Derakhim*), bk. 1, ch. 17 (fol. 25[b]): תאר עוגות ירדימו החולה כשיהיה בו סער חזק וחום חזק מחבור אצחק. → NM 4:138–9.

סְעָרָה › I. **discomfort:** كرب · Maimonides, *K. al-fuṣūl fī al-ṭibb* · trans. Zeraḥyah Ḥen (*Sefer ha-Peraqim*), 7.55: כשתאכל מזון ולא יקרה לך ממנו נפיחה ולא רעם ולא רפפות ולא שנגלוצו אבל יהיה מוצא אותך באסטומכתך סערה אין לך בו תועלת ויכבד באסטומכא. → NM 1:174.

· II. **disturbance**: a) Arab. قَلَق · Maimonides, *Šarḥ fuṣūl Abūqrāṭ* · trans. Moses ibn Tibbon (*Pirqei Abuqraṭ*), 1.22 (49): אמר המפרש: אמרו הרפואה רוצה בו המשלשל והחולי המסתער הוא אשר יהיו הליחות מסערות החולה הוסיפו אותו בחום יהיה להם והגרה מאבר אל אבר בתחלת החולי ויצערוהו ויחדשו לו סערה ולא יניחו לו לשקוט. → NM 3:170.

b) Arab. اضطراب · i. Maimonides, *K. al-fuṣūl fī al-ṭibb* · trans. Zeraḥyah Ḥen (*Sefer ha-Peraqim*), 6.86: הרעי אשר יהיה בו קצף יורה על אחד משני עניינים: או על חמימות מרובה תתיך הגוף ויתחדש הקצף בעבור הדבר אשר ירתיח לחויות הגוף אשר התיכם החמימות המרובה או על סערה מרובה מפני התנגד רוח עב ללחות. → NM 1:174.

· ii. Maimonides, *Šarḥ fuṣūl Abūqrāṭ* · trans. Zeraḥyah Ḥen (*Pirqei Abuqraṭ*), 2.13 (65): אמר המפרש: בהבדיל הטבע הדבר הרע מן הטוב והכנתו לדחות ולהוציא יתחדש מזה סערה. וראוי בהכרח בזמן הסערה שהחולה יצטער ויקשה עליו חליו. → NM 3:170.

[ספג] • *Hifʿil* **הִסְפִּיג** · I. **to loosen**: Arab. خلخل · Maimonides, *Šarḥ fuṣūl Abūqrāṭ* · trans. Anonymous (*Pirqei Abuqraṭ*), 1.1 (23): וכמו כן הפעולות הנמשכים לאלו הכחות ⟨...⟩ השניות כמו שהסם יקשה או ירכך או יספיג או יעבה. → NM 3:170.

· II. **to rarefy**: Arab. خفّف · Maimonides, *K. al-fuṣūl fī al-ṭibb* · trans. Zeraḥyah Ḥen (*Sefer ha-Peraqim*), 21.62: הרפואה המשככת לכאבים באמת יהיה סבת הכאב ליחה או רוח קרים או חמים באי זו עצם שתהיה הליחה הם הרפואה אשר חומה כחמימות הגוף או חמימות שיהיה בראשונה ויהיה עמו דקות עצם עד שתספיג ותדקדק ותבשל ותריק מה שנתבשל ויוציא מן הנקבים ועל כן ראוי שלא יהיה בו קיבוץ כלל. → NM 1:174–5.

ספוגות • **עשה ספוגות** → **עָשָׂה**.

סְפוֹגִי • **העצמים הספוגיים** → **עֶצֶם**.

סַפַּחַת · **eczema**: Arab. قوباء · Al-Zahrāwī, *K. al-taṣrīf li-man ʿağiza ʿan at-taʾlīf* · trans. Shem Tov ben Isaac (*Sefer ha-Shimmush*), bk. 27, fol. 138[b], col. b: ומועיל מן הספחת והנתק כשיוטח נו. → NM 4:139.

סְפִיגוּת · **looseness**: Arab. تخلخل · Maimonides, *Šarḥ fuṣūl Abūqrāṭ* · trans. Anonymous (*Pirqei Abuqraṭ*), 5.69 (289): אמר המפרש: הקור ימהר אל הגב יותר להיותו קר לרוב העצמות שיש לשם ומעוט הבשר והנשים יותר קרים מן האנשים והראיה על ספיגות העור מלפנים מצמיחת השערות. → NM 3:171.

[ספק] • *Puʿal* **סֻפַּק** • **סופק על** · **to be difficult for**: Arab. أشكل على · Galen, attr., *Prohibition of Burial* · trans. Judah al-Ḥarizi (*Sefer Issur ha-Qevurah le-Galienus*), par. 75: וזה החולי יסופק על הרופאים מאד כי אין לו הוראה מדפיקת עורק ויראה בעליו מת אמתי. → NM 4:139.

סָפֵק · **error**: Arab. وَهْم · Maimonides, *Šarḥ fuṣūl Abūqrāṭ* · trans. Zeraḥyah Ḥen (*Pirqei Abuqraṭ*), introduction (7): אלא שגאלינוס לא יורה זה ולא ירצה בשום פנים שיהיה בדברי אבוקרט ספק. → NM 3:171.

סֵפֶר • **ספר המבחרים** · ***The Epitomes***: Arab. المختصرات · Maimonides, *Šarḥ fuṣūl Abūqrāṭ* · trans. Anonymous (*Pirqei Abuqraṭ*), introduction (13): ואמנם כל פירוש שאזכור סתם הוא דבר גאלינוס ר״ל כונתו כאשר אני לא אשגיח לצמצם מלת לשונו ממש כמו שעשיתי בספר המבחרים. → NM 3:123.

סְפָרַד • **עפר ספרד** → **עָפָר**.

סְקִירָה · external angle of the eye: Arab. لَحَاظ · Ibn Sīnā, *K. al-Qānūn fī al-ṭibb* · trans. Nathan ha-Me'ati (*Sefer ha-Qanun*), bk. 1 (fol. 57[a]): והחלק השני עובר בנקב הנברא בעת הסקירה. → NM 4:139–40.

[סרח] • *Part. Hof'al* **מֻסְרָח** • **הגרגרים המוסרחים** → **גַּרְגַּר**.

סְתוּם • **סתום האף** · rheum: Arab. زكام · Maimonides, *Šarḥ fuṣūl Abūqrāṭ* · trans. Anonymous (*Pirqei Abuqraṭ*), 3.20 (126): והשלים זה הענין בשאמר שכבר יתחדש באביב אשר הוא המיושר והשוה שבפרקים חוליים שחוריים כמו הדאגה השחורי והשטות וחליים לבניים והנכפה וסתום האף ונמיכות הקול והשעול. → NM 3:171.

• **סתום הנחירים** · rheum: Arab. زكام / Gr. κόρυζα · Maimonides, *Šarḥ fuṣūl Abūqrāṭ* · trans. Anonymous (*Pirqei Abuqraṭ*), 3.14 (120): אמר אבוקרט: ואם יהיה צפוני ויבש יאות למי שטבעו רטוב ולנשים ואמנם שאר האנשים יקרה להם מורסת עין יבשה וקדחות חדות וסתום הנחירים ישנה ומהם מי שיקרה להם בלבול הדאגה השחורי שיארע מהמרה השחורה. → NM 3:171.

• *Plur.* **סתומים** · obstructions: Arab. سدّة, *Plur.* سدد · Ibn al-Jazzār, *Zād al-musāfir wa-qūt al-ḥādir* · trans. Moses ibn Tibbon (*Sefer Ṣedat ha-Derakhim*), introduction (fol. 3[b]): השער הב' בסתומים המתילדים בכבד. → NM 4:140.

סָתַם • *Part.* **סוֹתֵם** • **הסם הסותם** → **סַם**.

[סתר] • *Part. Nif'al* **נִסְתָּר** • **נסתר מן** · prevented from: Arab. محجوب عن · Ibn Sīnā, *K. al-Qānūn fī al-ṭibb* · trans. Nathan ha-Me'ati (*Sefer ha-Qanun*), bk. 1 (fol. 56[b]): והנה זכר לנפילת החתוך הזה תועלות שלשה אחד מהם שיהיה הרוח הנוזל אל אחת האישונים בלתי נסתר מהזיל אל האחרת. → NM 4:140.

• **מסבות נסתרות** → **סִבָּה**.

ע

עֶב • עב טיט · pus: Hippocrates, *Aphorisms* · trans. Do'eg ha-Edomi (*Sefer Agur*), 4.75 (212) (fol. 78a): תדין על המשתין עב טיט ודם כי חבורה או מספחת בכליות או במקום. → NM 3:172.

• **בלוי עב טיט** → **בְּלוּי**.

• **קבוץ עב טיט** → **קִבּוּץ**.

[עבד] • *Pi'el* **עִבֵּד** · to fortify; to tone: Arab. بدغ · Al-Zahrāwī, *K. al-taṣrīf li-man 'ağiza 'an at-ta'līf* · trans. Shem Tov ben Isaac (*Sefer ha-Shimmush*), bk. 27, fol. 137b, col. a: ואחרי כן מחזקים האסטומ' ומעבדים אותה מבלי מזיקים לעצביה. → NM 4:140.

• **עיבד האצטומכה** · to strengthen the stomach: Arab. دبغ المعدة · Al-Rāzī, *K. al-Manṣūrī* · trans. Shem Tov ben Isaac (*Sefer Almansur*), He 1 (30): הלילג השחור ובלעז מירבולנש אינדיש וב״מ הלילקים הודיים נאותים לטבעים כלם ולכל חולי ואין דבר בכלל יותר חשוב ולא יותר רב התועלת ממנו והוא ישלשל שלשול חלוש ויעבד האצטומכה ויועיל מן הטחורים. → NM 2:16.

[עבה] • *Pi'el* **עִבָּה** · to make rough: Arab. خشّن · Maimonides, *K. al-fuṣūl fī al-ṭibb* · trans. Zeraḥyah Ḥen (*Sefer ha-Peraqim*), 7.25: הליחות החדות או הרפואה המחודדת אשר יעבה האברים כשיהיה עמם מותר כח מרובה שיחום(?) באברים הבשריים חבלות ובעצמות נקירה. → NM 1:175.

• *Part. Pi'el* **מְעַבֶּה • מעבה דם** · blood clots: Hippocrates, *Aphorisms* · trans. Do'eg ha-Edomi (*Sefer Agur*), 4.80 (217) (fol. 78b): זרם שתן במעבה דם גם בתחתית הבטן ועל הערוה יכאב לאות כי זה יחול מן המקוה. → NM 3:134.

• **חסם המעבה** → **סַם**.

עִבּוּי · thickening: Arab. تغليظ · Maimonides, *K. al-fuṣūl fī al-ṭibb* · trans. Nathan ha-Me'ati (*Sefer ha-Peraqim*), 20.42: ואמנם החלב הנה הוא כאלו הוא מעבה ויותר מעבה מן החלב הגבינה והוא מן הדברים המעבים תכלית העבוי כשיאכל יבש. → NM 2:70.

עֹבִי · compactness; firmness; solidity: Arab. متانة · Ibn Sīnā, *K. al-adwiya al-qalbiya* · trans. Anonymous (*Sammim Libbiyim*), fol. 129a: כמתרי יש בו בשמיות וקביצות ועובי עצמיות. → NM 4:140.

עָבַר • עבר על · to be in accordance with: Arab. جرى على · Maimonides, *K. al-fuṣūl fī al-ṭibb* · trans. Nathan ha-Me'ati (*Sefer ha-Peraqim*), 25.37: וזה עובר על השרשים אשר הודיענו גאלינוס. → NM 2:70.

עֲגָבוֹת • עצם העגבות → **עֶצֶם**.

עָגוֹל → **עָגֹל**.

עָגוּל · eye-salve (collyrium): Arab. شياف · a) Ibn al-Jazzār, *Zād al-musāfir wa-qūt al-ḥāḍir* · trans. Moses ibn Tibbon (*Sefer Ṣedat ha-Derakhim*), bk. 2, ch. 1 (fol. 42b): ומזה תואר עגולים לבנים כוללים מועילים בע״ה לקצידה החמה והדפיקה. → NM 4:141.

b) Ibn al-Jazzār, *Zād al-musāfir wa-qūt al-ḥāḍir* · trans. Moses ibn Tibbon (*Sefer Ṣedat ha-Derakhim*), bk. 7, 15.3: וכאשר הריקונו כל הגוף נשוב אל הרפואות אשר יודעו במשככות והדוחות בהתחלה כמו שנדל ובול ארמיני ועגול ממיטא ואופי ומה שדומה לזה. → NM 1:63.

• **עגול הארכובה** › **patella**: Arab. رضفة · Ibn Sīnā, *K. al-Qānūn fī al-ṭibb* · trans. Nathan ha-Me'ati (*Sefer ha-Qanun*), bk. 1 (fol. 54[a]): ויש לו שתי קצוות אחד מהם בשריי ומתחבר בעגול הארכובה קודם שיהיה מיתר והאחר קרומיי מתחבר בקצה הפנימי משתי קצוות פחד הירך. → NM 4:141.

• **עגול העין** › **corona**: Arab. اكليل · Al-Zahrāwī, *K. al-taṣrīf li-man ʿağiza ʿan at-taʾlīf* · trans. Shem Tov ben Isaac (*Sefer ha-Shimmush*), bk. 30, 2.23 (fol. 212[a]): ואחר לשית פי המקדיח קרוב מעגול העין כעובי המכחל בלובן העין עצמו מצד זנבו. → NM 1:106.

• **העגול השחור שבבשר** › **jugular fossa**: Arab. لبّة / Gr. σφαγή / Lat. fossa iugularis · Ibn Sīnā, *K. al-Qānūn fī al-ṭibb* · trans. Nathan ha-Me'ati (*Sefer ha-Qanun*), bk. 1 (fol. 61[a]): אמנם החלק העולה משני חלקי האוריטי הנה הוא מתחלק לשני חלקים הגדול שבהם מתחיל עולה אצל סביב העגול השחור שבבשר הנקרא ליפה. → NM 4:141.

עגז › **sacrum**: Arab. عجز · Ibn Sīnā, *K. al-Qānūn fī al-ṭibb* · trans. Nathan ha-Me'ati (*Sefer ha-Qanun*), bk. 1 (fol. 35[b]): הפרק אחד עשר בנתוח העגז. → NM 4:141–2.

עגזי • **הוריד העגזי** → וְרִיד.

• **העצבים העגזיים** → עָצָב.

עָגֹל • **תולעים עגולים** → תּוֹלַעַת.

עָדַף • *Part.* **עוֹדֵף** › **epidemic**: Arab. وافد · Maimonides, *K. al-fuṣūl fī al-ṭibb* · trans. Zeraḥyah Ḥen (*Sefer ha-Peraqim*), 23.16: החליים הנקראים העודפים הם חליים כוללים מתחדשים ביושבי אחד מן המקומות ובקצת שנים והם נמשכים אחר שינוי מתחדש באויר או במים או במזונות המורגלים או בשלשתם. → NM 1:175.

• *Hifʿil* **הֶעֱדִיף** › **to stream**: Arab. فاض · Maimonides, *Šarḥ fuṣūl Abūqrāṭ* · trans. Anonymous (*Pirqei Abuqraṭ*), 7.11 (363): אמר המפרש: כשלא יספוק הליחה המתחדש לחולי הצד מקומה יעדיף ממנה דבר אל הריאה. → NM 3:172.

עֲדָשָׁה • *Plur.* **עדשים** • **עדשי המים** › **duckweed** [*Lemna* L.]: Arab. طحلب · Ibn al-Jazzār, *Zād al-musāfir wa-qūt al-ḥāḍir* · trans. Moses ibn Tibbon (*Sefer Ṣedat ha-Derakhim*), bk. 7, 15.4. → NM 1:71–2.

• **עדשי הפנים** › **freckles**: Arab. كلف · Ibn al-Jazzār, *Zād al-musāfir wa-qūt al-ḥāḍir* · trans. Moses ibn Tibbon (*Sefer Ṣedat ha-Derakhim*), introduction (Ms. Oxford, Bodleian Library, Poc. 353, Uri Heb. 314, fol. 1[b]): השער הכ״ה בעדשי הפנים והוא אלכלף. → NM 4:142.

עובי → עֹבִי.

[**עוג**] • *Hofʿal* **הוּעַג** › **to be kneaded**: Arab. عجن · Ibn Sīnā, *K. al-adwiya al-qalbiya* · trans. Anonymous (*Sammim Libbiyim*), fol. 134[b]: וישמר שיושמו הסמים האחרים על ענינם ויועג כמו שזכרנו. → NM 4:142.

עוּגָה › **pastille**: Arab. قرص · Ibn al-Jazzār, *Zād al-musāfir wa-qūt al-ḥāḍir* · trans. Moses ibn Tibbon (*Sefer Ṣedat ha-Derakhim*), bk. 7, 18.4: והנה יודק שורש אשקריולא מדברית ויולש בדבש ויעשה עוגות ויצניעם ויקח עוגה אחר עוגה ויתיכה במים ושלניטרי ויטוח אותה על הבהק וינקה אותו. → NM 1:63–4.

עוֹדֵף (*Part.*) → עָדַף.

עִוּוּת › 1. **colic**: a) Arab. مغص / Gr. στρόφος · Ibn al-Jazzār, *Zād al-musāfir wa-qūt al-ḥāḍir*

· trans. Moses ibn Tibbon (*Sefer Ṣedat ha-Derakhim*), introduction (fol. 3b): השער הי״ג בעוות והמשברים הוא אל מגת ובלע׳ טרנקדש. → NM 4:142.

b) Lat. torsio · Hippocrates, *Aphorisms* · trans. Hillel ben Samuel, 5.41 (261) (fol. 34b): אם תרצה לדעת אם האשה הרה תן לה לשתות מליקרטו כשהולכת לישן אם יעורר לה עוות בבטן היא הרה. → NM 3:172.

· II. **twitching:** Lat. tortura (Honofredi) · Ibn Zuhr, *Regimen of Health* · trans. Jacob ibn Tibbon (*Hanhagat ha-Beri'ut le-Abu 'Ali ben Zuhr*), ch. 28: עוות הפנים חזק הכח יבשר באלקוה שיקרב חדושה וראוי כאשר ירגיש זה שיעשה שלשול חזק ויחפף הפנים בחומץ ייין חזק כבר הורתח בהם פודנג׳ וימעט המזון וירחיק השתיה בכלל ויעשה גרגרים ועטושים. → NM 4:142–3.

• **עיוות הבטן** · **tenesmus:** Hippocrates, *Aphorisms* · trans. Do'eg ha-Edomi (*Sefer Agur*), 7.27 (379) (fol. 114b): אמר אפוקרט: כאשר יקרו שברים ועיוות הבטן לאשה הרה סבה להפיל העובר. → NM 3:172–3.

• **עוות ההבטה** · **squinting:** Lat. obliquitas aspectus · Al-Rāzī, attr., *On the Treatment of Small Children* · trans. Bonfos, ch. 11: מעוות ההבטה הנקרא אבליקוס. → NM 2:179.

• **אותם שיראו בעוות** → רָאָה.

עוֹמֵד (*Part.*) → עָמַד.

עוֹמֶק → עֹמֶק.

עוֹנָה · **attack; paroxysm (of a disease):** Arab. نوبة · a) Maimonides, *Šarḥ fuṣūl Abūqrāṭ* · trans. Moses ibn Tibbon (*Pirqei Abuqraṭ*), 2.13 (65): אמר אבקראט: מי שיבא לו הנקיון הנה יכבד עליו חליו בלילה אשר לפני עונת הקדחת אשר יבא בה הנקיון ובלילה אשר אחריו יהיה ברוב יותר קל. → NM 3:173.

b) Maimonides, *K. al-fuṣūl fī al-ṭibb* · trans. Zeraḥyah Ḥen (*Sefer ha-Peraqim*), 3.103: אותם שימותו בלא בחראן ימותו ביום העונה ויש מהם שימותו בתחלת עונות הקדחות ויוכל למות בעמידת העונה ויוכל למות בירידת העונה בהתיך הכח. → NM 1:175.

c) Maimonides, *K. al-fuṣūl fī al-ṭibb* · trans. Nathan ha-Me'ati (*Sefer ha-Peraqim*), 4.22: ועוד גם כן יהיה הדפק אם בתוספת אותם העונות ועליתם. → NM 2:70.

• **הקדחת שעונתה בכל יום** → קַדַּחַת.

עוֹנֶה (*Part.*) → עָנָה.

עוֹפֶרֶת • **קלפת עופרת** → קְלִפָּה.

עוֹצֶם → עֹצֶם.

עוֹצֵר (*Part.*) → עָצַר.

עוֹצֶר → עֹצֶר.

[עוק] • *Hif'il* הֵעִיק · **to prevent:** Arab. عاق · Maimonides, *Šarḥ fuṣūl Abūqrāṭ* · trans. Moses ibn Tibbon (*Pirqei Abuqraṭ*), 1.17 (44): ואם יעיקוהו עונות הקדחת ולא ימצא עתים רבים למזון תן אותו בפעמים מעטים. → NM 3:173.

עוֹקֵץ (*Part.*) → עָקַץ.

עוֹקֶץ → עֹקֶץ.

[עור] • *Pi'el* עוֹרֵר · **to irritate:** Arab. هاج / Gr. ἐρεθίζω · Maimonides, *Šarḥ fuṣūl Abūqrāṭ* · trans. Moses ibn Tibbon (*Pirqei Abuqraṭ*), 4.54 (191): אמר אבקראט: מי שקרה לו

בקדחת שורפת שעול רב יבש ואחר כן יהיה מעורר אותו מעט הנה הוא בלתי אפשר שיצמא. → NM 3:173.

• **עורר אסטנסות** · **to cause nausea**: Arab. أغثى · Maimonides, *K. al-fuṣūl fī al-ṭibb* · trans. Nathan ha-Me'ati (*Sefer ha-Peraqim*), 9.51: וכמו שכל המינים הנבאשים מהפכים הנפש ומעוררים אסטנסות כן כל המינים המבושמים טובי הריח מחזקים האסטומכה. → NM 2:30.

• **עורר התעוררות** · **to experiment**: Arab. أحدث حدثا / Gr. νεωτεροποιέω · Hippocrates, *Aphorisms* · trans. Nathan ha-Me'ati, 1.20 (47) (fol. 17ᵃ): אמר אבוקרט: הגופים אשר יבואם הגבול או שכבר בא להם הגבול על השלמות אין ראוי שתניע ולא שתעורר בהם שום התעוררות לא ברפואה משלשלת ולא בזולתה מהתעוררות אבל יונחו. → NM 3:174.

• *Inf. Hitpa'el* **הִתְעוֹרֵר** · **revival of strength**: Arab. إنعاش · Maimonides, *K. al-fuṣūl fī al-ṭibb* · trans. Nathan ha-Me'ati (*Sefer ha-Peraqim*), 20.30: כל מי שיצטרך להתעורר אין ראוי שישתה דבר לבד היין הרקיק הלבן הדק מעט סובל המים ואשר יש בו קביצות מעט. הנה זה הוא מהדברים היותר מועילים להם אם לא יהיה בהם קדחת. → NM 2:70.

עוֹר · **folio of pergament or paper**: Arab. جلد · Maimonides, *Šarḥ fuṣūl Abūqrāṭ* · trans. Moses ibn Tibbon (*Pirqei Abuqraṭ*), introduction (10): הנה ראיתי קצת המפרשים פירשו זה המאמר ממאמרי אבקראט והוא זה: וכאשר הגיע החולי לתכליתו אז ראוי שתהיה ההנהגה בתכלית האחרון מן הדקות שפירש אותו ביותר ממאה עורות בלא עניין ובלא סבה. → NM 3:174.

עִוֵּר • **המעי העור** → מְעִי.

עוֹרֵב • **חרטום העורב** → חַרְטוֹם.

עורף → עֹרֶף.

עוֹרֶק • **העורק התרדמיי** · **carotid artery**: Arab. العرق السباتي · Ibn Sīnā, *K. al-Qānūn fī al-ṭibb* · trans. Nathan ha-Me'ati (*Sefer ha-Qanun*), bk. 1 (fols. 56ᵇ–57ᵃ): שריג יוצא ממבוא העורק התרדמיי. → NM 4:143.

• *Plur.* **עורקים** • **העורקים הנחים** · **non-throbbing veins, vessels**: Arab. العروق الساكنة · Ibn Sīnā, *K. al-Qānūn fī al-ṭibb* · trans. Nathan ha-Me'ati (*Sefer ha-Qanun*), bk. 1 (fol. 63ᵃ): אמנם העורקים הנחים הנה צמיחת כלם מן הכבד. → NM 4:143.

• **נפיחת פיות העורקים מלמטה** → **נְפִיחָה**.

• **פיות עורקי הרחם** → **פֶּה**.

• **עורקים שוכנים** · **veins**: Arab. عروق ساكنة · Ibn Sīnā, *K. al-Qānūn fī al-ṭibb* · trans. Nathan ha-Me'ati (*Sefer ha-Qanun*), bk. 1 (fol. 60ᵃ): ויעברו עם שריגי אלה העצבים עורקים דופקים ושוכנים נכנסים במוצאיהם אל חוט השדרה. → NM 4:161.

• **תעלות העורקים** → **תְּעָלָה**.

[עות] • *Part. Pu'al* **מְעֻוָּת** • **מעוות הראות** · **squinting**: Arab. أحول, *Plur.* حول · Ibn Sīnā, *K. al-Qānūn fī al-ṭibb* · trans. Nathan ha-Me'ati (*Sefer ha-Qanun*), bk. 1 (fol. 56ᵇ): לכן יקרה למעוות הראות הנק' נירש שיראה הדבר כשני דברים בעת שתטה אחת האישונים למעלה או למטה. → NM 4:143.

עוֹתֵק (*Part.*) → עָתַק.

עִטוּף · **fainting**: Hippocrates, *Aphorisms* · trans. Do'eg ha-Edomi (*Sefer Agur*), 5.16 (236) (fol. 82ᵇ): אמר אפוקרט: ויפתחו וירחיבו המים החמים את גידי ההרגש ויסכלו הדעת ויעוררו זוב הדם גם יסבבו עטוף ופעמים יביאו בחומם המות. → NM 3:174.

עֲטָרָה • עטרת המלך · **king's clover; melilot** [*Melilotus officinalis*]: Arab. إكليل الملك · Maimonides, *K. al-fuṣūl fī al-ṭibb* · trans. Zeraḥyah Ḥen (*Sefer ha-Peraqim*), 21.69: הרפואות החמות בראשונה היבשות מאותן שמשמשין אותן שבעה ועשרים והם אורז ואנזרוט אשטוכדוס אסמרינו הנקרא בעברי עטרת המלך. → NM 4:143–4.

עטרי · **coronal**: Arab. إكليلي · Ibn Sīnā, *K. al-Qānūn fī al-ṭibb* · trans. Zeraḥyah Ḥen (*Sefer ha-Qanun*), bk. 1 (fol. 17[a]): ומן הראשונים חוליה משותפת עם המצח והוא עשוי (ונקרא העטרי בקשת וזה צורתו. → NM 4:144.

[עטש] • *Part. Hif'il* **מַעֲטִישׁ • דבר מעטיש** → **דָּבָר**.

עיוות → **עִוּוּת**.

עִיּוּן · I. **external angle of the eye**: Arab. لحاظ · Ibn Sīnā, *K. al-Qānūn fī al-ṭibb* · trans. Zeraḥyah Ḥen (*Sefer ha-Qanun*), bk. 1 (fol. 30[a]): והחלק השני יעבור בנקב הנברא במקום העיון. → NM 4:144.

· II. **intuition**: Arab. حدس · Maimonides, *Šarḥ fuṣūl Abūqrāṭ* · trans. Zeraḥyah Ḥen (*Pirqei Abuqraṭ*), 1.7 (21): ועל כן יצטרך להרגל ארוך בעניין הסימנים בכל אחת ואחת מהם ואז נוכל לדון במה שיתחדש בעיון טוב יהיה קרוב מן האמת. → NM 3:175.

• **דיבר בלא עיון** → **[דבר]**.

• **דבר נאמר בלי עיון** → **דָּבָר**.

• **רעיון נאמר בלי עיון** → **רַעְיוֹן**.

עַיֵּן • עין בעיון · **to regard**: Arab. لحظ · Maimonides, *K. al-fuṣūl fī al-ṭibb* · trans. Zeraḥyah Ḥen (*Sefer ha-Peraqim*), 25.59: וכל שכן אם היה אותו האיש נזדמן לו מזל מן המזלות הנחשבים ובני אדם עוינים אותו בעין הגדולה והמעלה וההקדם. → NM 1:176.

• *Part. Pi'el* **מְעַיֵּן** · **being indicative; [a day of] prognostic indication**: Hippocrates, *Aphorisms* · trans. Judah Shalom, 2.24 (76) (fols. 23[b]–24[a]): הרביעי הוא הוראה מהשביעי שלהם והשמיני התחלת השבוע האחר והמעיין הוא אחד עשר כי זה הוא רביעי מהשבוע השני והשבעה עשר גם כן מעיין כי הוא רביעי מארבעה עשר ושביעי מאחד עשר. → NM 3:135.

עַיִן • עין הארכובה · **patella**: Arab. عين الركبة · Ibn Sīnā, *K. al-Qānūn fī al-ṭibb* · trans. Zeraḥyah Ḥen (*Sefer ha-Qanun*), bk. 1 (fol. 22[b]): וראשה נעשה עם תחבולה ברצפה והיא עין הארכובה. → NM 4:144.

• **בת עין** → **בַּת**.

• **זנב העין** → **זָנָב**.

• **חיק העין** → **חֵיק**.

• **ירידת המים בעין** → **יְרִידָה**.

• **כלל העין** → **כְּלָל**.

• **עין הכתף** · **the process of the scapula that is shaped like the Arabic letter 'Ayin (i.e., the spine of the scapula)**: Arab. عين الكتف / Gr. σιγμοειδής · Ibn Sīnā, *K. al-Qānūn fī al-ṭibb* · trans. Nathan ha-Me'ati (*Sefer ha-Qanun*), bk. 1 (fol. 37[a]): והתוספת הזאת היא כמו הסנסן לחוליות נבראים לשמירה ונקרא עין הכתף. → NM 4:144–5.

• **מורסת העין** → **מֻרְסָא**.

• **הנצור אשר יהיה בדמע העין** → **נָצוּר**.

- עגול העין ← עִגּוּל.
- עין בעין ← עַיִן.
- צמח העין ← צֶמַח.
- קצה העין הגדול ← קָצֶה.
- קצה העין מצד האזן ← קָצֶה.
- קצוות העין ← קָצֶה.
- ראש העין ← רֹאשׁ.
- הרואה שלעין ← רוֹאֶה.
- תחתית העין ← תַּחְתִּית.
- תכליתיות בעין ← תַּכְלִיתִיּוּת.
- *Dual* **עֵינַיִם** · **the olecranon and coronoid fossa [of the humerus]**: Arab. عين, *Dual* عينان / Gr. βαθμίδες · Ibn Sīnā, *K. al-Qānūn fī al-ṭibb* · trans. Nathan ha-Me'ati (*Sefer ha-Qanun*), bk. 1 (fol. 38[a]): ואבוקראט קרא אלו שתי נקרות שני עינים. ← NM 4:145.
- אופל העינים ← אֹפֶל.
- אפר העינים ← אפר.
- לחבת העינים ← לֶהָבָה.
- לכלוך העינים ← לִכְלוּךְ.
- פתיחת העינים ← פְּתִיחָה.
- השנים אשר כנגד העינים ← שֵׁן.

עיצום ← עִצּוּם.

עיצור ← עִצּוּר.

עיקום ← עִקּוּם.

עיקר ← עִקָּר.

עירוב ← עֵרוּב.

[עכב] • *Part. Puʿal* **מְעֻכָּב** · **rare**: Arab. متفاوت · Maimonides, *K. al-fuṣūl fī al-ṭibb* · trans. Nathan ha-Me'ati (*Sefer ha-Peraqim*), 4.20: וכשילחוץ פי האסטומכה ויעסה אותו רוב מאכל או ליחות בלתי עוקצות ישפכו אליה אז ישוב הדפק מעוכב מאוחר וקטן וחלוש. ← NM 2:60–1.

עַכָּבִישׁ • אריגת העכביש ← אֲרִיגָה.

עַכְבָּר • **עכבר פרעה** · **weasel**: Arab. ابن عرس · Maimonides, *K. al-fuṣūl fī al-ṭibb* · trans. Nathan ha-Me'ati (*Sefer ha-Peraqim*), 21.54: ואבן ערס הוא עכבר פרעה אם ילקח אותו בעל החיים ויחפף בו עקיצתו יבריא מיד. ← NM 2:71.

עִכּוּב · **rarity**: Arab. تفاوت · Maimonides, *K. al-fuṣūl fī al-ṭibb* · trans. Nathan ha-Me'ati (*Sefer ha-Peraqim*), 4.6: עכוב הדפק או חולשתו או קטנו כל אחד משלשת המינים האלו כשיהיה בתכלית אשר אין אחריו תכלית הנה הוא מפוחד מאד ובעליו על צער גדול תמיד. ← NM 2:71.

- **עכוב השתן** · **dysuria**: Arab. عسر البول · Al-Zahrāwī, *K. al-taṣrīf li-man ʿağiza ʿan at-taʾlīf* · trans. Shem Tov ben Isaac (*Sefer ha-Shimmush*), bk. 27, fol. 136[a], col. a: ויש פחד מן הפטריות שאינם ממיתים שלא יקרה מהן חניקה וגנוח ועלוף וקרירות הידים והרגלים ועל הרוב ירדוף אותן שלשול וקיא חזקים ויתחדש מהן עכוב השתן גם כן. ← NM 4:145 (corr.).

עִכּוּל • העכול השני · **the second digestion (i.e., that in the liver):** Arab. الهضم الثاني · Al-Zahrāwī, *K. al-taṣrīf li-man ʿağiza ʿan at-ta'līf* · trans. Shem Tov ben Isaac (*Sefer ha-Shimmush*), bk. 27, fol. 135[a], col. b: והממעט מאכילתו חי אחר האכילה יתמעטו רוחותיו העת ההיא וירפה המעים ויעבור בקלות המזון בגידים ויחזק העכול השני אשר בכבד. → NM 4:145–6.

עֲכִירוּת · **sediment:** Arab. عكر · Maimonides, *K. al-fuṣūl fī al-ṭibb* · trans. Nathan ha-Me'ati (*Sefer ha-Peraqim*), 3.61: וגם ימצא לפעמים רבות במורסות הנקראות דבלות גשמים דומים לאבן ולחול ולחרס ולעץ ולפחם ולעכירות השמן ולשמרי היין ובזולת זה ממינים רבים. → NM 2:71.

• **עכירות הראות** · **clouded (blurred) vision:** Lat. obscuritas oculorum (Honofredi) · Ibn Zuhr, *Regimen of Health* · trans. Jacob ibn Tibbon (*Hanhagat ha-Beri'ut le-Abu ʿAli ben Zuhr*), 34: הרחיק עצמך מהאכילה מעכירות הראות בלילה. NM 4:146.

[עכל] • *Part. Pi'el* **מְעַכֵּל • הסם המעכל** → **סַם**.

עִלֵּג • העלג · **people who lisp:** Arab. الألثغ / Gr. τραυλός, *Plur.* τραυλοί · Maimonides, *Šarḥ fuṣūl Abūqrāṭ* · trans. Moses ibn Tibbon (*Pirqei Abuqraṭ*), 6.32 (324): אמר אבקראט: העלג יקרה להם בפרט שלשול ארוך. → NM 3:175–6.

עָלָה · **to culminate (disease; fever):** Hippocrates, *Aphorisms* · trans. Do'eg ha-Edomi (*Sefer Agur*), 1.10 (37) (fol. 24[b]): אמר אפוקרט: באשר ימהר החולי לעלות פתאום תרבה לדקדק מאכליו. → NM 3:176.

• **עלה בשנים** · **to be advanced in years; to be old:** Arab. مسنّ · Ibn al-Jazzār, *Zād al-musāfir wa-qūt al-ḥāḍir* · trans. Moses ibn Tibbon (*Sefer Ṣedat ha-Derakhim*) (Ms. Oxford, Bodleian Library, Poc. 353, Uri Heb. 314, fol. 10[a]): ואם עלה בשנים או היה חלוש ראוי שנזהר מהוצאת הדם ויסתפק על מה שזכרנו מהרפואה הכללית והפרטית. → NM 4:146.

• *Part. Pu'al* **מְעֻלֶּה • האיברים המעולים** → **אֵבֶר**.

עָלֶה • *Plur.* **עלים • אלף עלים** → **אֶלֶף**.

עָלֶה • העלה הרוחנית · **disorder of the spiritual members:** Armengaud Blaise, *Tabula Antidotarii* · trans. Estori ha-Parḥi (*Shemot ha-Mashqim*), 18 (57): ... דיאה קלמינטום בשעת שכיבה עם בשול ריגליסיאה מנוק⟨ה⟩ כנגד העלה הרוחנית. → NM 4:146.

עָלוּל · **patient:** Arab. عليل · Maimonides, *K. al-fuṣūl fī al-ṭibb* · trans. Nathan ha-Me'ati (*Sefer ha-Peraqim*), 7.50: העלול יוציא ברקיקה דבר מועט בשעול רב על שני פנים אם בסבת עובי הליחות ודבקותם וישתרגו ויסתבכו ויקשה המלטם ואם בסבת רקיקות הליחות. → NM 2:71.

עֲלוּקָה · **thick, clotted blood:** Arab. علق · Maimonides, *K. al-fuṣūl fī al-ṭibb* · trans. Nathan ha-Me'ati (*Sefer ha-Peraqim*), 6.91: הדם כשיקפה ויתקרש וישוב כעלוקה במקוה וכן אם יקפא במעים או באסטומכה או בחזה הנה הוא באלו יותר רע שאינו במקוה ויקרה לו בסבתו עלוף וכרכמות מראה וישוב הדפק קטן וחלוש ותכוף ויחם העלול ויתרפו אבריו. → NM 2:72.

עֲלִיָּה · **getting worse; increase (of a disease):** Arab. تزيّد · Maimonides, *K. al-fuṣūl fī al-ṭibb* · trans. Zeraḥyah Ḥen (*Sefer ha-Peraqim*), 9.20: ליתרגס ככלות עלייתו לך למשוח הגרון ברפואות חזקות וחריפות. → NM 1:176.

עֶלְיוֹן • חגיד העליון → **גִּיד.**
• **הזנאד העליון** → **זנאד.**
• **העומק אשר בעליון אחורי הצואר** → **עֹמֶק.**
• **העמוד העליון** → **עַמּוּד.**

עלייה → **עֲלִיָּה.**

עֲלִילָה ‣ **blemish; defect; fault:** Lat. vitium · Bruno Longobucco, *Cyrurgia Magna* · trans. Hillel ben Samuel (*Sefer Keritut*), fol. 104[a]: על כאב ועלילת הכבד תכוה על הכבד. → NM 1:34.

עַלְקָא (*Aram.*) ‣ **leech:** Arab. علق · Al-Zahrāwī, *K. al-taṣrīf li-man ʿağiza ʿan at-taʾlīf* · trans. Shem Tov ben Isaac (*Sefer ha-Shimmush*), bk. 27, fol. 126[b]. col. a: והנותן גריסיהם על מקום העלקא יפסיקו הדם. → NM 4:146.

עָמַד • *Part.* **עוֹמֵד** • **העצם העומד למטה מכל השדרה** → **עֶצֶם.**
• **העת העומד** → **עֵת.**
• *Hifʿil* **הֶעֱמִיד** ‣ **to set down in writing:** Arab. ثبّت · Maimonides, *K. al-fuṣūl fī al-ṭibb* · trans. Nathan ha-Me'ati (*Sefer ha-Peraqim*), introduction: ואלו הפרקים אשר העמדתים לא אומר שחברתים אבל אומר שבחרתים. → NM 2:72.

עַמּוּד • **העמוד העליון** ‣ **radius:** Arab. الزند الأعلى · Ibn Sīnā, *K. al-Qānūn fī al-ṭibb* · trans. Joseph Lorki (*Sefer ha-Qanun*), bk. 1 (fol. 12[b]): ואמנם פרק המרפק מתחבר מפרק העמוד העליון ופרק התחתון עם קנה הזרוע. → NM 4:146–7.
• **עצם העמוד** → **עֶצֶם.**
• **העמוד התחתון** ‣ **ulna:** Arab. الزند الأسفل · Ibn Sīnā, *K. al-Qānūn fī al-ṭibb* · trans. Joseph Lorki (*Sefer ha-Qanun*), bk. 1 (fol. 12[b]): ואמנם פרק המרפק מתחבר מפרק העמוד העליון ופרק התחתון עם קנה הזרוע. → NM 4:147.
• *Plur.* **עמודים** • **שני עמודים** ‣ **the two bones of the forearm (radius and ulna):** Arab. الزندان · Ibn Sīnā, *K. al-Qānūn fī al-ṭibb* · trans. Joseph Lorki (*Sefer ha-Qanun*), bk. 1 (fol. 12[b]): הזרוע מחובר משתי עצמות דבקות ונקראים שני עמודים. → NM 4:147.

עֲמִידָה ‣ I. **climax, culmination:** a) Arab. منتهى · Maimonides, *K. al-fuṣūl fī al-ṭibb* · trans. Zeraḥyah Ḥen (*Sefer ha-Peraqim*), 9.18: בעמידת מורסת המוח מי שתהיה חוליו עם תעורה וערבוב תשפוך על ראשו מישרת הפאפויר ותשים בקצה נחיריו ופניו מה שיקרר המוח. → NM 1:176.
b) Arab. انتهاء · Maimonides, *K. al-fuṣūl fī al-ṭibb* · trans. Zeraḥyah Ḥen (*Sefer ha-Peraqim*), 11.1: זמני החולי הכוללים הם ארבעה: התחלה ותוספת ועמידה וירידה ולפי עמוד על ידיעת הזמן ההווה מזמני החולי בהרגשה אמתית אי זה מזמניו הוא עתה. → NM 1:176.
‣ II. **maturity:** Arab. وقوف · Ibn Sīnā, *K. al-Qānūn fī al-ṭibb* · trans. Zeraḥyah Ḥen (*Sefer ha-Qanun*), bk. 1 (fol. 18[a]): וברוב הם צומחות באמצע זמן הגדול והוא אחר היותו רואה קרי עד שיגיע אל העמידה כי העמידה קרובה משלשים שנה ועל כן נקראות שני החלומות. → NM 4:147.
‣ III. **staying:** Arab. مكث · Maimonides, *K. al-fuṣūl fī al-ṭibb* · trans. Zeraḥyah Ḥen (*Sefer ha-Peraqim*), 9.97: חוליי פי הטבעת קשים להתרפא מפני ד׳ סבות והם ריבוי הרגש האבר והיותו מקום שיריקו בו המותרות נושכות ומיעוט עמידת הרפואה בו ומפני היות מזגו חם ולח. → NM 1:176.

[עמל] • *Nitpa'el* **נִתְעַמֵּל** · **to suffer from pain:** Arab. تعب / Gr. πονέω · Hippocrates, *Aphorisms* · trans. Nathan ha-Me'ati, 4.33 (170) (fol. 68[b]): אמר אבוקרט: ואם יהיה ג״כ כבר קדם ונתעמל אבר מן האברים קודם שיחלה בעליו הנה באבר ההוא יקבע החולי. → NM 3:176.

עָמָל · **pain:** Lat. labor / Arab. وجع · Hippocrates, *Aphorisms* · trans. Hillel ben Samuel, 2.1 (53) (fol. 7[b]): אמר אפוקרט: איזה מדוה שהשינה עושה עמל אות מות. → NM 3:177.

• **בלי עמל** · **spontaneous:** Gr. αὐτόματος · Hippocrates, *Aphorisms* · trans. Joseph Delmedigo, 2.5 (57): בלי עמל יגיעה מבשרת חלי. → NM 3:177.

• **בעלי העמל** → **בַּעַל**.

עֹמֶק • **העומק אשר בעליון אחורי הצואר** · **the nape of the neck:** Arab. نقرة / Lat. fovea nuchae · Ibn al-Jazzār, *Zād al-musāfir wa-qūt al-ḥādir* · trans. Moses ibn Tibbon (*Sefer Ṣedat ha-Derakhim*), bk. 1, ch. 10 (fol. 14[b]): ואם היה חלוש ולא תהיה בו קדחת נשים לו כוסות המציצה בחיצון כל אחד משוקיו גבוה טפח מן העקב או נשים כוסות המציצה בעומק אשר בעליון אחורי הצואר. → NM 4:147.

עמקי · **[growing] in the plains:** Arab. سهلي · Al-Zahrāwī, *K. al-taṣrīf li-man ʿağiza ʿan at-taʾlīf* · trans. Shem Tov ben Isaac (*Sefer ha-Shimmush*), fol. 135[a], col. b: האספרגוס שני מינים: עמקי והררי. → NM 4:148.

עֵנָב • *Plur.* **ענבים** · **berries:** Arab. حبّ · Al-Zahrāwī, *K. al-taṣrīf li-man ʿağiza ʿan at-taʾlīf* · trans. Shem Tov ben Isaac (*Sefer ha-Shimmush*), bk. 27, fol. 139[a]. col. b: עינבי ההדס הקרירות והיבישות גוברים עליהם. → NM 4:148.

• **תירוש ענבים קרוש בבשול** → **תִּירוֹשׁ**.

עִנְבִּי • **הענבית** · **the grapelike [tunic]:** Arab. العنبية / Lat. uveon · Ibn al-Jazzār, *Zād al-musāfir wa-qūt al-ḥādir* · trans. Moses ibn Tibbon (*Sefer Ṣedat ha-Derakhim*), bk. 2, ch. 6 (fol. 45[b]): ואם יהיה החולי מפני לחות עבה עומדת בין הכפורית והענבית ראוי שנצוה החולה להקיז הגיד העליון ויוציא מן הדם בשעור הצורך והכח. → NM 4:148.

• **הגלד הענבי** → **גֶּלֶד**.

[ענג] • *Part. Puʿal* **מְעֻנָּג** · I. **adolescent:** Arab. راهق · Ibn al-Jazzār, *Zād al-musāfir wa-qūt al-ḥādir* · trans. Moses ibn Tibbon (*Sefer Ṣedat ha-Derakhim*), bk. 1, ch. 6 (fol. 11[a]): ויעשה מאילו הטיחות מהם תאר טיחה מועלה בע״ה מן המוגלא והנגעים שיהיו בראש וכל שכן במעונגים והבחורים והוא מנוסה. → NM 4:148.

· II. **soft:** Lat. delicatus · Bruno Longobucco, *Cyrurgia Magna* · trans. Hillel ben Samuel (*Sefer Keritut*), 11[a]: וזכור כי כאשר יהיה האבר יותר נכבד ויותר מעונג כפי זה צריך שיתחברו חלקיו בעונג. → NM 1:30.

[ענה] • *Inf. Hitpaʿel* **הִתְעַנּוֹת** · **fasting:** Lat. ieiunium · Hippocrates, *Aphorisms* · trans. Hillel ben Samuel, 1.13 (40) (fol. 4[b]): א״א: הזקנים בקלות יוכלו להתענות ואחריהם הבחורים ופחות מהם הנערים ופחות מכלם הקטנים. → NM 3:177.

עָנָה · **to attack:** Arab. ناب · Maimonides, *K. al-fuṣūl fī al-ṭibb* · trans. Zeraḥyah Ḥen (*Sefer ha-Peraqim*), 25.24: אמר משה: המובן ממאמרו הראשון הוא שהליחה המתעפשת תחלה תהיה בתוך העורקים. וזמן המנוחה הוא הזמן אשר בין עיפוש חלק מזה הדבר ובין עיפוש מה שסמוך לו כמו שהומשל באשפה ותהיה הקדחת תענה והליחה מתעפשת בתוך העורקים כמו שאמר. → NM 1:176–7.

• *Part.* **עוֹנֶה** • **הקדחת העונה בכל יום** → **קַדַּחַת**.

עִיּוּן · **observation:** Arab. مباشرة · Maimonides, *Šarḥ fuṣūl Abūqrāṭ* · trans. Zeraḥyah Ḥen (*Pirqei Abuqraṭ*), 1.7 (21): ועל כן יצטרך להרגל ארוך בעניין הסימנים בכל אחת ואחת מהם ואז נוכל לדון במה שיתחדש בעיון טוב יהיה קרוב מן האמת. → NM 3:177.

עָנָן · **cloud in the eye; mist over the eyes:** Arab. ضبابة / Gr. νεφέλη · Ibn al-Jazzār, *Zād al-musāfir wa-qūt al-ḥāḍir* · trans. Moses ibn Tibbon (*Sefer Ṣedat ha-Derakhim*), bk. 2, ch. 6, fol. 46[b]: תאר עגולים טובים מועילים מן הענן והדמע והאכול ויובש העפעפים מסבות עשנים ברכומיים. → NM 4:148–9.

עִסּוּי · I. **evacuation; extraction:** Arab. عَصْر · Ibn Sīnā, *K. al-Qānūn fī al-ṭibb* · trans. Nathan ha-Me'ati (*Sefer ha-Qanun*), bk. 1 (fol. 52[a]): אמנם הבטן הנה עצליו שמנה ישתתפו בתועלות ומהם העזרה על עסוי איזה מה בקרבים מן היציאה והשתן. → NM 4:149.

· II. **tenesmus:** Arab. زحير · Hippocrates, *Aphorisms* · trans. Nathan ha-Me'ati, 7.27 (379) (fol. 132[a]): אמר אבוקרט: כשיתחדש במעוברות עסוי הנקר' זחיר יהיה סבה שתפיל. → NM 3:177.

עָסִיס · **rob (i.e., fruit juice boiled down to syrup):** Arab. رُبّ · Al-Zahrāwī, *K. al-taṣrīf li-man ʿağiza ʿan at-taʾlīf* · trans. Shem Tov ben Isaac (*Sefer ha-Shimmush*), bk. 27, fol. 132, col. b: ואחר להרגיל אחד מן העסיסים החמוצים אם הוא בעל מזג חם. → NM 4:149.

[עסק] • *Part. Nifʿal* **נֶעֱסָק** · **being treated (for an illness):** Hippocrates, *Aphorisms* · trans. Judah Shalom, 6.38 (330) (fol. 105[a]): באשר בו סרטן נסתר הוא יותר טוב שלא להתעסק כי הנעסקים ימותו יותר מהר והבלתי נעסקים נשארים זמן רב. → NM 3:178.

• *Hitpaʿel* **הִתְעַסֵּק** · **to be treated (for an illness):** Hippocrates, *Aphorisms* · trans. Judah Shalom, 6.38 (330) (fol. 105[a]): באשר בו סרטן נסתר הוא יותר טוב שלא להתעסק כי הנעסקים ימותו יותר מהר והבלתי נעסקים נשארים זמן רב. → NM 3:178.

עֲפִיצוּת · I. **acridity; bitterness:** Lat. pontificas · Ibn Sīnā, *K. al-adwiya al-qalbiya* · trans. Anonymous (*Sefer ha-Refuʾot ha-Libbiyot*), fol. 250[a]: מיראבולמש קיבולש ואינדיש קרים בראשונה ויבשים בשניה ולהם עפיצות שמורה על שיש לו קביצות עצמי. → NM 4:149.

· II. **astringency:** Lat. stipticitas · Ibn Sīnā, *K. al-adwiya al-qalbiya* · trans. Anonymous (*Sefer ha-Refuʾot ha-Libbiyot*), fol. 249[a]: ועם זה יש בו דקות והנה ניאות ברוח לריחניותו ועפיצותו. → NM 4:149.

עַפְעַף • *Plur.* **עפעפים** • **התפשט העפעפים** → **פָּשַׁט**.

עֲפִיצִי · **astringent:** Lat. stipticus · Ibn Sīnā, *K. al-adwiya al-qalbiya* · trans. Anonymous (*Sefer ha-Refuʾot ha-Libbiyot*), fols. 247[a–b]: אבל אותם שאומרים שהוא קר מתחלפים ג״כ שקצתם מניחים קרירותו בראשונה וקצתם בשניה אבל ידמה שהוא בסוף הראשונה ויובשו בשנית מפני זה הוא מהרפואות העפציות. → NM 4:149–50.

עָפָר • **עפר ספרד** · **Cimolian earth:** Arab. قيموليا · Ibn al-Jazzār, *Zād al-musāfir wa-qūt al-ḥāḍir* · trans. Moses ibn Tibbon (*Sefer Ṣedat ha-Derakhim*), bk. 7, 28.2. → NM 1:72.

[עפש] • *Part. Piʿel* **מְעַפֵּשׁ** • **הסם המעפש** → **סַם**.

עֵץ · **stalk; stem:** Arab. عود · Al-Zahrāwī, *K. al-taṣrīf li-man ʿağiza ʿan at-taʾlīf* · trans. Shem Tov ben Isaac (*Sefer ha-Shimmush*), bk. 27, fol. 127[a], col. b: ולתבל הבשר בכוסבר הלח ובצלים ועץ של שבת ושרשי כרשין וכשיצטמקו העדשים לשפוך מימיהם ולרחצם במים אחרים חמים. → NM 4:150.

עָצָב • העצב החוזר · **recurrent laryngeal nerve**: Arab. العصب الراجع · Ibn Sīnā, *K. al-Qānūn fī al-ṭibb* · trans. Zeraḥyah Ḥen (*Sefer ha-Qanun*), bk. 1 (fol. 30[b]): ועל כן נקרא העצב החוזר. → NM 4:150.

• **העצב החוזר למפרע** · **recurrent laryngeal nerve**: Arab. العصب الراجع · Ibn Sīnā, *K. al-Qānūn fī al-ṭibb* · trans. Nathan ha-Me'ati (*Sefer ha-Qanun*), bk. 1 (fol. 58[a]): ולכן נקר׳ העצב החוזר למפרע. → NM 4:151.

• **העצב אשר בו ילך השמע** · **the acoustic (auditory) nerve**: Arab. العصب الذي يجري فيه السمع · Ibn al-Jazzār, *Zād al-musāfir wa-qūt al-ḥādir* · trans. Moses ibn Tibbon (*Sefer Ṣedat ha-Derakhim*), bk. 2, ch. 7 (fol. 47[b]): ואם לא נראה דבר מזה וראינו נקב האזן בריא אין בו נזק ידענו כי העצב אשר בו ילך השמע כואב ואם היה כאב העצב השומע מפני מותר עב קר דבק או מפני רוח עבה או מורסא קרה ... אז ראוי לשלשל המותרות ההם. → NM 4:150.

• **העצב השומע** · **the acoustic (auditory) nerve**: Arab. العصبة السامعة · Ibn al-Jazzār, *Zād al-musāfir wa-qūt al-ḥādir* · trans. Moses ibn Tibbon (*Sefer Ṣedat ha-Derakhim*), bk. 2, ch. 7 (fol. 47[b]): ואם לא נראה דבר מזה וראינו נקב האזן בריא אין בו נזק ידענו כי העצב אשר בו ילך השמע כואב ואם היה כאב העצב השומע מפני מותר עב קר דבק או מפני רוח עבה או מורסא קרה ... אז ראוי לשלשל המותרות ההם. → NM 4:151.

• *Plur.* **עצבים • העצבים העגזיים** · **nerves of the sacrum; sacral nerves**: Arab. العصب العجزي · Ibn Sīnā, *K. al-Qānūn fī al-ṭibb* · trans. Nathan ha-Me'ati (*Sefer ha-Qanun*), bk. 1 (fol. 60[a]): הזוג הראשון מן העגזיים מתערב בקטניים כפי האמור. → NM 4:151.

• **העצבים הקטניים** · **nerves of the coccyx**: Arab. العصب القطني · Ibn Sīnā, *K. al-Qānūn fī al-ṭibb* · trans. Nathan ha-Me'ati (*Sefer ha-Qanun*), bk. 1 (fol. 60[a]): הזוג הראשון מן העגזיים מתערב בקטניים כפי האמור. → NM 4:151.

• **העצבים התנועיים** · **motor nerves**: Arab. الأعصاب الحركية · Ibn Sīnā, *K. al-Qānūn fī al-ṭibb* · trans. Nathan ha-Me'ati (*Sefer ha-Qanun*), bk. 1 (fol. 56[a]): ואמנם ⟨העצבים⟩ התנועיים הנה מגיעים אל המכוון. → NM 4:222.

עצביות · **having the property of a membrane, nerve**: Arab. عصبانية · Ibn Sīnā, *K. al-Qānūn fī al-ṭibb* · trans. Nathan ha-Me'ati (*Sefer ha-Qanun*), bk. 1 (fol. 50[a]): והאחר יותר קצר ממנו ופתיליו אל ההתרחבות וקצהו יותר חזק העצביות. → NM 4:151.

עָצָה · **coccyx**: Arab. عصعص · Al-Zahrāwī, *K. al-taṣrīf li-man ʿağiza ʿan at-taʾlīf* · trans. Shem Tov ben Isaac (*Sefer ha-Shimmush*), bk. 30, 2.96 (fol. 230[b]): והרבידא האחת הנתנת על העצה תועיל מטחורי פי הטבעת ומן השחין השפל ר״ל מן השחין אשר יהיה בירכים ולמטה. → NM 1:106.

עִצּוּם · I. **bearing down (i.e., contracting the abdominal muscles)**: Arab. تَزَحُّر · Al-Zahrāwī, *K. al-taṣrīf li-man ʿağiza ʿan at-taʾlīf* · trans. Shem Tov ben Isaac (*Sefer ha-Shimmush*), bk. 30, 2.75 (fol. 221[b]): ואם לא יצא העובר תקח רגליה ביחד ותנענעם בחזקה ואחר כך תסחוט למעלה מן החלציים מעט מעט עד שיעלה העובר למעלה ואחר תכניס המילדת ידה ותשוה העובר מעט מעט ותצוה האשה שתרגיל העיצום עד שיצא. → NM 1:107.

· II. **intestinal illness**: Arab. سَحْج / Gr. κοιλιακός · Al-Rāzī, *K. al-Manṣūrī* · trans. Shem Tov ben Isaac (*Sefer Almansur*), Bet 13 (20): בזרקטונא ובלעז שליום וכשישתה באישרוב גלאבי תכבה החום ותשקיט הלהבה ותרכך החזה ותועיל מן העיצום אשר יהיה במעים. → NM 2:16.

‣ III. **tenesmus:** Arab. زحير / Gr. τεινεσμός · Al-Zahrāwī, *K. al-taṣrīf li-man ʿağiza ʿan at-taʾlīf* · trans. Shem Tov ben Isaac (*Sefer ha-Shimmush*), bk. 27, fol. 146[b], col. a: חלב הבקר יותר עב מכל החלבים ויותר רחוק מן העכול והירידה ויותר כבד על האסטומ׳ ושלשולו הבטן יותר מועט אלא שהוא זן יותר מכל החלבים ועל כן חלבם מועיל מן השלשול המררי והעיצום הכרכומי. → NM 4:152.

• **העיצום וההפשטה** ‣ **intestinal abrasion:** Arab. سحوج الأمعاء / Gr. ἀπόσυρμα · Al-Zahrāwī, *K. al-taṣrīf li-man ʿağiza ʿan at-taʾlīf* · trans. Shem Tov ben Isaac (*Sefer ha-Shimmush*), bk. 27, fol. 125[a], col. b: הארז אמר אסחק כי הארז חם בתחלת המעלה הראשונה ואמר זולתו כי הוא קרוב מן השווי. והלחם העשוי ממנו יזון פחות מלחם החטה ויותר מתאחר להתעכל ועוצר המעים ומועיל מן העיצום וההפשטה ומן השחין המתהוה בהם. → NM 4:152.

עָצוּר (*Pass. Part.*) → **עָצַר**.

עִצּוּר ‣ I. **constipation:** Lat. constipatio · Al-Rāzī, attr., *On the Treatment of Small Children* · trans. Anonymous, 13: ואולי תקרה לקצת מהם קדחת וזחילת הבטן או עיצור. → NM 2:179.

‣ II. **cramps:** Arab. مغص · Ibn al-Jazzār, *Zād al-musāfir wa-qūt al-ḥādir* · trans. Moses ibn Tibbon (*Sefer Ṣedat ha-Derakhim*), bk. 7, 10.1: הנה יקרה למי שנשכו אפעה בתחלת הענין שישוב מראהו לבן ויתנפח ממנו מקום הנשיכה והנה גבה הנפח הרבה ויעשה המקום אבעבועות עד שיהיה דומה לשרפת אש ויקרה לו עלוף רב וסבוב וזיעה קרה ועוצר השתן ועצור ויקיא מרה כרכומית ואם לא ימהרו ברפואתו יגיע הארס אל הלב וימות. → NM 1:64.

‣ III. **pressure:** Arab. عصر · Ibn al-Jazzār, *Zād al-musāfir wa-qūt al-ḥādir* · trans. Moses ibn Tibbon (*Sefer Ṣedat ha-Derakhim*), bk. 7, 9.2: וכאשר הגיע אל האסטו׳ וקרה ממנו צער ודיות זיעה הוא רמויילאר עם קיא ונפח ושנוי מראה ופלצות ושרפה ועצור בפי האסטו׳ ומחשך הראות הנה אז ראוי למהרו ברפואה ואם לא ימות מהר. → NM 1:64.

• **עיצור הבטן** ‣ **constipation:** Hippocrates, *Aphorisms* · trans. Do'eg ha-Edomi (*Sefer Agur*), 3.5 (111) (fol. 50[b]): בתגבורת רוח צפונית יחול כאב הגרון ושעול ועצור הבטן וכאב הצלעות וקדחת באה עם קרירות. → NM 3:178–9.

• **עיצור המעים** ‣ **constipation:** Arab. حبس البطن · Al-Zahrāwī, *K. al-taṣrīf li-man ʿağiza ʿan at-taʾlīf* · trans. Shem Tov ben Isaac (*Sefer ha-Shimmush*), bk. 27, fol. 142[a], col. b: ותקונם ודחית נזקם לרוצה לתתם עוזרים לעצור המעים מבלי נזק לקלותם או לצלותם על האפר החם. → NM 4:152.

• **עיצור השתן** ‣ **dysuria:** Arab. عسر البول · Hippocrates, *Aphorisms* · trans. Do'eg ha-Edomi (*Sefer Agur*), 6.36 (328) (fol. 104[b]): כי תקיז דם מן המקורות הפנימיים ההקזה ההיא תרחיב עיצור השתן. → NM 3:179.

עֲצִירָה ‣ I. **binding:** Arab. حبس · Maimonides, *K. al-fuṣūl fī al-ṭibb* · trans. Nathan ha-Me'ati (*Sefer ha-Peraqim*), 13.28: השלשול אם יקובל תועלת בו אין ראוי שיפסק ואפילו במאכל אשר יש עמו כח מועט מעצירה וכל שכן הרפואות העוצרות כי אם יפסק תשוב הליחה הרעה למעלה ותוליד קדחת או מורסא בכבד ברוב או בשאר האברים. → NM 2:72.

‣ II. **constipation:** Lat. constipatio · Al-Rāzī, attr., *On the Treatment of Small Children* · trans. Bonfos, ch. 12: ואם יקרה להם שלשול הבטן יתרפא עם המשיחה אשר נאמר אחר זה וככה תעשה מהעצירה. → NM 2:72.

• **אופן העצירה** → אֹפֶן.

• **עצירת הבטן** ‣ **constipation**: Arab. احتباس الطبع · Maimonides, *K. al-fuṣūl fī al-ṭibb* · trans. Zeraḥyah Ḥen (*Sefer ha-Peraqim*), 8.27: ועצירת הבטן יעורר כל כאב מהליחות הגסות ויחליש כח הטבע ויפסיד הפעולות הנפשיות ויקרה ממנו התרדמה הכבדה והפסד הדעת. → NM 1:177.

• **עצירת השתן** ‣ **dysuria**: Arab. عسر البول / Gr. δυσουρία · Maimonides, *Šarḥ fuṣūl Abūqrāṭ* · trans. Moses ibn Tibbon (*Pirqei Abuqraṭ*), 3.5 (111): ואולם הרוח הצפוני יחדש שעול וכאב הגרון ויובש הבטן ועצירת השתן והפלצות וכאב בצלעות והחזה. → NM 3:179.

עָצָל • **העצל הישר מעצלי הבטן** ‣ **the rectus abdominis muscle**: Arab. العضل المستقيم من عضل البطن · Ibn Sīnā, *K. al-Qānūn fī al-ṭibb* · trans. Nathan ha-Me'ati (*Sefer ha-Qanun*), bk. 1 (fols. 48[b]–49[a]): ומזה זוג אצל קצוותיהם ומתדבק באמצע החזה מה שבין השחוס הנקר׳ אלחנגרי והתרקווה ומתדבק לעצל הישר מעצלי הבטן. → NM 4:153.

• **העצל המחזיר לאחור** ‣ **rotator muscles**: Arab. العضل المدير · Ibn Sīnā, K. al-Qānūn fī al-ṭibb · trans. Joseph Lorki (*Sefer ha-Qanun*), bk. 1 (fol. 16[a]): היותר גדולים בעצלי הירך הם המותחים אותו אח״כ אשר יקבצנו ... ואחריה העצל המרחיק ואחריו המקרב ואחריו המחזיר לאחור. → NM 4:153.

• **העצל המסבב** ‣ **rotator muscles**: Arab. العضل المدير · Ibn Sīnā, K. al-Qānūn fī al-ṭibb · trans. Nathan ha-Me'ati (*Sefer ha-Qanun*), bk. 1 (fol. 53[a]): הגדול שבעצלי פחד הירך הוא אותו אשר יפשיטהו ואחריו אותו אשר יקבצהו ... ואחריו העצל המרחיק ואחריו העצל המקרב ואחר העצל המסבב. → NM 4:153.

• **העצל המקרב** ‣ **adductor muscles**: Arab. العضل المقرب · Ibn Sīnā, K. al-Qānūn fī al-ṭibb · trans. Nathan ha-Me'ati (*Sefer ha-Qanun*), bk. 1 (fol. 53[a]): הגדול שבעצלי פחד הירך הוא אותו אשר יפשיטהו ואחריו אותו אשר יקבצהו ... ואחריו העצל המרחיק ואחריו העצל המקרב ואחר העצל המסבב. → NM 4:153.

• **העצל המרחיק** ‣ **abductor muscles**: Arab. العضل المبعد · Ibn Sīnā, K. al-Qānūn fī al-ṭibb · trans. Nathan ha-Me'ati (*Sefer ha-Qanun*), bk. 1 (fol. 53[a]): גדול שבעצלי פחד הירך הוא אותו אשר יפשיטהו ואחריו אותו אשר יקבצהו ... ואחריו העצל המרחיק ואחריו העצל המקרב ואחר העצל המסבב. → NM 4:153.

עַצְלָה ‣ I. **amentia**: Arab. بلادة · Ibn Sīnā, *K. al-adwiya al-qalbiya* · trans. Anonymous (*Sammim Libbiyim*), fol. 128[b]: כנדר: לבונה אליבנום חם בשניה יבש בראשונה מחזק הרוח אשר בלב ואשר במוח ולזה הוא מועיל מן העצלה והשכחה. → NM 4:153–4.

‣ II. **fatigue; weariness**: Arab. كلال · Ibn Sīnā, *K. al-adwiya al-qalbiya* · trans. Anonymous (*Sammim Libbiyim*), fol. 130[a]: נינופר: הוא קרוב במשפטו מן הכאמפור אלא שהוא יותר לח ולחותו תחדש ברוח אשר במוח עצלה ורפיון. → NM 4:154.

‣ III. **flabbiness**: Arab. رهل · Ibn al-Jazzār, *Zād al-musāfir wa-qūt al-ḥāḍir* · trans. Moses ibn Tibbon (*Sefer Ṣedat ha-Derakhim*), bk. 7, 15.2: והמורסא המתחדשת מליחה לבנה תקרא מורסא רפה ואותותיו לובן ורפיון וישאר מקום נעיצת האצבע עמוק ואין כאב עמו אבל לחות ועצלה. → NM 1:64.

[עצם] • *Hitpa'el* **הִתְעַצֵּם** ‣ **to bear down (i.e., to push, to contract the abdominal muscles and diaphragm during childbirth)**: Arab. تزحّر · Al-Zahrāwī, *K. al-taṣrīf li-*

man ʿağiza ʿan at-taʾlīf · trans. Shem Tov ben Isaac (*Sefer ha-Shimmush*), bk. 30, 2.75 (fol. 221b): ואחר כך תצוה שתתעצם ותעטישנה בחנינא כי העובר יצא. → NM 1:107.

עֶצֶם · consistency: Arab. قوام · Maimonides, *K. al-fuṣūl fī al-ṭibb* · trans. Nathan ha-Me'ati (*Sefer ha-Peraqim*), 5.12: וכשיהיה השתן דשן ומראהו ועצמו כמראה השמן הנה זה רע ממית. → NM 2:72.

• **עצם אבניי** · (lit., stony bone); the petrous part of the temporal bone: Arab. عظم حجري · Ibn Sīnā, *K. al-Qānūn fī al-ṭibb* · trans. Nathan ha-Me'ati (*Sefer ha-Qanun*), bk. 1 (fol. 57b): וגם המוצא אשר יש לו בעצם אבניי קשה סובל נקבים רבים. → NM 4:154.

• **העצם שעל האמה** · the hip bones; the pubic bones: Arab. إعظام العانة / Lat. ossa innominata; ossa pubis · Ibn Sīnā, *K. al-Qānūn fī al-ṭibb* · trans. Zeraḥyah Ḥen (*Sefer ha-Qanun*), bk. 1, ch. 25 (fol. 22a): הפרק הכ"ה בניתוח העצם שעל האמה. → NM 4:157.

• **בדק עצמו** → בָּדַק.

• **העצם הדומה ללמד בכתיבת היוונים** · the bone resembling the letter L in the Greek alphabet (i.e., the hyoid bone): Arab. العظم الشبيه اللام في كتابة اليونانيين · Ibn Sīnā, *K. al-Qānūn fī al-ṭibb* · trans. Nathan ha-Me'ati (*Sefer ha-Qanun*), bk. 1 (fol. 42b): הנה כל העצמות אם מנית אותם יהיו רמ"ח לבד השומשמניים ובלעדי העצם הדומה ללמד בכתיבת היוונים. → NM 4:154.

• **עצם דומה לעצמות הקוביא** · cuboid bone: Arab. نردي · Ibn Sīnā, *K. al-Qānūn fī al-ṭibb* · trans. Zeraḥyah Ḥen (*Sefer ha-Qanun*), bk. 1 (fol. 23a): ואחד מהם עצם דומה לעצמות הקוביא והוא עשוי בששה פנים מונחים על הצד החיצון. → NM 4:154.

• **עצם החזה** · sternum: Arab. قصّ · Ibn Sīnā, *K. al-Qānūn fī al-ṭibb* · trans. Zeraḥyah Ḥen (*Sefer ha-Qanun*), bk. 1, ch. 15 (fol. 20b): הפרק הט"ו בניתוח עצם האנצולא והוא עצם החזה. זה העצם הוא מחובר משבעה עצמות ולא מעצם אחד כמו שנודע בו בשאר המקומות מן התועלת. → NM 4:155.

• **עצם החלצים** · ilium: Arab. عظم الخاصرة · Ibn Sīnā, *K. al-Qānūn fī al-ṭibb* · trans. Zeraḥyah Ḥen (*Sefer ha-Qanun*), bk. 1 (fol. 22a): וכל אחד מהם יחלק אל ארבעה חלקים ומה שסמוך לצד חחיצון נקרא בער' אלכרקפה ועצם החלצים. → NM 4:155.

• **עצם הטבעת** · sacrum: Arab. عجز · Ibn Sīnā, *K. al-Qānūn fī al-ṭibb* · trans. Joseph Lorki (*Sefer ha-Qanun*), bk. 1 (fol. 12a): פרק י"א בנתוח עצם הטבעת. → NM 4:155.

• **עצם הכסל** · ilium: Arab. عظم الخاصرة · Ibn Sīnā, *K. al-Qānūn fī al-ṭibb* · trans. Nathan ha-Me'ati (*Sefer ha-Qanun*), bk. 1 (fol. 40a): וכל אחד מהם מתחלק לד' חלקים ואשר יטה לצד החיצונים נקרא אלחרכפא ועצם הכסל. → NM 4:155.

• **עצם הכתף** · scapula: Arab. عظم الكتف · Ibn Sīnā, *K. al-Qānūn fī al-ṭibb* · trans. Nathan ha-Me'ati (*Sefer ha-Qanun*), bk. 1 (fol. 49a): וחמשה עצלים צמיחתם מעצמות הכתף מהם עצל תולדתו מעצם הכתף ומתחבר מה שבין החוצץ והצלע העליון לכתף. → NM 4:155–6.

• **העצם הלמדי** · the hyoid bone: Arab. العظم اللامي · Ibn Sīnā, *K. al-Qānūn fī al-ṭibb* · trans. Nathan ha-Me'ati (*Sefer ha-Qanun*), bk. 1 (fol. 47b): העצלים המניעים הלשון הם תשעה שנים רחבים באים מהתוספות החיציות ומתחברים בצדדיו ושנים ארוכים צמיחתם מעליוני העצם הלמדי. → NM 4:156.

• **עצם מקום שער הרגלים** · hip bone; pubic bone: Arab. عظم العانة · Ibn Sīnā, *K. al-Qānūn fī al-ṭibb* · trans. Joseph Lorki (*Sefer ha-Qanun*), bk. 1 (fol. 18a): ולפי שאין לעצל הצומח מצד

מקום עצם שער הרגלים דרך אל הרגלים מאחורי הגוף ומפנימי הירכים לרוב מה ששם מהעצלים והגידים. → NM 4:156.

• **עצם העגבות** · **loins**: Arab. القطن · Maimonides, *K. al-fuṣūl fī al-ṭibb* · trans. Zeraḥyah Ḥen (*Sefer ha-Peraqim*), 16.5: העצר הוסת ברוב ירדפוהו מקרים רעים או כולם או קצתם ואילו הם כובד הגוף ונפילת תאות המזון ופלצות וכאב על עצם העגבות או הצואר או הקדקוד או הראש או שרשי העינים וקדחות שורפות ושתן במראה מעורב משחרות ואודם ויצא החלב מהשדים. → NM 1:177.

• **העצם העומד למטה מכל השדרה** · **loins**: Arab. القطن · Maimonides, *K. al-fuṣūl fī al-ṭibb* · trans. Zeraḥyah Ḥen (*Sefer ha-Peraqim*), 17.14: ואילו לפי דעתי צריכים להיותם מונעים עצמם מכל דבר שהוא מוליד הזרע ויאכלו מזון ורפואה שתכבה הזרע ויטריחו עליון גופם בשישחקו לכדור הקטון או הגדול או להעתיק האבנים וימשח העצם העומד למטה מכל השדרה הנקרא קוטון אחר צאתו מבית המרחץ במשיחות מקררות. → NM 1:177–8.

• **עצם העמוד** · **trochanter**: Arab. طروخانطير / Gr. τροχαντῆρ · Ibn Sīnā, *K. al-Qānūn fī al-ṭibb* · trans. Joseph Lorki (*Sefer ha-Qanun*), bk. 1 (fol. 16ᵃ): ומהם עצל תולדתו בכל שטח עצם עצמות הכסלים ויתדבק בעליון עצם העמוד הגדול. → NM 4:156.

• **עצם הערוה** · I. **lower abdomen**: Lat. pecten / Arab. ثنّة · Hippocrates, *Aphorisms* · trans. Hillel ben Samuel, 2.35 (87) (fol. 13ᵃ): א״א: בכל החלאים שיהיה מה שסמוך לטבור ולעצם הערוה עבים הוא טוב. → NM 3:180.

· II. **pubes**: Lat. pecten / Arab. عانة · Hippocrates, *Aphorisms* · trans. Hillel ben Samuel, 4.80 (217) (fol. 29ᵇ): ואותם שמשתינים דם עב ויש להם שטרנגוריאה רבה להם כאב בעצם הערוה ושפל הבטן מורה על חלי קרוב לשלפוחית. → NM 3:180.

• **העצם הרחב** · **sacrum**: Arab. العظم العريض · Ibn Sīnā, *K. al-Qānūn fī al-ṭibb* · trans. Nathan ha-Me'ati (*Sefer ha-Qanun*), bk. 1 (fol. 53ᵇ): ואמנם מטים לחוץ הם שני עצלים אחד מהן בא מן ⟨העצם⟩ הרחב. → NM 4:156–7.

• **העצם השוה** · **navicular or scaphoid bone**: Arab. الزورقي · Ibn Sīnā, *K. al-Qānūn fī al-ṭibb* · trans. Joseph Lorki (*Sefer ha-Qanun*), bk. 1 (fol. 13ᵇ): ועצמות כף הרגל כ״ו ... והעצם השוה ובו חלל הרגל הנקרא אכמץ. → NM 4:157.

• **העצם השפל** · **ulna**: Arab. الزند الأسفل · Ibn Sīnā, *K. al-Qānūn fī al-ṭibb* · trans. Zeraḥyah Ḥen (*Sefer ha-Qanun*), bk. 1 (fol. 21ᵃ): ואמנם פרק היד הוא מחובר מפרק הזינד העליון והוא העצם הסמוך לעצם השפל שניהם מחוברים יחד. → NM 4:157.

• **עצם תרדי** · **cuboid bone**: Arab. عظم نردي · Ibn Sīnā, *K. al-Qānūn fī al-ṭibb* · trans. Nathan ha-Me'ati (*Sefer ha-Qanun*), bk. 1 (fol. 41ᵇ): ואחד מהם ע⟨צ⟩ם תרדי כמשושה מונח על הצד החיצוני. → NM 4:157.

• *Plur.*[1] **עצמים** • **העצמים הספוגיים** · **ethmoid bones**: Arab. العظام المتخلخلة · Al-Zahrāwī, *K. al-taṣrīf li-man ʿağiza ʿan at-taʾlīf* · trans. Shem Tov ben Isaac (*Sefer ha-Shimmush*), bk. 30, 2.24 (fol. 212ᵇ): ואם לא יעבור הלחות על מה שראוי בידוע שבתוכו בשר מת בעליון העצמים הספוגיים לא השיגו הכלי לחתכו. → NM 1:107.

• *Plur.*[2] **עצמות** • **עצמות גב הערוה** · **the hip bones; the pubic bones**: Arab. إعظام العانة / Lat. ossa innominata; ossa pubis · Ibn Sīnā, *K. al-Qānūn fī al-ṭibb* · trans. Nathan ha-Me'ati (*Sefer ha-Qanun*), bk. 1, ch. 25 (fol. 40ᵃ): הפרק עשרים וחמש בנתוח עצמות גב הערוה. → NM 4:157–8.

• כאב קשרי העצמות → כְּאֵב.

• מחלת הדבקים וקשרי העצמות → מַחֲלָה.

• מחלת קשרי העצמות → מַחֲלָה.

• עצמות קטנים ‣ phalanges: Arab. سلاميات · Ibn Sīnā, *K. al-Qānūn fī al-ṭibb* · trans. Zeraḥyah Ḥen (*Sefer ha-Qanun*), bk. 1 (fol. 22ª): ונדבקו העצמות הקטנים הנקראים בער׳ סולימיית כלם בראשים מחודדים נכנס בהם אותם הראשים וביניהם לחות ויזקוסו. → NM 4:158.

• קשרי העצמות → קֶשֶׁר.

עֹצֶם ‣ largeness; size: Arab. عِظَم / Gr. μέγεθος · Hippocrates, *Aphorisms* · trans. Nathan ha-Me'ati, 2.54 (106) (fol. 40ª): אמר אבוקרט: עוצם הגוף בבחרותו לא תתעבהו אבל תאהבהו אלא שבעת הזקנה יכבד ויקשה עשייתו ויהיה יותר רע מן הגוף אשר הוא יותר חסר ממנו. → NM 3:179–180.

עַצְמוּת ‣ consistency: Arab. قوام · Maimonides, *K. al-fuṣūl fī al-ṭibb* · trans. Zeraḥyah Ḥen (*Sefer ha-Peraqim*), 2.14: ויהיה בעצמותו עובי והיא מתיילדת בגופות החולים לבד. → NM 1:178.

עַצְמִיּוּת ‣ existence: Arab. قوام · Maimonides, *K. al-fuṣūl fī al-ṭibb* · trans. Nathan ha-Me'ati (*Sefer ha-Peraqim*), 7.10: העלוף הוא נפילה יקרה לכחות בחדות ומהירות ועצמיות עצם הכחות וקיומם הוא בשווי הרוחות והליחות והאברים בכמותם ואיכותם. → NM 2:72–3.

עָצַר ‣ I. to be astringent: Arab. قبض · Maimonides, *K. al-fuṣūl fī al-ṭibb* · trans. Zeraḥyah Ḥen (*Sefer ha-Peraqim*), 7.34: סבת שברון השיניים והתפוצצם הוא בעבור חלקותם ומפני זה ראוי שתקשה אותם ותחזקם ברפואה העוצרת. → NM 1:178–9.

‣ II. to bind (tightly): Lat. stringere · Bruno Longobucco, *Cyrurgia Magna* · trans. Hillel ben Samuel (*Sefer Keritut*), fol. 56ᵇ: ואם יהיה השבר קרוב לכתף תעצרהו עמו. → NM 1:35.

‣ III. to be difficult: Arab. عسر · Maimonides, *K. al-fuṣūl fī al-ṭibb* · trans. Zeraḥyah Ḥen (*Sefer ha-Peraqim*), 6.94: ועל כן תהיה חולי השיתוק החזק ממית בהכרח והחלוש יעצור רפואתו כמו שאמר בוקראט. → NM 1:178.

• עצר עצמו מן ‣ to abstain from: Lat. abstinentia · Bruno Longobucco, *Cyrurgia Magna* · trans. Hillel ben Samuel (*Sefer Keritut*), fol. 82ᵇ: וצוה לחולה שיעצור עצמו מן המאכלים הרעים והמולידים אותה. → NM 1:35.

• *Part.* **עוֹצֵר** ‣ astringent; styptic: Lat. stipticus · a) Hippocrates, *Aphorisms* · trans. Hillel ben Samuel, 7.37 (389) (fol. 46ᵇ): א״א: כל דם אשר יקיאהו אדם בלי קדחת אין לירא ממנו וראוי שיתרפא בעוצרים הקרים. → NM 3:181–2.

b) Al-Rāzī, attr., *On the Treatment of Small Children* · trans. Anonymous, ch. 11: מחוליי העינים בנערים יקרה לנערים התחלפות חוליים בעינים ומהם הוא הנפח והסגר העפעפיים ואולי יקרה זה מרפואות עוצרות אשר הנשים משימות על ראשי הנערים. → NM 2:180.

• הכח העוצר → כֹּחַ.

• הסם העוצר → סַם.

• הסם העוצר הדם → סַם.

• הרפואות העוצרות → רְפוּאָה.

• *Pass. Part.* **עָצוּר** • עצור הבטן ‣ he who has constipated bowels: Arab. المعتقل البطن

· Maimonides, *Šarḥ fuṣūl Abūqrāṭ* · trans. Moses ibn Tibbon (*Pirqei Abuqraṭ*), 3.25 (131): ורוב מה שיתחדש הקווץ לשמן ולעצור הבטן לרבוי מותרי גופותם. → NM 3:179.

עֹצֶר • בעוצר · **difficult**: Hippocrates, *Aphorisms* · trans. Do'eg ha-Edomi (*Sefer Agur*), 5.55 (275) (fol. 91[b]): רעת קדחת לאשה הרה וחמום עצום בלא סבה אחרת לאות כי לידתה תהיה בעוצר או תפיל ותקרב למות. → NM 3:180–1.

• עוצר הבטן · **constipation**: a) Lat. ventres duri / Arab. البطون اليابسة · Hippocrates, *Aphorisms* · trans. Hillel ben Samuel, 3.5 (111) (fol. 16[b]): ואם תהיינה צפוניות עושות שעול ונחירות גרון ועוצר הבטן ועוצר השתן ורתת וכאב הצדדים והחזה. → NM 3:181.

b) Arab. احتباس البطن · Maimonides, *K. al-fuṣūl fī al-ṭibb* · trans. Zeraḥyah Ḥen (*Sefer ha-Peraqim*), 9.55: תקשה רפואת חולשת פי האסטומכה ומהירות הקרבונקלי עם עוצר הבטן כי מה שיתיר הבטן יביא הקרבונקלי ויהפך הנפש ואשר יחזק פי האסטומכה יעצור הבטן. → NM 1:178.

• עוצר הלידה · **difficult labor**: Hippocrates, *Aphorisms* · trans. Do'eg ha-Edomi (*Sefer Agur*), 5.35 (255) (fol. 86[b]): ממדוה הרחם או מעוצר הלידה אם יקרה אליה עטוש אות טוב הוא. → NM 3:181.

• עוצר הניפוש · **dyspnea**: Arab. عسر النفس · Maimonides, *K. al-fuṣūl fī al-ṭibb* · trans. Zeraḥyah Ḥen (*Sefer ha-Peraqim*), 23.79: החולי הנקרא צרות הניפוש ועוצר הניפוש בייחוד הוא החולי המתחדש מלחויות עבות דבקות עומדות בחלקי קנה הריאה וזה השם אמנם יפול על זה החולי ביחוד. → NM 1:178.

• עוצר השתן · **dysuria**: Arab. عسر البول / Gr. δυσουρία · Maimonides, *Šarḥ fuṣūl Abūqrāṭ* · trans. Moses ibn Tibbon (*Pirqei Abuqraṭ*), 6.36 (328): אמר אבקראט: הקזת העורק יתיך עוצר השתן וראוי שיחתכו העורקים הפנימיים. → NM 3:181.

עקב · **fibrous tissue; ligament**: Arab. عَقَب / Lat. nervi seu tendines, quibus chordae conficiuntur · Ibn Sīnā, *K. al-Qānūn fī al-ṭibb* · trans. Nathan ha-Me'ati (*Sefer ha-Qanun*), bk. 1 (fol. 42[b]): ודקדק הבורא והצמיח מן העצמות דבר דומה בעצבים נקרא עקבים וקשורים להתחברם עם העצבים ומסתבכים בו כדבר אחד. → NM 4:158.

עָקֵב · **calcaneus**: Arab. عَقِب · Ibn Sīnā, *K. al-Qānūn fī al-ṭibb* · trans. Nathan ha-Me'ati (*Sefer ha-Qanun*), bk. 1 (fol. 41[b]): עצמות כף הרגל ששה ... ועקב בו משען קיום. → NM 4:158.

עִקּוּם • חביט בעיקום → [נבט].

• עקום הפה · **paralysis of the facial nerve**: Arab. لقوة · Ibn al-Jazzār, *Zād al-musāfir wa-qūt al-ḥāḍir* · trans. Moses ibn Tibbon (*Sefer Ṣedat ha-Derakhim*), bk. 1, ch. 23 (fol. 34[a]): והקשה ממנו מה שיחשך בו הדבור ויקרה עמו עקום הפה. → NM 4:158–9.

עֲקִימָה • עקימת הפה · **paralysis of the facial nerve**: Judah ben Jacob, *Sefer Hanhagat ha-Beri'ut*, 8.5: אז ינקה הגוף ממנה בסמים המנקים אותה נפרדים או מורכבים פן תוליד בו בטול כל הגוף או חציו ועקימת הפה. → NM 4:159.

עֲקִיצָה · I. **biting, burning [pain]**: Arab. لذع · Al-Zahrāwī, *K. al-taṣrīf li-man ʿağiza ʿan at-taʾlīf* · trans. Shem Tov ben Isaac (*Sefer ha-Shimmush*), bk. 27, fol. 137[a], col. a: והם משקיטים העקיצה אשר תהיה באסטומכא. → NM 4:159.

· II. **colic**: Arab. مغص / Gr. στρόφος · Maimonides, *Šarḥ fuṣūl Abūqrāṭ* · trans. Zeraḥyah Ḥen (*Pirqei Abuqraṭ*), 5.41 (261): אמר בקראט: אם תרצה לדעת אם האשה הרה או אינה הרה תשקנה כשתרצה לישן מי הדבש ואם מצאה עקיצה בבטנה היא הרה ואם לא מצאה עקיצה אינה הרה. → NM 3:182.

‣ III. **disturbance**: Arab. قلق · Maimonides, *Šarḥ fuṣūl Abūqrāṭ* · trans. Anonymous (*Pirqei Abuqraṭ*), 1.22 (49): אמר המפרש: אמרו הרפואה ר״ל המשלשלת והחולי המתעורר הוא שיהיו הכימוסים עוקצים לחולה והזיקוהו בחום שיהיה להם בחוזק ונזילתם מאבר לאבר בתחלת החולי ויכאיבוהו ויחדשו לו עקיצה ולא יניחוהו לשקוט במקום אחד להיותם מתנועעים ונוזלים מאבר לאבר. → NM 3:182.

• **עקיצה בלב** ‣ **cardialgia**: Gr. καρδιωγμός · Hippocrates, *Aphorisms* · trans. Hillel ben Samuel, 4.17 (154) (fol. 21[b]): א״א: מי שיש לו קדחת ויש לו אסטניסות ועקיצה בלב ואופל העינים ומרירות בפה מורה שצריך אליו שינקהו מלמעלה. → NM 3:182–3.

• **עקיצה בפי האצטומ׳** ‣ **cardialgia**: Arab. نخس في الفؤاد / Gr. καρδιωγμός · Maimonides, *Šarḥ fuṣūl Abūqrāṭ* · trans. Zeraḥyah Ḥen (*Pirqei Abuqraṭ*), 4.17 (154): אמר בקראט: מי שאין בו קדחת והיה בו המנע מן המזון ועקיצה בפי האצטומ׳ וסתימה ומרירות בפה זה יורה על הרקתו ממעלה. → NM 3:183.

עָקַץ • *Part.* **עוֹקֵץ** • **הסם העוקץ** → **סַם**.

עֹקֶץ • **עוקץ החוטם** ‣ **the end of the nose**: Arab. طرف الأنف · Al-Zahrāwī, *K. al-taṣrīf li-man ʿağiza ʿan at-taʾlīf* · trans. Shem Tov ben Isaac (*Sefer ha-Shimmush*), bk. 30, 1.47 (208[a]): אמנם אם הגדמות כבר נתפרסם על החולה ויראה ראיה מבוארת ראוי אז לכוותו אלו הכויות הנזכרות בראש וכויה אחת על עוקץ החוטם. → NM 1:107–8.

עִקָּר ‣ **base; insertion; origin; the place of growth; root**: Arab. مغرز · Ibn Sīnā, *K. al-Qānūn fī al-ṭibb* · trans. Joseph Lorki (*Sefer ha-Qanun*), bk. 1 (fol. 14[a]): ואפשר שיקרב כנגד עקר האזן בקצת אנשים ויתדבק בו ומתחברים בו ויתנועע האזן. → NM 4:159.

• *Plur.* **עקרים** ‣ **origins**: Arab. مبادئ · Maimonides, *Šarḥ fuṣūl Abūqrāṭ* · trans. Moses ibn Tibbon (*Pirqei Abuqraṭ*), 4.49 (186): אמר המפרש: זה מבואר כי כאשר נראו אלו האותות עם חולשת הכח וקדמה הקדחת נודע כי היובש כבר גבר על עקרי העצבים ולכן התחדש העוות או זולתו ממה שזכר. → NM 3:183.

• **עיקרי הירכים** ‣ **groin**: Arab. أربيّة · Al-Zahrāwī, *K. al-taṣrīf li-man ʿağiza ʿan at-taʾlīf* · trans. Shem Tov ben Isaac (*Sefer ha-Shimmush*), bk. 30, 2.65 (fol. 220[a]): לפעמים תקרה הפיתקא בעיקרי הירכים כמו שאמרתי ויבלוט המקום. → NM 1:107.

[ערבב] • *Hitpaʿel* **הִתְעַרְבֵּב** • **התערבב השכל** ‣ **to suffer from mental confusion (delirium)**: Arab. اختلط الذهن · Maimonides, *Šarḥ fuṣūl Abūqrāṭ* · trans. Moses ibn Tibbon (*Pirqei Abuqraṭ*), 7.7 (359): אמר המפרש: התחבר הרתת עם הערבוב מעט שיקרה כי אם בקצת מרבים השכרות ויכבה החום הטבעי ויתחדש הרתת וימלא המוח מדם חם ואיד חם ויתערבב השכל. → NM 3:183.

עִרְבּוּב ‣ **dizziness**: Arab. سدر · Maimonides, *K. al-fuṣūl fī al-ṭibb* · trans. Nathan ha-Meʾati (*Sefer ha-Peraqim*), 25.11: מי שיהיה עלתו כאב ראש או סבובו או ערבובו אז ראוי שיוקז מן הרגל. → NM 2:73.

• **ערבוב שכל** ‣ **delirium**: a) Arab. تخليط · Ibn al-Jazzār, *Zād al-musāfir wa-qūt al-ḥāḍir* · trans. Moses ibn Tibbon (*Sefer Ṣedat ha-Derakhim*), bk. 7, 13.2: והמקרים אשר יקרו למי

שנשכו כלב שוטה אולם בהתחלה יחלום חלומות שאחריתם ערבוב שכל ופעמים יפחד תוך שנתו בעבור דבר שיפחידהו ויקרה לו בעת היקיצה כעס ויגון מבלתי סבה שתכעיסהו ואינו סובל לאדם שיביט אליו וירבה להביט סביבו. → NM 1:65.

b) Arab. اختلاط عقل · Maimonides, *K. al-fuṣūl fī al-ṭibb* · trans. Nathan ha-Me'ati (*Sefer ha-Peraqim*), 23.58: כשיגבר בראש לחות הנקרא מררות יתחדש מזה התעורה וערבוב שכל וכשיגבר בו ליחות עבות לבניות יתחדש מזה עם תרדמה הבהלה והבהלה הוא ערבוב שכל מועט. → NM 2:73–4.

• **הקדחת אשר יהיה עמה ערבוב השכל** → קַדַּחַת.

עֲרְבִי • **קוץ ערבי** → קוֹץ.

עֵרוּב • **עירוב חדם** · dysentery: Arab. اختلاف الدم / Gr. δυσεντερία · Maimonides, *Šarḥ fuṣūl Abūqrāṭ* · trans. Zeraḥyah Ḥen (*Pirqei Abuqraṭ*), 7.23 (375): אמר בקראט: ומהיציאה היחידה עירוב הדם. → NM 3:184.

עֶרְוָה • **בית הערוה** → בַּיִת.

• **גב הערוה** → גַּב.

• **גיד הערוה** → גִּיד.

• **מקום הערוה** → מָקוֹם.

• **עצם הערוה** → עֶצֶם.

• **עצמות גב הערוה** → עֶצֶם.

• **צמוח השיער בבית הערוה** → צָמַח.

• **צמיחת השער בגב הערוה** → צְמִיחָה.

• **צמיחת השער סביב הערוה** → צְמִיחָה.

• **קצה גיד הערוה** → קָצֶה.

• **השער סביב הערוה** → שֵׂעָר.

עָרוּם · malignant: Arab. خبيث · Al-Zahrāwī, *K. al-taṣrīf li-man ʿağiza ʿan at-taʾlīf* · trans. Shem Tov ben Isaac (*Sefer ha-Shimmush*), bk. 27, fol. 143[a], col. a: בשר התיש המוכלח מגונה המזון מוליד דם שחורי ומביא מתמידו אל חליים שחוריים וכל שכן מי שהוא מעותד להם כגון השוטים והנכפים ואל השחין הערום ודומיהם מן החליים הרעים. → NM 4:159–60.

עֲרִיפָה • **עריפת דם החוטם** · nosebleed: Arab. رعاف · Ibn al-Jazzār, *Zād al-musāfir wa-qūt al-ḥādir* · trans. Moses ibn Tibbon (*Sefer Ṣedat ha-Derakhim*), bk. 2, ch. 15 (fol. 55[b]): עריפת דם החוטם פעמים יהיה לטוב ופעמים לרע והמתהוה ממנו למה שהוא טוב כמו עריפת הדם אשר יהיה בקדחת השורפת וחולי מורסת הראש על דרך הנקיון. → NM 4:160.

• **עריפת דם הנחירים** · nosebleed: Arab. رعاف · Ibn al-Jazzār, *Zād al-musāfir wa-qūt al-ḥādir* · trans. Moses ibn Tibbon (*Sefer Ṣedat ha-Derakhim*), bk. 2, ch. 15 (fol. 55[a]): השער החמשה עשר בעריפת דם הנחירים. → NM 4:160.

עִרְעוּר · gargling: Arab. تغرغر · Al-Zahrāwī, *K. al-taṣrīf li-man ʿağiza ʿan at-taʾlīf* · trans. Shem Tov ben Isaac (*Sefer ha-Shimmush*), bk. 27, fol. 136[b], col. a: וערעור הגרון במים שנתבשלו בהם תאינים עוזר על התכת המורסות בקנה הריאה. → NM 4:160.

• *Plur.* **ערעורים** · gargling: Arab. غرغرة · Maimonides, *K. al-fuṣūl fī al-ṭibb* · trans. Nathan ha-Me'ati (*Sefer ha-Peraqim*), 3.87: כשתהיה ליחה חמה יורדת מן הראש אל העין

אז נתחיל בהרקת הגוף כוללת בהקזת העורק או בשלשול הבטן ואחר זה בהרקת הראש ביחוד בערעורים. → NM 2:74.

עַרְעָר · **artichoke** [*Cynara cardunculus* L.]: Arab. حرشف · Al-Zahrāwī, *K. al-taṣrīf li-man ʿağiza ʿan at-taʾlīf* · trans. Shem Tov ben Isaac (*Sefer ha-Shimmush*), bk. 27, fol. 135[b], col. b: הערער וב״ח העכביות יש ממנו שדי ויש ממנו פרדסי והפרדסי הוא הדרדר והשדי הוא הערער האמתי. → NM 4:160–1.

עֹרֶף • **השטיח על ערפו** → שָׁטַח.
• **חלל העורף** → חָלָל.
• **שטוח על ערפו** → שָׁטַח.
• **השטיחה על העורף** → שְׁטִיחָה.

עֲלוּקָה · **leeches**: Arab. علق · Al-Zahrāwī, *K. al-taṣrīf li-man ʿağiza ʿan at-taʾlīf* · trans. Shem Tov ben Isaac (*Sefer ha-Shimmush*), bk. 30, 2.97 (fol. 231[b]): הערקה תורגל ברוב הענינים באברים אשר לא תתכן בהם נתינת הרפידות. → NM 1:108.

עֵשֶׂב • **עשב הזכוכית** · **spreading pellitory** [*Parietaria ramiflora* L.]; **upright pellitory** [*Parietaria officinalis* L.]: Arab. حشيشة الزجاج · Ibn al-Jazzār, *Zād al-musāfir wa-qūt al-ḥādir* · trans. Moses ibn Tibbon (*Sefer Ṣedat ha-Derakhim*), bk. 1, ch. 7 (fol. 12[a]): או שישחק עמו קצת הסמים המנגבים כמו שיקח עשב הזכוכית. → NM 4:161.

עָשָׂה · I. **to apply (medicines)**: Arab. استعمل · Ibn al-Jazzār, *Zād al-musāfir wa-qūt al-ḥādir* · trans. Moses ibn Tibbon (*Sefer Ṣedat ha-Derakhim*), bk. 7, 9.3: והנה זכר גאליה ודיאשקורידוש רפואות יעשו בעת הפחד והיראה וינצל בלקיחתם מנזק הסמים הממיתים. → NM 1:65.

· II. **to consume; to take**: Arab. استعمل · Maimonides, *K. al-fuṣūl fī al-ṭibb* · trans. Zeraḥyah Ḥen (*Sefer ha-Peraqim*), 3.92: שים עינך והשגחתך שלא יתחדש בכבד ובטחול ובכליות קושי וברוב יקרו אילו המורסות הקשות למי שימצאנו מורסא חמה באחד מאילו השלשה אברים ואחר כן יעשה מאכלים שמולידים ליחות גסות או דבקות. → NM 1:179.

· III. **to use**: Arab. استعمل · Maimonides, *K. al-fuṣūl fī al-ṭibb* · trans. Nathan ha-Me'ati (*Sefer ha-Peraqim*), 8.56: ואמנם מי שגופו יבש וכחוש אז אין ראוי שיעשה חקנה. → NM 2:74.

• **עשה הנגע** · **to ulcerate**: Arab. أقرح · Ibn al-Jazzār, *Zād al-musāfir wa-qūt al-ḥādir* · trans. Moses ibn Tibbon (*Sefer Ṣedat ha-Derakhim*), bk. 7, 13.4: ואולם הרפואות אשר יעשו הנגע וירחיבוהו וימשכו הארס ממנו כמו שיקח שום ויכתוש אותו ויושם על המקום. → NM 1:65.

• **עשה ספוגות** · **to loosen**: Arab. خلخل · Maimonides, *Šarḥ fuṣūl Abūqrāṭ* · trans. Moses ibn Tibbon (*Pirqei Abuqraṭ*), 1.1 (23): וכן הפעולות הנמשכות אחר אלו הכוחות הראשונות הם אשר יקראו אותם הרופאים הכחות השניות כמו שיהיה הסם מקשה או מרפה או יעשה ספוגות או יעבה. → NM 3:170.

• **עשה הרפואה** · **to purge**: Arab. استعمل الدواء / Gr. φαρμακεύω · Maimonides, *Šarḥ fuṣūl Abūqrāṭ* · trans. Moses ibn Tibbon (*Pirqei Abuqraṭ*), 1.22 (49): אמר אבקראט: אמנם ראוי לך שתעשה הרפואה וההנעה אחר שיתבשל החולי אבל כל זמן שהוא נא ובתחלת החולי אין ראוי זה אם לא שיהיה החולי מסתער ואי אפשר ברוב הענין שיהיה החולי מסתער. → NM 3:184–5.

• *Inf.* **עשות** • **עשות מוגלא** · **empyema**: Arab. تقيّح / Gr. ἐμπύημα · Maimonides, *Šarḥ fuṣūl Abūqrāṭ* · trans. Moses ibn Tibbon (*Pirqei Abuqraṭ*), 5.8 (228): אמר אבקראט: מי שמצאהו חולי הצד ולא ינקה בארבעה עשר יום הנה יגיע עניינו לעשות מוגלא. → NM 3:184.

• **עשות מי רגלים** · **to pass water**: Arab. بال · Al-Zahrāwī, *K. al-taṣrīf li-man ʿağiza ʿan at-ta'līf* · trans. Shem Tov ben Isaac (*Sefer ha-Shimmush*), bk. 30, 3.18 (fol. 236ᵃ): וכשתרצה לעשות מי רגליה ראוי להסיר הצמר גפן בנחת ולהחזירו על הענין הנזכר. → NM 1:101.

עִשּׁוּן · **bath**: Lat. balneum · Bruno Longobucco, *Cyrurgia Magna* · trans. Hillel ben Samuel (*Sefer Keritut*), fol. 61ᵇ: ואם תרצה תניח עליו חלב מן האנטרי עם חמאה חם במזג וישאהו לפני העשון ואחר העשון. → NM 1:35.

עֲשִׂיָּה · **consumption; intake**: Arab. استعمال · Maimonides, *K. al-fuṣūl fī al-ṭibb* · trans. Nathan ha-Me'ati (*Sefer ha-Peraqim*), 3.91: הכבד והטחול הם האברים היותר מהירים והיותר מעותדים לקבל הקושי כשיִתרשל האדם בהם בעשית המאכלים הדבקים. → NM 2:74.

• **עשיית המוגלא** · **suppuration**: Arab. تقيّح · Maimonides, *Šarḥ fuṣūl Abūqrāṭ* · trans. Moses ibn Tibbon (*Pirqei Abuqraṭ*), 5.65 (285): והרבה פעמים ימצא בעל חולי הצד עשיית המוגלא. → NM 3:185.

• **עשיית הסם** · **purging**: Arab. استعمال الدواء · Maimonides, *Šarḥ fuṣūl Abūqrāṭ* · trans. Anonymous (*Pirqei Abuqraṭ*), 2.36 (89): אמר אבוקרט: מי שהיה גופו בריא עשית הסם בו יקשה. → NM 3:185.

• **עשיית הרפואה** · **purging**: Arab. استعمال الدواء / Gr. φαρμακεύω · Maimonides, *Šarḥ fuṣūl Abūqrāṭ* · trans. Moses ibn Tibbon (*Pirqei Abuqraṭ*), 2.36 (89): אמר אבקראט: מי שהיה גופו בריא הנה עשיית הרפואה בו קשה. → NM 3:185.

עשייה → עֲשִׂיָּה.

[עשן] • *Puʿal* עֻשַּׁן • **עושן במים** · I. **to be fomented**: Lat. fomentor · Bruno Longobucco, *Cyrurgia Magna* · trans. Hillel ben Samuel (*Sefer Keritut*), fol. 61ᵇ: ואם תכבד תנועתו אז יעושן במים חמים. → NM 1:35–6.

· II. **to be soaked in the bath**: Lat. humector in balneo · Bruno Longobucco, *Cyrurgia Magna* · trans. Hillel ben Samuel (*Sefer Keritut*), fol. 61ᵇ: ואם אחרי הבריאות ישאר כובד בתנועתו אז יעושן במים חמים. → NM 1:35.

עשנות · **smokiness**: Arab. دخانية · Al-Zahrāwī, *K. al-taṣrīf li-man ʿağiza ʿan at-ta'līf* · trans. Shem Tov ben Isaac (*Sefer ha-Shimmush*), bk. 27, fol. 147ᵃ, col. b: ותשוב בכלל הדברים החריפים תשתנה באסטומ׳ אל העשנות וסוג המרה הכרכומית ותעצור המעים עצירה חזקה. → NM 4:161.

עֲשָׁנִיּוֹת • **עשניות הדבש** · **honeycomb**: Lat. favositas mellis · Al-Rāzī, attr., *On the Treatment of Small Children* · trans. Bonfos, 1: ועשניות או אידיות הדבש הוא מין ממיני החולי הזה וימתיח על הנגע ותראה כמו קשקשים כי הוא מקשקש העור עם חכוך רב ומעט ממנו הוא כמו הדבש. → NM 2:180.

עֲשָׁשִׁית · **Pleiades**: Arab. ثريّا · Maimonides, *K. al-fuṣūl fī al-ṭibb* · trans. Zeraḥyah Ḥen (*Sefer ha-Peraqim*), 3.18: בעלות הכוכבים הנקראים עששית הוא תחלת הקיץ. → NM 1:179.

עֵת • **העת העומד** · **the current time (i.e., season)**: Arab. الوقت الحاضر · Maimonides, *Šarḥ fuṣūl Abūqrāṭ* · trans. Moses ibn Tibbon (*Pirqei Abuqraṭ*), 1.17 (44): אמר אבקראט: ראוי

שינתן לקצת החולים מזונם בפעם אחת ולקצתם בשתי פעמים וישים מה שיתן לו ממנו יותר או פחות וקצתם מעט מעט וראוי גם כן שינתן לעת העומד מזמני השנה חלקו מזה ולמנהג ולשנים. → NM 3:185–6.

[עתד] • *Part. Puʿal* **מְעֻתָּד** · **predisposed; susceptible**: Arab. مستعدّ · Al-Zahrāwī, *K. al-taṣrīf li-man ʿağiza ʿan at-taʾlīf* · trans. Shem Tov ben Isaac (*Sefer ha-Shimmush*), bk. 27, fol. 143[a], col. a: בשר התיש המוכלח מגונה המזון מוליד דם שחורי ומביא מתמידו אל חליים שחוריים וכל שכן מי שהוא מעותד להם כגון השוטים והנכפים ואל השחין הערום ודומיהם מן החליים הרעים. → NM 4:161–2.

עָתַק • *Part.* **עוֹתֵק** · **intermittent**: Arab. مقلع · Maimonides, *K. al-fuṣūl fī al-ṭibb* · trans. Zeraḥyah Ḥen (*Sefer ha-Peraqim*), 19.37: הזמנים המשובחים בהכנסת המרחץ בכל הקדחות שהם עותקות כשיהיה עובר היותו נכנס במרחץ הוא זמן שתתחיל הקדחת להתיר כי המרחץ אז יכין הגוף מיד ויתקנהו להתפרנס. → NM 1:175–6.

• *Part. Nifʿal* **נֶעֱתָק** · **relapsed**: Galen, *De diebus decretoriis* · trans. Shimshon ben Shlomo (*Qibbuṣei Maʾamarei Galenus bi-Yemei ha-Buḥran*), 3: ואמנם החליים שיארכו אחר ארבעה עשר עד שיגיעו אל הארבעים הנה יוחסו לחדות הנעתק. → NM 2:173.

פ

פַּגּוּת · **crudeness; rawness**: Arab. فجاجة · Maimonides, *Šarḥ fuṣūl Abūqrāṭ* · trans. Zeraḥyah Ḥen (*Pirqei Abuqraṭ*), 4.3 (174): אמר המפרש: חוזק הקדחת תכבה החמימות הטבעי ולא יתבשלו הליחות הקרות מאד אשר בנגלה הגוף אשר מהם תצא הזיעה הקרה וסימן פגות אילו הליחות וחוזק קרירותם היות חום הקדחת החזק לא תוכל לחמם מה שיצא ממנו. → NM 3:186.

פְּגִימָה · **trochlea [of humerus]**: Arab. حزّ · Ibn Sīnā, *K. al-Qānūn fī al-ṭibb* · trans. Nathan ha-Me'ati (*Sefer ha-Qanun*), bk. 1 (fol. 37b): וביניהם בלי ספק פגימה ובשתי קצוות אותה פגימה יש שתי נקרות מלמעלה לקדם ומתחת לאחור. → NM 4:162.

פָּגַשׁ · **to match**: Arab. لحق · Maimonides, *K. al-fuṣūl fī al-ṭibb* · trans. Nathan ha-Me'ati (*Sefer ha-Peraqim*), 16.20: מהירות הגדול בנשים יורה על שיש בהם חום נוסף פגש לחות גופותיהן. → NM 2:74–5.

פדלקון · **clyster**: Arab. محقن · Al-Zahrāwī, *K. al-taṣrīf li-man ʿağiza ʿan at-taʾlīf* · trans. Shem Tov ben Isaac (*Sefer ha-Shimmush*), bk. 30, 2.83 (fol. 223b): ראוי לעשות הפדלקון מכסף או מנחשת נתך. → NM 1:108.

• *Plur.* **פדלקונים** · **enemas**: Arab. حقن · Al-Rāzī, *K. al-Manṣūrī* · trans. Shem Tov ben Isaac (*Sefer Almansur*), Qof 15 (72): קרטאס הוא עלים עשויים מן האגמים לבן: כששורפין אותו יועיל אפרו משפיכת דם ויכנס בפדלקונים. → NM 2:16–7.

[פדלקן] • *Inf. Pi'el* **פדלקן** · **to irrigate**: Arab. حقن · Al-Zahrāwī, *K. al-taṣrīf li-man ʿağiza ʿan at-taʾlīf* · trans. Shem Tov ben Isaac (*Sefer ha-Shimmush*), bk. 30, 2.88 (fol. 226b): ואחר לקחת ממנו כפי הצורך ולטרפו במים ודבש ולפדלקן בו המחבוא. → NM 1:108.

פֶּה • **כבדי הפה** → **כָּבֵד**[2].

• **נגעי הפה** → **נֶגַע**.

• **נטית הפה** → **נְטִיָּה**.

• **נשיכה בפי האצטומכה** → **נְשִׁיכָה**.

• **פי העורב** · **(lit., crow's beak); coracoid process**: Arab. منقار الغراب · Ibn Sīnā, *K. al-Qānūn fī al-ṭibb* · trans. Zeraḥyah Ḥen (*Sefer ha-Qanun*), bk. 1 (fol. 20b): ולה שתי תוספות אחת מהן למעלה ומאחור ויקרא היותר משמש ופי העורב ובה קשרי הכתף עם העצם הנקר׳ קטולא. → NM 4:162.

• **עקום הפה** → **עִקּוּם**.

• **עקימת הפה** → **עִקּוּם**.

• **עקיצה בפי האצטומ׳** → **עֲקִיצָה**.

• **קצה פי הטבעת** → **קָצֶה**.

• **ריח הפה** → **רֵיחַ**.

• **השחין אשר בפה** → **שְׁחִין**.

• **שחיני הפה** → **שְׁחִין**.

• *Plur.* **פיות** • **פיות ורידי הרחם** · **cotyledons**: Lat. cotilidones · Hippocrates, *Aphorisms* · trans. Judah Shalom, 5.45 (265) (fol. 86a): כל מי שיש לה גוף ממוצע מפלת בחדש השני או בשלישי מבלתי סבה נגלית כאלו פיות ורידי הרחם הם מלאים מרירים ולא יוכלו להחזיק העובר בעבור הכבדות אבל ינותקו בקשרים. → NM 3:186–7.

• נפיחת פיות העורקים מלמטה → נְפִיחָה.

• פיות עורקי הרחם · **cotyledons**: Lat. cotilidones · Hippocrates, *Aphorisms* · trans. Hillel ben Samuel, 5.45 (265) (fol. 35ᵃ): א״א: אותן שגופן ממוצע ומפילות בחדש השני או השלישי בלי סבה ידועה הנה הן מלאות בפיות עורקי הרחם מליחות מרריות ולא יוכלו לסבול כובד העובר ונתקים. → NM 3:187.

• התוספות הדומות לפיות השדים → תּוֹסֶפֶת.

פִּהוּק · **eructation**: Arab. جشاء · Hippocrates, *Aphorisms* · trans. Nathan ha-Me'ati, 6.1 (293) (fol. 103ᵇ): אמר אבוקראט: כשיתחדש הפיהוק החמוץ הנקר׳ רוט בעלה הנקראת המעדת המעים אחר התארכו ולא היה בו קודם לכן הוא אות משובח. → NM 3:187.

[פוג] • *Part. Hif'il* מֵפִיג • סם המפיג → סַם.

פּוֹסֵק (*Part.*) → פָּסַק.

פּוּרְנִי (*Aram.*) · **brick oven fuelled with wood, similar to glass-making furnaces**: Arab. فرن / Gr. φοῦρνος · Al-Zahrāwī, *K. al-taṣrīf li-man ʿağiza ʿan at-ta'līf* · trans. Shem Tov ben Isaac (*Sefer ha-Shimmush*), bk. 27, fol. 125ᵃ, col. a: הלחם האפוי בתנור הוא יותר טוב מזה האפוי בפורני למהירות עכולו וצאתו מן האצטומכא. → NM 4:162–3.

• צלי הפורני → צָלִי.

פּוֹשֵׁר (*Part.*) → פָּשַׁר.

פּוֹתֵחַ (*Part.*) → פָּתַח.

[פזר] • *Part. Puʿal* מְפֻזָּר · I. **heterogeneous**: Arab. متشتّت · Maimonides, *Šarḥ fuṣūl Abūqrāṭ* · trans. Zeraḥyah Ḥen (*Pirqei Abuqraṭ*), 7.33 (385): אמר בקראט: מי שיהיה שתנו מפוזר יורה על שבגופו סערה חזקה. → NM 3:136.

· II. **porous**: Lat. rarus · Hippocrates, *Aphorisms* · trans. Hillel ben Samuel, 5.71 (291) (fol. 38ᵃ): א״א: אותם שעור בשרם נמתח ויבש וקשה ימותו מבלי שיזיעו אבל אותם שעורם רפה ומפוזר יתמו חלייהם עם זיעה. → NM 3:136 (corr.).

פָּחַד · **to expect**: Arab. توقّع / Gr. προσδέχομαι · Maimonides, *Šarḥ fuṣūl Abūqrāṭ* · trans. Moses ibn Tibbon (*Pirqei Abuqraṭ*), 3.6 (112): אמר אבקראט: כשיהיה הקייץ דומה לאביב ראוי שתפחד מהתחדש זיעה רבה בקדחות. → NM 3:187–8.

• *Part. Piʿel* מְפַחֵד · **to beware of**: Lat. timeo · Hippocrates, *Aphorisms* · trans. Judah Shalom, 4.6 (144) (fol. 53ᵇ): והקשים להקיא ובשריים הטב באמצעות ⟨ראוי לשלשל⟩ מלמטה ומפחדים בקייץ. → NM 3:188.

פַּחַד¹ · **danger**: Arab. خطر / Gr. σφαλερός · a) Maimonides, *K. al-fuṣūl fī al-ṭibb* · trans. Zeraḥyah Ḥen (*Sefer ha-Peraqim*), 12.38: וכשידוקר הגיד הדופק על רחבו בשני חציו אין בו פחד כי הוא יתקווץ כל אחד משני קצותיו אל הצד אשר הוא בו. → NM 1:179.

b) Maimonides, *Šarḥ fuṣūl Abūqrāṭ* · trans. Zeraḥyah Ḥen (*Pirqei Abuqraṭ*), 1.1 (14): הזמן קצר והמלאכה ארוכה והעת צר והנסיון פחד. → NM 3:188.

• פחד המים · **hydrophobia**: Arab. التفزّع من الماء · Al-Zahrāwī, *K. al-taṣrīf li-man ʿağiza ʿan at-ta'līf* · trans. Shem Tov ben Isaac (*Sefer ha-Shimmush*), bk. 27, fol. 143ᵇ, col. b: בשר הכלב חמימותו מרובה מבשר זכר הבקר ומועטה מבשר האריה ומי שנשכו כלב שוטה מאכילין אותו מכבד כלב צלוי כי הוא מועיל מפחד המים. → NM 4:163.

פַּחַד² · **femur; thigh**: Arab. فخذ · Ibn Sīnā, *K. al-Qānūn fī al-ṭibb* · trans. Nathan ha-Me'ati

(*Sefer ha-Qanun*), bk. 1 (fol. 67[a]): ומה שישאר מזה יבא אל הפחד ויתענף בו שריגים וענפים ואחד מהם מתחלק בעצלים אשר על מוקדם פחד הירדן. → NM 4:163.

• **פחד הירדן** · **femur; thigh**: Arab. فخذ · Ibn Sīnā, *K. al-Qānūn fī al-ṭibb* · trans. Nathan ha-Me'ati (*Sefer ha-Qanun*), bk. 1 (fol. 67[a]): ומה שישאר מזה יבא אל הפחד ויתענף בו שריגים וענפים ואחד מהם מתחלק בעצלים אשר על מוקדם פחד הירדן. → NM 4:163.

• *Plur.* **פחדים • פחדי הירכים** · **thighs**: Arab. فخذان / Gr. μηροί · Hippocrates, *Aphorisms* · trans. Nathan ha-Me'ati, 5.69 (289) (fol. 105[b]): אמר אבוקרט: הנה הרתת ברוב מתחיל בנשים מתחתית גב השדרה אל הגב עד הראש והוא באנשים מתחיל ברוב מאחור יותר שאינו מתחיל למקדם כמו מה שמתחיל מהזרועות ופחדי הירכים. → NM 3:188–9.

פָּחַת · **to be missing**: Arab. نقص · Maimonides, *Šarḥ fuṣūl Abūqrāṭ* · trans. Zeraḥyah Ḥen (*Pirqei Abuqraṭ*), 1.20 (47): ואמר גאלנוס כי אם יפחות אחת מאילו אינו בחראן אמיתי ושלם. → NM 3:189.

פטומת → **פְּטֹמֶת**.

פְּטֹמֶת • *Plur.* **פטומות • התוספות הדומות לשתי פטומות** → **תּוֹסֶפֶת**.

[פטר] • *Hif'il* **הִפְטִיר** · **to free**: Arab. خلّص · Al-Zahrāwī, *K. al-taṣrīf li-man 'ağiza 'an at-ta'līf* · trans. Shem Tov ben Isaac (*Sefer ha-Shimmush*), bk. 30, 2.94 (fol. 228[b]): ואם יהיו לו אזנים ונאחז בהם ראוי להפטיר הבשר המתעכב בהם מכל צד בכל ערמה שתתכן או להשתדל אם אין יכולת להפטיר הבשר לשבור האזנים ולפתול אותם עד שיפטרו. → NM 1:108–9.

פיהוק → **פִּהוּק**.

פִּיל • **חולי הפיל** → **חֳלִי**.

• **בני הפיל** → **בֵּן**[2].

• **מדוה הפיל** → **מַדְוֶה**.

• **מררת הפיל** → **מְרֵרָה**.

פירוך → **פֵּרוּךְ**.

פירוק → **פֵּרוּק**.

פישטולא · **fistula**: Lat. fistula · Bruno Longobucco, *Cyrurgia Magna* · trans. Hillel ben Samuel (*Sefer Keritut*), fol. 15[a]: ואם תתאחר רפואת החבלה בעניינים האלה אז תדע כמו שאמר אלבוקשין שכבר נעשה שם פישטולא והיא מכת הכבידות להרפא. → NM 1:45.

פִּיתְקָא (*Aram.*) (also: **פִּיתְקָה**) · **hernia**: a) Arab. فتوق · Al-Zahrāwī, *K. al-taṣrīf li-man 'ağiza 'an at-ta'līf* · trans. Shem Tov ben Isaac (*Sefer ha-Shimmush*), bk. 30, 1.45 (fol. fol. 202[b]): בבוית הפיתקא. → NM 1:109.

b) Arab. فتق · Al-Rāzī, *K. al-Manṣūrī* · trans. Shem Tov ben Isaac (*Sefer Almansur*), Gimel 13: גרא אלגלוד ובלע' גלות: טוב לשעפה והפיתקה ורקיקת הדם. → NM 2:17.

פיתקה → **פִּיתְקָא**.

פֶּלַח · 1. **cleft; fissure**: Arab. شقاق · Al-Zahrāwī, *K. al-taṣrīf li-man 'ağiza 'an at-ta'līf* · trans. Shem Tov ben Isaac (*Sefer ha-Shimmush*), bk. 30, 1.18 (fol. 205[a]): שער יח' בכוית פלחי השפתים יתחדש הרבה בשפה סדיקה תקרא השער וכל שכן בשפתי הנערים כשירפאו אלה הפלחים בסמים במה שזכרתי במאמר החלוקה ולא תצליח הרפואה ולא תשכיל ראוי לחמם מכוה קטן סכיני על זאת הצורה ולהיות גוף המכוה על דקות הסכין ואחר כך לחממו מהרה ולכוות בו הפלח עד שתגיע הכויה אל עומקו ואחר כך לרפאו בקירוטי עד שיבריא. → NM 1:109.

› II. half [of the head]: Arab. شقّ · Ibn al-Jazzār, *Zād al-musāfir wa-qūt al-ḥādir* · trans. Moses ibn Tibbon (*Sefer Ṣedat ha-Derakhim*), bk. 1, ch. 10 (fols. 13^b–14^a): ואם היה הכאב מתילד מפני המרה האדומה ימצא החולה חום חזק בראשו ויובש בנחיריו ולשונו וימצאהו תעורה וצמא ויהיה רוב כאבו בפלח הימין מן הראש. → NM 4:163–4.

• **פלח המח** › **cerebral hemisphere**: Arab. شقّ الدماغ · Ibn al-Jazzār, *Zād al-musāfir wa-qūt al-ḥādir* · trans. Moses ibn Tibbon (*Sefer Ṣedat ha-Derakhim*), bk. 1, ch. 23 (fol. 33^b): ואם הגיע החמר אל אחד מצדדי המוח ר״ל הפלח הימני או הפלח השמאלי יקרא הפלג ההוא חסר ויתיחס אל האבר אשר יסור הרגשו ותנועתו. → NM 4:164.

• *Plur.* **פלחים** • **פלחי השפתים** › **hare lip**: Arab. شقاق الشفة · Al-Zahrāwī, *K. al-taṣrīf li-man ʿağiza ʿan at-taʾlīf* · trans. Shem Tov ben Isaac (*Sefer ha-Shimmush*), bk. 30, 1.18 (fol. 205^a): שער יח׳ בכוית פלחי השפתים יתחדש הרבה בשפה סדיקה תקרא השער וכל שכן בשפתי הנערים כשירפאו אלה הפלחים בסמים במה שזכרתי במאמר החלוקה ולא תצליח הרפואה ולא תשכיל ראוי לחמם מכוה קטן סכיני על זאת הצורה ולהיות גוף המכוה על דקות הסכין ואחר כך לחממו מהרה ולכוות בו הפלח עד שתגיע הכויה אל עומקו ואחר כך לרפאו בקירוטי עד שיבריא. → NM 1:109.

פלחי • **הפלחי** › **migraine**: Arab. الشقيقة · Ibn al-Jazzār, *Zād al-musāfir wa-qūt al-ḥādir* · trans. Moses ibn Tibbon (*Sefer Ṣedat ha-Derakhim*), bk. 1, ch. 11 (fol. 19^a): וכשנרצה לרפאות הפלחי נעיין ואם היה מפני מותר חם והורה על זה מה שזכרנו כבר מאותות כאב הראש שסבתו חום. → NM 4:164.

פֶּלֶךְ • **פלך הארכובה** › **the patella of the knee**: Arab. فلكة الركبة · Al-Zahrāwī, *K. al-taṣrīf li-man ʿağiza ʿan at-taʾlīf* · trans. Shem Tov ben Isaac (*Sefer ha-Shimmush*), bk. 30, 3.15 (fol. 235^b): פלך הארכובה לא יקרה בו שבר אלא על המעט. → NM 1:109–10.

פִּלְפֵּל • *Plur.* **פלפלין** • **שלשת הפלפלין** → **שְׁלֹשָׁה**.

פלפלי • **הפלפליי** › **the pepper [stomachic]**: Arab. الفلافلي · Ibn Sīnā, *K. al-adwiya al-qalbiya* · trans. Anonymous (*Sammim Libbiyim*), fol. 133^a: עוד החולקים מן הרופאים יחשבו שיש מן הטריאק והמטרידיטוס חום עובר הגבול ויעמדו מלהשתמש בשעור חצי משקל ממנו ולא יעמדו מלחשתמש בארבעה משקלים הכמוני ומן הפלפליי. → NM 4:165.

[פלץ] • *Hitpaʿel* **הִתְפַּלֵּץ** › **to shiver; to suffer from rigor**: Lat. rigeo (Honofredi) · Ibn Zuhr, *Regimen of Health* · trans. Jacob ibn Tibbon (*Hanhagat ha-Beriʾut le-Abu ʿAli ben Zuhr*), ch. 27: שער כ״ז בשווי הישיבות והטיולים ראוי שלא יהיה אל אלו המקומות מחום מה שיזיע בו הגוף או [...] ולא גם כן מהקור מה שיתפלץ עמו הגוף. → NM 4:165.

פַּלָּצוּת › **rigor; shivering**: a) Arab. نافض · Maimonides, *Šarḥ fuṣūl Abūqrāṭ* · trans. Moses ibn Tibbon (*Pirqei Abuqraṭ*), 4.46 (183): אמר אבקראט: כשיקרה פלצות בקדחת בלתי נפסקת למי שכבר נחלש הנה היא מאותות המות. → NM 3:189.

b) Arab. اقشعرار / Gr. φρίκη · Maimonides, *Šarḥ fuṣūl Abūqrāṭ* · trans. Moses ibn Tibbon (*Pirqei Abuqraṭ*), 7.4 (356): אמר אבקראט: כשיתחדש עם הזיעה פלצות אין זה אות טוב. → NM 3:189.

פָּנוּי • **המקום הפנוי** → **מָקוֹם**.

פָּנִים › **cheek**: Arab. خدّ · Ibn Sīnā, *K. al-Qānūn fī al-ṭibb* · trans. Zeraḥyah Ḥen (*Sefer ha-Qanun*), bk. 1 (fol. 24^a): הפרק הששי בניתוח המושקלי של הפנים. הפנים לו שתי תנועות. → NM 4:165.

• עדשי הפנים ← עֲדָשָׁה.

• תמונת הפנים ← תְּמוּנָה.

פְּנִים • המסך אשר בפנים ← מָסָךְ.

פְּנִימִי • **הפנימי** · **vena cava**: Arab. الأجوف · Ibn Sīnā, *K. al-Qānūn fī al-ṭibb* · trans. Joseph Lorki (*Sefer ha-Qanun*), bk. 1 (fol. 19[b]): פרק ה׳ בנתוח הוריד הפמימי היורד כבר השלמנו מאמרינו בחלק העולה מ⟨ה⟩פנימי והוא היותר קטון שבשני חלקיו. → NM 4:165–6.

• האברים הפנימיים ← אֵבֶר.

• הוריד הפנימי ← וְרִיד.

• הוריד הפנימי היורד ← וְרִיד.

• המסך הפנימי ← מָסָךְ.

• הקנה הפנימי ← קָנֶה.

• הקרום הפנימי ← קְרוּם.

פניס · **sugar candy; a sweetmeat**: Arab. فانيد / Pers. پانيد; پانيذ · Al-Zahrāwī, *K. al-taṣrīf li-man ʿağiza ʿan at-taʾlīf* · trans. Shem Tov ben Isaac (*Sefer ha-Shimmush*), bk. 27, fol. 141[b], col. a: ודחית נזקם לאכלם על הצום ולאכול אחריהם בעל הלחה הלבנה מן הדבש ובעל החמימות מן הסוכר או מן הפניס. → NM 4:166.

פִּסְחוּת · **lameness**: Arab. عرج · Maimonides, *Šarḥ fuṣūl Abūqrāṭ* · trans. Zeraḥyah Ḥen (*Pirqei Abuqraṭ*), 6.60 (352): אמר המפרש: אותם הלחויות יתייבשו בכויה וכשלא יתיבשו אותן הלחויות בכויה יתחדש הפסחות ולא יתפרנס הרגל לפי מנהגו ויכחש. → NM 3:189–90.

פָּסַק • *Part.* **פוֹסֵק** • הקדחות הפוסקות ← קַדַּחַת.

• *Part. Nifʿal* **נִפְסָק** · **intermittent**: Arab. مفارق · Maimonides, *K. al-fuṣūl fī al-ṭibb* · trans. Zeraḥyah Ḥen (*Sefer ha-Peraqim*), 25.23: כי הקדחות הנפסקות והם אשר הפסקם מבואר מורגש אמנם יהיה זה בהיות הליחה המולידה לקדחת מתחרף רץ בגוף כולו. → NM 1:180.

• *Hifʿil* **הִפְסִיק** · **to dissolve**: Arab. قطع · Ibn al-Jazzār, *Zād al-musāfir wa-qūt al-ḥādir* · trans. Moses ibn Tibbon (*Sefer Ṣedat ha-Derakhim*), bk. 7, 19.2: וראוי לרפאת המין הראשון מן הקובא בהוצאת הדם בהקזה אם עזר הזמן והשנים והמנהג ואחר כן בשלשול ברפואות אשר יפסיקו חומר השריפה. → NM 1:65.

פֶּסֶק • התיר הפסק דין ← [נתר].

פַּעַם • *Plur.* **פעמים** · **cycles**: Hippocrates, *Aphorisms* · trans. Do'eg ha-Edomi (*Sefer Agur*), 4.59 (196) (fol. 73[b]): צרודה קדחת שלישית על הסובל עד תעבור עליו ז׳ פעמים. → NM 3:190.

פקעיות · **non-alcoholic beer**: Arab. فقاع · Al-Zahrāwī, *K. al-taṣrīf li-man ʿağiza ʿan at-taʾlīf* · trans. Shem Tov ben Isaac (*Sefer ha-Shimmush*), bk. 27, fol. 128[a]: השער השני במימות והשלג והמים הקפוים ומיני היין והשכר והפקעיות. → NM 4:166.

פֵּרוּד • **פרוד (ה)דבוק** · **the dissolution of continuity**: a) Arab. انحلال الاتّصال · Ibn al-Jazzār, *Zād al-musāfir wa-qūt al-ḥādir* · trans. Moses ibn Tibbon (*Sefer Ṣedat ha-Derakhim*), bk. 7, 14.3: ואולם הכאב הנה הוא שנוי פתאום יהיה מן מזג חם או קר או מפרוד דבוק. → NM 1:66.

b) Arab. تفرّق الاتّصال · Ibn al-Jazzār, *Zād al-musāfir wa-qūt al-ḥādir* · trans. Moses ibn Tibbon (*Sefer Ṣedat ha-Derakhim*), bk. 7, 25.1: כשיתחדש פרוד הדבוק בעצם הנה הכונה ברפואתו הדביק העצם. → NM 1:66.

פֵּרוּךְ · **massage**: Judah ben Jacob, *Sefer Hanhagat ha-Beri'ut*, 9.2: ודע כי מיני הפירוך וחלקיהם רבים ממנו חזק וממנו רפה ואמצעי ביניהם. → NM 4:166.

פרונקא (*Aram.*) • *Plur.* **פרונקות** (*Aram.* **פרונקאות**) · **cloth**: Arab. خرق · Al-Zahrāwī, *K. al-taṣrīf li-man ʿağiza ʿan at-taʾlīf* · trans. Shem Tov ben Isaac (*Sefer ha-Shimmush*), bk. 30, 2.10 (fol. 210[b]): ואם לא יראה השרנאק בתחלת הביקוע ראוי להוסיף בביקוע מעט בנחת עד שיבלוט ואחר למשכו כמו שאמרתי ולטבול אחרי כן פרונקות בחומץ ומים ולתתם על המקום ולהדקו בכלונסה. → NM 1:110.

פֵּרוּק • **פירוק חבור** · **dissolution of continuity**: Arab. تفرّق الاتّصال · Maimonides, *K. al-fuṣūl fī al-ṭibb* · trans. Nathan ha-Me'ati (*Sefer ha-Peraqim*), 25.21: כבר עיין זולתנו ורבים מהרופאים דבר ג'אלינוס בסבות הכאב ומצאנו במקומות רבים שמשים סבתו סבה אחת והוא פירוק חבור לבד. → NM 2:75.

פֶּרַח • **פרח המלח** · **salt efflorescence; salt scum**: Arab. زهرة الملح · Ibn al-Jazzār, *Zād al-musāfir wa-qūt al-ḥādir* · trans. Moses ibn Tibbon (*Sefer Ṣedat ha-Derakhim*), bk. 1, ch. 24 (fol. 40[a]): וירחץ במים שנתבשלו בהם סמים חמים וימשח במה שזכרנו מן השמנים אחר שיצא ממים חמים שהושלך בהם פרח המלח. → NM 4:166.

• **פרח הנחשת** · **verdigris**: Lat. flos eris · Bruno Longobucco, *Cyrurgia Magna* · trans. Hillel ben Samuel (*Sefer Keritut*), fol. 14[b]: ושמור שלא תרגיל בו נקיון חזק כמו פרח הנחשת. → NM 1:36.

• *Plur.* **פרחים** · **menstrual blood; menstruation**: Hippocrates, *Aphorisms* · trans. Do'eg ha-Edomi (*Sefer Agur*), 5.39 (259) (fol. 87[b]): אמר אפוקרט: סימן האשה שאינה הרה ולא מיניקת בהיות לה חלב שיפסקו פרחיה. → NM 3:190.

[פרנס] • *Piʿel* **פִּרְנֵס** · **to feed**: Arab. غذا · a) Maimonides, *K. al-fuṣūl fī al-ṭibb* · trans. Zeraḥyah Ḥen (*Sefer ha-Peraqim*), 9.47: המילוי אשר ישתלשל עמו הטבע עד שיתרבה ויחטוף הכח תפרנסנו בדברים עוצרים בסדר והרבה פעמים תפול תאות המזון עם אחד ממיני השלשול הנק' דרב וצריך שיקח החולה מרקחת החבושים ודומיהו. → NM 1:180.

b) Maimonides, *K. al-fuṣūl fī al-ṭibb* · trans. Zeraḥyah Ḥen (*Sefer ha-Peraqim*), 9.124: הנהגת שיברון העצם אחר מה שתצטרך ממלאכת חיד הוא שתנהיג החולה בהנהגה מדקדקת בתכלית והרבה פעמים תצטרך אל שלשול הבטן ברפואה ובהתחלה אבל אחר כן תפרנסהו במזון טוב הכימוס והרבה יהיה פרנסתו ושיהיה בו דבקות. → NM 1:180.

• *Part. Piʿel* **מְפַרְנֵס** • **הכח המפרנס** → **כֹּחַ**.

• *Part. Hitpaʿel* **מִתְפַּרְנֵס** • **היה מתפרנס** · **to be nourished**: Arab. اغتذى · Maimonides, *K. al-fuṣūl fī al-ṭibb* · trans. Zeraḥyah Ḥen (*Sefer ha-Peraqim*), 1.56: האסטומכא והמעים יהיו מתפרנסים בשני דברים: האחד מהם המזון אשר ילך בהם ויתעכל בהם והאחר מה שימשכו מן הכבד. → NM 1:180.

פַּרְנָסָה · **nourishment**: Arab. غذاء · Maimonides, *K. al-fuṣūl fī al-ṭibb* · trans. Zeraḥyah Ḥen (*Sefer ha-Peraqim*), 9.124: הנהגת שיברון העצם אחר מה שתצטרך ממלאכת היד הוא שתנהיג החולה בהנהגה מדקדקת בתכלית והרבה פעמים תצטרך אל שלשול הבטן ברפואה ובהתחלה אבל אחר כן תפרנסהו במזון טוב הכימוס והרבה יהיה פרנסתו ושיהיה בו דבקות. → NM 1:180.

פַּרְסִי • **האש הפרסי** → **אֵשׁ**.

פַּרְעֹה • עכבר פרעה → **עַכְבָּר**.

[פרק] • *Puʿal* **פֹּרַק • או שיפורק חבורו** · **or its continuity is broken up**: Lat. aut eius continuitas solvatur / Arab. وإمّا بأن يتفرّق اتّصاله · Galen, *De inaequali intemperie* · trans. David Caslari (*Sefer Roʿa Mezeg Mitḥallef*), 3.4: וכל אחד ואחד שתרצה מהאברים לא ישתנה ולא יצא מטבעו ולא יפסד אם לא יחומם או לא יקורר או לא יתלחלח או לא ינוגב או שיפורק חבורו. → NM 2:167–8.

פֶּרֶק • פרק היד · **(lit., joint of the hand); wrist**: Lat. iunctura manus · Bruno Longobucco, *Cyrurgia Magna* · trans. Hillel ben Samuel (*Sefer Keritut*), fol. 61[b]: וישתוה עוד שיונח פרק היד על שום לוח ויפשטנו בפשוט ראוי. → NM 1:36.

• **פרק המרפק** · **humerus**: Arab. عضد · Al-Zahrāwī, *K. al-taṣrīf li-man ʿağiza ʿan at-taʾlīf* · trans. Shem Tov ben Isaac (*Sefer ha-Shimmush*), bk. 30, 3.11 (fol. 235[a]): שער י״א בחבוש שבר ⟨פרק⟩ המרפק הנקרא בלשונם אל עצ׳ד זה הפרק הוא בין המרפק אל ראש הכתף. → NM 1:110.

• **פרק קנה הזרוע הסמוך ליד** · **wrist**: Arab. معصم · Al-Zahrāwī, *K. al-taṣrīf li-man ʿağiza ʿan at-taʾlīf* · trans. Shem Tov ben Isaac (*Sefer ha-Shimmush*), bk. 30, 3.28 (fol. 237[b]): שער כ״ח ברפואת שמיטת פרק קנה הזרוע הסמוך ליד. → NM 1:110.

• *Plur.* **פרקים • פרקי האצבעות** · **phalanges**: Arab. سلاميات · Ibn Sīnā, *K. al-Qānūn fī al-ṭibb* · trans. Nathan ha-Meʾati (*Sefer ha-Qanun*), bk. 1 (fol. 40[a]): ונתחברו פרקי האצבעות כלם בזיזים ונקרות נכנסים ביניהם לחות דבקה. → NM 4:166–7.

• **הקעת הפרקים** → **הֲקָעָה**.

פִּרְקִי · **articular**: Arab. مفصلي · Ibn Sīnā, *K. al-Qānūn fī al-ṭibb* · trans. Nathan ha-Meʾati (*Sefer ha-Qanun*), bk. 1 (fol. 32[b]): והתוספות הפרקיות גם כן ענינם זה כי הוא מהודק קצתם בקצתם הדוק חזק בקשורים ומאסרים מכל הצדדים. → NM 4:167.

פֶּרֶשׁ • *Plur.* **פרשות • בית הפרשות** → **בַּיִת**.

• **סוף הפרשות** → **סוֹף**.

פָּשׁוּט (*Pass. Part.*) → **פָּשַׁט**.

פָּשַׁט · **to expand**: Arab. بسط · Ibn Sīnā, *K. al-Qānūn fī al-ṭibb* · trans. Zeraḥyah Ḥen (*Sefer ha-Qanun*), bk. 1 (fol. 26[a]): אלו הם המושקלי הפושטים. → NM 4:167.

• **פשט הרוח** · **to dilate the pneuma**: Arab. بسط الروح · Ibn Sīnā, *K. al-adwiya al-qalbiya* · trans. Anonymous (*Sammim Libbiyim*), fols. 124[b]–125[a]: ולו סגולה לשמוח הלב ולחזקו ויעזור בזה דקדוקו ויפשט הרוח ויקשרהו וינגבהו ויזככהו. → NM 4:167.

• *Pass. Part.* **פָּשׁוּט** · **unmixed**: Arab. صرف · Maimonides, *Šarḥ fuṣūl Abūqrāṭ* · trans. Moses ibn Tibbon (*Pirqei Abuqraṭ*), 7.23 (375): אמר אבקראט: ומהצואה הפשוטה שלשול הדם. → NM 3:190.

• *Nifʿal* **נִפְשַׁט** · **to ulcerate**: Lat. ulcerari · Bruno Longobucco, *Cyrurgia Magna* · trans. Hillel ben Samuel (*Sefer Keritut*), fol. 43[b]: אבל אם הסרטן נפשט לא יתרפא בדברים הקרים אבל צריך שיחתוך ויאומנו בו רפואות חמות מאד כמו הכויה באש. → NM 1:36.

• *Piʿel* **פִּשֵּׁט • פשט המעים** · **to excoriate the intestines**: Lat. excoriare intestina · Bruno Longobucco, *Cyrurgia Magna* · trans. Hillel ben Samuel (*Sefer Keritut*), fol. 86[a]: וזה כמו שאמר ב״ס שזאת הרפואה אינה מחממת ולא מפשטת המעים. → NM 1:36.

• *Inf. Hitpaʿel* **הִתְפַּשֵּׁט** • **התפשט העפעפים** › **ptillosis**: Arab. سلاق · Maimonides, *K. al-fuṣūl fī al-ṭibb* · trans. Nathan ha-Me'ati (*Sefer ha-Peraqim*), 23.71: והעפעפים אשר יתעבו ויתקשו וישוב מראיהם אדום וישרו הריסים הוא העלה הנקראת סלאק כלומ׳ התפשט העפעפים. → NM 2:75.

• *Part. Hitpaʿel* **מִתְפַּשֵּׁט** • **החבלות המתפשטות** → **חַבָּלָה**.

• *Hifʿil* **הִפְשִׁיט** › I. **to abrade**: Arab. سحج · Maimonides, *K. al-fuṣūl fī al-ṭibb* · trans. Nathan ha-Me'ati (*Sefer ha-Peraqim*), 6.90: לפעמים יקרה בתחלת שלשול הדם הסרת התאוה ואין זה אות רע כי חליחות האדומיות הנשפכות מן הכבד אל המעים ויפשיטום ישפך מהם אל האסטומכה ואז תפול התאוה. → NM 2:75.

› II. **to extend; to stretch**: Arab. بسط · Ibn Sīnā, *K. al-Qānūn fī al-ṭibb* · trans. Nathan ha-Me'ati (*Sefer ha-Qanun*), bk. 1 (fol. 50[a]): וכשיתנועעו אלו השנים יפשיט⟨ו⟩ הרסג פשוט עם מעט קבוב. → NM 4:168.

› III. **to rarefy**: Arab. بسط · Ibn Sīnā, *K. al-adwiya al-qalbiya* · trans. Anonymous (*Sammim Libbiyim*), fol. 126[a]: ויש לו עם זה דקות והוא בסבת הבושמיות אשר בו נאות לעצם הרוח [ו]למה שיש בו מן הקביצות עם הדקות מקשר אותו מנקה לעצמיותו מפשיט אותו. → NM 4:167–8.

• *Part. Hofʿal* **מֻפְשָׁט** › **ulcerated**: Lat. ulceratus · Bruno Longobucco, *Cyrurgia Magna* · trans. Hillel ben Samuel (*Sefer Keritut*), 81[a]: המקום מופשט לא תקררנו אלא ואם כל זה אם מסביב. → NM 1:31.

פְּשִׁירָה › **abatement**: Arab. فترة · Maimonides, *K. al-fuṣūl fī al-ṭibb* · trans. Nathan ha-Me'ati (*Sefer ha-Peraqim*), 25.24: המובן מדברו הראשון הוא הליחה המתעפשת מעט מעט שתהיה בתוך העורקים. וזמן הפשירה הוא המנוחה הוא הזמן אשר בין עפוש חלק מאותו דבר ובין עפוש השכן אליו כמו שתראה בדמיון זה באשפה. → NM 2:76.

פָּשַׁר • *Part.* **פּוֹשֵׁר** • **היה פושר** › **to be weak**: Arab. فتر · Maimonides, *K. al-fuṣūl fī al-ṭibb* · trans. Zeraḥyah Ḥen (*Sefer ha-Peraqim*), 1.32: פעולות המושקולי כולם בזמן השינה יהיו פושרים. → NM 1:179.

פַּת • **פת הדראה** › **whole wheat bread**: Arab. خبز الخشكار · Al Zahrāwī, *K. al-taṣrīf li-man ʿağiza ʿan at-taʾlīf* · trans. Shem Tov ben Isaac (*Sefer ha-Shimmush*), bk. 27, fol. 123[a], col. b: המאמר בלחם הלחם העשוי מן החטה הוא בטבעו על הכלל חם ויבש במעלה השניה לקנותו זה מן האש והקמח הנלקח מן החטה לעשות ממנו הלחם שלשה מינים הסלת והקמח הדק הנבדל מן הסלת הנקרא בלשונם דרמך ובי״ל פלור והקמח האדום אשר יעשה ממנו פת הדראה. → NM 4:41–42.

פָּתַח › I. **to break forth**: Arab. انفجر · Maimonides, *Šarḥ fuṣūl Abūqrāṭ* · trans. Zeraḥyah Ḥen (*Pirqei Abuqraṭ*), 5.15 (235): אמר המפרש: אם לא יצא החומר אשר פתח והגיע בחלל החזה יתעפש ותתחדד ותנגע הריאה.→ NM 3:190–1.

› II. **to incise**: Arab. شقّ · Maimonides, *K. al-fuṣūl fī al-ṭibb* · trans. Zeraḥyah Ḥen (*Sefer ha-Peraqim*), 15.48: כשתראה הרפואה לא תהיה לה יכולת להתיר הטרי כולו אבל יגבר עליה הטרי ונצח אותה ראוי שתפתח אותו הצמח ותפתחנו במקום העליון שבו והיותר דק ועשה שיהיה הטרי ניגר ושים מה שייבש מבלתי עקיצה. → NM 1:181.

› III. **to lance**: Arab. بطّ · Maimonides, *K. al-fuṣūl fī al-ṭibb* · trans. Zeraḥyah Ḥen

החולי שבעין הנקרא ברדה צריכה לחיתוך וכן הטרי המקובץ בעין (*Sefer ha-Peraqim*), 15.25: בחולי הנקרא אלכמנא ברוב תרופא ברפואה מתירה לא בדבר שמייבש יובש חזק כי הוא יריק הרוב ויקפיא הנשאר ואנחנו הריקונו זה הטרי כשפתחנו הקרום הנקרא קרנית במקום האכליל. → NM 1:181.

• *Part.* פּוֹתֵחַ • הסם הפותח → סַם.

פְּתִיחָה ‣ I. **deobstruent property (of a remedy)**: Arab. تفتيح · Ibn Sīnā, *K. al-adwiya al-qalbiya* · trans. Anonymous (*Sammim Libbiyim*), fol. 126[b]: בהמן: הוא באם חם בשנית יבש בראשונה וממנו לבן ואדום והאדום יותר חזק החום ובשניהם יחד קביצות עם דקדוק ופתיחה. → NM 4:168.

‣ II. **incision**: Arab. بطّ · Maimonides, *K. al-fuṣūl fī al-ṭibb*· trans. Zeraḥyah Ḥen (*Sefer ha-Peraqim*), 15.49: וכשליחות ישתעפו באבר בין האברים המתדמים חלקיהם ויתחייב שתריק מן האבר בעצמו ראוי שתשים על אותו האבר רפואה תדחה מה שירוץ לו. וההרקה תהיה עם הפתיחה ועם הרפואה המתירה וכל שכן אם תרגיש שיהיה בין האברים המתדמים החלקים דבר עצור וכלוא. → NM 1:181.

• **פתיחת האזן** ‣ **the external acoustic meatus; the inner cavity of the ear; the middle ear; the tympanic cavity**: Arab. صماخ · Ibn Sīnā, *K. al-Qānūn fī al-ṭibb* · trans. Joseph Lorki (*Sefer ha-Qanun*), bk. 1 (fol. 17[a]): והחלק הראשון מכל זוג ממנו יכוון אל הקרום ⟨...⟩ פתיחת האזן. → NM 4:168.

• **פתיחת העינים** ‣ **staring eyes**: Arab. شخوص العينين · Galen, attr., *Prohibition of Burial* · trans. Judah al-Ḥarizi (*Sefer Issur ha-Qevurah le-Galienus*), par. 15: ואולם בסוף זאת העלה יקרה לבעליה פתיחת העינים. → NM 4:168.

פְּתִיל • *Plur.* **פתילים** ‣ I. **fibers**: Arab. شظايا · Maimonides, *K. al-fuṣūl fī al-ṭibb* · trans. Nathan ha-Me'ati (*Sefer ha-Peraqim*), 1.74: הפתילים שבכל אחד מן המעים עגולים ונכרכים ברחב בשני עורותיהם יחד. → NM 2:76.

‣ II. **tendrils**: Arab. خيوط · Ibn al-Jazzār, *Zād al-musāfir wa-qūt al-ḥāḍir* · trans. Moses ibn Tibbon (*Sefer Ṣedat ha-Derakhim*), bk. 1, ch. 10 (Ms. Oxford, Bodleian Library, Poc. 353, Uri Heb. 314, fol. 4[b]): וזכר גם כן שאם יכתשו עלי הגפנים ופתיליהם ויעשה מהם רטיה יועיל מכאב הראש הכרכומי. → NM 4:168.

פְּתִילָה ‣ **suppository**: Arab. شيافة · Al-Zahrāwī, *K. al-taṣrīf li-man ʿağiza ʿan at-taʾlīf* · trans. Shem Tov ben Isaac (*Sefer ha-Shimmush*), bk. 27, fol. 144[a], col. a: ואם יתחדש בבטן הברה ואומץ המעים ראוי לעשות לו פתילה מורידה הצואה או פדלקון בבורית וחלב פקועות ופניס וכיוצא בהם. → NM 4:169.

פתלתוליות ‣ **a griping or wringing**: Lat. tortio (h.l., cramps) · Al-Rāzī, attr., *On the Treatment of Small Children* · trans. Bonfos, 15: משלשול בטן הנערים. ימשך שלשול בטן הילדים לפעמים יקרה שלשול חוץ מצמיחת השינים כמו שאמרנו או בסבת קרירות ובעבור זה לא יקשר הילד או יקרה בסבת הפסד החלב או בסבת הליחה הלבנה או בסבת ליחה אדומה ואותות האדומה כאשר יבא ביציאת הילד כרכומיות או ירוקיות או שיצא תכף אחר שינק בלי שום איחור ואותות הקרירות והלבנה הוא שיהיה לחולה לובן ופתלתוליות בבטן. → NM 2:180.

צ

צֵאָה · **emptying; excrement; voiding (h.l., stools):** a) Lat. egestio · Al-Rāzī, attr., *On the Treatment of Small Children* · trans. Anonymous, ch. 16: מזחילת הבטן בילדים פעמים רבות תקרה לילדים זחילה בעבור תולדת השינים כאשר אמרנו או בעבור קרירות כשיוחתל הנער או בעבור הפסד החלב ממרירה או מליחה ואות המרירה הוא שימצא צהובות ביציאת הילד או חידוד והיציאה יוצאת בלי עיכוב ואות הקור והליחה הוא הלובן בציאה והכאב בבטן כשהיא יוצאת. → NM 2:181.

b) Arab. براز / Gr. ὑποχώρησις · i. Maimonides, *Šarḥ fuṣūl Abūqrāṭ* · trans. Zeraḥyah Ḥen (*Pirqei Abuqraṭ*), 4.83 (220): אמר בקראט: מי שישתין בלילה שתן הרבה יורה זה כי צאתו תמעט. → NM 3:191.

· ii. Maimonides, *K. al-fuṣūl fī al-ṭibb* · trans. Nathan ha-Me'ati (*Sefer ha-Peraqim*), 6.75: הציאה הרקיקה המחוברת אשר תצא בעת המנהג כשתהיה פחות מן הראוי בערך אל מה שילקח מן המזון הנה זה מורה שהוא נשארה ממנו שארית בקצת המעים וזה רע באיזה צד שיהיה. → NM 2:76.

צֹאָה • **צואת העין** · **a humor that gathers in the corner of the eye; rheum:** Arab. رمص / Gr. λήμη · Al-Rāzī, *K. al-Manṣūrī* · trans. Shem Tov ben Isaac (*Sefer Almansur*), Alef 17 (16): אנזרות: טוב לצואת העין והאפר והחבורות הטריות. → NM 2:17.

צבא → **צבה**.

צבה • **הצבא** · [the illness called] **flatulent, gassy, windy:** Arab. النافخة / Gr. φυσώδης · Ibn al-Jazzār, *Zād al-musāfir wa-qūt al-ḥāḍir* · trans. Moses ibn Tibbon (*Sefer Ṣedat ha-Derakhim*), bk. 1, ch. 18 (fol. 27[b]): כמו אשר יקרה זה בחולי אשר יקרא הצבא אלנפכא בערבי. → NM 4:169.

צְבוּת • **צבות חמה** · **(lit., hot swelling); effusion:** Arab. ورم حارّ · Al-Zahrāwī, *K. al-taṣrīf li-man ʿağiza ʿan at-taʾlīf* · trans. Shem Tov ben Isaac (*Sefer ha-Shimmush*), bk. 30, 2.4 (fol. 209[b]): ולשית עליו כלונסה טבולה ביין ושמן או חומץ ויין כדי שלא תתחדש צבות חמה. → NM 1:110–1.

צֶבַע • *Plur.* **צבעים** · **kinds:** Arab. ألوان · Maimonides, *Šarḥ fuṣūl Abūqrāṭ* · trans. Moses ibn Tibbon (*Pirqei Abuqraṭ*), 2.14 (66): אמר המפרש: כי רבוי צבעיו יורה על הרקת מינים רבים מן הליחות. → NM 3:191.

צַד • **בעלת הצד** → **בַּעֲלָה**.

• **חולי הצד** → **חֳלִי**.

• **מדוה הצד** → **מַדְוֶה**.

• **קצה העין מצד האזן** → **קָצֶה**.

• *Plur.*[1] **צדים** • **צדי האמה** · **ureter:** Arab. حالب · Galen, attr., *Prohibition of Burial* · trans. Judah al-Ḥarizi (*Sefer Issur ha-Qevurah le-Galienus*), par. 31: והמקום השלישי העורך בין צדי האמה והאמה כשיהודקו הדוק חזק ירגיש האדם כמו התלהבות האש ואם תראה זה הנה הוא חי. → NM 4:169.

• **מה שלמטה מצדי הכסלים** → **מַטָּה**.

• *Plur.*[2] **צדדים** • **כאב הצדדים** → **כְּאֵב**.

צְהוּב · **hairy surface of a fabric**: Arab. زِئْبِر · Al-Zahrāwī, *K. al-taṣrīf li-man ʿağiza ʿan at-ta'līf* · trans. Shem Tov ben Isaac (*Sefer ha-Shimmush*), bk. 27, fol. 150, col. b: כל לבוש מתלהט חלק חומו בכלל לגופות יותר מועט משאר הלבוש וראוי ללבוש אותו בקיץ ומה שיש לו כובד או ציהוב והיתה אריגתו מתחלחלת או שיהיה עב בלתי מתלהט הוא מחמם הגוף יותר וראוי ללבשו בסתו. → NM 4:171.

• **על גבו ציהוב** · **covered with yellow fuzz**: Arab. مزغب الجسم · Al-Zahrāwī, *K. al-taṣrīf li-man ʿağiza ʿan at-ta'līf* · trans. Shem Tov ben Isaac (*Sefer ha-Shimmush*), bk. 27, fol. 138ᵇ, col. a: ויש ממנו מין לבן רב החמימות ועל גבו ציהוב והוא בלתי מתפלח. → NM 4: 170–1.

צוֹאה → צֹאָה.

צָוָּאר • **העומק אשר בעליון אחורי הצואר** → עֹמֶק.

צוֹלֵל (*Part.*) → צָלַל.

צוֹלֵעַ (*Part.*) → צָלַע.

[**צום**] • **המעי הצם** → מְעִי.

צוּף • **צוף הדבש** · **honeycomb**: Lat. favositas mellis · Arab. شهدة · Al-Rāzī, attr., *On the Treatment of Small Children* · trans. Anonymous, ch. 1: צוף הדבש נקרא חלי אחד אשר הוא מן ספאטי ואז ייראו על המכות כמו קשקשים והעור הוא מתפוצץ עם חיכוך חזק ויזוב מהם כמו דבש. → NM 2:180.

צוֹפֵד (*Part.*) → צָפַד.

צַחְצוּחַ • *Plur.* **צחצוחים** • **צחצוחי חלב** · **beestings; colostrum; first milk**: Arab. لِبًا · Al-Zahrāwī, *K. al-taṣrīf li-man ʿağiza ʿan at-ta'līf* · trans. Shem Tov ben Isaac (*Sefer ha-Shimmush*), bk. 27, fol. 147ᵇ, col. a: צחצוחי חלב יותר עבים מהגבנה ויותר מתאחרים להתעכל ויותר רחוקים לרדת. → NM 4:170.

ציאה → צֵאָה.

ציהוב → צִהוּב.

צילבחא → צלבחא.

צילחתא → צִלְחָתָא.

ציני → צִנִּי.

ציפורן → צִפּוֹרֶן.

צִיר • *Plur.* **צירים** · **colic**: Arab. مغص / Gr. στρόφος · Maimonides, *Šarḥ fuṣūl Abūqrāṭ* · trans. Moses ibn Tibbon (*Pirqei Abuqraṭ*), 4.11 (148): אמר אבקראט: מי שהיו בו צירים וכאב תחת הטבור וכאב בשפל הבטן תמיד ולא יסורו ברפואה משלשלת ולא בזולתה הנה ענינו יבוא אל השקוי היבש. → NM 3:191–2.

• **צירים בבטן** · **colics**: Arab. مغص, *Plur.* أمغاص · Al-Zahrāwī, *K. al-taṣrīf li-man ʿağiza ʿan at-ta'līf* · trans. Shem Tov ben Isaac (*Sefer ha-Shimmush*), bk. 27, fol. 143ᵇ, col. b: בשר הזאב יותר חם מבשר הכלב אלא שהוא עב וקשה להתעכל מאד ומוליד צירים בבטן. → NM 4: 170.

• **צירים וחבלים** · **colic**: Arab. مغس · Al-Zahrāwī, *K. al-taṣrīf li-man ʿağiza ʿan at-ta'līf* · trans. Shem Tov ben Isaac (*Sefer ha-Shimmush*), bk. 27, fol. 142ᵃ, col. a: ותקונם ודחית נזקם למי שיולידו לו צירים וחבלים באצטומכא למצוץ עליהם מן הרמונים הקוססים. → NM 4:170–1.

צלבחא (*Aram.*) ‣ **eel**: Arab. سلباح · Al-Zahrāwī, *K. al-taṣrīf li-man ʿağiza ʿan at-taʾlīf* · trans. Shem Tov ben Isaac (*Sefer ha-Shimmush*), bk. 27, fol. 150^{a}, col. a: הצילבחא היא מין הדגים אלא שהיא מתילד במקומות מעופשים וביצה. → NM 4:171.

צְלוֹבְחָא → צלבחא.

צְלוֹפְחָא → צלבחא.

צִלְחָתָא (*Aram.*) ‣ **migraine**: Arab. شقيقة · Al-Zahrāwī, *K. al-taṣrīf li-man ʿağiza ʿan at-taʾlīf* · trans. Shem Tov ben Isaac (*Sefer ha-Shimmush*), bk. 30, 1.3 (fol. 203^{b}): השער השלישי בכוית הצילחתא החדשה. → NM 1:111.

צָלִי • צלי אש ‣ **a dish of fried meat, which has been diced or sliced and fried with onion, a small amount of vinegar or *murrī* (liquid fermented sauce) and some spices and herbs**: Arab. القليّة المشوية · Ibn al-Jazzār, *Zād al-musāfir wa-qūt al-ḥādir* · trans. Moses ibn Tibbon (*Sefer Ṣedat ha-Derakhim*), bk. 1, ch. 19 (29^{b}): ויהיה מזונו צלי קדר וצלי אש וכרוב מבושל בבשר צאן או כרוב שלוק מתוקן במוריס ושמן טוב. → NM 4:171.

• צלי הפורני ‣ **(lit., [a dish of meat] roasted in the oven); a dish consisting of meat, onions, honey, rosewater, coriander, a lot of saffron, and a few cooked almonds**: Arab. شوي الفرن · Al-Zahrāwī, *K. al-taṣrīf li-man ʿağiza ʿan at-taʾlīf* · trans. Shem Tov ben Isaac (*Sefer ha-Shimmush*), bk. 27, fol. 145^{b}: צלי הפורני רב המזון קשה להתעכל ולרדת מן האסטומ׳ נוטה להוליד המרה השחורה. → NM 4:171.

• צלי קדר ‣ **a dish of sliced and braised red meat of quadrupeds, marinated in sauce, and slowly simmered in a small amount of liquid with oil, spices, and herbs, and sometimes vegetables**: Arab. طباهجة · Ibn al-Jazzār, *Zād al-musāfir wa-qūt al-ḥādir* · trans. Moses ibn Tibbon (*Sefer Ṣedat ha-Derakhim*), bk. 1, ch. 19 (fol. 29^{b}): ויהיה מזונו צלי קדר וצלי אש וכרוב מבושל בבשר צאן או כרוב שלוק מתוקן במוריס ושמן טוב. → NM 4:171–2.

צְלִילָה ‣ **ringing in the ears (tinnitus)**: Arab. دويّ / Gr. ἦχος · Ibn al-Jazzār, *Zād al-musāfir wa-qūt al-ḥādir* · trans. Moses ibn Tibbon (*Sefer Ṣedat ha-Derakhim*), bk. 2, ch. 8 (fol. 49^{a}): ואם היתה הצלילה מפני חולי שהחליש האבר חנח יועילחו חומץ חם עם סחיטת אישנץ. → NM 4:172.

צְלִיעָה ‣ **lameness**: Arab. عَرَج · Maimonides, *Šarḥ fuṣūl Abūqrāṭ* · trans. Anonymous (*Pirqei Abuqraṭ*), 6.60 (352): אמר המפרש: נגוב זה הרטיבות הרירי הוא בכויה וכשלא יתנגב זה הרטיבות בכויה יתחדש הצליעה ולא יזונו הרגלים על מנהגם ויצטמקו. → NM 3:192.

צָלַל • *Part.* **צוֹלֵל • היה צולל** ‣ **to form a sediment**: Arab. رسب / Gr. ὑφίσταμαι · Maimonides, *Šarḥ fuṣūl Abūqrāṭ* · trans. Moses ibn Tibbon (*Pirqei Abuqraṭ*), 4.79 (216): אמר אבקראט: מי שהיה צולל בשתנו דבר דומה לחול אבן יתילד לו במקוה. → NM 3:192.

צָלַע • *Part.* **צוֹלֵעַ • היה צולע** ‣ **to become lame**: Arab. عرج · Maimonides, *Šarḥ fuṣūl Abūqrāṭ* · trans. Anonymous (*Pirqei Abuqraṭ*), 6.60 (352): אמר אבוקרט: מי שבאתהו כאב מיושן בירכיו ונשמטה ירכו ודאי יצטמק רגלו מכל וכל ואם לא יכוה יהיה צולע. → NM 3:192.

צֵלָע • *Plur.*[1] **צלעים • תחת הצלעים** → תַּחַת.

• *Plur.*[2] **צלעות • צלעות אמצע החזה** ‣ **false ribs**: Arab. أضلاع الزور · Ibn Sīnā, *K. al-Qānūn fī al-ṭibb* · trans. Joseph Lorki (*Sefer ha-Qanun*), bk. 1 (fol. 12^{a}): ואמנם הה׳ הקצרים

הנשארים הם עצמות האחור וצלעות אמצע החזה נבראו ראשיהם דבקים נבדלים כדי להיות בטוחים מהשבירה בשעת ההכאה. → NM 4:172.

• **כאב תחת הצלעות** → **כְּאֵב**.

• **צלעות כוזבות** · **false ribs**: Arab. أضلاع الزور · Ibn Sīnā, *K. al-Qānūn fī al-ṭibb* · trans. Nathan ha-Me'ati (*Sefer ha-Qanun*), bk. 1 (fol. 36[b]): ואמנם החמשה המקוצרות הנשארות הנה הם עצמות האחור וצלעות הכוזבות נבראו ראשיהם מחוברים בשחוסים לבטוח מן ההשבר בעת הנגיפה. → NM 4:172–3.

• **מה שתחת הצלעות** → **תַּחַת**.

צַלְעוּת · **lameness**: Arab. عرج · Al-Zahrāwī, *K. al-taṣrīf li-man ʿağiza ʿan at-taʾlīf* · trans. Shem Tov ben Isaac (*Sefer ha-Shimmush*), bk. 30, 3.14 (fol. 235[b]): ואם יחובש אחד מהם מבלי התחבר אליו השוק האחר על כל פנים יקרה לבעליו צלעות מתמיד. → NM 1:111.

צִמּוּק · **marasmus**: Arab. ذبول · Maimonides, *K. al-fuṣūl fī al-ṭibb* · trans. Nathan ha-Me'ati (*Sefer ha-Peraqim*), 22.44: וקרבת החתולים ועורותיהם מוריש הצמוק והשדפון. → NM 2:76–7.

• **קדחות הצמוק והכחש** → **קַדַּחַת**.

• *Plur.* **צמוקים** (also: **צמוקין**) • **צמוקי ההר** · **(lit., mountain raisins); (seeds of) stavesacre** [***Delphinium staphisagria*** **L.;** ***Ranunculaceae***]: a) Arab. زبيب الجبل · Ibn al-Jazzār, *Zād al-musāfir wa-qūt al-ḥādir* · trans. Moses ibn Tibbon (*Sefer Ṣedat ha-Derakhim*), bk. 1, ch. 1 (fol. 6[b]): או יטוח אותו בבשר קולוקונטידא אחר שיודק בחומץ ושמן או יטוח בצמוקי ההר כמו כן. → NM 4:173.

b) Arab. حبّ الرأس · Al-Rāzī, *K. al-Manṣūrī* · trans. Shem Tov ben Isaac (*Sefer Almansur*), Mem 14 (52): מיובזג ובלע' אישטאפיזקרא או קפאפורגא והוא חב ⟨א⟩ל ראס והוא צמוקי ההר. → NM 2:17.

• **הצמוקין השמשיים** · **raisins**: Lat. uvae passae (Honofredi) · Ibn Zuhr, *Regimen of Health* · trans. Jacob ibn Tibbon (*Hanhagat ha-Beri'ut le-Abu ʿAli ben Zuhr*), ch. 10: אולם שמירת האצטומ' יהיה בעשית הקיא פעם אחת בחדש שהוא ינקה אותה ממותרי המאכל ומהליחות הרעות, ובאכילת הצמוקין השמשיים בגרעיניו על הצום שהוא יחזק אותה ויתקן המזגים הרעים אשר בה. → NM 4:173.

צָמַח · **to grow [together again]**: Lat. augeor (Articella); cresco (Ravenna) · Hippocrates, *Aphorisms* · trans. Hillel ben Samuel, 7.28 (380) (fol. 46[a]): א"א: כל עצם או תנוך נשבר בגוף לא יצמח. → NM 3:193.

• *Inf.* **צְמֹחַ** • **צמוח השיער בבית הערוה** · **puberty**: Arab. نبات الشعر في العانة · Maimonides, *Šarḥ fuṣūl Abūqrāṭ* · trans. Zeraḥyah Ḥen (*Pirqei Abuqraṭ*), 5.7 (227): אמר בקראט: מי שמצאו הויציאו הנק' בערבי אלצרע קודם צמוח השיער בבית הערוה יתחדש לו העתק. → NM 3:193.

• **צמח השער בשפל הבטן** · **puberty**: Arab. إنبات الشعر في العانة / Gr. ἥβη · Maimonides, *Šarḥ fuṣūl Abūqrāṭ* · trans. Moses ibn Tibbon (*Pirqei Abuqraṭ*), 3.28 (134): אמר אבקראט: ורוב מה שיקרה לנערים מן החליים יבא בקצתו הנקיון בארבעים יום ובקצתו בשבעה חדשים ובקצתו בשבע שנים ובקצתו כאשר גמרו לצמח השער בשפל הבטן ואולם מה שישאר מן החליים שלא יתך בזמן הצמיחה או בנקבות בעת שיגר מהן דם הנדות הנה מדרכם שיאריכו. → NM 3:193–4.

צֶמַח ‣ I. **abscess; imposthume; the separation of corrupt matter into an ulcer**: a) Lat. apostema / Gr. ἀπόστημα · Bruno Longobucco, *Cyrurgia Magna* · trans. Hillel ben Samuel (*Sefer Keritut*), fol. 45[a]: עוד בעבור שכל כאב מקבץ הריאומה ששם נעשה הנפח והצמח שבעבורם יבוא הקווץ אל נקלה. → NM 1:36–7.

b) Arab. خراج · Al-Zahrāwī, *K. al-taṣrīf li-man ʿağiza ʿan at-taʾlīf* · trans. Shem Tov ben Isaac (*Sefer ha-Shimmush*), bk. 30, 2.45 (fol. 216[a]): ואומר כי הצמח יהיה עמו חמימות וקדחת ומכאובים מקיפים אותו מפה ומפה עד שתשקוט רתיחת המותר ויגמר העפוש ואז תשקוט הקדחת והחמימות. → NM 1:111.

‣ II. **inflammation**: Hippocrates, *Aphorisms* · trans. Doʾeg ha-Edomi (*Sefer Agur*), 3.24 (130) (fol. 56[a]): אמר אפוקרט: קטנים ונערים ויונקי שדיים יחול עליהם שחין צומח בפה ובחך ועל שפתם קיח ושעול ותעורה ופחד קבוץ לחות וצמח בטבורם גם באזניהם. → NM 3:194.

‣ III. **pustule**: Arab. بثر · Maimonides, *K. al-fuṣūl fī al-ṭibb* · trans. Nathan ha-Meʾati (*Sefer ha-Peraqim*), 6.71: מי שיהיו בו נגעי המעים ויקרה לו צמא חזק ויתראה אחורי אזניו צמח שחור דומה לגרגיר הכרסינה ימות. → NM 2:77.

• **צמח אדום** ‣ **erysipelas**: Hippocrates, *Aphorisms* · trans. Doʾeg ha-Edomi (*Sefer Agur*), 5.43 (263) (fol. 88[b]): עלה צמח אדום ברחם אשה הרה אות רע הוא. → NM 3:194.

• **צמח בבשר דומה לדמיון הבשר** ‣ **buboes**: Hippocrates, *Aphorisms* · trans. Doʾeg ha-Edomi (*Sefer Agur*), 4.55 (192) (fol. 72[b]): פעמים יקרה לעלות עם קדחת צמח בבשר דומה לדמיון הבשר אות רע אם לא תהיה קדחת יום. → NM 3:195.

• **צמח חזירי** ‣ **scrofulous tumor**: Arab. ورم خنزيري · Al-Zahrāwī, *K. al-taṣrīf li-man ʿağiza ʿan at-taʾlīf* · trans. Shem Tov ben Isaac (*Sefer ha-Shimmush*), bk. 30, introduction (fol. 201[b]): וזה שראיתי רופא איש בער לא ידע וכסיל לא יבין את זאת שבקע על צמח חזירי בצואר אשה וחתך בבערותו קצת ורידי הצואר והוא לא ידע והרעיף דם האשה עד שנפלה בין ידיו ומתה. → NM 1:111.

• **צמח במוח** ‣ **phrenitis**: Arab. برسام · Maimonides, *Šarḥ fuṣūl Abūqrāṭ* · trans. Anonymous (*Pirqei Abuqraṭ*), 7.12 (364): אמר אבוקרט: ומן מדוה הריאה מדוח חשרסם חוא צמח במוח. → NM 3:195.

• **צמח אשר צמח במוח הראש** ‣ **an inflammation of the brain (phrenitis)**: Hippocrates, *Aphorisms* · trans. Doʾeg ha-Edomi (*Sefer Agur*), 4.72 (209) (fol. 77[a]): שב השתן להיות לבן רע הוא ואף כי בסובלי קדחת הבאה מצמח אשר צמח במוח הראש. → NM 3:194–5.

• **נתבעבע הצמח** → [**בעבע**].

• **צמח העין** ‣ **ophthalmia**: Arab. رمد · Maimonides, *Šarḥ fuṣūl Abūqrāṭ* · trans. Anonymous (*Pirqei Abuqraṭ*), 6.17 (309): כשהיה באדם צמח העין הנקרא רמד בער׳ ובאתהו שלשול זהו משובח. → NM 3:195.

צְמִיחָה ‣ **swelling**: Arab. ورم · Maimonides, *Šarḥ fuṣūl Abūqrāṭ* · trans. Anonymous (*Pirqei Abuqraṭ*), 4.55 (192): אמר המפרש: כשהיתה סבת הקדחת מורסת ההאלבין והדומה לו מן הבשר הרך יהיה קדחת יומית. אמנם כשהיתה לקדחת סבה אחרת ונתחבר עמה צמיחת ההאלבין והדומה לו אז הוא אות רע. → NM 3:195–6.

• **צמיחת השער בגב הערוה** ‣ **puberty**: Arab. نبات الشعر في العانة · Hippocrates, *Aphorisms* ·

trans. Nathan ha-Me'ati, 5.7 (227) (fol. 86[b]): אמר אבוקרט: מי שימצאהו כפיון קודם צמיחת השער בגב הערוה הנה יתחדש לו העתק. → NM 3:196.

• **צמיחת השער סביב הערוה** · **puberty**: Arab. نبات الشعر في العانة · Maimonides, *Šarḥ fuṣūl Abūqrāṭ* · trans. Moses ibn Tibbon (*Pirqei Abuqraṭ*), 5.7 (227): אמר אבקראט: מי שמצאו חולי הנופל קודם צמיחת השער סביב הערוה הנה יתחדש לו העתק. → NM 3:196.

• **צמיחת השער בתחתון** · **puberty**: Hippocrates, *Aphorisms* · trans. Judah Shalom, 3.28 (134) (Ms. Paris, BN, héb. 1113, fol. 47[b]): ורבים מחוליי הילדים יוגבלו קצתם בארבעים יום וקצתם בשבעה חדשים וקצתם בשבע שנים וקצתם יבואו אל צמיחת השער בתחתון וכל אחד מן החליים הנשארים בילדים שיהיו בלתי נתכים בעת צמיחת התחתון או בנשים בעת הגרת הוסת דרכם להאריך מאד. → NM 3:196.

[צמק] • *Part. Pu'al* **מְצֻמָּק** · **suffering from marasmus**: Arab. مذبول · Maimonides, *K. al-fuṣūl fī al-ṭibb* · trans. Nathan ha-Me'ati (*Sefer ha-Peraqim*), 19.34: המצומקים וכל מי שיגבר עליו היובש אינו צריך במרחץ לאויר חם אבל אל מי האמבטי אשר בתכלית השווי. → NM 2:61.

• *Hitpa'el* **הִצְטַמֵּק** · **to boil down; to thicken**: Arab. طبخ · Al-Zahrāwī, *K. al-taṣrīf li-man 'ağiza 'an at-ta'līf* · trans. Shem Tov ben Isaac (*Sefer ha-Shimmush*), bk. 27, fol. 127[a], col. b: העדשים המבושלים בבשר החי ראוי לבשלם על זה התאר והוא לקחת מן הבשר השמן ולבשלו במה שיכסהו מן המים שתי פעמים ולהסיר חלאתו ולבשל מן העדשים הלבנים הקלופים בעשרה כמותם ממים מתוקים בקדרה אחרת ולתבל הבשר בכוסבר הלח ובצלים ועץ של שבת ושרשי כרשין וכשיצטמקו העדשים לשפוך מימיהם ולרחצם במים אחרים חמים. → NM 4:173–4.

צֶמֶר • **זוהמת הצמר** → זֻהֲמָה.

צִנּוֹר • **צנור הכיור** · **spout**: Arab. أنبوب · Ibn al-Jazzār, *Zād al-musāfir wa-qūt al-ḥādir* · trans. Moses ibn Tibbon (*Sefer Ṣedat ha-Derakhim*), bk. 1, ch. 10 (fol. 16[b]): וירחץ הראש במים שנתבשלו בהם קמומילא ואניט וקורונא ריאל ותהיה יציאת המים מצנור הכיור כדי שיפליג תוך הראש יותר. → NM 4:174.

• *Plur.* **צנורות** • **צנורות הגידים** · **mesentery**: Arab. جداول العروق · Ibn Sīnā, *K. al-Qānūn fī al-ṭibb* · trans. Joseph Lorki (*Sefer ha-Qanun*), bk. 1 (fol. 18[b]): ואח״כ יחלק מן הגיד הדופק הגדול הזה שני גידים דופקים יפרדו בצנורות הגידים אשר סביב המעי הישר. → NM 4:174.

צִנִּי • **ציניי ותריסי** · **shield-shaped; thyroid [cartilage]**: Arab. درقي · Ibn Sīnā, *K. al-Qānūn fī al-ṭibb* · trans. Nathan ha-Me'ati (*Sefer ha-Qanun*), bk. 1 (fol. 46[b]): והוא מחובר משחוסים שלשה אחד מהם שחוס אשר ישיגהו החוש קדם הגרון ותחת הזקן ונקרא הדרקי הציניי והתריסי בהיות מקוער מפנים מגובן החוץ ודומה הצנה והתריס. → NM 4:174.

[צער] • *Part. Hitpa'el* **מִצְטַעֵר** • **תנועה מצטערת** → תְּנוּעָה.

צַעַר · I. **disturbance**: Arab. اضطراب / Gr. ταραχή · Maimonides, *Šarḥ fuṣūl Abūqrāṭ* · trans. Moses ibn Tibbon (*Pirqei Abuqraṭ*), 7.33 (385): אמר אבקראט: מי שהיה שתנו משובש יורה כי בגופו צער חזק. → NM 3:196–7.

· II. **sleeplessness**: Arab. أرق · Ibn al-Jazzār, *Zād al-musāfir wa-qūt al-ḥādir* · trans. Moses ibn Tibbon (*Sefer Ṣedat ha-Derakhim*), bk. 1, ch. 18 (fol. 26[a]): מורסת הראש במאמר מוחלט היא מורסא חמה תקרה בקצת קרומות המוח ישיגהו תמיד צער ושגעון וערבוב השכל. → NM 4:175.

• **צער באסטומכא** · an upset stomach: Arab. قلق في المعدة · Al-Zahrāwī, *K. al-taṣrīf li-man ʿağiza ʿan at-taʾlīf* · trans. Shem Tov ben Isaac (*Sefer ha-Shimmush*), bk. 27, fol. 144[a], col. a: ואם לא יתעכל וירגיש בכבדות וצער באסטומכא וגעש נפסד ותעורה וצרות הנשימה ורוגז ראוי לעורר הקיא. → NM 4:175.

צָפַד • *Part.* **צוֹפֵד** · agglutinant; gluey: Lat. glutinativus · Armengaud Blaise, *Tabula Antidotarii* · trans. Estori ha-Parḥi (*Shemot ha-Mashqim*), 19 (59): דיאה דרגאגן דרגאגאן שרף קר בשנייה לח בראשונה צופד ומדבק. → NM 4:175.

צִפּוֹר • *Plur.* **צפרים** · sparrows: Arab. عصافير · Maimonides, *K. al-fuṣūl fī al-ṭibb* · trans. Nathan ha-Me'ati (*Sefer ha-Peraqim*), 20.69: הצפרים מועילים מן הרפיון והפאלג והלקוה וכאיבי השקוי ומוסיפים בחוזק המשגל. → NM 2:77.

צפורן → **צִפֹּרֶן**.

צִפֹּרֶן · ungula (i.e., pterygium): Arab. ظفرة · a) Al-Zahrāwī, *K. al-taṣrīf li-man ʿağiza ʿan at-taʾlīf* · trans. Shem Tov ben Isaac (*Sefer ha-Shimmush*), bk. 30, 2.16 (fol. 211[a]): הצפורן תהיה על שני מינים עצביית דומה לקרום דק או בלתי עצביית דומה ללחות קפוי לבן. → NM 1:111–2.

b) Maimonides, *K. al-fuṣūl fī al-ṭibb* · trans. Zeraḥyah Ḥen (*Sefer ha-Peraqim*), 15.24: רפואת הציפורן אשר תהיה בעין בעודנו קטון יהיה בדברים מטהרים כרפואת הגרב כשתוסיף ותתקשה אז תרפא בברזל. → NM 1:182.

• **צפורן סוסית** · coltsfoot [*Tussilago farfara* L.]: Lat. ungula caballina · Armengaud Blaise, *Tabula Antidotarii* · trans. Estori ha-Parḥi (*Shemot ha-Mashqim*), 26 (73): נינופארנום נינופאר פרח צפורן סוסית קרה ולחה בשלישית. → NM 4:175.

• *Plur.* **צפרנים** • **לובן הצפרנים** → **לֹבֶן**.

• **סיג הצפרנים** → **סִיג**.

צָרֶבֶת · eschar: Arab. خشكريشة · Maimonides, *K. al-fuṣūl fī al-ṭibb* · trans. Nathan ha-Me'ati (*Sefer ha-Peraqim*), 15.9: וגם יאותו הרפואות האלה לעלה הידועה בגחלת כשיונחו על מקום הכשברישה הוא הצרבת כי זה המקום אשר יגיעהו העפוש שאין ראוי שיונחו על מה שהוא סביביו. → NM 2:77–8.

[צרד] • *Hifʿil* **הִצְרִיד** · to make [the voice] hoarse: Lat. rautifico (Honofredi) · Ibn Zuhr, *Regimen of Health* · trans. Jacob ibn Tibbon (*Hanhagat ha-Beri'ut le-Abu ʿAli ben Zuhr*), ch. 9: ואמרו הרופאים: אכילת אזביב השמשיים בבלתי גרעין על הצום יחזק קנה שלו ובהרחקת תבשילים מלוחים מאד שהם ישאירו לכלוך בקנה ויצרידו הקול. → NM 4:175–6.

צָרוּת • **צרות הניפוש** · orthopnea: Arab. ضيق النفس · a) Maimonides, *K. al-fuṣūl fī al-ṭibb* · trans. Zeraḥyah Ḥen (*Sefer ha-Peraqim*), 3.76: החליים הארוכים כמו צרות הניפוש והחול והטחורים באף והחבלות הרעות ודומיהם כי רוב אילו הכאבים אשר יתילדו לנערים ולילדים יתרפאו עד מ׳ יום. → NM 1:182.

b) Maimonides, *K. al-fuṣūl fī al-ṭibb* · trans. Zeraḥyah Ḥen (*Sefer ha-Peraqim*), 23.79: החולי הנקרא צרות הניפוש ועוצר הניפוש בייחוד הוא החולי המתחדש מלחויות עבות דבקות עומדות בחלקי קנה הריאה וזה השם אמנם יפול על זה החולי ביחוד. → NM 1:182.

• **צרות הנשימה** · orthopnea: Arab. ضيق النفس · Al-Zahrāwī, *K. al-taṣrīf li-man ʿağiza ʿan* *at-ta'līf* · trans. Shem Tov ben Isaac (*Sefer ha-Shimmush*), bk. 27, fol. 132[a], col. b: והחוג והרעישה וכבדות כל הגוף וצרות הנשימה הממית בעליו באורך הזמן. → NM 4:176.

צֳרִי · **antidote; theriac**: Lat. tiriaca · Ibn Sīnā, *K. al-adwiya al-qalbiya* · trans. Anonymous (*Sefer ha-Refu'ot ha-Libbiyot*), fols. 248[b]–249[a]: דרוניקש: חם ויבש בתחלת המדרגה השנית ובו סגולה חזקה מאד בחזוק הלב ולשמחו ולה אינו מנגד שום הפעולות ועוזרת בצריותו ומה שיש בו מעפיצות דק ומפני זה הוא צרי כל הארסים. → NM 4:176.

• סַם → **הסם הצרי**.

צְרִידוּת • **צרידות קול** · **hoarseness**: Arab. بحوحة · Hippocrates, *Aphorisms* · trans. Nathan ha-Me'ati, 2.40 (92) (fol. 36[a]): אמר אבוקרט: מי שיקרה לו צרידות קול ונזלים לזקן התש כח לא יחשב שיתבשל. → NM 3:197.

צֳרִיּוּת · **having theriacal (antidotal) property**: Lat. tiriacalitas · Ibn Sīnā, *K. al-adwiya al-qalbiya* · trans. Anonymous (*Sefer ha-Refu'ot ha-Libbiyot*), fol. 246[b]: והסמים המחזקים לצריותם נכנסים בכל רפואת הלב לפי שהם נאותים בסגולה לטבע האנושי. → NM 4:176.

צָרַעַת • **הצרעת הגדמיית** · **elephantiasis**: Arab. الجذام · Maimonides, *K. al-fuṣūl fī al-ṭibb* · trans. Nathan ha-Me'ati (*Sefer ha-Peraqim*), 9.98: מן החליים השחוריים המתחדשים בעור הגרב והתקלפות העור וכשיתחדש בבשר או בעורקים יקרא סרטאן. והצרעת הגדמיית גם כן רוב התחדשותה מדם שחוריי. → NM 2:78.

ק

[קבב] • *Piʿel* קִבֵּב ‧ I. **to bend one's head**: Arab. انكبّ ‧ Ibn al-Jazzār, *Zād al-musāfir wa-qūt al-ḥādir* ‧ trans. Moses ibn Tibbon (*Sefer Ṣedat ha-Derakhim*), bk. 2, ch. 14 (fol. 54^b): ואם היה מפני חום נצוה החולה לעשות דברים קרים דקים כמו קבוב על אד המים שנתבשל בהם קאממילא ורדים והדס או יקבב על עשן אבן מחוממת אחר שיזה עליו חומץ יין. → NM 4:176–7.

‧ II. **to produce pronation**: Arab. أكبّ ‧ Ibn Sīnā, *K. al-Qānūn fī al-ṭibb* ‧ trans. Nathan ha-Me'ati (*Sefer ha-Qanun*), bk. 1 (fol. 50^a): ואמנם המקבב הוא זוג המונח מחוץ. → NM 4:177.

קֵבָה • קיבת האשה ‧ **female pudenda**: Arab. فرج المرأة ‧ Al-Zahrāwī, *K. al-taṣrīf li-man ʿağiza ʿan at-taʾlīf* ‧ trans. Shem Tov ben Isaac (*Sefer ha-Shimmush*), bk. 30, 3.18 (fol. 236^a): שער י״ח בשבר קיבת האשה ועצם הזקן התחתון ואמת האיש. → NM 1:112.

• כאב הקיבה → כְּאֵב.

קִבּוּב ‧ **pronation**: Arab. كبّ ‧ Ibn Sīnā, *K. al-Qānūn fī al-ṭibb* ‧ trans. Nathan ha-Me'ati (*Sefer ha-Qanun*), bk. 1 (fol. 50^a): וכשיתנועעו אלו השנים יפשיט⟨ו⟩ הרסג פשוט עם מעט קבוב. → NM 4:177.

קָבוּץ (*Pass. Part.*) → קָבַץ.

קִבּוּץ ‧ I. **astringency**: Arab. قبْض ‧ a) Ibn al-Jazzār, *Zād al-musāfir wa-qūt al-ḥādir* ‧ trans. Moses ibn Tibbon (*Sefer Ṣedat ha-Derakhim*), bk. 7, 26.2: וזאת ההרכבה נאותה לגופות הקשים כשיצטרכו מן הקבוץ אל שעור יותר נוסף. → NM 1:66.

b) Maimonides, *K. al-fuṣūl fī al-ṭibb*‧ trans. Zeraḥyah Ḥen (*Sefer ha-Peraqim*), 13.45: מדבריו: כל המשלשלים כל אשר תרחצם יפחות פעולתם וכן כשתרתיחם. וכל אשר תשחקם היטב יהיה הזקם יותר מתועלתם בפעולת השלשול ואם המשלשל יהיה בטוח ירבה השתן וכל העוצרים יהיו הפך כי כל אשר תרחץ המשלשל והארכת בישולו תוסיף קיבוץ וכן כל אשר תשחקנו יוסיף קביצה ועוצר לשתן כמו כן. → NM 1:182.

‧ II. **collection (accumulation [of residues])**: Lat. collectio / Arab. جمْع ‧ Galen, *De inaequali intemperie* ‧ trans. David Caslari (*Sefer Roʿa Mezeg Mitḥallef*), 3.2: אמנם אחר בישול אותו המותר ימשכו שני אלו עניינים: האחד הוא התילדות מוגלא ואחר קיבוץ. → NM 2:168.

‧ III. **density**: Arab. كثافة ‧ Maimonides, *K. al-fuṣūl fī al-ṭibb* ‧ trans. Nathan ha-Me'ati (*Sefer ha-Peraqim*), 7.40: הרפרוף סבתו רוח עב נעצר במקום סתום הנקבים שלא ימצא מקום להמלט ולא יוכל להיות נתך בשביל עביו ולא ימצא מקום להמלט ולצאת בשביל קבוץ חלקי הגשמים המקיפים אותו. → NM 2:78.

‧ IV. **flexion**: Arab. انقباض ‧ Ibn Sīnā, *K. al-Qānūn fī al-ṭibb* ‧ trans. Zeraḥyah Ḥen (*Sefer ha-Qanun*), bk. 1 (fol. 27^b): והושם האצבע מקצר בקבוץ על מושקלי אחד. → NM 4:177.

• **קבוץ הגידים** ‧ **spasm**: Hippocrates, *Aphorisms* ‧ trans. Do'eg ha-Edomi (*Sefer Agur*), 2.26 (78) (fol. 73^a): יעיד קבוץ הגידים בבוא קדחת אחריהם טוב וההפך רע. → NM 3:197.

• **קבוץ עב טיט** ‧ **empyema**: Hippocrates, *Aphorisms* ‧ trans. Do'eg ha-Edomi (*Sefer

הנצל מחולי הגרון זהו אשקננציאה אם יהפך לבוא אל הריאה לז' :(Agur), 5.10 (230) (fol. 82[b]) ימים ימות ואם יעברם נעשה אמפיסיש זהו קבוץ עב טיט. → NM 3:197.

קְבִיצָה · **astringency**: Arab. قبّض · Maimonides, *K. al-fuṣūl fī al-ṭibb* · trans. Zeraḥyah Ḥen (*Sefer ha-Peraqim*), 13.45: מדבריו: כל המשלשלים כל אשר תרחצם יפחות פעולתם וכן כשתרתיחם. וכל אשר תשחקם היטב יהיה הזקם יותר מתועלתם בפעולת השלשול ואם המשלשל יהיה בטוח ירבה השתן וכל העוצרים יהיו הפך כי כל אשר תרחץ המשלשל והארכת בישולו תוסיף קיבוץ וכן כל אשר תשחקנו יוסיף קביצה ועוצר לשתן כמו כן. → NM 1:183.

קְבִיצוּת · I. **astringency**: Arab. قبض · Maimonides, *K. al-fuṣūl fī al-ṭibb* · trans. Nathan ha-Me'ati (*Sefer ha-Peraqim*), 9.71: ההנדבי המדברי והגניי הגובר על מזגם קור מועט ובהם יש עם זה מעט ממרירות שני המינים יחד קובצים קביצות שוה. → NM 2:78.

· II. **flexion**: Arab. قبض · Ibn Sīnā, *K. al-Qānūn fī al-ṭibb* · trans. Nathan ha-Me'ati (*Sefer ha-Qanun*), bk. 1 (fol. 51[b]): ואמנם התחתון ממנו הנה קביצותם עם ירידה והשפלה ואמנם העליון הנה קביצותו עם מעט הגבהה והרמה. → NM 4:177.

[קבל] • *Pu'al* **קֻבַּל** • **קובל מופת על** · **to be concluded to**: Arab. استدلّ على · Hippocrates, *Aphorisms* · trans. Nathan ha-Me'ati, 1.23 (50) (fol. 18[a]): אמר אבוקרט: אין ראוי שיקובל מופת על שעור מה שראוי שיורק מן הגוף מרבויו. → NM 3:197–8.

קַבָּלָה · **flexion**: Arab. قبض · Ibn Sīnā, *K. al-Qānūn fī al-ṭibb* · trans. Zeraḥyah Ḥen (*Sefer ha-Qanun*), bk. 1 (fol. 27[b]): והנמוך מהם קבלתו עם הכנעה וחוסר והעליון קבלתו עם מעט הרמה ונשיאות. → NM 4:177.

[קבס] • *Part. Nif'al* **נִקְבָּס** · **someone suffering from indigestion**: Arab. المتخوم · Al-Zahrāwī, *K. al-taṣrīf li-man 'ağiza 'an at-ta'līf* · trans. Shem Tov ben Isaac (*Sefer ha-Shimmush*), bk. 30, 2.95 (fol. 230[a]): ואין ראוי להקיז הנקבס עד סור הקבסתו. → NM 1:112.

קִבְסָא (*Aram.*) (also: **קִבְסָה**) · I. **dyspepsia; indigestion**: Arab. تخمة · Maimonides, *K. al-fuṣūl fī al-ṭibb* · trans. Nathan ha-Me'ati (*Sefer ha-Peraqim*), 2.24: הקבסא הרצופה זו אחר זו היא גדולת הכח להוליד הכימוסים ולהוליד החוליים בין שתהיה הקבסא ממאכלים טובי הכימוס ובין שתהיה מרעי הכימוס. → NM 2:78–9.

· II. **eructation**: Arab. جشاء / Gr. ὀξυρεγμία · Maimonides, *Šarḥ fuṣūl Abūqrāṭ* · trans. Moses ibn Tibbon (*Pirqei Abuqraṭ*), 6.1 (293): אמר אבקראט: כשתתחדש הקבסה החמוצה בחולי אשר תקרא קלוח המעים אחר הארכו ולא היתה כן קודם זה הנה היא אות טוב. → NM 3:198.

· III. **nausea**: Arab. غثيان · Ibn al-Jazzār, *Zād al-musāfir wa-qūt al-ḥāḍir* · trans. Moses ibn Tibbon (*Sefer Ṣedat ha-Derakhim*), bk. 7, 9.4: וזאת הרפואה כשישתה אותה ולא יקח אחריה סם המות תעמוד במקומה ואם ישתה אחריה סם ממית תחדש קבסא ויצטרך הסם הממית אשר שתה לצאת בקיא מכח המרקחת. → NM 1:66.

• **גורם קבסא** → **גֹּרֵם**.

קִבְסָה → **קִבְסָא**.

[קבע] • *Part. Nif'al* **נִקְבָּע** • **הקדחת הנקבעת** → **קַדַּחַת**.

קָבַץ · I. **to be astringent**: Arab. قبض · Maimonides, *K. al-fuṣūl fī al-ṭibb* · trans. Nathan ha-Me'ati (*Sefer ha-Peraqim*), 9.48: כשיותר הטבע מבעל הקבסא בפתילה או בחוקן אז תזון העלול מיד בשעתו במה שלא יקבץ כלל. → NM 2:79.

‣ II. **to draw together; to flex**: Arab. قبض · Ibn Sīnā, *K. al-Qānūn fī al-ṭibb* · trans. Nathan ha-Me'ati (*Sefer ha-Qanun*), bk. 1 (fol. 55[a]): ואמנם העצלים המניעים האצבעות בקובצים. → NM 4:178.

• *Part.* **קוֹבֵץ** ‣ **astringent**: Arab. قابض · a) Maimonides, *K. al-fuṣūl fī al-ṭibb* · trans. Zeraḥyah Ḥen (*Sefer ha-Peraqim*), 8.63: האסטומכא והכבד יותר צריכים משאר האברים אל דברים קובצים. → NM 1:183; corr. 2:198.

b) Maimonides, *K. al-fuṣūl fī al-ṭibb* · trans. Nathan ha-Me'ati (*Sefer ha-Peraqim*), 9.37: רפואות רקיקת הדם הם אותם שיחוברו מסמנים מנגבים מבלי עקיצה וסמנים יש בהם קצת המעדה וסמנים קובצים. → NM 2:81.

• **הסם הקובץ** → **סַם**.

• *Pass. Part.* **קָבוּץ** ‣ **contracted; shrivelled**: Arab. منقبض · Ibn al-Jazzār, *Zād al-musāfir wa-qūt al-ḥādir* · trans. Moses ibn Tibbon (*Sefer Ṣedat ha-Derakhim*), bk. 2, ch. 17 (fol. 57[a]): ואם ראינו הלשון אדומה מאד הנה הוא אות חום ואם לבנה מאד הנה הוא אות הקור ואם תהיה רכה עם לחות הרבה בה הוא אות לחות ואם היתה נגובה מאד קבוצה הוא אות יובש. → NM 4:178.

• *Pi'el* **קִבֵּץ** ‣ I. **to brace**: Arab. جمع / Gr. συνίστημι · Maimonides, *Šarḥ fuṣūl Abūqrāṭ* · trans. Moses ibn Tibbon (*Pirqei Abuqraṭ*), 3.17 (123): אמר אבקראט: ואולם עניני האויר בכל יום ויום מה שהיה מהם צפוני הנה הוא יקבץ הגופות ויאמצם ויחזקם ויחזק תנועותיהם ויפה מראיהם ויזכך השמע להם וייבש הבטן ויחדש בעיניים עקיצה. → NM 3:198–9.

‣ II. **to draw together; to flex**: Arab. قبض · Ibn Sīnā, *K. al-Qānūn fī al-ṭibb* · trans. Nathan ha-Me'ati (*Sefer ha-Qanun*), bk. 1 (fol. 49[b]): העצלים המניעים הקנה יש מהם שיקבצוהו ומהם שימתחוהו. → NM 4:178.

• *Part. Pu'al* **מְקֻבָּץ** • **מקובץ החלקים** ‣ **dense**: Arab. متكاثف · Hippocrates, *Aphorisms* · trans. Nathan ha-Me'ati, 5.62 (282) (fol. 101[a]): אמר אבוקרט: כשיהיה רחם האשה קר ומקובץ החלקים אז לא תתעבר. → NM 3:138.

קָבָר • **לחם קיבר** → **לֶחֶם**.

קַדַּחַת • **הקדחת הבאה בכל יום** ‣ **quotidian fever**: Arab. الحمّى النائبة في كلّ يوم · Maimonides, *K. al-fuṣūl fī al-ṭibb* · trans. Nathan ha-Me'ati (*Sefer ha-Peraqim*), 10.19: מיני הקדחות הפוסקות המסתלקות סלוק נרגש הם שלשה והם השלישית והבאה בכל יום הנקראת תמידית כלומר קוטידיאנא והרביעית. → NM 2:79.

• **הקדחת הדבקה** ‣ **continuous fever**: Arab. الحمّى الدائمة · Maimonides, *K. al-fuṣūl fī al-ṭibb* · trans. Nathan ha-Me'ati (*Sefer ha-Peraqim*), 10.21: הקדחת הדבקה אע״פ שתנועתה כבדה ומתפשטת לארבעים יום אז היא גם כן נמנית מן החליים החדים. → NM 2:79; corr. 3:268.

• **קדחת דקה** ‣ **hectic fever**: Arab. حمّى الدقّ · Maimonides, *K. al-fuṣūl fī al-ṭibb* · trans. Nathan ha-Me'ati (*Sefer ha-Peraqim*), 3.27: רוע מזג המתחלף לפעמים יהיה בגוף כלו כשקוי הבשרי ובקדחות כלם לבד קדחת דקה. → NM 2:79–80.

• **וסתות הקדחת** → **וֶסֶת**.

• **קדחת חצי שלישית** ‣ **semi-tertian fever**: Arab. حمّى شطر الغبّ · Maimonides, *Šarḥ fuṣūl Abūqrāṭ* · trans. Moses ibn Tibbon (*Pirqei Abuqraṭ*), 4.43 (180): אמר המפרש: זאת אשר היא תמידית ותתחזק ותשוב שלישית אשר בה סכנה היא חצי שלישית. → NM 3:199.

• קדחת יום · **ephemeral fever**: Arab. حمّى يوم · Maimonides, *K. al-fuṣūl fī al-ṭibb* · trans. Nathan ha-Me'ati (*Sefer ha-Peraqim*), 4.23: וכשיהיה הדפק חזק וגדול נעדר הקושי הנה זה הוראה מבוארת שהיא קדחת יום. → NM 2:80.

• הקדחת הנקבעת · **the stable fever**: Lat. febris fixa / Arab. الحمّى المعروفة بالثابتة · Galen, *De inaequali intemperie* · trans. David Caslari (*Sefer Ro'a Mezeg Mitḥallef*), 1.1: אמר גליאינוס רוע מזג מתחלף לפעמ׳ יהיה בכל הגוף החי כמו מה שיקרה לאיזה איש באחד ממיני השיקוי, לא בכל שיקוי אלא באחד ממיניו ר״ל בבשרי ובאות(ה) הקדחת שיסבול החולה קור וחום בתכונה אחת שקורין היוונים אֵיפִּלא ובהרבה מהקדחות אחרות זולת הקדחת הנקבעת הנקראת שידפון. → NM 2:168.

• הקדחת העונה בכל יום · **quotidian fever**: Arab. الحمّى النائبة كلّ يوم · Maimonides, *K. al-fuṣūl fī al-ṭibb* · trans. Zeraḥyah Ḥen (*Sefer ha-Peraqim*), 8.65: אמנם הקדחת העונה בכל יום אי אפשר שתתחדש אלא עם חולי באסטומכא כמו שהרביעית אי אפשר שתתחדש אלא עם חולי הטחול. → NM 1:183.

• הקדחת שעונתה בכל יום · **quotidian fever**: Arab. الحمّى النائبة كلّ يوم · Maimonides, *K. al-fuṣūl fī al-ṭibb* (Medical *Aphorisms*)) · trans. Nathan ha-Me'ati (*Sefer ha-Peraqim*), 8.65: אמנם הקדחת שעונתה בכל יום לא יחשב שתתחדש אלא עם עלה באסטומכה כמו שהרביעית לא יחשב שתתחדש אלא עם עלת הטחול. → NM 2:80.

• הקדחת אשר יהיה עמה ערבוב השכל · **fever associated with mental confusion (phrenitis)**: Arab. الحمّى التي يكون معها اختلاط العقل / Gr. φρενῖτις · Maimonides, *Šarḥ fuṣūl Abūqrāṭ* · trans. Moses ibn Tibbon (*Pirqei Abuqraṭ*), 3.30 (136): אמר אבקראט: ואולם מי שעבר אלו השנים הנה יקרה לו הרנפלי וחלי הצד וחלי הריאה והקדחת אשר תהיה עמה היקיצה והקדחת אשר יהיה עמה ערבוב השכל והקדחת השורפת והשפיכה והשלשול הארוך וחמרמרות המעים וקלוח המעים ופתיחת פיות העורקים מלמטה. → NM 3:199.

• הקדחת הקיימת · **fixed fever (i.e., hectic fever)**: Lat. febris fixa / Arab. الحمّى الثابتة · Galen, *De inaequali intemperie* · trans. David Caslari (*Sefer Ro'a Mezeg Mitḥallef*), 6.4: ואולם אותה הקדחת הקיימת אשר היא מבנשאה(?) קיימת קיום חזק לא ירגישנה מי שיסבול אותה. → NM 2:169.

• קדחת רביעית · **quartan fever**: a) Hippocrates, *Aphorisms* · trans. Do'eg ha-Edomi (*Sefer Agur*), 2.25 (77) (fol. 40ª): יקל מדוה קדחת רביעית להרפא בקייץ ובחורף יארך עד הגיע ימי החום. → NM 3:199–200.

b) Arab. حمّى الربع · Maimonides, *K. al-fuṣūl fī al-ṭibb* · trans. Nathan ha-Me'ati (*Sefer ha-Peraqim*), 10.19: מיני הקדחות הפוסקות המסתלקות סלוק נרגש הם שלשה והם השלישית והבאה בכל יום הנקראת תמידית כלומר קוטידיאנא והרביעית. → NM 2:80.

• קדחת השדפון · **hectic fever**: Lat. febris etica / Arab. حمّى اقطيقوس · Galen, *De inaequali intemperie* · trans. David Caslari (*Sefer Ro'a Mezeg Mitḥallef*), 5.3: ולזה הוא שאין בעל אחת הקדחות מזה הסוג שקדם זכרה בסמוך ר״ל קדחת השדפון מרגיש בכאב וחולי ואין החולה מרגיש בה כלל. → NM 2:169.

• קדחת שדפונית · **febris fixa (i.e., hectic fever)**: Lat. febris fixa / Arab. الحمّى الثابتة · Galen, *De inaequali intemperie* · trans. David Caslari (*Sefer Ro'a Mezeg Mitḥallef*), 7.3: ובאמת

מהדברים שאינם למטה מזה בבאור שכל הקדחות המתארכות ימשך אחריהם קדחת שדפונית. → NM 2:169.

• **קדחת שלישית** › **tertian fever:** a) Hippocrates, *Aphorisms* · trans. Do'eg ha-Edomi (*Sefer Agur*), 4.59 (196) (fol. 73[b]): צרודה קדחת שלישית על הסובל עד תעבור עליו ז' פעמים ואם לא תעבור תתארך מאד. → NM 3:200.

b) Arab. حمّى الغبّ · Maimonides, *K. al-fuṣūl fī al-ṭibb* · trans. Nathan ha-Me'ati (*Sefer ha-Peraqim*), 10.19: מיני הקדחות הפוסקות המסתלקות סלוק נרגש הם שלשה והם השלישית והבאה בכל יום הנקראת תמידית כלומר קוטידיאנא והרביעית. → NM 2:80.

• *Plur.* **קדחות** • **קדחות מעורבות** › **mixed (irregular) fevers:** Arab. حمّيات مختلطة / Gr. πλάνητες · Maimonides, *Šarḥ fuṣūl Abūqrāṭ* · trans. Moses ibn Tibbon (*Pirqei Abuqraṭ*), 3.22 (128): אמר אבקראט: ואולם החורף הנה יקרה בו רוב חליי הקיץ וקדחות רבעיות ‹ו›מעורבות. → NM 3:200.

• **קדחות נבוכות** › **mixed (irregular) fevers:** Lat. febres errantes · Hippocrates, *Aphorisms* · trans. Hillel ben Samuel, 3.22 (128) (fol. 18[b]): א"א: בחרף יולדו מחליי הקיץ הרבה וקדחות רביעיות ונבוכות. → NM 3:200.

• **הקדחות הפוסקות** › **intermittent fevers:** Arab. الحمّيات المفارقة · Maimonides, *K. al-fuṣūl fī al-ṭibb* · trans. Nathan ha-Me'ati (*Sefer ha-Peraqim*), 10.19: מיני הקדחות הפוסקות המסתלקות סלוק נרגש הם שלשה והם השלישית והבאה בכל יום הנקראת תמידית כלומר קוטידיאנא והרביעית. → NM 2:80.

• **קדחות הצמוק והכחש** › **marasmic fevers:** Arab. حمّيات الذبول · Maimonides, *K. al-fuṣūl fī al-ṭibb* · trans. Nathan ha-Me'ati (*Sefer ha-Peraqim*), 10.60: ברוב אנחנו מוצאים שקדחות דקות וקדחות הצמוק והכחש מתחדשות כשיהיה הפגע באמת דבק בלב ובעורקי הכבד ואחריהם האסטומכה. → NM 2:80–1.

קָדַם • *Part.* **קוֹדֵם** • **הקודם מן הראש** › **the front of the head:** Arab. مقدّم الرأس · Ibn al-Jazzār, *Zād al-musāfir wa-qūt al-ḥāḍir* · trans. Moses ibn Tibbon (*Sefer Ṣedat ha-Derakhim*), bk. 1, ch. 10 (fol. 16[b]): ואם היה כאב הראש מחום השמש ושריפתו ראוי שיוצק על הקודם מן הראש שמן ורדים מעורב במים קר"ט או בחומץ יין. → NM 4:179.

• *Hif'il* **הִקְדִּים** › **to order:** Arab. تقدّم · Maimonides, *K. al-fuṣūl fī al-ṭibb* · trans. Zeraḥyah Ḥen (*Sefer ha-Peraqim*), 9.48: ותעשה זה ביום השני ותקדים החולה בהכנסת המרחץ. → NM 1:183.

• *Inf. Hif'il* **הַקְדִּים** • **הקדים הגזר דין** › **to predict:** Arab. التقدّم بالقضية · Maimonides, *Šarḥ fuṣūl Abūqrāṭ* · trans. Zeraḥyah Ḥen (*Pirqei Abuqraṭ*), 2.19 (71): להקדים הגזר דין בחליים החדים על מות או על בריאות אינך בו על תכלית הבטחון. → NM 3:200–1.

[קדר] • *Hif'il* **הִקְדִּיר** › **to benumb; to have a narcotic effect:** Arab. خدّر · Al-Rāzī, *K. al-Manṣūrī* · trans. Shem Tov ben Isaac (*Sefer Almansur*), Bet 2 (18): בנג: מחמם ומקדיר והשחור יותר חזק ואפשר שימית והדך אותו ומחבש בו המורסות החזקות הדפיקה מקדיר אותם ומשקיטם. → NM 2:17–8.

קֵדָר • **צלי קדר** → **צְלִי**.

קְדֵרָה › **skull:** Arab. قحف · Ibn Sīnā, *K. al-Qānūn fī al-ṭibb* · trans. Nathan ha-Me'ati (*Sefer ha-Qanun*), bk. 1 (fol. 28[b]): הפרק השני בנתוח קדרת המוח. → NM 4:178.

קובדי • כפל הקובדי → **כֶּפֶל**.

קוביא • עצם דומה לעצמות הקוביא → **עֶצֶם**.

קוֹבֵץ (*Part.*) → **קָבַץ**.

קוֹדֵם (*Part.*) → **קָדַם**.

קִוּוּץ (see also: **כִּוּוּץ**) ‣ I. **contraction**: Arab. تقبّض · Ibn al-Jazzār, *Zād al-musāfir wa-qūt al-ḥādir* · trans. Moses ibn Tibbon (*Sefer Ṣedat ha-Derakhim*), bk. 7, 17.2: ואם יתילד החולי הזה מפני שרפת מרה כרכומית הנה אותותיו כרכומית המראה ויובש החזה וסדיקת הידים והרגלים וקווץ ויבשות ויגלה מעט מעט בשעור מן הזמן. → NM 1:67.

‣ II. **disrupture**: Arab. فسخ · Ibn al-Jazzār, *Zād al-musāfir wa-qūt al-ḥādir* · trans. Moses ibn Tibbon (*Sefer Ṣedat ha-Derakhim*), bk. 7, 14.3: ופעמים שיתחדש הכאב מסבות מחוץ ולא הרגיש בהם החולה והוא שיהיה כבר העמיד האבר ההוא אשר התחדש לו בו הכאב בעת נומו בתכונה בלתי ראויה או שעותו פתאום וכל שכן אם קרהו קור עד שיתחדש בו קווץ. → NM 1:66–7.

‣ III. **spasm**: a) Lat. spasmus · Bruno Longobucco, *Cyrurgia Magna* · trans. Hillel ben Samuel (*Sefer Keritut*), fol. 15[a]: אמר גלינו ושאר החכמים התרת הדבקות בגידים מרוב הרגשתם והדבקתם במוח ממהרות להביא הקווץ. → NM 1:37.

b) Arab. كزاز / Gr. σπάσμα; σπάσμος; τέτανος · Ibn al-Jazzār, *Zād al-musāfir wa-qūt al-ḥādir* · trans. Moses ibn Tibbon (*Sefer Ṣedat ha-Derakhim*), bk. 1, ch. 23 (fol. 35[a]): תאר גרגרי קבאשיה לפי מה שתקנתיהו ונסיתיהו והוא מועיל מן הפלג ועקום הפה ומן הקווץ והוא אלכזאז ומכל חולי שסבתו קור ומהנקרס והקולון והרוחות העבות. → NM 4:179.

c) Arab. تشنّج · i. Ibn al-Jazzār, *Zād al-musāfir wa-qūt al-ḥādir* · trans. Moses ibn Tibbon (*Sefer Ṣedat ha-Derakhim*), bk. 7, 9.2: וכאשר יקרה ממשוש מזון או משקה שרפה או תרדמה או קווץ בצפרנים או נפח לאצבע הנה ראוי להשמר ממנו כי בו סם המות. → NM 1:66.

· ii. Maimonides, *K. al-fuṣūl fī al-ṭibb* · trans. Zeraḥyah Ḥen (*Sefer ha-Peraqim*), 3.10: הגופות שהם מקבלים מהר הקיווץ ומוכנים לו הם גופות הנערים מפני חולשת עצם העצבים בהם. → NM 1:157.

קול • אפיסת הקול → **אֲפִיסָה**.

• **הפסד הקול** → **הֶפְסֵד**.

• **ניחור הקול** → **נִחוּר**.

• **נמיכות הקול** → **נְמִיכוּת**.

• **צרידות קול** → **צְרִידוּת**.

• **שפלות הקול** → **שִׁפְלוּת**.

קולון ‣ **colic**: Arab. قولنج · Maimonides, *Šarḥ fuṣūl Abūqrāṭ* · trans. Moses ibn Tibbon (*Pirqei Abuqraṭ*), 3.22 (128): אמר אבקראט: ואולם החורף הנה יקרה בו רוב חליי הקיץ וקדחות רבעיות מעורבות וחליי הטחול ושקוי ושדפון וטפטוף השתן ושלשול הדם וקלוח המעים וכאב הירך והאסכרא והרבקיי והקולון החזק אשר יקראוהו היונים אילאוס והחולי הנופל והשטות והוסואס השחורי. → NM 3:201.

[קום] • *Part.* **קָם** • **הקם מן החולי** ‣ **convalescent**: Arab. الناقه / Gr. ἐκ νούσου … · Maimonides,

Šarḥ fuṣūl Abūqrāṭ · trans. Moses ibn Tibbon (*Pirqei Abuqraṭ*), 2.8 (60): אמר אבקראט: הקם מן החולי כאשר יקח מן המזון ולא יתחזק הנה זה יורה שהוא אוכל ממנו יותר ממה שיסבול ואם היה זה והוא לא יקח מן המזון יותר מדי סבלו הורה שגופו צריך אל הנקוי. → NM 3:202–3.

• *Pi'el* קִיֵּם • **קיים במקומו** · **to record**: Arab. ثبّت · Maimonides, *K. al-fuṣūl fī al-ṭibb* · trans. Nathan ha-Me'ati (*Sefer ha-Peraqim*), introduction: ואני הטבתי לבחון אותו הענין שנכפל זכרונו הרבה בדבריו במקום מאותם המקומות וקימתיו במקומו. → NM 2:81.

• *Pol'el* קוֹמֵם · **to counteract**: Arab. قاوم · Maimonides, *K. al-fuṣūl fī al-ṭibb* · trans. Nathan ha-Me'ati (*Sefer ha-Peraqim*), 21.51: וכמו שדוחה המרקחת הזה הפגעים הקורים לגוף כן מועיל לפגעי הנפש ויקומם המרה השחורה עצמה ומסיר המרה כמו שמסיר רעת הארסים מהרמשים. → NM 2:81.

קוֹסֵס (*Part.*) → קָסַס.

קוססות · **having a taste between sweet and sour**: Arab. مزازة · Al-Zahrāwī, *K. al-taṣrīf li-man 'ağiza 'an at-ta'līf* · trans. Shem Tov ben Isaac (*Sefer ha-Shimmush*), bk. 27, fol. 138[a], col. b: והחשוב שבמין האגס מה שיהיה ממנו בעל בשר דק הקלפה ושיש בטעמו מעט קוססות וקביצות. → NM 4:179.

קוֹץ • **קוץ ערבי** · **(lit., Arabian thorn); thistle**: *Anonymous Glossary*, Ms. Oxford, Bodleian Library, Mich. Add. 22, fol. 5[b]: איברא קוץ הרועה קוץ ערבי. → NM 4:180.

• **קוץ הרועה** · **(lit., needle of the shepherd); thistle**: *Anonymous Glossary*, Ms. Oxford, Bodleian Library, Mich. Add. 22, fol. 5[b]: איברא קוץ הרועה קוץ ערבי. → NM 4:180.

• *Plur.* **קוצים** · **spines (i.e., spinous processes)**: Arab. شوك · Ibn Sīnā, *K. al-Qānūn fī al-ṭibb* · trans. Nathan ha-Me'ati (*Sefer ha-Qanun*), bk. 1 (fol. 32[a]): ובעד השנית שהשדרה מחסה ומגן לאיברים הנכבדים המונחים לפניה ולכן ברא לה קוצים וסנסנים. → NM 4:179–80.

קוצר → קֹצֶר.

קור → קֹר.

קושי → קֹשִׁי.

קטורת → קְטֹרֶת.

קטן · **loins**: Arab. قطن · Ibn Sīnā, *K. al-Qānūn fī al-ṭibb* · trans. Nathan ha-Me'ati (*Sefer ha-Qanun*), bk. 1 (fol. 35[b]): והקטן עם העגז הוא כמושב כן לשדרה כלה והוא משענת ונושא לעצם הערוה עאנה ומקום צמיחת עצבי הרגל. → NM 4:180.

קָטָן • **האבר הקטן** → אֵבֶר.

• **אצבע קטנה** → אֶצְבַּע.

• **מרק תרנגולים קטנים** → מָרָק.

• **עצמות קטנים** → עֶצֶם.

• **הקנה הקטן** → קָנֶה.

• **התולעים הקטנים** → תּוֹלַעַת.

קטני • **העצבים הקטניים** → עָצָב.

[קטר] • *Hif'il* הִקְטִיר • **הקטיר האף בדבר** · **to apply a certain ingredient as an errhine**: Al-Rāzī, *K. al-Manṣūrī* · trans. Shem Tov ben Isaac (*Sefer Almansur*), Pe 6 (64): פאוניא ובלעז פאווינה: טוב לפחד הנערים כשתולין אותו עליהם ו⟨כש⟩מקטירין בו האף. → NM 2:18 (corr.).

קְטֹרֶת · **soot**: Arab. دخان · Al-Rāzī, *K. al-Manṣūrī* · trans. Shem Tov ben Isaac (*Sefer Almansur*), Dalet 7 (28): דכאן ר״ל קטרת: קטורת הדברים תשוב אל פעולת מה שיצמח ממנה. → NM 2:18.

קִיא • חפץ הקיא → חֵפֶץ.
• ריצון קיא → רָצוֹן.
• שלשול היוצא הקיא → שִׁלְשׁוּל.
• שלשול וקיא → שִׁלְשׁוּל.

קיבה → קֵבָה.

קיבר → קִבֵּר.

קִיּוּם · **compactness; firmness; solidity**: a) Arab. ثبات · Ibn al-Jazzār, *Zād al-musāfir wa-qūt al-ḥādir* · trans. Moses ibn Tibbon (*Sefer Ṣedat ha-Derakhim*), bk. 1, ch. 14 (fols. 20[b]–21[a]): השער הארבעה עשר בחולי השכחה: טוב השמירה וקלות הזכרנות הדברים ההוים בנפש יורה כי עצם החלק האחרון מן המוח אשר יקראוהו הרופאים הזכרון הוא עצם יש לו קיום ושווי ואם יהיה עצמו נגר שלא יהיה לו קיום יהיה בעליו שכחן גדול עם רוחק ההבנה והסח הדעת ואיחור השכל. → NM 4:181.

b) Lat. soliditas · Ibn Sīnā, *K. al-adwiya al-qalbiya* · trans. Anonymous (*Sefer ha-Refu'ot ha-Libbiyot*), fol. 246[a]: הסם העוצר והמדביק נכנס ברפואות הלב שהם יתנו לעצם הרוח קיום ודבוק נאות. → NM 4:180–1.

קִיטוֹר · I. **bad breath**: Arab. بَخَر · Al-Rāzī, *K. al-Manṣūrī* · trans. Shem Tov ben Isaac (*Sefer Almansur*), Samekh 14 (58): סעד ובלעז סיפרום אורטירגאנגלי וב״ח סיגלי: חם יבש מחמם האצטומכה והכבד ומפרך החצץ טוב לקיטור והעיפוש בפה או באף. → NM 2:18; corr. 3:268.

· II. **vapor**: a) Arab. بخار · Al-Zahrāwī, *K. al-taṣrīf li-man ʿağiza ʿan at-ta'līf* · trans. Shem Tov ben Isaac (*Sefer ha-Shimmush*), bk. 27, fol. 127[a], col. a: והמזון המתילד מהם על הכלל עב קשה להתעכל מתאחר לרדת מולידים דם שחורי וכל שכן כשיאכלו בקליפיהם ולפיכך הם ממלאים מוח מתמידם מקטורים עבים שחוריים מכאיבים. → NM 4:181.

b) Lat. vapor · Ibn Sīnā, *K. al-adwiya al-qalbiya* · trans. Anonymous (*Sefer ha-Refu'ot ha-Libbiyot*), fol. 250[a]: לאפיש ארמיני: יש לו סגולה לחזק הלב ולשמחו מפריד ביותר הקיטור השחוריי והעשני מהרוח וגם מנקה הגוף מליחה שחוריית. → NM 4:181.

קיים → קַיָּם.

קילור • *Plur.* קילורים · **eye lotions**: Arab. شيافات · Al-Zahrāwī, *K. al-taṣrīf li-man ʿağiza ʿan at-ta'līf* · trans. Shem Tov ben Isaac (*Sefer ha-Shimmush*), bk. 30, 2.15 (fol. 211[a]): ולהפריד בין העפעף והעין בפתילה של פשתן ולשית מִמעלה על העין ספוג טבול בחלבוני בצים ואחר שלשה ימים ראוי להרגיל הקילורים המגלידים עד שיבריא. → NM 1:112.

קַיָּם • הקדחת הקיימת → קַדַּחַת.

קיפאל • הקיפאל · **the cephalic vein**: Arab. القيفال · Ibn Sīnā, *K. al-Qānūn fī al-ṭibb* · trans. Nathan ha-Me'ati (*Sefer ha-Qanun*), bk. 1 (fol. 66[a]): והרביעי והוא הגדול שבהם והוא אותו אשר יראה ויעלה וישתלח ענף מאסף עמו שריג מן הקיפאל ויתהוה ממנו האכחל ושאריתו הוא הבאסליק. → NM 4:181–2.

קיפל → קיפאל.

[קיץ] • *Part. Hof'al* מֻקָץ · **being awake, esp., a kind of illness that arouses and keeps**

awake: Arab. منبّه / Lat. quas expergefacio · Ibn al-Jazzār, *Zād al-musāfir wa-qūt al-ḥādir* · trans. Moses ibn Tibbon (*Sefer Ṣedat ha-Derakhim*), bk. 1, ch. 15 (fols. 22ᵃ–22ᵇ): השער הט״ו בחולי הנקרא המוקץ כשיתחדש במאוחר מן המוח ליחה לבנה עם מרה אדומה וימזגו יחד יקרה מזה שיהיה החולה מושלך על ערפו כמת ועיניו פתוחות עד אצל שלא יגיע ממנו אל הנפש נזק ולא צער ויהיה שקט החולה ומנוחתו מפני קור הליחה הלבנה ולחותה ויהיה תעורתו והקצתו מפני יובש המרה האדומה וחדודה ולכן אמר גאלינוס כי הכונה ברפואת החולי הזה הנקרא המוקץ נקוי המוח משתי אלו הליחות המתהפכות בעצמיהם ר״ל ליחה לבנה ומרה אדומה. → NM 4:182–3.

קישור → קֶשֶׁר.

קְלוֹחַ · **clyster**: Arab. حقنة · Ibn al-Jazzār, *Zād al-musāfir wa-qūt al-ḥādir* · trans. Moses ibn Tibbon (*Sefer Ṣedat ha-Derakhim*), bk. 1, ch. 15 (fols. 22ᵇ–23ᵃ): ואם תהיה המרה האדומה יותר גוברת ירבה מן השמנים הקרים וימעיט מן החמים ואם הליחה הלבנה יותר גוברת ירבה מן השמנים החמים וימעיט מן הקרים ויקח זה למשל ולדמיון בכל מה שירפאו בו החולי הזה מקלוח הנקרא קלישטירי או פתילות אם נעצר הטבע או רפואה משלשלת או משקה או מזון. → NM 4:183.

• **קלוח הבטן** · **lientery**: Hippocrates, *Aphorisms* · trans. Judah Shalom, 4.12 (149) (fol. 54ᵇ): בכל מי שיהיה קלוח הבטן בסתו הוא רע להריק מלמעלה. → NM 3:201.

• **קלוח המעים** · **lientery**: Arab. زلق الأمعاء / Gr. λειεντερία · Maimonides, *Šarḥ fuṣūl Abūqrāṭ* · trans. Moses ibn Tibbon (*Pirqei Abuqraṭ*), 3.30 (136): אמר אבקראט: ואולם מי שעבר אלו השנים הנה יקרה לו הרנפלי וחלי הצד וחלי הריאה והקדחת אשר תהיה עמה היקיצה והקדחת אשר יהיה עמה ערבוב השכל והקדחת השורפת והשפיכה והשלשול הארוך וחמרמרות המעים וקלוח המעים ופתיחת פיות העורקים מלמטה. → NM 3:201–2.

• *Plur.* **קלוחים** · **clysters**: Arab. حقن · Ibn al-Jazzār, *Zād al-musāfir wa-qūt al-ḥādir* · trans. Moses ibn Tibbon (*Sefer Ṣedat ha-Derakhim*), bk. 7, 9.7: וכאשר נדע שהאסטו׳ כבר נקתה ולא ימצא בה מן הסם עקיצה ולא שרפה ולא צער אז נצוה לשלשל הטבע בקלוחים ממוצעי החום כדי שישלשלו מה שהגיע מן הסם אל המעים. → NM 1:67.

קָלוּי · **frying**: Arab. قلي · Maimonides, *K. al fuṣūl fī al ṭibb* · trans. Zeraḥyah Ḥen (*Sefer ha-Peraqim*), 20.64: ראוי שתתנהג בכלל המזונות בכלל כי מה שיהיה מהם חריף ומחודד או מר יהיה מזונו מעט ומה שיהיה מהם אין טעם לו מה שהגיע ממזונו אל הגוף מרובה וברוב מה שיהיה מתוק וכל שכן אם יהיה גרם קשה בין שיהיה אילו הטעמים והמאכלים בטבע או נקנים במלאכה כלומר בבישול ובצלי אש ובקלוי ובשרוי במים ודומה לאילו. → NM 1:183–4.

[קלח] • *Part. Piʿel* **מְקַלֵּחַ** • *Plur.* **מקלחים** · **clysters**: Arab. حقن · Ibn al-Jazzār, *Zād al-musāfir wa-qūt al-ḥādir* · trans. Moses ibn Tibbon (*Sefer Ṣedat ha-Derakhim*), bk. 1, ch. 23 (Ms. Oxford, Bodleian Library, Poc. 353, Uri Heb. 314, fol. 10ᵃ): ואם יצטרך למקלחים יעשה להם קלוחים בסמים חמים. → NM 4:104.

קָלִי • **קמח קלי** → קֶמַח.

קליבוסתא (*Aram.*) · **coccyx; femur**: Lat. ancha · Bruno Longobucco, *Cyrurgia Magna* · trans. Hillel ben Samuel (*Sefer Keritut*), fol. 62ᵇ: השמטת הקליבוסתא היא מד׳ פנים א׳ שיושמט מצד פְּנים ב׳ מצד חוץ ג׳ מצד פָּנים ד׳ מצד אחור. → NM 1:37.

קליפה → קְלִפָּה.

קְלָף · **folio:** Arab. جلد · Maimonides, *Šarḥ fuṣūl Abūqrāṭ* · trans. Anonymous (*Pirqei Abuqraṭ*), introduction (10): כבר ראיתי קצת המפרשים פירשו זה המאמר ממאמרי אבוקרט והוא זה: וכאשר הגיע החולי לתכליתו אז צריך שיהיה ההנהגה בקצה האחרון מן הדקות וכי הוא פי' זה ביותר ממאה קלפים בלא ענין וללא סבה. → NM 3:202.

קְלִפָּה · I. **squamous (aquamosal) suture:** Arab. الدرز القشري · Ibn Sīnā, *K. al-Qānūn fī al-ṭibb* · trans. Nathan ha-Me'ati (*Sefer ha-Qanun*), bk. 1 (fol. 29[a]): ואמנם שני השלבים הכוזבים המה לוקחים באורך הראש על נכחיות החציי משני צדדים ואינם שוקעים בעצם תכלית השקיעה ואלו השנים נקראים שתי קלפות. → NM 4:183.

· II. **tunic:** Arab. طبقة · Maimonides, *K. al-fuṣūl fī al-ṭibb* · trans. Zeraḥyah Ḥen (*Sefer ha-Peraqim*), 3.52: הלחות הכפורי והביציי הזכוכיי וכן הכת הקרניי אין בו גידים בשום פנים אבל תתפרנס הלחות הזכוכיי בהזיע הלחות הכפוריי והזכוכיית במה שיגיע לה מן הקלפה השכבית אשר היא מרובה בגידים הדופקים ובלתי דופקים. → NM 1:184.

• **קלפת נחשת** · **copper filings:** Arab. قشور النحاس · Ibn al-Jazzār, *Zād al-musāfir wa-qūt al-ḥāḍir* · trans. Moses ibn Tibbon (*Sefer Ṣedat ha-Derakhim*), bk. 7, 16.2. → NM 1:72.

• **קלפת עופרת** · **dross of lead:** Lat. scoria plumbi · Bruno Longobucco, *Cyrurgia Magna* · trans. Hillel ben Samuel (*Sefer Keritut*), fol. 25[b]. → NM 1:37.

• *Plur.* **קליפות** · I. **epithelial debris; scales:** Arab. قشور · Maimonides, *K. al-fuṣūl fī al-ṭibb* · trans. Nathan ha-Me'ati (*Sefer ha-Peraqim*), 13.37: החוקן במים ומלח אנחנו עושים אותו במי שיהיה במעיו שחינים ונגעים מעופשים ותרחוץ כל מה שכבר נתעפש ויצאו קלפות אינם קטנות. → NM 2:82.

· II. **eschar:** Arab. خشكريشة / Gr. ἐσχάρα · Al-Zahrāwī, *K. al-taṣrīf li-man ʿağiza ʿan at-ta'līf* · trans. Shem Tov ben Isaac (*Sefer ha-Shimmush*), bk. 30, 1.52 (fol. 208[a]): ואחרי כן להשהותו שלשה ימים ואחר לתת על המקומות הנכוים גפרית שחוק עם שמן זית עד שינתקו הקליפות כלן. → NM 1:112–3.

· III. **scabs:** Arab. قشور · Ibn al-Jazzār, *Zād al-musāfir wa-qūt al-ḥāḍir* · trans. Moses ibn Tibbon (*Sefer Ṣedat ha-Derakhim*), bk. 7, 22.1: ואם יהיה עם ליחה לבנה יוליד נגעים לחים עם קליפות לבנות. → NM 1:67.

· IV. **scales:** Hippocrates, *Aphorisms* · trans. Do'eg ha-Edomi (*Sefer Agur*), 4.81 (218) (fol. 79[a]): קבוץ עב טיט ודם בתוך השתן גם מראה הקליפות וריח קשה כל זה יעיד על חבורת המקוה. → NM 3:202.

· V. **tunics:** Arab. صفاقات · Maimonides, *K. al-fuṣūl fī al-ṭibb* · trans. Zeraḥyah Ḥen (*Sefer ha-Peraqim*), 3.53: כמו שיכלול החוש לעור ... כן ירגשו כמו כן הקרומות והקליפות והגידים הדופקים ובלתי דופקים והרחם והמיעים והשלפוחית והאסטומכא וכל הקרביים ואע״פ שיהיה בעצבים שני הכחות יחד וכלי התנועה היא המושקולי. → NM 1:184.

קְלָפִי · **cartiliginous:** Arab. غضروفي · Ibn Sīnā, *K. al-Qānūn fī al-ṭibb* · trans. Zeraḥyah Ḥen (*Sefer ha-Qanun*), bk. 1 (fol. 20[a]): עצם העצה מחובר מחוליות שלשה קלפיי אין לו תוספת. → NM 4:183–4.

• **החוליה הקלפית** → חֻלְיָה.

קְלָפִי • **השלב הקלפיי** → שָׁלָב.

קָם (*Part.*) → [קום].

קֶמַח • **קמח אורובי** · **meal of bitter vetch:** Lat. farina orobi · Bruno Longobucco, *Cyrurgia Magna*· trans. Hillel ben Samuel (*Sefer Keritut*), fol. 24[b]. → NM 1:45.

• **קמח לופיני** · **meal of lupines:** Lat. farina lupinorum · Bruno Longobucco, *Cyrurgia Magna* · trans. Hillel ben Samuel (*Sefer Keritut*), fol. 24[b]. → NM 1:46.

• **קמח קלי** · **semolina:** Arab. سويق · Maimonides, *K. al-fuṣūl fī al-ṭibb* · trans. Nathan ha-Me'ati (*Sefer ha-Peraqim*), 9.4: וכן תשרה להם לחם או קמח קלי ביין חי כי בהתערב היין החי במאכל תבטח מעלות ממנו אידים חמים יזיקו אל המקום הכואב. → NM 2:82.

קֶמֶט • *Plur.* **קמטים** • **קמטי האסטוכמה** · **the lining of the stomach:** Arab. خمل المعدة · Maimonides, *K. al-fuṣūl fī al-ṭibb* · trans. Nathan ha-Me'ati (*Sefer ha-Peraqim*), 2.20: וכשתהיה זאת הליחה העוקצת כרתית או חמוצה או מלוחה הנה היא שוקעת בחללי קמטי האסטוכמה. → NM 2:82.

קנדי → **כנדי.**

[קנה] • *Part. Nif'al* **נִקְנֶה** · **(lit., had by [someone]); having; suffering from:** Lat. habitus / Gr. ἐχόμενος · Hippocrates, *Aphorisms* · trans. Judah Shalom, 4.57 (194) (fol. 60[b]): הקווץ או המשיכה הנקנית הקדחת הבא עליהם תתיך החולי. → NM 3:203.

קָנֶה · **forearm:** Arab. ساعد · Ibn Sīnā, *K. al-Qānūn fī al-ṭibb* · trans. Nathan ha-Me'ati (*Sefer ha-Qanun*), bk. 1 (fol. 37[b]): והנקרה החיצונית היא הגדולה ממנה ומה שנלוה לנקרה הפנימי בלתי חלק ובלתי עגול החפירה אבל כגדר הישר עד שיתנועע בו תוספת הקנה אל הצד החיצוני יגיע אליו ויעמד אצלו. → NM 4:184.

• **הקנה הגדול** · **tibia:** Arab. القصبة الكبرى · Ibn Sīnā, *K. al-Qānūn fī al-ṭibb* · trans. Nathan ha-Me'ati (*Sefer ha-Qanun*), bk. 1 (fol. 41[a]): השוק היא כמו הקנה מחוברת משני עצמים אחד מהם יותר גדול ויותר ארוך והוא פנימי ונקרא הקנה הגדול והשני יותר קטון ויותר קצר ... ונקרא הקנה הקטון. → NM 4:184.

• **קנה החוטם** · **(lit., tube(s) of the nose); nostril(s):** Arab. قصبة الأنف / Lat. canales narium · Ibn al-Jazzār, *Zād al-musāfir wa-qūt al-ḥāḍir* · trans. Moses ibn Tibbon (*Sefer Ṣedat ha-Derakhim*), bk. 1, ch. 21 (Ms. Oxford, Bodleian Library, Poc. 353, Uri Heb. 314, fol. 9[a]): ופעמים יבא פתאום מבלתי חולי וזה כי קנה חוטם האדם קצר ויגיעו בעבור זה מהר דברים מזיקים מחוץ למוח כמו אבק ועשן וקור חזק וזריחת השמש ומה שדומה להם. → NM 4:184–5.

• **הקנה החיצוני** · **fibula:** Arab. القصبة الوحشية · Ibn Sīnā, *K. al-Qānūn fī al-ṭibb* · trans. Nathan ha-Me'ati (*Sefer ha-Qanun*), bk. 1 (fol. 54[b]): ועצל מסתבך ממנו שני מיתרים אחד מהם מקבץ כף הרגל והשני מפשיט הבהן וזה שהעצל הזה צמיחתו מראש הקנה הפנימי מקום שפוגע החיצוני וימשך ביניהם ומשתרג לשני מיתרים. → NM 4:185.

• **קנה הטוב** · **lemon grass [*Cymbopogon martini*]:** Arab. قصب الذريرة; قصب الطيب / Gr. κάλαμος ἀρωματικός · Ibn Zuhr, *Regimen of Health* · trans. Jacob ibn Tibbon (*Hanhagat ha-Beri'ut le-Abu 'Ali ben Zuhr*), ch. 5: והתמדת הרחת המוסרחים והעכורים יעכירו הרוח הנפשי וינצחו אותו ולזה יתחיב להריח הריח הטוב ולהתמידו ולהתעשן בעשן הבשמים כעשן הליגנאלובין והענבר וקנה הטוב. → NM 4:185.

• **הקנה הימני** · **fibula:** Arab. القصبة الوحشية · Ibn Sīnā, *K. al-Qānūn fī al-ṭibb* · trans. Joseph Lorki (*Sefer ha-Qanun*), bk. 1 (fol. 16[b]): ועצל אחד ישתרגו ממנו שני יתרים האחד מהם יקבץ

הרגל והשני יפשט הבהן וזה ⟨ש⟩העצל הזה תולדתו מראש הקנה השמאלי באיזה מקום שפוגע הימני ויולד ממנו וישתרג לשני יתרים. → NM 4:185.

• **הקנה הפנימי** · **tibia**: Arab. القصبة الانسية · Ibn Sīnā, *K. al-Qānūn fī al-ṭibb* · trans. Nathan ha-Me'ati (*Sefer ha-Qanun*), bk. 1 (fol. 54[b]): אמנם המגביהים יש מהם עצל גדול מונח קדם הקנה הפנימי. → NM 4:186.

• **פרק קנה הזרוע הסמוך ליד** → **פֶּרֶק**.

• **הקנה הקטן** · **fibula**: Arab. القصبة الصغرى · Ibn Sīnā, *K. al-Qānūn fī al-ṭibb* · trans. Nathan ha-Me'ati (*Sefer ha-Qanun*), bk. 1 (fol. 41[a]): השוק היא כמו הקנה מחוברת משני עצמים אחד מהם יותר גדול ויותר ארוך והוא פנימי ונקרא הקנה הגדול והשני יותר קטון ויותר קצר ... ונקרא הקנה הקטון. → NM 4:186.

• **קנה הריאה** · **windpipe (trachea)**: a) Arab. قصبة الرئة · Maimonides, *Šarḥ fuṣūl Abūqrāṭ* · trans. Moses ibn Tibbon (*Pirqei Abuqraṭ*), 4.54 (191): אמר ג'אלינוס: אי אפשר בשעול ואפילו לא ירוק כלום שלא יתלחלחו קני הריאה ממה שימשך אליו עם השעול ולכן לא יצמא. → NM 3:203–4.

b) Maimonides, *K. al-fuṣūl fī al-ṭibb* · trans. Nathan ha-Me'ati (*Sefer ha-Peraqim*), 23.76: נקרא קנה הריאה חלקום והוא הגרגרת בלשוננו. → NM 2:82–3.

• **הקנה השמאלי** · **tibia**: Arab. القصبة الانسية · Ibn Sīnā, *K. al-Qānūn fī al-ṭibb* · trans. Joseph Lorki (*Sefer ha-Qanun*), bk. 1 (fol. 16[b]): ואמנם המרימים מהם עצל גדול מונח לפני הקנה השמאלי. → NM 4:186.

• *Plur.* **קנים** • **שני הקנים** · **the two bones [of the leg] (i.e., tibia and fibula)**: Arab. القصبتان · Ibn Sīnā, *K. al-Qānūn fī al-ṭibb* · trans. Nathan ha-Me'ati (*Sefer ha-Qanun*), bk. 1 (fol. 42[a]): והקרסול מונח בין שתי הקצות הבולטים משני הקנים מקיפים עליו מצדדיו ר"ל מעליונו ותחתיתו. → NM 4:186–7.

• **קני הסוכר** · **sugar canes**: Arab. قصب السكّر · Al-Zahrāwī, *K. al-taṣrīf li-man ʿağiza ʿan at-ta'līf* · trans. Shem Tov ben Isaac (*Sefer ha-Shimmush*), bk. 27, fol. 139[b], col. b: קני הסוכר בטבעם ומזגם קרובים מטבע המוזי. → NM 4:186.

קִנְיָן · **constitution**: Lat. habitudo (Constantine) / Gr. ἕξις · Hippocrates, *Aphorisms* · trans. Judah Shalom, 2.34 (86) (fol. 29[a]): בכל החליים פחות יסתכנו החולים כשהם מאותו הטבע מהשנים והקנין והעת אשר יהיה בהם החולי ויותר מזה כל אשר אינו מסכים לאחד מהם. → NM 3:204.

קָסַס • *Part.* **קוֹסֵס** · **having a taste between sweet and sour**: Arab. مُزّ · Al-Zahrāwī, *K. al-taṣrīf li-man ʿağiza ʿan at-ta'līf* · trans. Shem Tov ben Isaac (*Sefer ha-Shimmush*), bk. 27, fol. 137[b], col. b: והמבושל ישתנה בפעולתו כפי טעמו כי יש ממנו עפוץ ויש ממנו חמוץ ויש ממנו קוסס ויש ממנו מתוק ויש ממנו תפל. → NM 4:187.

קַעֲרוּרִית • **קערורית האצטומכא** · **the concave part (bottom) of the stomach**: Lat. fundus stomaci (Honofredi) · Ibn Zuhr, *Regimen of Health* · trans. Jacob ibn Tibbon (*Hanhagat ha-Beri'ut le-Abu ʿAli ben Zuhr*), ch. 8: והרחקת אכילת העצמים הדקים כמו עצם העוף והפרדייץ והצפרים והתרנגולים ואכילת הדגים הקוציים זולת עצמי השיות והתישים הסריסים כאשר יותך מהם לעיסותם ממה שירכך הקנה והאוילה וירכך הושט וישלשל המעברות ויעזור לירידת המאכל בקערורית האצטומכא. → NM 4:187.

קָפָא • *Pass. Part.* **קָפוּא** · **solid**: Arab. جامد · Maimonides, *Šarḥ fuṣūl Abūqrāṭ* · trans. Moses ibn Tibbon (*Pirqei Abuqraṭ*), 2.7 (59): אמר המפרש: וזה כי הגופות אשר ירזו בזמן מועט אמנם התחדש להם הרזון ההוא והכחש מהרקת הלחויות לא מהתכת האיברים הקפואים. → NM 3:204.

• *Part. Nif'al* **נִקְפָּא** · **solid**: Arab. جامد · Maimonides, *Šarḥ fuṣūl Abūqrāṭ* · trans. Zeraḥyah Ḥen (*Pirqei Abuqraṭ*), 2.7 (59): אמר המפרש: זה בעבור כי הגופות אשר יקחם הרזון בזמן מועט אמנם נתחדש להם זה הכחש והרזון מהרקת הלחויות לא מהתכת האיברים הנקפאים. → NM 3:163.

קִפָּאוֹן · **catalepsy**: Arab. جمود · Maimonides, *K. al-fuṣūl fī al-ṭibb* · trans. Nathan ha-Me'ati (*Sefer ha-Peraqim*), 23.59: כשיחזק על המוח הקור ויתערב בו לחות יתחדש ממנו הברסם הקר והוא ליתרגס ונקרא בלשונם ליטרג׳יאה וכשיתערב עם הקור יובש יתחדש ממנו הקפאון. → NM 2:83.

קָפוּא (*Pass. Part.*) → **קָפָא**.

קְפִיאָה · **catalepsy**: Arab. جمود · Maimonides, *K. al-fuṣūl fī al-ṭibb* · trans. Nathan ha-Me'ati (*Sefer ha-Peraqim*), 23.64: בטול הדמיונות יאמר לו השקיעה והקפיאה. → NM 2:83.

קֵץ · **culmination**: Arab. منتهى / Gr. ἀκμή · Maimonides, *Šarḥ fuṣūl Abūqrāṭ* · trans. Zeraḥyah Ḥen (*Pirqei Abuqraṭ*), 1.10 (37): אמר בקראט: ואותם יבואם קץ חלים תחילה ראוי שינהגו בהנהגה הדקה תחילה. → NM 3:204–5.

קָצֶה • **קצה האמה** · **urethra**: Arab. إحليل · Maimonides, *Šarḥ fuṣūl Abūqrāṭ* · trans. Zeraḥyah Ḥen (*Pirqei Abuqraṭ*), 4.82 (219): אמר בקראט: מי שיצאה בתור בקצה האמה שלו כשתפתח יסור חליו. → NM 3:205.

• **קצה הגיד** · **foreskin**: Arab. قلفة · Maimonides, *Šarḥ fuṣūl Abūqrāṭ* · trans. Moses ibn Tibbon (*Pirqei Abuqraṭ*), 6.19 (311): אמר אבקראט: כאשר נחתך עצם או אליל או עצב או המקום הדק מן הלחי או קצה הגיד לא יצמח ולא יתחבר. → NM 3:205.

• **קצה גיד הערוה** · **rectum**: Hippocrates, *Aphorisms* · trans. Do'eg ha-Edomi (*Sefer Agur*), 5.58 (278) (fol. 92[a]): שמור בעלות צמח בקצה גיד הערוה או בפי הרחם כי יחול מזה הטפת השתן במכאוב ופוקות. → NM 3:205.

• **קצה העין הגדול** · **the inner angle of the eye**: Arab. المأق الأكبر · Maimonides, *K. al-fuṣūl fī al-ṭibb* · trans. Nathan ha-Me'ati (*Sefer ha-Peraqim*), 23.71: והסרת הבשר אשר בקצה העין הגדול הנקרא מאק הגדול יאמר לעלה הזאת דמעה. → NM 2:83.

• **קצה העין מצד האזן** · **external angle of the eye**: Arab. لحاظ · Ibn Sīnā, *K. al-Qānūn fī al-ṭibb* · trans. Joseph Lorki (*Sefer ha-Qanun*), bk. 1 (fol. 17[a]): והחלק הב׳ עובר בנקב הנברא אצל קצה העין מצד האזן. → NM 4:187.

• **קצה פי הטבעת** · **rectum**: Arab. طرف الدبر · Maimonides, *Šarḥ fuṣūl Abūqrāṭ* · trans. Moses ibn Tibbon (*Pirqei Abuqraṭ*), 5.58 (278): אמר אבקראט: כשיקרה בקצה פי הטבעת או ברחם מורסא ימשך אחריו הטפת השתן. → NM 3:205.

• *Plur.* **קצוות** • **הקצוות אשר הדמע יורד מהן** · **the inner and outer angle (canthi) of the eye**: Arab. مأقان · Ibn Sīnā, *K. al-Qānūn fī al-ṭibb* · trans. Zeraḥyah Ḥen (*Sefer ha-Qanun*), bk. 1 (fol. 23[b]): אמנם זה המושקולי ד׳ מהם בצדדיו הד׳ למעלה ולמטה ושתי הקצוות אשר הדמע יורד מהן הנקרא בערבי מאקין. → NM 4:188.

• **קצוות העין** · **the inner and outer angle (canthi) of the eye**: Arab. مأقان · Ibn Sīnā, *K. al-Qānūn fī al-ṭibb* · trans. Nathan ha-Me'ati (*Sefer ha-Qanun*), bk. 1 (fol. 43[a]): הפרק הרביעי בנתוח עצלי כלל העין ואמנם העצלים המניעים לכלל העין הם עצלים ששה ארבעה מהם בצד הם הארבעה למעלה ולמטה בשתי קצוות העין הנקרא מאקים. → NM 4:188.

קָצָוִי • *Plur.* **קצויות** · **wisdom teeth**: Arab. ناجذ, *Plur.* نواجذ · Ibn Sīnā, *K. al-Qānūn fī al-ṭibb* · trans. Nathan ha-Me'ati (*Sefer ha-Qanun*), bk. 1 (fol. 31[b]): והקצויות יצמחו ברוב באמצע זמן הגדול והוא אחר ההמרצה אל ההעמדה וזה כי ההעמדה קרובה מל׳ שנה ולכן נקראים שני אלחלם כלו׳ החלימה. → NM 4:188.

קִצּוּר • *Plur.* **קצורים** · ***Epitomes***: Arab. مختصرات · Maimonides, *Šarḥ fuṣūl Abūqrāṭ* · trans. Moses ibn Tibbon (*Pirqei Abuqraṭ*), introduction (13): אבל כל פירוש שאזכרהו סתם הנה הוא דברי ג׳אלינוס ר״ל עניינו כי אני לא שמתי כונתי ללקוט דבריו במילותיו כמו שעשיתי בקצורים. → NM 3:205–6.

קצידה · **ophthalmia**: Arab. رمد · Maimonides, *Šarḥ fuṣūl Abūqrāṭ* · trans. Moses ibn Tibbon (*Pirqei Abuqraṭ*), 3.21 (127): אמר אבקראט: ואולם בקיץ הנה יקרה קצת אלו החליים וקדחות מתמידות והשורפות ושלישית הרבה וקיא ושלשול וקצידה וכאב באזן ונגעים בפה ועפוש בנגעים. → NM 3:206.

• **לפלוף הוא קצידה** → **לִפְלוּף**.

קְצִירָה → **קצידה**.

[קצף] • *Part. Pu'al* **מְקֻצָּף** • **דבש מקוצף** → **דְּבַשׁ**.

קֶצֶף • **קצף הים** · **sepiolite** [*Spuma maris*]: Arab. زبد البحر · Ibn al-Jazzār, *Zād al-musāfir wa-qūt al-ḥādir* · trans. Moses ibn Tibbon (*Sefer Ṣedat ha-Derakhim*), bk. 7, 16.3. → NM 1:72.

קֹצֶר • **קוצר הרוח** · **despondency**: Lat. pusillanimitas · Hippocrates, *Aphorisms* · trans. Hillel ben Samuel, 6.23 (315) (fol. 40[b]): היראה וקוצר הרוח המתמידים בלא סבה ידועה ר״ל מקרית יורה על כי האיש ההוא יפול בחלי המלנקוניאה. → NM 3:206–7.

קַר • **זרעים קרים** → **זֶרַע**.

קֹר · **winter**: Arab. شتاء · Maimonides, *Šarḥ fuṣūl Abūqrāṭ* · trans. Zeraḥyah Ḥen (*Pirqei Abuqraṭ*), 1.12 (39): וכן זמני השנה כי קדחת הרביעית הבאה בקיץ תהיה קצרה ברוב הענינים והבאה בימי החורף תהיה ארוכה ברוב וכל שכן כשתהיה סמוכה בקור. → NM 3:207.

• **זמן הקור** → **זְמַן**.

• **ימי הקור** → **יוֹם**.

קָרָא • **קרא על** · **to study under**: Arab. قرأ على · Maimonides, *K. al-fuṣūl fī al-ṭibb* · trans. Zeraḥyah Ḥen (*Sefer ha-Peraqim*), 8.69: אמר משה וכן אני לא ראיתיהו במערב ולא אמר שום אחד מאותם הזקנים אשר קראתי עליהם שהוא ראם. → NM 1:184.

[קרב] • *Part. Pi'el* **מְקָרֵב** • **העצל המקרב** → **עָצָל**.

קֶרֶב · I. **belly**: Hippocrates, *Aphorisms* · trans. Do'eg ha-Edomi (*Sefer Agur*), 7.26 (378) (fol. 114[b]): יתקררו הקצוות עם כאב חזק על הקרב אות רע הוא. → NM 3:207–8.

· II. **cavity**: a) Hippocrates, *Aphorisms* · trans. Do'eg ha-Edomi (*Sefer Agur*), 7.38 (390) (fol. 117[a]): סבב זוב הנחירים לרדת אל הקרב העליון יבלה וישוב להיות עב טיט עד עשרים יום. → NM 3:208.

b) Lat. venter · Hippocrates, *Aphorisms* · trans. Hillel ben Samuel, 7.54 (406) (fol. 47[b]): כל אותם שתעצר להם ליחה לבנה בין הכליות והבטן ותכאיב אין לה מוצא בקרבים אם תגר אל השלפוחית יסור הכאב. → NM 3:208.

· III. **diaphragm**: Hippocrates, *Aphorisms* · trans. Do'eg ha-Edomi (*Sefer Agur*), 4.18 (155) (fol. 62[b]): הכאב שהוא למעלה מן הקרב יאות לטהרו למעלה, ההוא אשר למטה מן הקרב יאות לטהר למטה. → NM 3:207.

• **קרב בעל השתים עשרה אצבעות** · **duodenum**: Judah ben Jacob, *Sefer Hanhagat ha-Beri'ut*, 8.1: ונקרא הקרב הזה הדבק בשוער בעל שתים עשרה אצבעות כי שעורו מכל אדם שתים עשרה אצבעות מאצבעות ידיו. → NM 4:188–9.

• **החלב המכסה (את) הקרב** → **חֵלֶב**.

• **החלב אשר על הקרב** → **חֵלֶב**.

• *Plur.* **קרבים** · **hypochondrium**: Hippocrates, *Aphorisms* · trans. Judah Shalom, 6.40 (332) (fols. 106[a]): באשר יתהווה כאב אצל הקרבים בלי פליגמון הקדחת הבא עליו יתיך הכאב. → NM 3:208.

קרדום → **קֻרְדֹּם**.

קֻרְדֹּם · **occipital protuberance**: Arab. فأس · Maimonides, *K. al-fuṣūl fī al-ṭibb* · trans. Nathan ha-Me'ati (*Sefer ha-Peraqim*), 3.107: כשתתלה קרן המציצה על העורף במקום העצם הנקרא הקרדום יהיה מהדברים היותר חזקי התועלת מלמנוע שפיכת הליחות אל העין. → NM 2:83.

קָרוּי • **בלתי קרוי** · **roofless**: Arab. لا سقف له · Galen, attr., *Prohibition of Burial* · trans. Judah al-Ḥarizi (*Sefer Issur ha-Qevurah le-Galienus*), par. 45: ויכניסו החולה ויסגרו בעדו בבית בלתי קרוי. → NM 4:189.

קְרוּם · **siphac (peritoneum)**: Lat. siphac / Arab. صفاق · Galen, *De inaequali intemperie* · trans. David Caslari (*Sefer Ro'a Mezeg Mithallef*), 3.3: אמנם הקיבוץ המתהווה בקרום הנקרא ציפאק הוא רע. → NM 2:169.

• **קרום הלב** · **pericardium**: Arab. حجاب القلب · Galen, attr., *Prohibition of Burial* · trans. Judah al-Ḥarizi (*Sefer Issur ha-Qevurah le-Galienus*), par. 187: והמין האחר מפני השינה וזה שהאדם רב המילוי ממאכלים או מהדברים הלחים ויכבד זה על טבעו וישן על צדו האחד ויטו המאכלים והכימוסים אל ⟨הלב⟩ וילחצו קרומו. → NM 4:189.

• **קרום מכסה** · I. **membrane; peritoneum**: Arab. صفاق · Maimonides, *K. al-fuṣūl fī al-ṭibb* · trans. Nathan ha-Me'ati (*Sefer ha-Peraqim*), 15.36: הרקת המים הנעצרים בבטן בעל השקוי הנודי תהיה ממנו אם ברפואות מתיכות ואם בנקיבת הקרום המכסה הנקרא ציפאק בברזל. → NM 2:83–4.

· II. **pannus**: Lat. pannus · Bruno Longobucco, *Cyrurgia Magna* · trans. Hillel ben Samuel (*Sefer Keritut*), fol. 64[b]: חליי העינים מתהפכים כי מהן חוליי הדמעות ומהן אודם ומהן קרום מכסה. → NM 1:38.

• **הקרום הפנימי** · **omentum**: Hippocrates, *Aphorisms* · trans. Do'eg ha-Edomi (*Sefer Agur*), 7.55 (407) (fol. 120[b]): שטף מים רבים בעברו דרך הכבד ומשם יעבור אל הקרום הפנימי אז ימלאו הבטן ויביאו המות. → NM 3:208–9.

• **הקרום הקשה** · **the hard membrane (i.e., dura mater)**: Arab. الغشاء الصلب · Ibn Sīnā, *K.*

al-Qānūn fī al-ṭibb · trans. Nathan ha-Me'ati (*Sefer ha-Qanun*), bk. 1 (fol. 65[b]): ומתפרד ממנו שריגים בשני קרומי המוח לזונם ושיקשר הקרום הקשה במה שסביבותיו ולמעלה הימנו. → NM 4:189.

• *Plur.* **קרומים • קרומי המוח** · **meninges**: Arab. حجب الدماغ · Al-Zahrāwī, *K. al-taṣrīf li-man ʿağiza ʿan at-taʾlīf* · trans. Shem Tov ben Isaac (*Sefer ha-Shimmush*), bk. 27, fol. 127[a], col. b: ומחדשים חלומות רעים וממלאים האסטומ׳ והמעים רוחות מנפחות ומולידים סתומים ומתיחה ועצירת הבטן ומזיקים אל הריאה והטרפשה ואל קרומ⟨י⟩ המוח ויתר העצבים והקרומות. → NM 4:189.

• **מורסות קרומי המוח** → **מֻרְסָא**.

קָרוּשׁ (*Pass. Part.*) → **קָרַשׁ**.

קָרְחוּת · **baldness caused by sores on the head**: Arab. قرع · Maimonides, *Šarḥ fuṣūl Abūqrāṭ* · trans. Moses ibn Tibbon (*Pirqei Abuqraṭ*), 6.34 (326): יאמר ג׳אלינוס: רוצה בכאן הקרחות וכאשר נעתקה הליחה ההיא הרעה למטה יתחדש הדליות ויצמח השער. → NM 3:209.

קְרִירוּת · **rigor**: Arab. نافض · Maimonides, *K. al-fuṣūl fī al-ṭibb* · trans. Zeraḥyah Ḥen (*Sefer ha-Peraqim*), 7.23: יתקבץ בגוף ליחה פליאומטיקא זכוכיית ולא תתעפש ותחדש ריגור ימים רבים זו אחר זו וכל זמן היות האדם נח ולא יתנועע כלל וינוח הקרירות ההוא. → NM 1:185.

קֶרֶן • *Plur.* **קרנים** · **clitoris**: Arab. بظر · Al-Zahrāwī, *K. al-taṣrīf li-man ʿağiza ʿan at-taʾlīf* · trans. Shem Tov ben Isaac (*Sefer ha-Shimmush*), bk. 30, 2.71 (fol. 220[b]): שער ע״א בחתוך קרני הרחם הנקרא בלשונם אל בטר ובשר הבולט בקיבות הנשים. הקרנים לפעמים יוסיף שעורם על המנהג הטבעי עד שוב הרחם מכוער המראה. → NM 1:113.

• **קרני המציצה** · **cupping glasses**: Arab. محجمة · Hippocrates, *Aphorisms* · trans. Nathan ha-Me'ati, 5.50 (270): אמר אבוקרט: כשתרצה לעצור דם הנדות באשה אז תשים אצל כל אחד משני שדיה קרני המציצה מהיותר גדולים שיהיו. → NM 3:209.

• **קרני הראש** · **the frontal prominences**: Arab. قرنا الرأس · Al-Zahrāwī, *K. al-taṣrīf li-man ʿağiza ʿan at-taʾlīf* · trans. Shem Tov ben Isaac (*Sefer ha-Shimmush*), bk. 30, 1.2 (fol. 203[a–b]): ועתיד אני לזכור עוד זאת הכויה במקומה וראוי להיות המכוה שמכ⟨וים⟩ בו קרני הראש ואחוריו יותר דק מן המכוה שמכוים בה אמצע הראש. → NM 1:113.

• **קרני הרחם** · **clitoris**: Arab. بظر · Al-Zahrāwī, *K. al-taṣrīf li-man ʿağiza ʿan at-taʾlīf* · trans. Shem Tov ben Isaac (*Sefer ha-Shimmush*), bk. 30, 2.71 (fol. 220[b]): שער ע״א בחתוך קרני הרחם הנקרא בלשונם אל בטר ובשר הבולט בקיבות הנשים. הקרנים לפעמים יוסיף שעורם על המנהג הטבעי עד שוב הרחם מכוער המראה. → NM 1:113.

קרנייי • **הכת הקרנייי** → **כַּת**.

קרסול → **קַרְסֹל**.

קַרְסֹל · **anklebone; astragalus; talus**: Arab. كعب · Ibn Sīnā, *K. al-Qānūn fī al-ṭibb* · trans. Nathan ha-Me'ati (*Sefer ha-Qanun*), bk. 1 (fol. 41[b]): עצמות כף הרגל ששה קרסול שבו ישלם הפרק עם השוק. → NM 4:190.

קָרַע · **to dissect**: Arab. شقّ · Maimonides, *K. al-fuṣūl fī al-ṭibb* · trans. Zeraḥyah Ḥen (*Sefer ha-Peraqim*), 15.31: כשתהיה קורע הקרום הקרני יהיה תחלת מה שיפגושך הלחות הדק הדקיק ויהיה ניגר וזב והוא הלחות אשר הרבה פעמים אנו רואים שיגר ויצא מן הנקב אשר ינקב בעין אשר ימחט המים. ואחרי כן יתכווץ העין בעצמו. → NM 1:185.

קִרְקוּר · [intestinal] rumbling(s): Arab. قرقرة / Gr. διαβορβωρύζω · a) Maimonides, *Šarḥ fuṣūl Abūqrāṭ* · trans. Moses ibn Tibbon (*Pirqei Abuqraṭ*), 4.73 (210): אמר אבקראט: מי שהיו המקומות אשר למטה מחלציו ממנו נפוחים ובהם קרקור ואחר כן התחדש לו כאב בשפל שדרתו הנה בטנו יתרכך אם לא שיצאו ממנו רוחות רבות או שישתין שתן רב. → NM 3:209–10.

b) Maimonides, *K. al-fuṣūl fī al-ṭibb* · trans. Nathan ha-Me'ati (*Sefer ha-Peraqim*), 7.55: כשתאכל מאכל ולא יקרה לך ממנו קרקור ולא נפח ולא רפרוף ולא פוקות אך שימצאך באסטומכה מצוק אין הרגלך בו בכיוצא בו ויכבד עליך אותו המאכל ותשתקק שירד או שיתחדש לך גיעוש הנקרא רוט ותמצא עם זה בקצת העתים צרות הנשימה אין ספק אז שהאסטומכה כבר נתקבצה על המאכל על צד ההתגעשות. → NM 2:84.

[קרקר] • *Part. Pi'el* **מְקַרְקֵר** · **suffering from [intestinal] rumblings**: Hippocrates, *Aphorisms* · trans. Judah Shalom, 4.73 (210) (fol. 71[a]): כאשר הקרבים נפוחים מקרקרים בבא על זה כאב הכסלים הנה ירוכך הבטן אם לא שיוציא רוחיות אם יהיה לו רבוי השתן. → NM 3:210.

[קרר] • *Part. Pi'el* **מְקָרֵר** • **אבק מקרר** → **אָבָק**.

קָרֵשׁ • *Pass. Part.* **קָרוּשׁ** • **דם קרוש** → **דָּם**.

• **חחלב הקרוש** → **חָלָב**.

• **תירוש ענבים קרוש בבשול** → **תִּירוֹשׁ**.

קָשֶׁה · **dense**: Arab. متكاثف / Gr. πυκνός · Maimonides, *Šarḥ fuṣūl Abūqrāṭ* · trans. Moses ibn Tibbon (*Pirqei Abuqraṭ*), 5.62 (282): כשיהיה רחם האשה קר קשה לא תתעבר. → NM 3:210.

• **סוכר קשה** → **סֻכָּר**.

• **הקרום הקשה** → **קְרוּם**.

קִשּׁוּא • *Plur.* **קשואים** • **קשואים מרים** · **squirting cucumber** [*Ecballium Elaterium* L.]: Arab. قثّاء الحمار · Ibn al-Jazzār, *Zād al-musāfir wa-qūt al-ḥāḍir* · trans. Moses ibn Tibbon (*Sefer Ṣedat ha-Derakhim*), bk. 2, ch. 18 (fol. 61[a]): תואר רפואה חברתיה ונסיתיה ומצאתיה מועילה לכאב השנים והטוחנות מקור ורוח עבה ערובו יקח פליטרי ואישוף ופולי ושרש קשואים מרים. → NM 4:190.

קֶשֶׁר · **ligament**: Arab. رباط · Maimonides, *K. al-fuṣūl fī al-ṭibb* · trans. Zeraḥyah Ḥen (*Sefer ha-Peraqim*), 1.8: העצבים לא יהיה דבק שום דבר מהם בתנוד בלעז קרטילייני ולא בקישור ולא בשמן ולא בעצם אלא בשניים לבדם מן כל העצמות כי הם יתדבקו בשרשיהם עצבים חלקים. → NM 1:185–6.

• *Plur.* **קשורים** • **קשורי השוליא** · **cotyledons**: Gr. κοτυληδών, *Plur.* κοτυληδόνες · Hippocrates, *Aphorisms* · trans. Joseph Delmedigo, 5.45 (265): והממוצעות בבשר אם מפילות בחדש השני או השלישי בלי סבה מבוארת תדע שכוסות הרחם מליאים מליחה דבקיית ואינן יכולים להחזיק העובר מפני הכובד וקשורי השוליא נפרקים. → NM 3:210–1.

קֹשִׁי · 1. **erection**: Arab. إنعاظ · a) Al-Zahrāwī, *K. al-taṣrīf li-man ʿağiza ʿan at-ta'līf* · trans. Shem Tov ben Isaac (*Sefer ha-Shimmush*), bk. 27, fol. 131[b], col. b: שכר החטה: יש ששותים אותו מתוק חדש ויש ששותים אותו ישן והמתוק רב המזון קשה להתעכל רב הרוחות והנפח ומוסיף בתאות המשגל והקושי תוספת גדולה. → NM 4:190.

b) Maimonides, *Šarḥ fuṣūl Abūqrāṭ* · trans. Moses ibn Tibbon (*Pirqei Abuqraṭ*), 6.30 (322): וכאשר הזיק המשגל בעצבים בכלל בעבור הרקת רוחו והקרו אותו יהיה נזק

זה בעצבי הרגלים יותר חזק. ואנחנו נראה תמיד כי כאשר יתקררו הרגלים ילד הקושי. → NM 3:211.

c) Maimonides, *K. al-fuṣūl fī al-ṭibb* · trans. Zeraḥyah Ḥen (*Sefer ha-Peraqim*), 22.61: וכשתשחק זרע האורוגא והושמה בבצים שאינם מבושלים אלא מעט עם מעט מלח האשטינק ויעשה מהם חסו יוסיף בזרע ויחזק הקושי מאד. → NM 1:186.

d) Maimonides, *K. al-fuṣūl fī al-ṭibb* · trans. Nathan ha-Me'ati (*Sefer ha-Peraqim*), 22.61: ואם ישחק זרע גרגיר ויושם בביצה נמרשת עם מעט מלח אשטינקוש ויגמע יוסיף בזרע ויחזק הקושי מאד. → NM 2:84.

‣ II. **tension**: Arab. توتّر · Maimonides, *Šarḥ fuṣūl Abūqrāṭ* · trans. Moses ibn Tibbon (*Pirqei Abuqraṭ*), 5.49 (269): אמר המפרש: כדי שיתחדש לבטן משיכה וקושי ויעזור על נפילת השליא. → NM 3:211.

• **קושי החשתנה** ‣ **dysuria**: Arab. عسر البول · Maimonides, *Šarḥ fuṣūl Abūqrāṭ* · trans. Anonymous (*Pirqei Abuqraṭ*), 3.5 (111): ואמנם הצפונים יחדשו שעול וכאב הגרון ויובש הבטן וקושי ההשתנה והסמור וכאב הצלעות והחזה. → NM 3:211.

• **קשי יציאת השתן** ‣ **dysuria**: Arab. عسر البول · Hippocrates, *Aphorisms* · trans. Nathan ha-Me'ati, 6.36 (328) (Ms. Paris, BN, héb. 1108, fol. 94[b]): אמר אבוקראט: הקזת העורק מתיך קשי יציאת השתן וראוי שיחתכו העורקים הפנימיים. → NM 3:211.

• **קושי השתן** ‣ I. **difficult urination (dysuria)**: a) Lat. difficultas urinandi (Honofredi) · Galen, attr., *Prohibition of Burial* · trans. Judah al-Ḥarizi (*Sefer Issur ha-Qevurah le-Galienus*), par. 26: ואין ראוי שיעצר דבר מן השתן כי עצירת השתן מביא קושי השתן וחולי במקוה ורפיונה. → NM 4:190–1.

b) Arab. عسر البول · Maimonides, *Šarḥ fuṣūl Abūqrāṭ* · trans. Anonymous (*Pirqei Abuqraṭ*), 6.36 (328): אמר אבוקרט: הקזת העורקים מתיר קושי השתן ⟨ו⟩ראוי שיחתכו העורקים הפנימיים. → NM 3:212.

‣ II. **strangury**: Arab. تقطير البول · Maimonides, *Šarḥ fuṣūl Abūqrāṭ* · trans. Anonymous (*Pirqei Abuqraṭ*), 3.16 (122): ואמנם התחלואים המתחדשים בעבור מיעוט המטר הם הכליה ומורסת העין וכאב הפרקים וקושי השתן ושלשול הדם. → NM 3:211–2.

קְשִׁירָה ‣ **ligament**: Arab. رباط · a) Maimonides, *K. al-fuṣūl fī al-ṭibb* · trans. Zeraḥyah Ḥen (*Sefer ha-Peraqim*), 15.29: הרפואה הלחה הניגרת לא תעמוד אלא בקשר ועל כן תשים רפואת הגרב יבישה כי הקשירה צריכה להיות על העין כולו. → NM 1:186.

b) Maimonides, *K. al-fuṣūl fī al-ṭibb* · trans. Nathan ha-Me'ati (*Sefer ha-Peraqim*), 15.29: הרפואה הרטובה הנזולה לא תתעכב אלא בקשירה ולכן תשים רפואות אלגרב יבשות כי הקשירה צריכה שתהיה על העין כלה והעין אינה סובלת שתקשור בקשירה שלא תפרד ממנה מימים רבים בשעור שיתחיל בה הנאצור. → NM 2:84.

• *Plur.* **קשירות** ‣ **bandage**: Lat. ligatura · Bruno Longobucco, *Cyrurgia Magna* · trans. Hillel ben Samuel (*Sefer Keritut*), fol. 61[b]: ואם לאו תוסיף לעשות התחבושת והקשירות עד שיתחזק. → NM 1:38.

‣ II. **ligaments**: Lat. ligamenta · Bruno Longobucco, *Cyrurgia Magna* · trans. Hillel ben Samuel (*Sefer Keritut*), fol. 61[a]: ההשמטה מן הגומברו היא יותר חזקה מן השאר ודומה גם כן השבתו ויהיה מחוזק הקשירות וקטנם ומהתנגדות גוממותו. → NM 1:38.

קַשִּׁישׁ • *Plur.* **קשישים** • **splints**: Arab. جبائر • Al-Zahrāwī, *K. al-taṣrīf li-man ʿağiza ʿan at-ta'līf* • trans. Shem Tov ben Isaac (*Sefer ha-Shimmush*), bk. 30, introduction (fol. 201[b]): וראיתי אחר מתעסק בזאת המלאכה בכדי חייו אצל קצת קציני ארצותינו ונתחדש לסריס שחור שנשבר שוקו קרוב מן הערקוב ונתחדשה בו חבורה ומהר הסכל בסכלותו והדק השבר על החבורה בבלונסות ובקשישים. → NM 1:113.

קַשְׁקַשׁ • **splint**: Arab. جبيرة • Al-Zahrāwī, *K. al-taṣrīf li-man ʿağiza ʿan at-ta'līf* • trans. Shem Tov ben Isaac (*Sefer ha-Shimmush*), bk. 30, 3.4 (fol. 234[a]): ואחר לתת על הלחי הנשבר הקירותי ואחר כך לתת עליו בגד גס ולתת על הבגד קשקש גדול עשוי בחכמה. → NM 1:113.

קַשְׂקַשִׂי • **הקשקשי** • **that which has scales; that which is scaly**: Arab. ما له فلوس • Al-Zahrāwī, *K. al-taṣrīf li-man ʿağiza ʿan at-ta'līf* • trans. Shem Tov ben Isaac (*Sefer ha-Shimmush*), bk. 27, fol. 149[b], col. b: והקשקשי הוא בכלל יותר חשוב ממה שאין לו קשקשת. → NM 4:191.

[קשר] • *Part. Piʿel* **מְקַשֵּׁר** • **fortifying**: Arab. مُمَتِّن • Ibn Sīnā, *K. al-adwiya al-qalbiya* • trans. Anonymous (*Sammim Libbiyim*), fol. 125[a]: ויהיה סם מקשר לרוח. → NM 4:191.

• *Hitpaʿel* **הִתְקַשֵּׁר** • **to congeal**: Arab. انعقد / Gr. συστρέφω • Hippocrates, *Aphorisms* • trans. Nathan ha-Me'ati, 5.40 (260) (fol. 95[b]): אמר אבוקרט: מי שיתקשר דם בשדי האשה מורה זה בענינה על שטות. → NM 3:214.

קֶשֶׁר • **bandage**: Lat. ligatura • Bruno Longobucco, *Cyrurgia Magna* • trans. Hillel ben Samuel (*Sefer Keritut*), fol. 61[b]: ויתלה זרועו אל צוארו ויונח כן כמה ימים אחר כן תתיר ואם תראה שנתחזק הדבק במקומו אז תתיר הקשר. → NM 1:38.

• **קשר הזרוע** • **elbow**: Lat. cubitus • Hippocrates, *Aphorisms* • trans. Hillel ben Samuel, 6.22 (314) (fol. 40[a]): א"א: כל כאב עובר מהגב לקשר הזרוע ההקזה תרפאו. → NM 3:212.

• *Plur.* **קשרים** • I. **bandage**: Arab. رباط • Ibn al-Jazzār, *Zād al-musāfir wa-qūt al-ḥāḍir* • trans. Moses ibn Tibbon (*Sefer Ṣedat ha-Derakhim*), bk. 7, 15.5: ואם התילדה המורסא מפני ליחה לבנה והיא אשר תקרא מורסא רפה הנה ראוי להשקות החולה הרפואות אשר יורידו ליחה לבנה ואחרי כן יושם עליה אספוג בלול במים שנתערב עמהם חומץ ויקשור האספוג בקשרים תחיה תחלתם מלמטה ותכליתם למעלה. → NM 1:68.

• II. **joints**: Hippocrates, *Aphorisms* • trans. Do'eg ha-Edomi (*Sefer Agur*), 4.45 (182) (fol. 69[a]): נדין על אשר צמחו בבשרו צמחים או כאב בין הקשרים אחרי קדחת כי ישוב לאכל יותר על משאו. → NM 3:212.

• III. **ligaments**: Arab. رباط • Maimonides, *K. al-fuṣūl fī al-ṭibb* • trans. Zeraḥyah Ḥen (*Sefer ha-Peraqim*), 1.7: הקשרים העגולים והיתרים יחשוב מי שאין לו עיון בניתוח שהן עצבים. → NM 1:186.

• IV. **tumors**: Arab. عُقَد / Gr. συστροφή • a) Ibn al-Jazzār, *Zād al-musāfir wa-qūt al-ḥāḍir* • trans. Moses ibn Tibbon (*Sefer Ṣedat ha-Derakhim*), bk. 2, ch. 13 (fol. 53[b]): או יקח מן הרפואה הזאת כי היא תמהר בריאות הנואסיר והקשרים המתהוים בחוטם. → NM 4:191.

b) Ibn al-Jazzār, *Zād al-musāfir wa-qūt al-ḥāḍir* • trans. Moses ibn Tibbon (*Sefer Ṣedat ha-Derakhim*), bk. 7, 23.1: וזכר גם כן כי פגי תאנים כשיבושלו ויעשה מהם תחבושת ירכך הקשרים והחזירים ויתיכם. → NM 1:68.

• **קשרי האצבעות** • **joints**: Hippocrates, *Aphorisms* • trans. Do'eg ha-Edomi (*Sefer Agur*),

אמר אפוקרט: נכון כל גוף אשר תקרהו קדחת ארוכה שיצמחו בבשרו צמחים 4.44 (181) (fol. 69[a]):
או כאב בין קשרי אצבעותיו. → NM 3:212–3.

• **קשרי הדבקים** · **joints**: Hippocrates, *Aphorisms* · trans. Do'eg ha-Edomi (*Sefer Agur*), 3.16 (122) (fol. 53[b]): אמר אפוקרט: כח יבשות האויר בהמנע הגשם יוליד תחלואי העיניים כאב קשרי הדבקים כובד הזלת השתן ונזילת דם. → NM 3:213.

• **קשרי הזרועות** · **forearms**: Lat. cubiti / Arab. ساعدان · Hippocrates, *Aphorisms* · trans. Hillel ben Samuel, 5.69 (289) (fol. 37[b]): א״א: הפלצות מתחיל לנשים בחלצים ומהגב ועולה אל הראש וכן לאנשים יותר מאחור מאשר הוא מפנים או מקשרי הזרועות והירכים. → NM 3:213.

• **כאב קשרי העצמות** → **כְּאֵב**.

• **מחלת הדבקים וקשרי העצמות** → **מַחֲלָה**.

• **מחלת קשרי העצמות** → **מַחֲלָה**.

• **קשרי העצמות** · **joints**: Hippocrates, *Aphorisms* · trans. Do'eg ha-Edomi (*Sefer Agur*), 4.31 (168) (fol. 66[a]): יעיד על בעלי היגיעה הסובלים קדחת כי רוב הצמחים אשר יצמחו בהם יהיו במקום קשרי העצמות או על צדי לחיתם. → NM 3:213.

ר

רָאָה • ראה בדעת · to think: Arab. رأى · Maimonides, *Šarḥ fuṣūl Abūqrāṭ* · trans. Zeraḥyah Ḥen (*Pirqei Abuqraṭ*), 2.29 (81): כל זמן שיהיה החולי בהתחלתו אם תראה בדעתך להניע שום דבר תניעהו. → NM 3:214.

• **אותם שיראו בעוות** · squinting: Arab. أحول, *Plur.* حول · Ibn Sīnā, *K. al-Qānūn fī al-ṭibb* · trans. Zeraḥyah Ḥen (*Sefer ha-Qanun*), bk. 1 (fol. 30[a]): ועל כן יקרה לאותם שיראו בעוות שיראו הדבר שני דברים בסור אחת משתי הבבות לצד מעלה או לצד מטה. → NM 4:143.

• *Part. Nif'al* **נִרְאֶה** · clear; evident: Arab. ظاهر · Ibn al-Jazzār, *Zād al-musāfir wa-qūt al-ḥādir* · trans. Moses ibn Tibbon (*Sefer Ṣedat ha-Derakhim*), bk. 2, ch. 17 (fol. 57[b]): ואם קרה העדר התנועה והפסק הדבור מן הלשון מבלתי שאר אברי הגוף ולא נראה בלשון חולי נראה ידענו כי זה מפני כאב העצב אשר יעבור בו כח התנועה מן המוח אל הלשון. → NM 4:191.

רֵאָה • בעלת הריאה → בַּעֲלָה.

• **חולי הריאה** → חֳלִי.

• **כאב הריאה** → כְּאֵב.

• **מדוה הריאה** → מַדְוֶה.

• **מורסת הריאה** → מֻרְסָא.

• **נזילה על הריאה** → נְזִילָה.

• **קנה הריאה** → קָנֶה.

רָאוּי • היה ראוי · to remain: Arab. لزم · Maimonides, *K. al-fuṣūl fī al-ṭibb* · trans. Zeraḥyah Ḥen (*Sefer ha-Peraqim*), introduction: כי אני אלו התרתיו על אחד מאותן המקומות היתה ראויה אותה הקושיא בעצמה. → NM 1:186.

רְאוּת · pupil: Arab. ناظر · a) Al-Zahrāwī, *K. al-taṣrīf li-man 'ağiza 'an at-ta'līf* · trans. Shem Tov ben Isaac (*Sefer ha-Shimmush*), bk. 30, 2.23 (fol. 212[a]): וראוי לתת שעור הכנסת המקדיח כעין שעור הרוחק אשר יהיה מן הנער אל סוף השחרות והוא עגול העין כי נחשת המקדיח יראה בעצם הראות היטב לזכות הקרום הקרני. → NM 1:113–4.

b) Ibn al Jazzār, *Zād al musāfir wa qūt al ḥādir* · trans. Moses ibn Tibbon (*Sefer Ṣedat ha-Derakhim*), bk. 2, ch. 4 (fol. 45[a]): תאר אבק יחזק הראות ויסיר הדמע. → NM 4:191–2.

• **כאב הראות** → כְּאֵב.

• **מעוות הראות** → [עות].

• **עכירות הראות** → עֲכִירוּת.

רְאָיָה · sign: Arab. دليل · Maimonides, *Šarḥ fuṣūl Abūqrāṭ* · trans. Moses ibn Tibbon (*Pirqei Abuqraṭ*), 7.41 (393): אמר אבקראט: כשיתחדש בישישים בסבת הרקת שלשול או קיא ⟨או⟩ פיהוק אין זה ראיה טובה. → NM 3:214.

• **לקח ראיה על** → לָקַח.

ראש · root [of a tooth]: Arab. رأس · Ibn Sīnā, *K. al-Qānūn fī al-ṭibb* · trans. Nathan ha-Me'ati (*Sefer ha-Qanun*), bk. 1 (fol. 31[b]): ואמנם המלתעות הנעוצות בלחי בתחתון הפחות שיהיה לכל אחד מהם שני ראשים ולפעמים יותר. → NM 4:192.

• **ראש האמה** · foreskin: Hippocrates, *Aphorisms* · trans. Judah Shalom, 6.19 (311) (fol. 100[a]): כאשר נחתך עצם או שחוס או עצב או מקום הדק מהלחי או ראש האמה לא יצמח ולא יתדבק. → NM 3:215.

• **בלבול בראש** → **בִּלְבּוּל**.

• **בלבול הראש השחור** → **בִּלְבּוּל**.

• **גיד הראש** → **גִּיד**.

• **גיד הראש הנקרא אכחל** → **גִּיד**.

• **גלגול הראש** → **גִּלְגּוּל**.

• **הזולות הראש** → **הַזָּלָה**.

• **ראש הכתף** · **acromion process; superior process of scapula**: Arab. رأس الكتف / Gr. ἀκρώμιον · Ibn Sīnā, *K. al-Qānūn fī al-ṭibb* · trans. Nathan ha-Me'ati (*Sefer ha-Qanun*), bk. 1 (fol. 37[a]): ונוטה אל הצד החיצוני ומחוברת בראש הכתף ונקשרת בה הכתף ובהם יחדו נקשר הזרוע. → NM 4:192.

• **ראש הלב** · **the apex of the heart**: Arab. رأس القلب · Ibn Sīnā, *K. al-Qānūn fī al-ṭibb* · trans. Nathan ha-Me'ati (*Sefer ha-Qanun*), bk. 1 (fol. 62[a]): ואמנם החלק היורד מן אוריטי הנה הוא הולך תחלה אל יושר עד שיסמך אל החוליא החמשית כי היא הנחתה נכח הנחת ראש הלב. → NM 4:192.

• **מורסת הראש** → **מֻרְסָא**.

• **מחוג הראש** → **מָחוֹג**.

• **נשירות שער הראש** → **נְשִׁירוּת**.

• **ראש העין** · **[inner] angle of the eye**: Arab. مأق العين · Al-Zahrāwī, *K. al-taṣrīf li-man ʿağiza ʿan at-taʾlīf* · trans. Shem Tov ben Isaac (*Sefer ha-Shimmush*), bk. 30, 1.17 (fol. 201[b]): י״ז בכוית הגרגתני אשר יקרה בראש העין. → NM 1:114.

• **צמח אשר צמח במוח הראש** → **צֶמַח**.

• **קרני הראש** → **קֶרֶן**.

• **ריבועי הראש** → **רִבּוּעַ**.

• *Plur.* **ראשים** • **ראשי הירכים** · **groin**: Arab. أربيّة · Al-Zahrāwī, *K. al-taṣrīf li-man ʿağiza ʿan at-taʾlīf* · trans. Shem Tov ben Isaac (*Sefer ha-Shimmush*), bk. 30, 2.40 (fol. 215[a]): ויש מהם מה שצריך לבקעו בקוע בעל שלש זויות ⟨ומה שצריך⟩ לחתוך ממנו כתבנית עלה ההדס כמו צמח ראשי הירכים. → NM 1:114.

• **התוספות הדומים בשני ראשי השדים** → **תּוֹסֶפֶת**.

רַב • **אבר שיש לו מתרים רבים** → **אֵבֶר**.

• **רבח** · **gum tragacanth**: Arab. كثيراء · Al-Zahrāwī, *K. al-taṣrīf li-man ʿağiza ʿan at-taʾlīf* · trans. Shem Tov ben Isaac (*Sefer ha-Shimmush*), bk. 27, fol. 123[b], col. a: ומתועלות הקמח הדק על דרך הסם כי כשלשין אותו מבלי מלח היטב כראוי ורוחצין אותו במים עד שיצא חלבו וכחו ואחר כן מבשלין החלב ההוא היטב בשזיפין ורבה עד שובם בגדר המזון. → NM 4:192.

רִבּוּעַ • *Plur.* **ריבועים** • **ריבועי הראש** · **the prominence of the head**: Lat. cornu capitis · Bruno Longobucco, *Cyrurgia Magna* · trans. Hillel ben Samuel (*Sefer Keritut*), fol. 103[b]: על חולי הישן מכאב הראש תכוה על כל ריבועי הראש. → NM 1:39.

רבידא (*Aram.*) · **cupping vessel**: Arab. محجمة · Al-Zahrāwī, *K. al-taṣrīf li-man ʿağiza ʿan *at-ta'līf* · trans. Shem Tov ben Isaac (*Sefer ha-Shimmush*), bk. 30, 3.8 (fol. 234[b]): ואמרו קצתם שראוי לתת על המקום רבידא. → NM 1:114.

• *Plur.* **רבידות** · **cupping vessels**: Al-Zahrāwī, *K. al-taṣrīf li-man 'ağiza 'an at-ta'līf* · trans. Shem Tov ben Isaac (*Sefer ha-Shimmush*), bk. 30, 2.96 (fol. 230[b]): הרבידות נעשות מן הקרנות ומן העצים ומן הנחשת ומן הזכוכית. → NM 1:114.

רְבִיכָה • *Plur.* **רביכות** · **a dish consisting of broken pieces of bread sopped in broth with meat and/or vegetables**: Arab. ثرائد, *Sing.* ثريدة; ثريد · Al-Zahrāwī, *K. al-taṣrīf li-man 'ağiza 'an at-ta'līf* · trans. Shem Tov ben Isaac (*Sefer ha-Shimmush*), bk. 27, fol. 123[b], col. 2–124[a], col. 1: הרביכות: הרביכה זנה מועט וממהרת להתעכל ולרדת מן האסטומ' יותר מן הלחם הטבול במרק ולפי כך ראוי להנזר מן הרביכות בעלי היגיעה והטיול והרוצה להנעים גופו. → NM 4:192–3.

רְבִיעִי • **רְבִיעִית** · **quartan fever**: Arab. ربع · Maimonides, *Šarḥ fuṣūl Abūqrāṭ* · trans. Zeraḥyah Ḥen (*Pirqei Abuqraṭ*), 4.59 (196) אמר גאלנוס: הנה מצאנו הבחראן ברביעית ומצאנוהו שהוא לפי מנין ההקפות לא לפי מספר הימים. → NM 3:215.

• **קדחת רביעית** → **קַדַּחַת**.

[רבע] • *Part. Pu'al* **מְרֻבָּע** · **cross-legged**: Arab. متربّع · Al-Zahrāwī, *K. al-taṣrīf li-man 'ağiza 'an at-ta'līf* · trans. Shem Tov ben Isaac (*Sefer ha-Shimmush*), bk. 30, 3.13 (fol. 235[b]): וכשיקרה אל המסרק שבר או ריסוק ראוי להושיב החולה מרובע ולפניו כסא ולתת היד על הכסא פתוחה. → NM 1:105.

רֹגֶז · **distress**: Arab. كرب · Al-Zahrāwī, *K. al-taṣrīf li-man 'ağiza 'an at-ta'līf* · trans. Shem Tov ben Isaac (*Sefer ha-Shimmush*), bk. 27, fol. 136[a], col. a: אם יקרה מאכילתן צרות הנשימה ורגז ועלוף ראוי למהר ולשתות מן המוריס ומן הבורית ואחר ממי הדבש. → NM 4:193.

רָגִיל · **having skill (i.e., skilled)**: Arab. حاذق · Al-Zahrāwī, *K. al-taṣrīf li-man 'ağiza 'an at-ta'līf* · trans. Shem Tov ben Isaac (*Sefer ha-Shimmush*), bk. 30, 2.86 (fol. 225[b]): ורפאוהו רבים מן הרופאים קרוב משתי שנים ולא היה בהם רגיל במלאכת היד. → NM 1:114.

• **היה רגיל** · **to apply; to use**: Lat. uti · Bruno Longobucco, *Cyrurgia Magna* · trans. Hillel ben Samuel (*Sefer Keritut*), fol. 51[b]: ונחבוש תחבושות משיבות חשבר וחחשמטח בלי גמורה והוא אותו שהיו בו רגילין הקדמונים מאבק הרחים. → NM 1:39.

[רגל] • *Hif'il* **הִרְגִּיל** · 1. **to administer; to apply; to use**: a) Lat. administrare · Bruno Longobucco, *Cyrurgia Magna* · trans. Hillel ben Samuel (*Sefer Keritut*), fol. 12[b]: ואם התולה יהיה מעט בשום פנים לא תחתכנו והרפואה המצמיחה תרגיל שם. → NM 1:39.

b) Arab. استعمل · i. Al-Zahrāwī, *K. al-taṣrīf li-man 'ağiza 'an at-ta'līf* · trans. Shem Tov ben Isaac (*Sefer ha-Shimmush*), bk. 30, 1.3 (fol. 203[b]): כשיתחדש בחצי הראש כאב חזק נמשך אל העין ראוי להריק החולה בסמים המנקים הראש ולהרגיל יתר הרפואות אשר זכרתי בחלוקות החליים. → NM 1:114–5.

· ii. Ibn al-Jazzār, *Zād al-musāfir wa-qūt al-ḥādir* · trans. Moses ibn Tibbon (*Sefer Ṣedat ha-Derakhim*), bk. 2, ch. 4 (fol. 44[b]): והעושה הגרגרים ימשח ידו בשמן ורדים וירגיל בהם. → NM 4:193–4.

· iii. Al-Rāzī, *K. al-Manṣūrī* · trans. Shem Tov ben Isaac (*Sefer Almansur*), Zayin 12 (34): זנגופר ובלעז וירמליון וב"מ ששר: חם יכנס אל הרטיות יועיל אל

החבורות המעופשות תועלת גדולה והרוצה להרגילו צריך לשחקו ולזרותו על האיכולים כי הוא מנגבם ומנגב כל שחין מעופש. → NM 2:18–9.

c) Lat. uti · Al-Rāzī, attr., *On the Treatment of Small Children* · trans. Bonfos, ch. 23: וירגיל זה השמן תמיד. → NM 2:181.

· II. **to take**: a) Arab. استعمل · Maimonides, *K. al-fuṣūl fī al-ṭibb* · trans. Nathan ha-Me'ati (*Sefer ha-Peraqim*), 3.92: ורוב מה שיקרו אלו המורסות הקשות למי שימצאהו מורסא חמה באחד מאלו האברים השלשה ואחר ירגיל מאכלים מולידים ליחות עבות או דבקות. → NM 2:84–5.

b) Hippocrates, *Aphorisms* · trans. Judah Shalom, 4.45 (182) (fol. 64[a]): בכל מי אשר יהיו צמחים בפרקים או יגיעות הנעשים אחר קדחות ארוכות יורה כי אלו ירגילו מזונות יותר מן הראוי. → NM 3:215.

• **הרגיל במרחץ** · **to bathe in the bathhouse; to take a bath**: Lat. uti balneo · Bruno Longobucco, *Cyrurgia Magna* · trans. Hillel ben Samuel (*Sefer Keritut*), fol. 82[b]: וישמור החולה שלא ירגיל מאד במרחץ בעבור שהוא מתיך החומר הדק ומקשה העב. → NM 1:39.

רֶגֶל • **רגל יונים** · **(lit., pigeon's foot); alkanet** [*Alkanna tinctoria* L.; *Anchusa tinctoria* L.]: *Anonymous Glossary*, Ms. Vatican, Biblioteca Apostolica, ebr. 361, fol. 181[a]: רגל יונים ע׳ רג׳ל חמאמה לע׳ פיקולומין. → NM 4:194.

• **מסרק הרגל** → **מַסְרֵק**.

• *Plur.* **רגלים** • **בא לו חולי הרגלים** → [**בוא**].

• **חולי הרגלים** → **חֳלִי**.

• **עצם מקום שער הרגלים** → **עֶצֶם**.

• **עשות מי רגלים** → **עָשָׂה**.

• **שפולי הרגלים** → **שִׁפּוּל**.

[רגע] • *Nif'al* **נִרְגַּע אל** · **נרגע אל** · **to find relief in**: Arab. استراح إلى · Maimonides, *K. al-fuṣūl fī al-ṭibb* · trans. Nathan ha-Me'ati (*Sefer ha-Peraqim*), 13.31: אנשים רבים ירגעו במהירות הענין אל ההרקה החזקה וישקטו בה. → NM 2:85.

[רגש] • *Part. Hitpa'el* **מִתְרַגֵּשׁ** · **epidemic**: Arab. وافد · Maimonides, *K. al-fuṣūl fī al-ṭibb* · trans. Nathan ha-Me'ati (*Sefer ha-Peraqim*), 23.16: החלאים הנקראים המתרגשים הם חלאים כוללים מתחדשים באנשי ארץ מה בקצת השנים. → NM 2:64.

[רדם] • *Part. Nif'al* **נִרְדָּם** • **השריינים הנרדמים** → **שרין**.

• *Part. Hif'il* **מַרְדִּים** · I. **having a narcotic effect; narcotic**: Arab. مخدّر · Ibn al-Jazzār, *Zād al-musāfir wa-qūt al-ḥādir* · trans. Moses ibn Tibbon (*Sefer Ṣedat ha-Derakhim*), bk. 2, ch. 18 (fol. 61[a]): ואם לא ינוח הכאב במה שזכרנו ויביא הצורך אל רפואות יותר חזקות נצוה החולה שיתמיד להניח פלוניה או שכאזניא או תריאק על השן הכואבת ואם לא ינוח הכאב עם זה ראוי שיעשה רפואות מרדימות. → NM 4:104–5.

· II. **soporific**: Arab. مرقد · Ibn al-Jazzār, *Zād al-musāfir wa-qūt al-ḥādir* · trans. Moses ibn Tibbon (*Sefer Ṣedat ha-Derakhim*), bk. 1, ch. 17 (fol. 25[a]): ואם נתחדשה התעורה מפני מזונות חמים או סמים חמים יתרפא במה שזכרנו לפי מה שיטה אליו מזגו ויעשה מאלו הרפואות. מזה תואר מרדים מחבור אסחק בן עמרן שירדים בהריח אותו. → NM 4:104.

• סם המרדים → סַם.

• *Plur.* מרדימים › narcotics: Arab. مخدّرات · Maimonides, *K. al-fuṣūl fī al-ṭibb* · trans. Nathan ha-Me'ati (*Sefer ha-Peraqim*), 8.39: אלו הרפואות המחוברות להשקיט הכאבים שנכנס בהם המרדימים ראוי לאדם שיכוון בחבורם לשלשה ענינים. → NM 2:62.

• *Hof'al* הָרְדַם › to turn numb: Arab. خدر · Maimonides, *K. al-fuṣūl fī al-ṭibb* · trans. Nathan ha-Me'ati (*Sefer ha-Peraqim*), 23.23: אלכדר כלו' תרדמת האברים הוא דבר מורכב מקשי ההרגש וכובד התנועה ויהיה מקור האויר ומלחיצת הגשמים העצביים ומנגיעת בעל החיים הימיי. והאברים יקרה להם תחלה שיורדמו ואחר ישובו שלא יהיה בהם לא הרגש ולא תנועה ויאמר לזה המין מן ההיזק רפיון. → NM 2:85.

רוֹאֶה › pupil: Arab. ناظر · Maimonides, *K. al-fuṣūl fī al-ṭibb* · trans. Nathan ha-Me'ati (*Sefer ha-Peraqim*), 15.30: המים אחר שירדו ויזלו בפני הרואה ראוי שתאחז המקדה זמן ארוך במקומות אשר ירצה שינוחו המים כדי שישתרגו בו. → NM 2:85.

• הרואה שלעין › pupil: Arab. حدقة · Maimonides, *K. al-fuṣūl fī al-ṭibb* · trans. Zeraḥyah Ḥen (*Sefer ha-Peraqim*), 25.17: אמר משה זה תמה כי המים היורדים בעין וחבלת הקרנית העמוקה בהיותה נכח הרואה שלעין ואחר כן עלתה בשר תזיק בחוש הראות תחלה ואי זו חולי שבא לעצב אשר יהיה בו חוש הראות באילו החליים ודומיהם. → NM 1:186–7.

רוּחַ • איברי הרוח → אֵבֶר.

• המתיח הרוח → [מתח].

• הרוח החיה › the vital pneuma: Judah ben Jacob, *Sefer Hanhagat ha-Beri'ut*, 2.1 (117): גם הכח המוליד לא יהיה תמיד תמים פעלו זולתו כי הוא צריך אל הרוח החיה ואל החום הטבעי. → NM 4:194.

• חיסר הרוח → [חסר].

• חסרון הרוח → חֶסְרוֹן.

• הסם המשבר הרוח → סַם.

• הסם חשובר רוח → סַם.

• פשט הרוח → פָּשַׁט.

• *Plur.* רוחות › intestinal rumbling: Arab. قرقرة · Maimonides, *Šarḥ fuṣūl Abūqrāṭ* · trans. Zeraḥyah Ḥen (*Pirqei Abuqraṭ*), 4.73 (210): אמר בקראט: מי שהיה בו במקומות אשר מתחת הצלעות רוחות גוברות ואחר כן נתחדש בו כאב בסוף גבו למטה בטנו ישתלשל אלא אם ישולחו ממנו רוחות הרבה או ישתין שתן מרובה וזה בקדחות. → NM 3:215–6.

• סכסוך הרוחות → סִכְסוּךְ.

רוֹחַב → רֹחַב.

רוּחִי • האיברים הרוחיים → אֵבֶר.

• האשך הרוחיי → אֶשֶׁךְ.

רוּחָנִי • האברים הרוחניים → אֵבֶר.

• העלה הרוחנית → עִלָּה.

רוֹחֵץ (*Part.*) → רָחַץ.

רוט • גיעוש הנקרא רוט → גְּעוּשׁ.

רוע → רַע.

רוֹעֶה • מטה הרועה → מַטֶּה.

• מקל הרועה → מַקֵּל.

• קוץ הרועה → קוֹץ.

רושד • דבש רושד → דְּבַשׁ.

רושם → רֹשֶׁם.

[רחב] • *Part. Nif'al* **נִרְחָב** · **supinated:** Arab. باطح · Ibn Sīnā, *K. al-Qānūn fī al-ṭibb* · trans. Joseph Lorki (*Sefer ha-Qanun*), bk. 1 (fol. 15ᵇ): ואם יעזור אותו עצל הבוהן אשר נזכור אותו אחר זה ישלים הפכת ⟨בהן⟩ הכף נרחב. → NM 4:194.

• *Hitpa'el* **הִתְרַחֵב** • **נגעים אשר יתרחבו** → נֶגַע.

• *Part. Hitpa'el* **מִתְרַחֵב** • **המורסא המתרחבת** → מֻרְסָא.

• **הנגעים המתרחבים** → נֶגַע.

• **השחינים המתרחבים** → שְׁחִין.

• *Hif'il* **הִרְחִיב** · **to supinate:** Arab. بطح · Ibn Sīnā, *K. al-Qānūn fī al-ṭibb* · trans. Joseph Lorki (*Sefer ha-Qanun*), bk. 1 (fol. 15ᵇ): ואמנם המרחיב הזרוע זוג האחד ממנו מונח מחוץ בין שני העמודים הנקראים זנדין. → NM 4:194.

• **הרחיב הנפש** · **to dilate the soul (i.e., to rejoice the soul):** Arab. بسط النفس · Ibn al-Jazzār, *Zād al-musāfir wa-qūt al-ḥādir* · trans. Moses ibn Tibbon (*Sefer Ṣedat ha-Derakhim*), bk. 1, ch. 20 (fol. 30ᵇ): ואמר רופוש אין היין לבדו כשישתה בשווי מרחיב הנפש ומסיר ממנה הדאגה. → NM 4:194–5.

רָחָב • **מקום רחב** → מָקוֹם.

• **העצם הרחב** → עֶצֶם.

רֹחַב · **supination:** Arab. بَطْحٌ · Ibn Sīnā, *K. al-Qānūn fī al-ṭibb* · trans. Joseph Lorki (*Sefer ha-Qanun*), bk. 1 (fol. 15ᵇ): ואלו הקובצים והמותחים הם עצמם פועלים השפוע והרחב. → NM 4:195.

• **רוחב החדר** · **cavity:** Arab. فضاء · Maimonides, *Šarḥ fuṣūl Abūqrāṭ* · trans. Anonymous (*Pirqei Abuqraṭ*), 6.27 (319): אמר המפרש: בלויים יקראו כל מי שהיה בו מוגלא ברוחב החדר אשר בין החזה והריאה ויצטרך שיכוה סובל זה החולי ליבש זה הרטיבות כשנלאו לצאת ברקיקה. → NM 3:216.

• **החוליא החולכת ברוחב** → חֻלְיָה.

רָחְבִּי • **השלב הרחבי** → שָׁלָב.

רָחוּץ (*Pass. Part.*) → רָחַץ.

רֵחַיִם · **(lit., millstone); a hard formation in a woman's womb:** Arab. رحا / Gr. μύλη ·
a) Maimonides, *K. al-fuṣūl fī al-ṭibb* · trans. Zeraḥyah Ḥen (*Sefer ha-Peraqim*), 23.97: הרחים הנולדים ברחמי הנשים הוא בשר יולידהו האשה אין צורה לו. → NM 1:187.

b) Maimonides, *K. al-fuṣūl fī al-ṭibb* · trans. Nathan ha-Me'ati (*Sefer ha-Peraqim*), 23.97: הרחים המתילד ברחמי הנשים הוא בשר שתלד האשה שאין לו צורה. → NM 2:86.

רְחִיצָה · **extraction:** Arab. غسالة · a) Maimonides, *K. al-fuṣūl fī al-ṭibb* · trans. Zeraḥyah Ḥen (*Sefer ha-Peraqim*), 2.2: כמו שימצא בגוף לחות מימיי כאלו הוא רחיצת החלק הגס אשר בו כן ימצא בכל הליחות לחות מימיי רקיק. → NM 1:187.

b) Maimonides, *K. al-fuṣūl fī al-ṭibb* · trans. Nathan ha-Me'ati (*Sefer ha-Peraqim*),

2.2: כמו שימצא בחלב לחות מימיית כאלו הוא רחיצת החלק העב אשר בו כן ימצא בכל הליחות לחות מימיית רקיקה. → NM 2:85–6.

רֶחֶם • בליטת הרחם → בְּלִיטָה.

• התחנקות הרחם → הִתְחַנְּקוּת.

• חניקת הרחם → חֲנִיקָה.

• כוסות הרחם → כּוֹס.

• מחנק הרחם → מַחֲנָק.

• פיות ורידי הרחם → פֶּה.

• פיות עורקי הרחם → פֶּה.

• קרני הרחם → קֶרֶן.

• תחתית הרחם → תַּחְתִּית.

• תיק הרחם → תִּיק.

רָחַץ • *Part.* רוֹחֵץ • הסם הרוחץ → סַם.

• *Pass. Part.* רָחוּץ • הלחם הרחוץ → לֶחֶם.

[רחק] • *Part. Hif'il* מַרְחִיק • העצל המרחיק → עָצֵל.

רָטֹב • סכר הרטוב → סֻכָּר.

רטוב → רָטֹב.

רְטִיָּה · **fomentation; fomenting:** Arab. تكميد · Maimonides, *Šarḥ fuṣūl Abūqrāṭ* · trans. Moses ibn Tibbon (*Pirqei Abuqraṭ*), 6.31 (323): אמר אבקראט: כאיבי העינים יתיכו אותם שתית היין החי או המרחץ והרטיה או הקזת העורק או שתית המשלשל. → NM 3:216.

ריאה → רֵאָה.

ריאומה · **catarrh; rheum:** Lat. reuma · Bruno Longobucco, *Cyrurgia Magna* · trans. Hillel ben Samuel (*Sefer Keritut*), fol. 45[a]: עוד בעבור שכל כאב מקבץ הריאומה ששם נעשה הנפח והצמח שבעבורם יבוא הקווץ אל נקלה. → NM 1:45.

רִיבְדָּא → רבידא.

ריבוע → רִבּוּעַ.

רֵיחַ • ריח דבק · **fragrant smell:** Arab. رائحة تعبق · Maimonides, *K. al fuṣūl fī al ṭibb* (Medical *Aphorisms*)) · trans. Nathan ha-Me'ati (*Sefer ha-Peraqim*), 9.53: ונריח לו בשר חזיר צלי ומבושל ובכלל כל מה שיזון ממה שיש לו ריח דבק. → NM 2:36.

• ריח הפה · **bad breath:** Arab. بخر · Lat. foetor oris · Ibn al-Jazzār, *Zād al-musāfir wa-qūt al-ḥādir* · trans. Moses ibn Tibbon (*Sefer Ṣedat ha-Derakhim*), introduction (fol. 2[b]): השער הכ״ג בריח הפה. → NM 4:195.

רֵיחָנִיּוּת · **aroma; fragrance:** Lat. aromaticitas · Ibn Sīnā, *K. al-adwiya al-qalbiya* · trans. Anonymous (*Sefer ha-Refu'ot ha-Libbiyot*), 249[a]: ועם זה יש בו דקות והנה ניאות ברוח לריחניותו ועפיצותו. → NM 4:195.

ריסוק → רִסּוּק.

ריעוע → רִעוּעַ.

[ריק] • *Hif'il* הֵרִיק · **to apply a purgative:** Hippocrates, *Aphorisms* · trans. Judah Shalom, 4.1 (138) (fol. 51[a]): ההרות אם יתעוררו הליחות ראוי להריק מן החדש הרביעי עד השביעי. → NM 3:216.

רֵיק • המקום הריק → **מָקוֹם**.

ריקוח → **רִקּוּחַ**.

רֵיקוּת ‧ I. **perineum**: Arab. فضاء ‧ Al-Zahrāwī, *K. al-taṣrīf li-man ʿağiza ʿan at-taʾlīf* ‧ trans. Shem Tov ben Isaac (*Sefer ha-Shimmush*), bk. 30, 2.70 (fol. 220[b]): שער ע׳ ברפואת האנדרוגירוס. האנדרוגינוס יהיה בזכרים על שני מינים האחד מהם שיראה במה שימשך אל הריקות או בעור הבצים במה שיש בין הבצים תבנית דומה לקיבת אשה יש בו שער. → NM 1:115.

‧ II. **purgation**: Hippocrates, *Aphorisms* ‧ trans. Judah Shalom, 2.35 (87) (fol. 29[b]): בכל חולי היות במה שאצל הטבור וגב הערוה עובי הוא יותר טוב ודק מאד וכחוש רע ובכמו זה סכנה אל אותם הרקות אשר מלמטה. → NM 3:216–7.

• **בריקות נפש** ‧ **on an empty stomach**: Arab. على الريق ‧ Maimonides, *K. al-fuṣūl fī al-ṭibb* ‧ trans. Nathan ha-Me'ati (*Sefer ha-Peraqim*), 22.36: שתית תשעה גרגרים מן הפטדה הוא זמרד שחוקה ומנופה בגמיעת מים בריקות נפש מפסיק פגע הארסים. → NM 2:86.

רִיר ‧ **mucilage**: Arab. لعاب ‧ Ibn al-Jazzār, *Zād al-musāfir wa-qūt al-ḥādir* ‧ trans. Moses ibn Tibbon (*Sefer Ṣedat ha-Derakhim*), bk. 7, 8.5: ואם יצא ממנו דבר בפה ימשחהו בריר שיליום עם ריר זרע חבושים ומעט שמן ורדים. → NM 1:68.

רַךְ • מורסת הבשר הרך → **מֻרְסָא**.

רִמּוֹן • *Plur.* **רמונים • תבשיל הרמונים** → **תַּבְשִׁיל**.

רָמַז ‧ **to advise**: Arab. أشار ‧ Maimonides, *K. al-fuṣūl fī al-ṭibb* ‧ trans. Zeraḥyah Ḥen (*Sefer ha-Peraqim*), 3.85: ולא ארמוז בהזרתו לעולם אלא לעתים רחוקות שנזיר במעט הזרה כשלא יהיה שם כאב ויהיה הגוף נקי. → NM 1:187.

רנפלי ‧ **asthma**: Arab. ربو ‧ Al-Rāzī, *K. al-Manṣūrī* ‧ trans. Shem Tov ben Isaac (*Sefer Almansur*), Alef 8 (14): אשקיל: חם חד חריף מועיל מן הכפיון וגודל הטחול ולחישת האפעה והרנפלי הישן. → NM 2:19.

רסג ‧ **carpus; tarsus**: Arab. رسغ ‧ Ibn Sīnā, *K. al-Qānūn fī al-ṭibb* ‧ trans. Nathan ha-Me'ati (*Sefer ha-Qanun*), bk. 1 (fol. 38[b]): הרסג מחובר מעצמים רבים שלא יכללהו פגע. → NM 4:195.

רִסּוּק ‧ I. **bruise; bruising**: a) Arab. وثء ‧ i. Al-Zahrāwī, *K. al-taṣrīf li-man ʿağiza ʿan at-taʾlīf* ‧ trans. Shem Tov ben Isaac (*Sefer ha-Shimmush*), bk. 30, 2.89 (fol. 227[a]): ואם תקרה אל הצפורן מכה או ריסוק ונתחדש בה כאב חזק ראוי להקיז החולה בתחלה. → NM 1:115.

‧ ii. Ibn al-Jazzār, *Zād al-musāfir wa-qūt al-ḥādir* ‧ trans. Moses ibn Tibbon (*Sefer Ṣedat ha-Derakhim*), bk. 7, 25.4: ומזה רפואה תועיל מן השבר והרסוק. → NM 1:68.

b) Arab. فسخ ‧ Maimonides, *Šarḥ fuṣūl Abūqrāṭ* ‧ trans. Moses ibn Tibbon (*Pirqei Abuqraṭ*), 2.6 (58): אמר המפרש: רוצה בכאב בכאן סבת הכאב כמו שיהיה בחולה מורסא חמה או חומרא והנגע והרסוק והכתישה ומה שדומה לזה והיה בלתי מרגיש בו שכלו מעורבב. → NM 3:217.

‧ II. **contusion**: Arab. وثء ‧ Al-Zahrāwī, *K. al-taṣrīf li-man ʿağiza ʿan at-taʾlīf* ‧ trans. Shem Tov ben Isaac (*Sefer ha-Shimmush*), bk. 30, 1.46 (fol. 207[b]): שער מו׳ בכוית הריסוק. → NM 1:115.

רַע • אפיסת המים הרעים → **אֲפִיסָה**.

• חולי המים הרעים → חֳלִי.

• המים הרעים → מַיִם.

רֹעַ • **רוע בשול** · **indigestion**: Lat. indigestio (Honofredi) · Ibn Zuhr, *Regimen of Health* · trans. Jacob ibn Tibbon (*Hanhagat ha-Beri'ut le-Abu 'Ali ben Zuhr*), ch. 24: וראוי שירחיק רוע בשול וימעט המאכל ביום ההוא ויקל המזון כאשר ימשך. → NM 4:195.

• **רוע בשול האצטומכא** · **indigestion**: Arab. تخم / Gr. ἀπεψία · Ibn al-Jazzār, *Zād al-musāfir wa-qūt al-ḥādir* · trans. Moses ibn Tibbon (*Sefer Ṣedat ha-Derakhim*), introduction (fols. 3[a–b]): השער הט׳ ברוע בשול האצטומכא הוא אלתכם. → NM 4:195–6.

• **רוע הניפוש** · **shortness of breath**: Arab. رداءة التنفّس · Maimonides, *Šarḥ fuṣūl Abūqrāṭ* · trans. Zeraḥyah Ḥen (*Pirqei Abuqraṭ*), 3.31 (137): אמר בקראט: אמנם הזקנים יקרה להם רוע הניפוש. → NM 3:217.

• **רוע נפש** · **despondency**: Arab. خبث نفس · Maimonides, *Šarḥ fuṣūl Abūqrāṭ* · trans. Moses ibn Tibbon (*Pirqei Abuqraṭ*), 5.61 (281): אמר אבקראט: כשלא יגר דם נדות האשה בעונותיו ולא יתחדש בה פלצות ולא קדחת אבל יקרה לה צער ועלוף ורוע נפש דע שהיא כבר נתעברה. → NM 3:218.

• **רוע הנשימה** · I. **asthma**: Gr. ἄσθμα · Hippocrates, *Aphorisms* · trans. Joseph Delmedigo, 3.26 (132): וליותר גדולים יקרו מורסות הגרון ודחיית חוליות הצואר לפנים ורוע הנשימה והולדת האבן במקוה והתולעים העגולים והדקים והיבלת התלויה וצמחים קשים באחורי האזנים וטפטוף השתן והחזירים ושאר צמחים אבל ביותר אלו הנזכרים. → NM 3:217–8.

· II. **shortness of breath**: Arab. رداءة التنفّس / Gr. δύσπνοια · Maimonides, *Šarḥ fuṣūl Abūqrāṭ* · trans. Moses ibn Tibbon (*Pirqei Abuqraṭ*), 3.31 (137): אמר אבקראט: ואולם הישישים הנה יקרה להם רוע הנשימה. → NM 3:217.

[רעד] • *Part. Nif'al* **נִרְעָד** · **vibratory**: Arab. مرتعد · Maimonides, *K. al-fuṣūl fī al-ṭibb* · trans. Nathan ha-Me'ati (*Sefer ha-Peraqim*), 4.37: כשיהיה הכח חזק וגרם העורק קשה והצורך מכריח הרבה יהיה הדפק נרעד וכשיחסר אחד מאלו הענינים אז לא יהיה הדפק נרעד. → NM 2:69.

רַעַד · **twitching of muscles and their tendons**: Arab. اختلاج / Lat. subsultus tendinum · Ibn al-Jazzār, *Zād al-musāfir wa-qūt al-ḥādir* · trans. Moses ibn Tibbon (*Sefer Ṣedat ha-Derakhim*), bk. 1, ch. 24 (fol. 39[b]): ואולם הרעד הנקרא בערבי איכתילאג׳ הוא התפשטות יוצא מן הטבע ויתחדש בכל האיברים אשר מדרכם שיתפשטו. → NM 4:196.

רָעָה • **רעת הליחה השחורה** · **melancholic delusion**: Hippocrates, *Aphorisms* · trans. Do'eg ha-Edomi (*Sefer Agur*), 3.22 (128) (fol. 55[b]): אמר אבוקרט: פגרי החורף להביא על הגופים קצת המדוים אשר באו עליו בימי הקייץ פרצת קדחת רביעית נפח טחול אפיסת המים הרעים החולי היבש יציאת השתן במכאוב הזלת הבטן והדם וכאב הירכים פוקות מיני השעול וכאב המעי הגדול והחולי המפיל רעת הליחה השחורה וכאב הגרון. → NM 3:219.

רִעוּעַ · **affliction**: Arab. آفة · Maimonides, *Šarḥ fuṣūl Abūqrāṭ* · trans. Moses ibn Tibbon (*Pirqei Abuqraṭ*), 6.45 (337): אמר המפרש: רוב מה שיארך זמן הנגע מפני ריעוע שהשיג העצם וכשיצא העצם הנפסד יתרפא וישאר המקום עמוק. → NM 3:218–9.

רַעְיוֹן • **רעיון נאמר בלי עיון** · **error**: Arab. وَهْم · Maimonides, *Šarḥ fuṣūl Abūqrāṭ* · trans. Moses ibn Tibbon (*Pirqei Abuqraṭ*), introduction (13): ופרקי אבקראט אלו יש מהם פרקים

מסופקים צריכים לפירוש ומהם מבוארים בעצמם ומהם כפולים ומהם מה שלא יועיל במלאכת הרפואות ומהם רעיון פשוט נאמר בלי עיון. → NM 3:175.

רְעִיפָה • רעיפת הדם · **hemorrhage**: Arab. نزف · Al-Zahrāwī, *K. al-taṣrīf li-man ʿağiza ʿan at-taʾlīf* · trans. Shem Tov ben Isaac (*Sefer ha-Shimmush*), bk. 30, 2.55 (fol. 217b): ולהשמר בעת המלאכה מרעיפת הדם שהיא תקרה הרבה ואם תקרה ראוי להרגיל מה שיפסיקנו ולרפא החבורה עד שתבריא. → NM 1:115.

• **רעיפת דם מן החוטם** · **nosebleed**: Arab. رعاف · Hippocrates, *Aphorisms* · trans. Hillel ben Samuel, 3.27 (133) (fol. 19a): א״א: אבל העוברים השנים האלה לזמן הבגרות יבואו להם הרבה מאלו וקדחות ארוכות ורעיפת דם מן החוטם. → NM 3:219.

• **רעיפת דם מן הנחירים** · **nosebleed**: Arab. رعاف · Hippocrates, *Aphorisms* · trans. Nathan ha-Me'ati, 3.27 (133) (fols. 55a–b): אמר אבוקרט: ואמנם מי שיעבור אלו השנים ויקרב שיצמח לו שער בגב הערוה הנקרא עאנה בערבי אז יקרה לו הרבה מאלו החליים וקדחות יותר ארוכות ורעיפת דם מן הנחירים. → NM 3:219.

רְעִישָׁה · **tremor**: a) Arab. ارتعاش · Al-Zahrāwī, *K. al-taṣrīf li-man ʿağiza ʿan at-taʾlīf* · trans. Shem Tov ben Isaac (*Sefer ha-Shimmush*), bk. 27, fol. 134b, col. b: ומתועלותיו גם כן על דרך הסם שהוא מועיל מן הרעישה וחולשת הראות. → NM 4:196.

b) Arab. رعشة · Maimonides, *Šarḥ fuṣūl Abūqrāṭ* · trans. Anonymous (*Pirqei Abuqraṭ*), 6.26 (318): אמר אבוקרט: מי שקרה לו בקדחת השורפת רעישה אז ערבוב השכל יתירנה ממנו. → NM 3:220.

רַעַם · **intestinal rumblings**: Arab. قرقرة · Maimonides, *K. al-fuṣūl fī al-ṭibb* · trans. Zeraḥyah Ḥen (*Sefer ha-Peraqim*), 7.55: כשתאכל מזון ולא יקרה לך ממנו נפיחה ולא רעם ולא רפפות ולא שונגלוצו ... אין ספק שבזה האסטומכא נתקבצה על המזון על דרך הרעש. → NM 1:187–8.

[רעע] • *Hitpaʿel* **הִתְרוֹעֵעַ** · **to suffer from a colic**: Hippocrates, *Aphorisms* · trans. Do'eg ha-Edomi (*Sefer Agur*), 5.41 (261) (fol. 88a): שמת לבך לדעת מאשה אם היא הרה ואם לא השקה אותה בעת שכיבה מים ודבש ואם יתרועעו מעיה לאות כי הרה. → NM 3:220.

[רעף] • *Hifʿil* **הִרְעִיף • הרעיף דם** · **to have a nosebleed**: Arab. رعف / Gr. αἱμορραγέω ἐκ τῶν ῥινῶν · Maimonides, *Šarḥ fuṣūl Abūqrāṭ* · trans. Anonymous (*Pirqei Abuqraṭ*), 4.74 (211): ואם הרעיף דם יהיה תכלית חליו עם זה במהרה לאלתר. → NM 3:220.

רַעַשׁ · **tremor**: Hippocrates, *Aphorisms* · trans. Do'eg ha-Edomi (*Sefer Agur*), 6.26 (318) (fol. 101b): טירוף הדעת אל הסובל קדחת דולקת ⟨ו⟩רעש באיברים אות רפואה הוא. → NM 3:220–1.

[רפא] • *Piʿel* **רִפֵּא** · I. **to practise**: Arab. عالج · Maimonides, *K. al-fuṣūl fī al-ṭibb* · trans. Zeraḥyah Ḥen (*Sefer ha-Peraqim*), 20.62: המזון שהוא קשה להתיר והוא מזון הדברים שהם עבים ודבקים כמו מזון בשר החזיר והלחם הטוב הנקי ושלא יתקרב בו שום טורח ויתמיד לעשות זה המזון ימהר לו החולי ממילוי כמו שמי שירפא הטורח ויתמיד להיות ניזון עם הירקות ומי השעורים יפסיד גופו וימהר אליו הטיצי. → NM 1:188.

· II. **to purge**: Lat. medico · Hippocrates, *Aphorisms* · trans. Hillel ben Samuel, 1.22 (49) (fol. 6b): הענינים המבושלים ראוי לרפאת ולהניע והפגים לא יניע בהתחלה אם אינם הומיים והרוב באמת אינם הומיים. → NM 3:221.

[רפה] • *Hif'il* **הִרְפָּה** · to loosen: Arab. خلخل · Maimonides, *Šarḥ fuṣūl Abūqrāṭ* · trans. Zeraḥyah Ḥen (*Pirqei Abuqraṭ*), 1.1 (23): וכן הפעולות הנמשכות לאלו הכוחות הראשונות והם אשר יקראום הרופאים הכוחות השניות כמו שתהיה הרפואה תקשה או תחליק או תרפה או תקבץ. → NM 3:221.

• *Part. Hif'il* **מַרְפֶּה** • **חסם המרפה** → **סַם**.

• **סמים מרפים ומחלחלים** → **סַם**.

רָפֶה • **מורסת הבשר הרפה** → **מֻרְסָא**.

• **רפה הנקבים** · porous: Arab. متخلخل / Gr. χαλαρός · Hippocrates, *Aphorisms* · trans. Nathan ha-Me'ati, 5.71 (291) (fol. 106[a]): אמר אבוקרט: מי שיהיה עורו מתוח נגוב וקשה הנה הוא ימות מבלי זיעה ומי שיהיה עורו רך ורפה הנקבים הנה הוא ימות עם זיעה. → NM 3:221.

רְפוּאָה • **השקה הרפואה** → **[שקה]**.

• **השתדלות הרפואה** → **הִשְׁתַּדְּלוּת**.

• **התעסקות הרפואה** → **הִתְעַסְּקוּת**.

• **רפואה מחברת** · **incarnative medicine**: Lat. medicamen incarnativum · Bruno Longobucco, *Cyrurgia Magna* · trans. Hillel ben Samuel (*Sefer Keritut*), fol. 21[a–b]: הרפואה המחברת כמו שאמר ב"צ היא מה שמקבץ בין שני חלקים רחוקים. → NM 1:25.

• **רפואה מחליקה** · **detergent remedy**: Lat. medicina abstersiva · Bruno Longobucco, *Cyrurgia Magna* · trans. Hillel ben Samuel (*Sefer Keritut*), fol. 26[b]: ויש לך לדעת שהמכות הנמסות הטריות צריכות רפואה מחליקה יותר מאותה שמניחין בשאר המכות. → NM 1:26.

• **רפואה מתאימה** · **a consolidative remedy**: Lat. medicamen consolidativum · Bruno Longobucco, *Cyrurgia Magna* · trans. Hillel ben Samuel (*Sefer Keritut*), fol. 21[b]: והרפואה המתאימה היא אותה שמיבשת שטח המכה עד שיעשה שם קליפה שישמרנה מן הדברים המזיקים. → NM 1:41.

• **רפואה מתירה** · **dissolving medications**: Arab. أدوية تحلّل · Maimonides, *K. al-fuṣūl fī al-ṭibb*· trans. Zeraḥyah Ḥen (*Sefer ha-Peraqim*), 15.25: החולי שבעין הנקרא ברדה צריכה לחיתוך וכן הטרי המקובץ בעין בחולי הנקרא אלכמנא ברוב תרופא ברפואה מתירה לא בדבר שמייבש יובש חזק כי חוא ירק חרוב ויקפיא הנשאר. ← NM 1:179 (corr.).

• **נתן הרפואה** → **נָתַן**.

• **עשה הרפואה** → **עָשָׂה**.

• **עשיית הרפואה** → **עֲשִׂיָּה**.

• **שתיית הרפואה** → **שְׁתִיָּה**.

• *Plur.* **רפואות** • **רפואות הברזל** · **operative treatment**: Arab. علاج الحديد · Maimonides, *K. al-fuṣūl fī al-ṭibb* · trans. Nathan ha-Me'ati (*Sefer ha-Peraqim*), 8.43: הדרך אשר תלך בה תמיד הוא שתשתדל להריק ולהתיך מה שהוא יוצא מן הטבע ואם אי אפשר שישלם זה בסבת טבע האבר או בסבת שהעלה עלה שלא תבריא ותמגל כלומר שתסבב שישוב מוגלא אותו הדבר היוצא חוץ מן הטבע ותעפשהו ואם לא יצליח נחתכהו ונשרש אותו אם ברפואות הברזל ואם ברפואות השורפות והכוות. → NM 2:33.

• **הרפואות אשר יודעו במשככות** · **remedies which are known as restraining**: Arab. الأدوية التي تعرف بالرداعة · Ibn al-Jazzār, *Zād al-musāfir wa-qūt al-ḥāḍir* · trans. Moses ibn Tibbon (*Sefer Ṣedat ha-Derakhim*), bk. 7, 15.3: וכאשר הריקונו כל הגוף נשוב אל הרפואות אשר יודעו במשככות והדוחות בהתחלה. → NM 1:61–2.

• **הרפואות העוצרות** · **binding drugs**: Arab. الأدوية الحابسة · Maimonides, *K. al-fuṣūl fī al-ṭibb* · trans. Nathan ha-Me'ati (*Sefer ha-Peraqim*), 13.28: השלשול אם יקובל תועלת בו אין ראוי שיפסק ואפילו במאכל אשר יש עמו כח מועט מעצירה וכל שכן הרפואות העוצרות כי אם יפסק תשוב הליחה הרעה למעלה ותוליד קדחת או מורסא בכבד ברוב או בשאר האברים. → NM 2:73.

רְפִידָה · *Plur.* **רפידות** · **pads**: Arab. رفائد · a) Maimonides, *K. al-fuṣūl fī al-ṭibb* · trans. Zeraḥyah Ḥen (*Sefer ha-Peraqim*), 15.65: בהיות העצם נשבר תשים הרפידות טבולות ביין קובץ ושחור וכל שכן בקייץ כי אתה אם תעשה בקיץ השמן או הקירוטי יתחדש באברים עיפוש. → NM 1:188.

b) Maimonides, *K. al-fuṣūl fī al-ṭibb* · trans. Nathan ha-Me'ati (*Sefer ha-Peraqim*), 15.69: ואם כן יהיה כל מה שמקיף באבר ארבע דברים: הקשירה הנוגעת האבר והרפידות והקשירה אשר עליהן והחבישות. → NM 2:86–7.

רִפְיוֹן · **looseness**: Arab. تخلخل · Maimonides, *Šarḥ fuṣūl Abūqrāṭ* · trans. Moses ibn Tibbon (*Pirqei Abuqraṭ*), 5.69 (289): יבא מהר לגב להיותו יותר קר לרוב העצמות שם ומיעוט הבשר והנשים יותר קרות מן האנשים והביא ראיה מרפיון הקודם מצמיחת השער שם. → NM 3:222.

• **רפיון האברים** · **shivers**: Arab. كزاز · Maimonides, *K. al-fuṣūl fī al-ṭibb* · trans. Nathan ha-Me'ati (*Sefer ha-Peraqim*), 22.16: והקשטור מועיל מרפיון האברים תועלת מבוארת. → NM 2:87.

רְפָפוּת · **palpitation**: Arab. اختلاج · Maimonides, *K. al-fuṣūl fī al-ṭibb* · trans. Zeraḥyah Ḥen (*Sefer ha-Peraqim*), 7.40: הרפפות סבתו רוח עב כלוא במקום קשה לא ימצא מקום שיצא ממנו. → NM 1:188–9.

רִפְרוּף · **twitching**: Arab. اختلاج · Maimonides, *K. al-fuṣūl fī al-ṭibb* · trans. Nathan ha-Me'ati (*Sefer ha-Peraqim*), 3.55: הרפרוף מתחדש בכל האברים שאפשר שיתפשטו. → NM 2:87.

רַפְשִׁי · **turbid**: Arab. كدر / Gr. βορβορώδης · Hippocrates, *Aphorisms* · trans. Nathan ha-Me'ati, 7.44 (396) (fol. 136[a]): אמר אבוקרט: מי שירוק מבעלי המוגלא ויצא ממנו מוגלא לבנה בבת אחת הנה הוא ישלם וימלט ואם יצא ממנו מוגלא רפשיית סרוחה הנה הוא ימות. → NM 3:222.

רָצוֹן • **הגרת הזרע מבלי רצון** → הֲגָרָה.

• **רצון קיא** · **nausea**: Arab. تهوّع · Maimonides, *K. al-fuṣūl fī al-ṭibb* · trans. Zeraḥyah Ḥen (*Sefer ha-Peraqim*), 6.34: ומי שיקרה לו השקוטומיאה מפני פי האסטומכא יקדים לו דפיקת הלב ורצון קיא. → NM 1:189.

רצפה · **patella**: Arab. رضفة · Ibn Sīnā, *K. al-Qānūn fī al-ṭibb* · trans. Zeraḥyah Ḥen (*Sefer ha-Qanun*), bk. 1 (fol. 28[b]): ולו שני קצוות האחד מהם בשריי ויתדבק ברצפה קודם היותו יתר והאחר קרומי יתחבר בקצה הפנימי מקצויי הירך. → NM 4:196–7.

[רצץ] • *Pu'al* **רֻצַּץ** · **to be crushed**: Arab. رُضَّ · Ibn al-Jazzār, *Zād al-musāfir wa-qūt al-ḥāḍir* · trans. Moses ibn Tibbon (*Sefer Ṣedat ha-Derakhim*), bk. 1, ch. 23 (fol. 37[a]): ירוצץ כל זה ויושם בשמן וירתיחהו על האש עד שיקח השמן כח הסמים. → NM 4:197.

רַקָּה · **cheek**: Arab. خدّ · Ibn Sīnā, *K. al-Qānūn fī al-ṭibb* · trans. Nathan ha-Me'ati (*Sefer ha-Qanun*), bk. 1 (fol. 44[a]): הפרק הששי בנתוח עצלי הרקה. הרקה יש לה שתי תנועות. → NM 4:197.

• **בליטת הרקה** → בְּלִיטָה.

רְקוּחַ · **composition (of a remedy)**: Arab. تأليف · Ibn al-Jazzār, *Zād al-musāfir wa-qūt al-ḥādir* · trans. Moses ibn Tibbon (*Sefer Ṣedat ha-Derakhim*), bk. 7, 26.1: והנה זכר גליאה בספר תחבולות הבריאות כי זאת הרפואה תהיה רקוחה על שלשה מינים. → NM 1:68.

• *Plur.* **רקוחים** · **stomachics**: Arab. جوارشن, *Plur.* جوارشنات · Ibn Sīnā, *K. al-adwiya al-qalbiya* · trans. Anonymous (*Sammim Libbiyim*), fol. 133ª: ואולם אשר בו רוע מזג חם ובמזגים החמים והארצות החמות הנה לא יקל אליהם בהם ולא בשאר המרקחות והריקוחים החמים אלא בעת ההכרח הנגלה. → NM 4:197.

רְקוּק · **expectoration**: Arab. نفث · Maimonides, *K. al-fuṣūl fī al-ṭibb* · trans. Nathan ha-Me'ati (*Sefer ha-Peraqim*), 21.21: סכנג׳בין חזק החמיצות אם שינגב הליחות ויוסיף בדביקותם והתלותם שיקשה רקוקם. → NM 2:87.

רקות → רֵיקוּת.

רְקִיקָה • **רקיקת הדם** · **hemoptysis**: Arab. نفث الدم / Gr. ἅιματος πτύσις · Maimonides, *Šarḥ fuṣūl Abūqrāṭ* · trans. Moses ibn Tibbon (*Pirqei Abuqraṭ*), 3.29 (135): אמר אבקראט: ואולם הבחורים הנה יקרה להם רקיקת הדם והשדפון והקדחות החדות וחולי הנופל ושאר החליים אבל כי רוב מה שיקרה להם מה שזכרנוהו. → NM 3:222–3.

[רקק] • *Hif'il* **הִרְקִיק** · **to purify**: Arab. روّق · Maimonides, *K. al-fuṣūl fī al-ṭibb* · trans. Zeraḥyah Ḥen (*Sefer ha-Peraqim*), 7.15: והרוח החיונית בישרון האויר היוצא ולפתוח סתמי העור ולנקות כלי הניפוש מן העובי ומן הדבקות ולפתוח סתמיהם ושיכניס בגופו דברים שירקיקו דם הלב ויסירו העבירות מרוחו עם הרפואות. → NM 1:189.

רֹשֶׁם • **מקום הרושם** → מָקוֹם.

[רתע] • *Hif'il* **הִרְתִּיעַ** · **to restrain; to subdue; to suppress**: Arab. قمع · Al-Zahrāwī, *K. al-taṣrīf li-man ʿağiza ʿan at-ta'līf* · trans. Shem Tov ben Isaac (*Sefer ha-Shimmush*), bk. 27, fol. 137ᵇ, col. b: ומסגלתו שהוא מדקדק החלטים ומגיר השתן בדקות ומרתיע המרה הכרכומית. → NM 4:197–8.

• **הרתיע לאחור** · **to repel; to restrain**: Arab. ردع · Al-Zahrāwī, *K. al-taṣrīf li-man ʿağiza ʿan at-ta'līf* · trans. Shem Tov ben Isaac (*Sefer ha-Shimmush*), bk. 30, 2.87 (fol. 226ᵇ): והשתדלתי להרתיע לאחור המותר ההוא במה שנתתי על היד מן חסמים אחר חרקת הגוף ולא נרתע לאחור המותר. → NM 1:116 (corr.).

• *Part. Hif'il* **מַרְתִּיעַ** • **הסם המרתיע** → סַם.

רֶתֶת · **rigor**: Hippocrates, *Aphorisms* · trans. Do'eg ha-Edomi (*Sefer Agur*), 4.46 (183) (fol. 69ᵇ): נכר וידוע על כל סובל קדחת התמיד אם יקרהו קור ורתת והוא חלוש כי אות מות הוא. → NM 3:223.

ש

שָׁאַף · **to inhale through the nose**: Arab. استنشق · Maimonides, *K. al-fuṣūl fī al-ṭibb* · trans. Zeraḥyah Ḥen (*Sefer ha-Peraqim*), 9.6: בהיות המותרות הניגרים מן האף מימיות בלתי מבושלים היותינו מתקנים אותם יהיה בדברים אשר תטבול הראש כדי שיחמם המוח ועם הדברים אשר תשאף ואשר יריק באוזן. → NM 1:189.

שְׁבָב • *Plur.* **שבבים** · **fragments**: Arab. شظايا · Al-Zahrāwī, *K. al-taṣrīf li-man ʿağiza ʿan at-taʾlīf* · trans. Shem Tov ben Isaac (*Sefer ha-Shimmush*), bk. 30, 2.84 (fol. 224[b]): ואם עשתה רושם בעצם וחתכה ממנו שבבים. → NM 1:116.

שבוטא → שִׁיבּוּטָא.

שבולת → שִׁבֹּלֶת.

שְׁבִיל • **שביל השתן** · **urethra**: Gr. οὐρήθρα · Hippocrates, *Aphorisms* · trans. Joseph Delmedigo, 4.82 (219): מי שנולדה לו צמיחה בשביל השתן כשיבא לידי מורסא ויבקע מתרפא. → NM 3:223.

שְׁבִירָה · **hernia**: Lat. crepatura · Al-Rāzī, attr., *On the Treatment of Small Children* · trans. Anonymous, ch. 22: כבר אמרנו למעלה בכמה פנים תקרה השבירה ועתה אין אנו צריכין לומר זולתי הרפואות ההכרחיות. ונאמר ראשונה תחבושת מועיל לילדים בשבירתם מהשבירה. → NM 2:181.

שְׂבָכָה · **rete mirabile**: Arab. شبكة · Ibn Sīnā, *K. al-Qānūn fī al-ṭibb* · trans. Nathan ha-Me'ati (*Sefer ha-Qanun*), bk. 1 (fol. 62[a]): ולכן נפרשה השבכה תחת המוח להחזיר הדם השרייני והרוח בו ויתדמה במזג המוחיי אחרי הבשול. → NM 4:198.

• **השבכה השליית** · **choroid plexus**: Arab. الشبكة المشيمية · Ibn Sīnā, *K. al-Qānūn fī al-ṭibb* · trans. Nathan ha-Me'ati (*Sefer ha-Qanun*), bk. 1 (fol. 65[b]): ואחר נמתח מן החדר האמצעי אל שני החדרים המוקדמים ופוגע בעורקים הדופקים העולים שם ומתארג הקרום ⟨הידוע⟩ כשבכה השליית. → NM 4:198.

שִׁבֹּלֶת • **שבולת הזקן** · **chin**: Arab. ذقن · Al-Zahrāwī, *K. al-taṣrīf li-man ʿağiza ʿan at-taʾlīf* · trans. Shem Tov ben Isaac (*Sefer ha-Shimmush*), bk. 30, 2.96 (fol. 231[a]): ונתינת הרבידות מתחת שבולת הזקן מועילות מן השחין הדק אשר בפה הנקרא בלשונם אל קלאע. → NM 1:116.

שָׁבַר • *Part.* **שׁוֹבֵר** • **הסם השובר רוח** → סַם.

• *Inf. Nifʿal* **הִשָּׁבֵר** · **(lit., to be broken); to abate; to cease**: Arab. انكسر · Ibn al-Jazzār, *Zād al-musāfir wa-qūt al-ḥāḍir* · trans. Moses ibn Tibbon (*Sefer Ṣedat ha-Derakhim*), bk. 1, ch. 18 (fol. 26[b]): ואולם אשר יתערבב שכלם בסבת כאב המוח לבד הנה ערבובם יתוסף ויגדל מעט מעט ויתמיד בהם אחר מנוחת הכאב והשבר הקדחת ולא יפסק כלל כי החולי במוח עצמו. → NM 4:198.

• *Part. Piʿel* **מְשַׁבֵּר** • **הסם המשבר הרוח** → סַם.

שֶׁבֶר • *Plur.* **שברים** • **חשבת השברים** → הֲשָׁבָה.

שִׁבָּרוֹן · **pain**: Arab. كلال / Gr. πόνος · Maimonides, *Šarḥ fuṣūl Abūqrāṭ* · trans. Moses ibn Tibbon (*Pirqei Abuqraṭ*), 4.44 (181): אמר אבקראט: מי שמצאהו קדחת ארוכה הנה יקרה לו אם יציאות ואם שברון בפרקיו. → NM 3:223.

[שבש] • *Part. Puʿal* **מְשֻׁבָּשׁ** · **heterogeneous**: Arab. متشتّت / Gr. διεστηκώς · Maimonides,

Šarḥ fuṣūl Abūqrāṭ · trans. Moses ibn Tibbon (*Pirqei Abuqraṭ*), 7.33 (385): אמר אבקראט: מי שהיה שתנו משובש יורה כי בגופו צער חזק. → NM 3:145.

שָׁגַל · **to have sexual intercourse**: Arab. جامع · Galen, attr., *Prohibition of Burial* · trans. Judah al-Ḥarizi (*Sefer Issur ha-Qevurah le-Galienus*), par. 109: והמין האחר הוא מפני אכילת המטעמים אשר לא נאכלו מזמן ארוך כמי שחסר לו לחם ימים רבים ואחר אכלו או מפני המשגל שעמד זמן ארוך ואחר שגל. → NM 4:198–9.

שִׁגָּעוֹן · **raving**: Arab. هذيان · Ibn al-Jazzār, *Zād al-musāfir wa-qūt al-ḥādir* · trans. Moses ibn Tibbon (*Sefer Ṣedat ha-Derakhim*), bk. 1, ch. 18 (fol. 26[a]): מורסת הראש במאמר מוחלט היא מורסא חמה תקרה בקצת קרומות המוח ישיגהו תמיד צער ושגעון וערבוב השכל. → NM 4:199; cf. *Sefer ha-Yosher* (Ms. Oxford, Bodleian Library, Opp. 180 (cat. Neubauer 2134), fol. 7[b]): השער מן מילאוקוניא הוא החולה השגעון.

• **השגעון השחור** · **melancholic delusion**: Arab. الوسواس السوداوي · Ibn al-Jazzār, *Zād al-musāfir wa-qūt al-ḥādir* · trans. Moses ibn Tibbon (*Sefer Ṣedat ha-Derakhim*), bk. 1, ch. 18 (fol. 26[b]): וכבר זכר גאלינוס שכל הערבובים נמשכים אחר הליחות החדות העוקצות ואין דבר מהם שתהיה הסבה בו ליחה קרה זולת הערבוב אשר יקרא השגעון השחור והוא בערבי אלוסואס אלסודאוי. → NM 4:199.

שַׁד • *Dual* **שָׁדַיִם** • **התוספות הדומות לפיות חשדים** → **תּוֹסֶפֶת**.

• **התוספות הדומים בשני ראשי השדים** → **תּוֹסֶפֶת**.

שָׁדוּף (*Pass. Part.*) → **שָׁדַף**.

שָׂדִי · **wild**: Arab. بري · Al-Zahrāwī, *K. al-taṣrīf li-man ʿağiza ʿan at-taʾlīf* · trans. Shem Tov ben Isaac (*Sefer ha-Shimmush*), bk. 27, fol. 126[b], col. b: השדיים מכל מיני האפונין פעולותיהם יותר חזקים מן הפרדסיים. → NM 4:199.

שָׁדַף • *Pass. Part.* **שָׁדוּף** · **ill**: Arab. سقيم · Maimonides, *K. al-fuṣūl fī al-ṭibb* · trans. Zeraḥyah Ḥen (*Sefer ha-Peraqim*), 8.14: אבל כשיהיו אותם האברים שדופים החולי לקח חוקו מעצם הגוף והפחד עליו מרובה ואי אפשר שיתרפא החולה עד שתשוב אל האברים השרשיים כחם המיוחד בהם. → NM 1:190.

• *Hitpaʿel* **הִשְׁתַּדֵּף** · I. **to waste away**: Arab. ذبل / Gr. ἀναλίσκομαι · Maimonides, *Šarḥ fuṣūl Abūqrāṭ* · trans. Moses ibn Tibbon (*Pirqei Abuqraṭ*), 1.14 (41): אמר אבקראט: מה שהיה מן הגופות בגדול הנה החום הטבעי בו בתכלית מה שיהיה מן הרבוי ויצטרך בעבור זה מן המזון ליותר ממה שיצטרך אליו שאר הגופים שאם לא יאכל מן המזון מה שיצטרך אליו ישתדף גופו ויחסר. → NM 3:224.

· II. **to wither**: Arab. ذبل · Al-Zahrāwī, *K. al-taṣrīf li-man ʿağiza ʿan at-taʾlīf* · trans. Shem Tov ben Isaac (*Sefer ha-Shimmush*), bk. 30, 2.64 (fol. 220[a]): ואם תקרה הזמורה לכל הכיסים ראוי להוציא אחד מן הבצים מן הכיסים פן תעדר הביצה מזון מפני חתוך הכיסים ותשתדף ולא יהיה בה תועלת. → NM 1:116.

• *Part. Hitpaʿel* **מִשְׁתַּדֵּף** · **meager**: Arab. ضامر · Al-Zahrāwī, *K. al-taṣrīf li-man ʿağiza ʿan at-taʾlīf* · trans. Shem Tov ben Isaac (*Sefer ha-Shimmush*), bk. 27, fol. 125[b], col. a: ויש ממנו מין שלישי דק משתדף עב מעט הלובן לא נתבשל בשבלים כל צרכו וזה המין מגונה מאד לא יאות לעשות ממנו שרף ולא לחם כלל. → NM 4:199–200.

שִׁדָּפוֹן · **phthisis**: Arab. سلّ · a) Maimonides, *K. al-fuṣūl fī al-ṭibb* · trans. Nathan ha-

Me'ati (*Sefer ha-Peraqim*), 22.44: וקרבת החתולים ועורותיהם מוריש הצמוק והשדפון. → NM 2:87.

b) Maimonides, *Šarḥ fuṣūl Abūqrāṭ* · trans. Moses ibn Tibbon (*Pirqei Abuqraṭ*), 3.29 (135): אמר אבקראט: ואולם הבחורים הנה יקרה להם רקיקת הדם והשדפון והקדחות החדות וחולי הנופל ושאר החליים אבל כי רוב מה שיקרה להם מה שזכרנוהו. → NM 3:224.

• **קדחת השדפון** → **קַדַּחַת**.

שדפוני • **קדחת שדפונית** → **קַדַּחַת**.

שְׁדֵרָה • **חוט השדרה** → **חוּט**.

• **מוחיות השדרה** → **מֹחִיּוּת**.

• **שפל השדרה** → **שֵׁפֶל**.

• **תחתית השדרה** → **תַּחְתִּית**.

[שוב] • **שב חגר** · **to become lame**: Arab. عرج / Gr. χωλόομαι · Maimonides, *Šarḥ fuṣūl Abūqrāṭ* · trans. Moses ibn Tibbon (*Pirqei Abuqraṭ*), 6.60 (352): אמר אבקראט: מי שקרהו כאב הירך זמן גדול והיתה ירכו נוקעת הנה כל רגלו תצמוק וישוב חגר אם לא יכוה. → NM 3:79–80.

• **יין מבושל עד ששב כדבש** → **יַיִן**.

• *Hifʿil* **הֵשִׁיב** · **to accustom**: Arab. عوّد · Maimonides, *K. al-fuṣūl fī al-ṭibb* · trans. Zeraḥyah Ḥen (*Sefer ha-Peraqim*), 7.51: כשירצה האדם לרומם קולו ראוי לו שישיב רוחו ויפתח פיו מאד עד שיכנס בו אויר מרובה ירחיב הגרון ויהיה הקול גדול. → NM 1:190.

שׁוֹבֵר (*Part.*) → **שָׁבַר**.

שָׁוֶה • **העצם השוה** → **עֶצֶם**.

שׁוֹטֶה • **כלב שוטה** → **כֶּלֶב**.

• *Plur.* **שוטים** · **[those suffering from] melancholy**: Arab. (ذو) المالنخوليا · Al-Zahrāwī, *K. al-taṣrīf li-man ʿağiza ʿan at-taʾlīf* · trans. Shem Tov ben Isaac (*Sefer ha-Shimmush*), bk. 27, fol. 143ª, col. a: בשר התיש המוכלח מגונה המזון מוליד דם שחורי ומביא מתמידו אל חליים שחוריים וכל שכן מי שהוא מעותד להם כגון השוטים והנכפים ואל השחין הערום ודומיהם מן החליים הרעים. → NM 4:200.

שׁוֹכֵן (*Part.*) → **שָׁכַן**.

שׁוּלְיָא • **קשורי השוליא** → **קֶשֶׁר**.

שׁוֹמֵעַ (*Part.*) → **שָׁמַע**.

שׁוֹמֵר · **pupil**: Arab. ناظر · Maimonides, *K. al-fuṣūl fī al-ṭibb* · trans. Zeraḥyah Ḥen (*Sefer ha-Peraqim*), 15.30: המים אחר שירד ויפחות מפני השומר ראוי שתחזיק אותו עם המחט שעה גדולה במקומות אשר ירצה שינוח בו כדי שיתאחז בו. → NM 1:190.

שומשמני → **שֻׁמְשְׁמָנִי**.

שׁוּעָל • **אילן השועל** → **אִילָן**.

• **אשכי השועל** → **אֶשֶׁךְ**.

• **חולי השועל** → **חֳלִי**.

• **מדוה השועל** → **מַדְוֶה**.

שׁוֹעֵר (*Part.*) → **שָׁעַר**.

שׁוֹקֵד (*Part.*) → **שָׁקַד**.

שׁוֹר • שור הבר · wild cow (ox): Arab. البقر الوحشية · Al-Zahrāwī, *K. al-taṣrīf li-man ʿağiza ʿan at-taʾlīf* · trans. Shem Tov ben Isaac (*Sefer ha-Shimmush*), bk. 27, fol. 143[b], col. a: וכן צריך לעשות בכל בשר עב כבשר שור הבר. → NM 4:200.

שׁוֹרֵף (*Part.*) → **שָׂרַף.**

שׁוֹרֵץ (*Part.*) → **שָׁרַץ.**

שותפות → **שֻׁתָּפוּת.**

שׁוֹתֵת (*Part.*) → **שָׁתַת.**

שָׁחוּן · ulcerous: Lat. vulneratus · Hippocrates, *Aphorisms* · trans. Judah Shalom, 5.23 (243) (fol. 80[b]): ובארישפילא הבלתי שחונה כי הוא מזיק לשחונה. → NM 3:224–5.

שחוס • למטה משחוס החזה → **מַטָּה.**

שחוסי · cartiliginous: Arab. غضروفي · Ibn Sīnā, *K. al-Qānūn fī al-ṭibb* · trans. Nathan ha-Me'ati (*Sefer ha-Qanun*), bk. 1 (fol. 35[b]): העצה מחובר מחוליות שחוסיים אין תוספות אליהם. → NM 4:201.

שחור → **שָׁחֹר.**

שחורה → **שְׁחֹרָה.**

שְׁחוֹרִי · black bilious; melancholic: Arab. سوداوي · Al-Zahrāwī, *K. al-taṣrīf li-man ʿağiza ʿan at-taʾlīf* · trans. Shem Tov ben Isaac (*Sefer ha-Shimmush*), bk. 27, fol. 131[b], col. b: שכר התמרים עב מוליד דם שחורי. → NM 4:201.

• **הבלבול השחורי** → **בִּלְבּוּל.**

• **בלבול השכל השחורי** → **בִּלְבּוּל.**

• **הדאגה השחורי** → **דְּאָגָה.**

• **החשתוממות השחורי** → **הִשְׁתּוֹמְמוּת.**

שֶׁחִי • תחת השחי → **תַּחַת.**

שְׁחִיטָה · angina: Arab. ذبحة / Gr. κυνάγχη · Maimonides, *Šarḥ fuṣūl Abūqrāṭ* · trans. Anonymous (*Pirqei Abuqraṭ*), 5.10 (230): אמר אבוקרט: מי שקרתהו שחיטה הנקרא אסכרה וימלט ממנו ונטה החומר אל ריאתו הוא ימות בשבעה ימים. ואם יעברם יחזור להוצאת מוגלא. → NM 3:225.

שחיי • השחיי · the axillary vein: Arab. الابطي · Ibn Sīnā, *K. al-Qānūn fī al-ṭibb* · trans. Zeraḥyah Ḥen (*Sefer ha-Qanun*), bk. 1 (fol. 34[b]): והשני ישתלח אל מקום כפל הקוברי בנראה של הזרוע ויתערבו בו שעיפים מן השחיי. → NM 4:201.

שְׁחִין · pustule: Arab. بثر / Gr. ἐξάνθημα · Ibn al-Jazzār, *Zād al-musāfir wa-qūt al-ḥāḍir* · trans. Moses ibn Tibbon (*Sefer Ṣedat ha-Derakhim*), bk. 2, ch. 1 (fol. 42[b]): תאר עגולים שלישיים לבנים מועילים מן הנגעים והקצידא והשחין וכבר נסיתים. → NM 4:202.

• **שחין דק** · I. aphthae: Arab. قلاع / Gr. ἄφθα, *Plur.* ἄφθαι · Al-Zahrāwī, *K. al-taṣrīf li-man ʿağiza ʿan at-taʾlīf* · trans. Shem Tov ben Isaac (*Sefer ha-Shimmush*), bk. 27, fol. 141[a], col. a: ומזיקים אל הדרדני ומחדדים שחין דק בפה ומולידים האפר בעינים. → NM 4:202.

· II. pustules: Arab. بثر, *Plur.* بثور · a) Al-Zahrāwī, *K. al-taṣrīf li-man ʿağiza ʿan at-taʾlīf* · trans. Shem Tov ben Isaac (*Sefer ha-Shimmush*), bk. 27, fol. 147[b], col. a: קום החלב משלשל המרה הכרכומית ומועיל מן הבהק והגרב והשחין הדק. → NM 4:202.

b) Al-Zahrāwī, *K. al-taṣrīf li-man ʿağiza ʿan at-taʾlīf* · trans. Shem Tov ben Isaac

(*Sefer ha-Shimmush*), bk. 30, 1.55 (fol. 208ᵇ): יתחדש בגוף שחין דק מכוער מחמרים קרים עבים נפסדים. → NM 1:116–7.

• **השחין אשר בפה** › **aphthae**: Arab. قلاع / Gr. ἄφθα, *Plur.* ἄφθαι · Maimonides, *Šarḥ fuṣūl Abūqrāṭ* · trans. Moses ibn Tibbon (*Pirqei Abuqraṭ*), 3.24 (130): ואולם בשנים הנה יקרו אלו החליים: בילדים הקטנים בעת שיולדו יקרה להם השחין אשר בפה והקיא והשעול והיקיצה והפחד ומורסת הטבור ולחות האזנים. → NM 3:225.

• *Plur.* **שחינים** • **השחינים המתרחבים** › **herpes**: Arab. القروح التي تسعى · Hippocrates, *Aphorisms* · trans. Nathan ha-Me'ati, 5.22 (242) (fol. 90ᵇ): והוא מהיותר נאות שבדברים לשבר העצמות וכ״ש לאותם שהם ערומים מבשר ויותר מיוחד מזה לעצמות הראש ובכל מה שהמיתו הקור או השחינו ולשחינים המתרחבים. → NM 3:225–6.

• **שחיני הפה** › **aphthae**: Hippocrates, *Aphorisms* · trans. Judah Shalom, 3.24 (130) (fol. 47ᵃ): ובשנים אלו לקטנים הילדים הנולדים מחדש שחיני הפה. → NM 3:226.

שְׁחִיקָה • **שחיקת הגריסים** › **coarse meal**: Arab. سويق الجريش · Maimonides, *Šarḥ fuṣūl Abūqrāṭ* · trans. Anonymous (*Pirqei Abuqraṭ*), 7.31 (383): מי שהיה לו קדחת ויצלול בשתנו שמרים דומים לשחיקת הגריסים יורה על אורך החולי. → NM 3:227.

[שחן] • *Part. Hif'il* **מַשְׁחִין** • **הסם המשחין** → **סַם**.

[שחף] • *Part. Pu'al* **מְשֻׁחָף** • *Plur.* **משוחפין** › **people suffering from phthisis**: Arab. مسلول, *Plur.* مسلولين · Al-Zahrāwī, *K. al-taṣrīf li-man ʿağiza ʿan at-taʾlīf* · trans. Shem Tov ben Isaac (*Sefer ha-Shimmush*), bk. 27, fol. 125ᵇ, col. b: ומתועלתיו על דרך הסם כי כשיעשה ממנו שרף מבושל היטב ויורגל בשמן שקדים מתוקים או בחמאה יועיל למשוחפין ובבעלי השעול היבש. → NM 4:108.

שַׁחֶפֶת › **wasting**: Arab. سلّ · Al-Zahrāwī, *K. al-taṣrīf li-man ʿağiza ʿan at-taʾlīf* · trans. Shem Tov ben Isaac (*Sefer ha-Shimmush*), bk. 30, 1.24 (fol. 205ᵇ): כשיהיה השעול וחלי הריאה מלחויות קרות ולא תהיה אל החולה קדחת ולא שחפת ויהיה החלי ישן. → NM 1:117.

שָׁחֹר • **בלבול הראש השחור** → **בִּלְבּוּל**.

• **העגול השחור שבבשר** → **עִגּוּל**.

• **רעת הליחה השחורה** → **רָעָה**.

• **השגעון השחור** → **שִׁגָּעוֹן**.

שְׁחֹרָה › **melancholy (i.e., black bile)**: Lat. melancolia / Arab. سوداء · Galen, *De inaequali intemperie* · trans. David Caslari (*Sefer Ro'a Mezeg Mitḥallef*), 4.3: והאבר גם כן אשר בו המורסא או הוא קרוב לאברים אשר הם רבי הדם או רחוק מהם ועוד כי הדם שתגבר בו האדומ׳ או השחורה או הליחה או הרוח. → NM 2:170.

• **הבלבול הקורה מן השחורה** → **בִּלְבּוּל**.

• **חולי השחורה** → **חֳלִי**.

• **תחלוא השחורה** → **תַּחֲלוּא**.

[שחת] • *Part. Hof'al* **מֻשְׁחָת** • **מושחת מחולי** › **suffering from phthisis**: Arab. مسلول · Maimonides, *Šarḥ fuṣūl Abūqrāṭ* · trans. Moses ibn Tibbon (*Pirqei Abuqraṭ*), 3.10 (116): אמר המפרש: להיותו קר יבש מתחלף המזג הנה הוא יזיק המושחתים מחולי מאד. → NM 3:146.

שָׁטוּחַ (*Pass. Part.*) → **שָׁטַח**.

שְׁטוּת · I. **delirium; delusion; mental confusion:** a) Arab. وسواس · Al-Rāzī, *K. al-Manṣūrī* · trans. Shem Tov ben Isaac (*Sefer Almansur*), Bet 12 (20): בלאדור: חם יבש מאד יועיל מן החליים הקרים ⟨ו⟩השכחה אלא שהוא ישרוף הדם ואפשר שיעורר שטות. → NM 2:19.

b) Arab. اختلاط · Maimonides, *Šarḥ fuṣūl Abūqrāṭ* · trans. Moses ibn Tibbon (*Pirqei Abuqraṭ*), 6.53 (345): אין ממיני השטות דבר טוב והיותר רע מהם מה שהיה עמו הקדמה להלחם וחטיפה והוא השטות. → NM 3:226–7.

c) Lat. desipientia · Hippocrates, *Aphorisms* · trans. Hillel ben Samuel, 6.53 (345) (fol. 43[b]): א"א: השטות עם שחוק הוא בטוח אבל אותו אשר עם אבל הוא כבד. → NM 3:226.

· II. **melancholy:** Arab. مالنخوليا · Al-Zahrāwī, *K. al-taṣrīf li-man ʿağiza ʿan at-taʾlīf* · trans. Shem Tov ben Isaac (*Sefer ha-Shimmush*), bk. 30, 1.11 (fol. 204[a]): שער י"א בכוית השטות. כשתהיה סבתו לחויות נפסדות ולחה לבנה עבה ראוי לכוותו הכויות אשר זכרתי בבעל הפלג. → NM 1:117.

· III. **rabies:** Arab. كَلَب · Ibn al-Jazzār, *Zād al-musāfir wa-qūt al-ḥāḍir* · trans. Moses ibn Tibbon (*Sefer Ṣedat ha-Derakhim*), bk. 7, 13.1: הכלב בטבעו קר ויבש גוברת עליו מרה שחורה ולשפעת הליחה הזאת השחורית בו והיותה גוברת עליו תתעפש ותכלול הפסדה כל גופו ויוציאהו זה אל השטות. → NM 1:69.

שָׁטַח · **to plaster; to rub; to smear:** Arab. طلى · Ibn al-Jazzār, *Zād al-musāfir wa-qūt al-ḥāḍir* · trans. Moses ibn Tibbon (*Sefer Ṣedat ha-Derakhim*), bk. 1, ch. 1 (fol. 6[b]): או יקח רודא מדברית או גרעיניה וישחק בחומץ יין ויטוח בו או יטוח בליברוס לבן או שחור או בשל ניטרי אחר שישחק בחומץ יין וישטחהו עליו שעה אחר שעה ואחר כך יקנחהו במטלית. → NM 4:203.

• *Pass. Part.* **שָׁטוּחַ** • **שטוח על ערפו** · **supinated:** Arab. باطح · Ibn Sīnā, *K. al-Qānūn fī al-ṭibb* · trans. Nathan ha-Me'ati (*Sefer ha-Qanun*), bk. 1 (fol. 50[b]): ואם יעזרהו עצל הבוהן אשר נזכיר אחר זה ישלם הפוך הכף שטוח על ערפו. → NM 4:202.

• *Hifʿil* **הִשְׁטִיחַ** · I. **to expand:** Arab. بسط · Ibn Sīnā, *K. al-Qānūn fī al-ṭibb* · trans. Nathan ha-Me'ati (*Sefer ha-Qanun*), bk. 1 (fol. 48[a]): אלו הם העצלים המשטיחות. → NM 4:203.

· II. **to rejoice:** Arab. بسط · Maimonides, *K. al-fuṣūl fī al-ṭibb* · trans. Nathan ha-Me'ati (*Sefer ha-Peraqim*), 8.32: לחשב בדברים המשמחים משטיח הנפש ומזרזה ויתפשט בזה החום הטבעי. → NM 2:87.

· III. **to spread:** Arab. طلى · Al-Zahrāwī, *K. al-taṣrīf li-man ʿağiza ʿan at-taʾlīf* · trans. Shem Tov ben Isaac (*Sefer ha-Shimmush*), bk. 30, 1.49 (fol. 208[a]): ואחרי כן לרפאתה בקמח עדשים עם שמן ורד ועלי לשון טלה ודם יונה ודם תחמס מכל אחד חלק שוה ולערב את הכל ולהשטיחם על בגד ולתתו על המקום עד שיבריא. → NM 1:117.

• **השטיח על ערפו** · **to supinate:** Arab. بطح · Ibn Sīnā, *K. al-Qānūn fī al-ṭibb* · trans. Nathan ha-Me'ati (*Sefer ha-Qanun*), bk. 1 (fol. 49[b]): ואמנם המשטיח לקנה על ערפו הוא זוג אחד נפרד ומונח מחוץ בין שני הזנאדים. → NM 4:203.

שְׁטִיחָה • **השטיחה על העורף** · **supination:** Arab. بَطْح · Ibn Sīnā, *K. al-Qānūn fī al-ṭibb* · trans. Nathan ha-Me'ati (*Sefer ha-Qanun*), bk. 1 (fol. 50[b]): ואלו המקבצים והמפשיטים הם בעצמם פועלים הקבוב והשטיחה על העורף. → NM 4:203.

שָׂטָן • **זבל שטן** → זֶבֶל.

שיבא (*Aram.*) ‣ **splinter**: Arab. شظية · Al-Zahrāwī, *K. al-taṣrīf li-man ʿağiza ʿan at-taʾlīf* · trans. Shem Tov ben Isaac (*Sefer ha-Shimmush*), bk. 30, 3.6 (fol. 234[b]): ואם יפרד מן העצם שִׁיבָּא ותהיה עוקצת מתחת העור ראוי לבקע עליה ולהסירה. → NM 1:118.

שִׁיבּוּטָא (*Aram.*) ‣ **fish of uncertain identity**: Arab. شبّوط · Al-Zahrāwī, *K. al-taṣrīf li-man ʿağiza ʿan at-taʾlīf* · trans. Shem Tov ben Isaac (*Sefer ha-Shimmush*), bk. 27, fol. 149[b], col. b: החשוב יותר ממיני הדג הוא המין הנודע בשבוטא הנקרא אצל המצריים אל בלטי. → NM 4:203–4.

שילוח → שִׁלּוּחַ.

[שים] • *Hofʿal* **הושם** • **הושם בנחיריו** ‣ **to be applied as an errhine**: Arab. سعط · Ibn al-Jazzār, *Zād al-musāfir wa-qūt al-ḥādir* · trans. Moses ibn Tibbon (*Sefer Ṣedat ha-Derakhim*), bk. 1, ch. 10 (fol. 15[b]): ויושם בנחיריו מיץ מברילה עם חלב אשה ילדה בת ושמן ורדים או שמן ויאולד. → NM 4:204.

שינוי → שִׁנּוּי.

שיעור → שִׁעוּר.

שיער → שֵׂעָר.

שיפוע → שִׁפּוּעַ.

שִׁכְחָה ‣ **lethargus**: Hippocrates, *Aphorisms* · trans. Judah Shalom, 3.30 (136) (fol. 49[b]): ובאותם אשר על אלו השנים יקרה אשמא ופלברשין ומורסת הריאה ופרנשין ושכחה וקבשו' ואדומה ודיאריאה ארוכה וזחיר וחלקות הבטן וטחורים. → NM 3:227.

שְׁכִיבָה ‣ **alleviation**: Lat. sedari · Bruno Longobucco, *Cyrurgia Magna* · trans. Hillel ben Samuel (*Sefer Keritut*), fol. 79[a]: ואותות המורסא הקשה הוראה עליה שכיבת הכאב וקושי מתרבה. → NM 1:40.

שְׁכִינָה ‣ **rest**: Arab. سكون · Maimonides, *K. al-fuṣūl fī al-ṭibb* · trans. Zeraḥyah Ḥen (*Sefer ha-Peraqim*), 1.27: אבל מי שהוא ישן ויש בו שכרות או טורח חזק או חולשה הוא ירפה כל אברי גופו בתכלית הרפיון וישיב המושקולי בצורה הממוצעת ויהיה שוכן שכינה שלמה בהיותו ישן. → NM 1:191.

[שכך] • *Part. Piʿel* מְשַׁכֵּךְ • **הרפואות אשר יודעו במשככות** → רְפוּאָה.

שֵׂכֶל • **בלבול השכל** → בִּלְבּוּל.

• **בלבול השכל השחורי** → בִּלְבּוּל.

• **התערבב השכל** → [ערבב].

• **ערבוב שכל** → עִרְבּוּב.

• **הקדחת אשר יהיה עמה ערבוב השכל** → קַדַּחַת.

שֶׁכֶם ‣ **collarbone (clavicle)**: Arab. ترقوة · Ibn Sīnā, *K. al-Qānūn fī al-ṭibb* · trans. Joseph Lorki (*Sefer ha-Qanun*), bk. 1 (fol. 12[a]): פרק י״ו בנתוח השכם. השכם עצם מונח על כל אחד משני צדי עליון החזה. → NM 4:204.

שָׁכַן • *Part.* שׁוֹכֵן ‣ **motionless**: Arab. ساكن · Maimonides, *K. al-fuṣūl fī al-ṭibb* · trans. Zeraḥyah Ḥen (*Sefer ha-Peraqim*), 1.15: ורוב אברי הפנים יתנועעו ברצון והעצמות שוכנות ואינם צריכים ליתרים. → NM 1:190.

• **עורקים שוכנים** → עוֹרֵק.

[שכר] • *Part. Puʿal* **מְשֻׁכָּר** › **drunk; intoxicated:** Arab. مخمور · Ibn al-Jazzār, *Zād al-musāfir wa-qūt al-ḥādir* · trans. Moses ibn Tibbon (*Sefer Ṣedat ha-Derakhim*), bk. 1, ch. 19 (fol. 29ᵃ): וראוי שיתרפא מזה אחר שיעיין שאם היה המשוכר בעל מזג חם נשים על ראשו שמנים קרים. → NM 4:109.

שִׁכָּרוֹן › **intoxication:** Ibn Zuhr, *Regimen of Health* · trans. Jacob ibn Tibbon (*Hanhagat ha-Beri'ut le-Abu ʿAli ben Zuhr*), ch. 24: וראוי לו שלא ידחה האכילה כאשר תבא התאוה אם לא שתהיה התאוה כוזבת כאשר התעורר בשכרון לבעלי הקבסא. → NM 4:204.

[שכשך] • *Part. Puʿal* **מְשֻׁכְשָׁךְ** • **החלב המשוכשך** → **חָלָב**.

שָׁלָב • **השלב הארוכיי** › **the longitudinal suture:** Arab. الدرز الطولي · Ibn Sīnā, *K. al-Qānūn fī al-ṭibb* · trans. Nathan ha-Me'ati (*Sefer ha-Qanun*), bk. 1 (fol. 29ᵃ): ויהיה השלב הרחבי באמצע הרוחב מן האוזן אל האזן כמו שהשלב הארוכיי באמצע האורך. → NM 4:204.

• **השלב הקלפיי** › **the squamosal suture:** Arab. الدرز القشري · Ibn Sīnā, *K. al-Qānūn fī al-ṭibb* · trans. Nathan ha-Me'ati (*Sefer ha-Qanun*), bk. 1 (fol. 29ᵇ): ושני הגדרים אשר ימין ושמאל הם העצמות אשר יש בהם האזנים הנקראים אלחגריין כלומ' האבנים לקשים כאבן ונאחז כל אחד מהם מלמעלה השלב הקלפיי. → NM 4:205.

• **השלב הרחבי** › **the transverse suture:** Arab. الدرز العردي · Ibn Sīnā, *K. al-Qānūn fī al-ṭibb* · trans. Nathan ha-Me'ati (*Sefer ha-Qanun*), bk. 1 (fol. 29ᵃ): ויהיה השלב הרחבי באמצע הרוחב מן האוזן אל האזן כמו שהשלב הארוכיי באמצע האורך. → NM 4:205.

• *Plur.* **שלבים** › **cranial sutures:** Arab. شأن, *Plur.* شؤون · Ibn Sīnā, *K. al-Qānūn fī al-ṭibb* · trans. Nathan ha-Me'ati (*Sefer ha-Qanun*), bk. 1 (fol. 28ᵇ): ולכמו התבנית הזה יש שלבים ג' אמתיים ושני שלבים כוזבים. → NM 4:205.

שַׁלְהֶבֶת › I. **heat:** Hippocrates, *Aphorisms* · trans. Do'eg ha-Edomi (*Sefer Agur*), 4.65 (202) (fol. 75ᵃ): דמה לעלות שלהבת בקרב העליון ואפיסת הלב עם קדחת אות רע הוא. → NM 3:227.

› II. **temperature:** Arab. لهيب · Ibn al-Jazzār, *Zād al-musāfir wa-qūt al-ḥādir* · trans. Moses ibn Tibbon (*Sefer Ṣedat ha-Derakhim*), bk. 7, 15.4: וכאשר שככה שלהבת האבר החולה נחבשחו קודם שישוב ירוק. → NM 1:69.

שָׁלוּחַ (*Pass. Part.*) → **שָׁלַח**.

שִׁלּוּחַ • **שילוח הדם** › **hemorrhage:** Arab. انبعاث الدم · Maimonides, *K. al-fuṣūl fī al-ṭibb* · trans. Zeraḥyah Ḥen (*Sefer ha-Peraqim*), 15.41: יכריחנו העניין אל הכויה בהיות שילוח הדם בעבור חולי שנפל באבר או בעבור עיפוש שקרהו. → NM 1:191.

שָׁלוּק (*Pass. Part.*) → **שָׁלַק**.

שָׁלוֹשׁ → **שְׁלֹשָׁה**.

שלושה → **שְׁלֹשָׁה**.

שָׁלַח • *Pass. Part.* **שָׁלוּחַ** • **שלוח מן** › **coming from:** Arab. منبعث من · Ibn al-Jazzār, *Zād al-musāfir wa-qūt al-ḥādir* · trans. Moses ibn Tibbon (*Sefer Ṣedat ha-Derakhim*), bk. 2, ch. 17: ואם היה החולי מן המוח והורה על זה המופת אשר הקדמנו או מפני העצב השלוח מן המוח אשר יעבור בו כח התנועה אל הלשון נצוה החולה שישתה הגיראש הגדולות אשר דרכם לנקות המוח. → NM 4:205.

שִׁלְיָה › **afterbirth (fetal membranes, placenta, umbilical cord); chorioid plexus; chorion:** Arab. مشيمة · Ibn Sīnā, *K. al-Qānūn fī al-ṭibb* · trans. Nathan ha-Me'ati (*Sefer *ha-Qanun*), bk. 1 (63^a): והנוטה אל האצילי ושני הנרדמים מקום שיתפרדו בשבכה ובשליה. → NM 4:205–6.

שליי • השבכה השליית → שְׂבָכָה.

שְׁלִישִׁי • קדחת חצי שלישית → קַדַּחַת.

• קדחת שלישית → קַדַּחַת.

[שלך] • *Part. Hif'il* **מַשְׁלִיךְ • הכח המשליך** → כֹּחַ.

שָׁלֵם ‧ I. **to grow [together again]**: Arab. نمى · Maimonides, *Šarḥ fuṣūl Abūqrāṭ* · trans. Moses ibn Tibbon (*Pirqei Abuqraṭ*), 7.28 (380): אמר אבקראט: כאשר נחתך דבר מן העצם או מן האליל לא ישלם. → NM 3:228.

‧ II. **to reach a crisis**: Hippocrates, *Aphorisms* · trans. Do'eg ha-Edomi (*Sefer Agur*), 3.28 (134) (fol. 57^b): אמר אפוקרט: שלמו ימי המדוים האלה לקץ ארבעה זמנים זמן ראשון ארבעים יום שני לקץ שבעה חדשים שלישי לשבע שנים שנת צמיחת הזקן לאנשים ולנשים בעת נדתם. → NM 3:227–8.

• שלם על ‧ **to contain**: Arab. اشتمل على · Maimonides, *K. al-fuṣūl fī al-ṭibb* · trans. Zeraḥyah Ḥen (*Sefer ha-Peraqim*), introduction: המאמר הראשון ישלם על פרקים יהיו נתלים בהנחת המלאכה כלומר צורת אברי גוף האדם ופעולותיו וכוחותיו. → NM 1:191.

• זיעה שלמה → זֵיעָה.

שָׁלַק • *Pass. Part.* **שָׁלוּק • הבשר השלוק** → בָּשָׂר.

שְׁלֹשָׁה • שלשת הפלפלין ‧ **dyatrion pipereon**: Lat. dyatrion pipereon · Ibn Sīnā, *K. al-adwiya al-qalbiya* · trans. Anonymous (*Sefer ha-Refu'ot ha-Libbiyot*), fol. 252^a: והרופאים הסכלים עדיין חושבים שיש למטרודיטוס ולתריאק חום גובר ומפני זה בורחים לתת ממנה שעור חצי זהוב ואמנם לא יהיו נסוגים מלתת ד' זהובים מהדיאסימינום ומרקחת שלשת הפלפלין. → NM 4:164 (corr.).

שִׁלְשׁוּל ‧ **purgation**: Arab. إسهال · a) Ibn al-Jazzār, *Zād al-musāfir wa-qūt al-ḥāḍir* · trans. Moses ibn Tibbon (*Sefer Ṣedat ha-Derakhim*), bk. 2, ch. 1 (fol. 41^b): וירגיל להכנס במרחץ אחר נקוי הגוף אם בהקזה או בשלשול. → NM 4:206.

b) Maimonides, *K. al-fuṣūl fī al-ṭibb* · trans. Nathan ha-Me'ati (*Sefer ha-Peraqim*), 3.110: לא תקרר ולא תרתיע המורסא הנקראת חמרא עד שיורק כלל הגוף בשלשול הבטן ברפואה מוציאה האדומה. → NM 2:88.

• שלשול הבטן ‧ **diarrhea**: Lat. fluxus ventris · Hippocrates, *Aphorisms* · trans. Hillel ben Samuel, 2.14 (66) (fol. 9^a): בשלשול הבטן שנוי הציאות מועיל אם לא ישתנו לרע. → NM 3:228.

• שלשול (ה)דם ‧ **dysentery**: Arab. اختلاف دم · Maimonides, *Šarḥ fuṣūl Abūqrāṭ* · trans. Moses ibn Tibbon (*Pirqei Abuqraṭ*), 3.11 (117): אמר אבקראט: ואולם בזמני השנה אומר כי כשיהיה הסתו מעט מטר צפוני ויהיה האביב ממטיר דרומי יתחייב בהכרח שיתחדשו בקיץ קדחות חדות וקצידה בעינים ושלשול דם ורוב מה שיקרה שלשול הדם לנשים ולבעלי הטבע הלח. → NM 3:228.

• שלשול עם דם ‧ **dysentery**: Hippocrates, *Aphorisms* · trans. Do'eg ha-Edomi (*Sefer Agur*), 4.24 (161) (fol. 64^a): חרדת השלשול עם דם אם יהיו תוצאות הדם מתולדת המרה השחורה הוא אות רע. → NM 3:229–30.

• שלשול היוצא הקיא · cholera: Arab. هيضة · Maimonides, *Šarḥ fuṣūl Abūqrāṭ* · trans. Anonymous (*Pirqei Abuqraṭ*), 3.30 (136): אמר אבוקרט: מי שעבר אלו השנים יקרה לו נזילה על הריאה וחולי הצד וחולי הריאה ושכחה והקדחת אשר תהיה עמה התעורה והקדחת אשר יהיה עמה ערבוב השכל וקדחת השורפת ושלשול היוצא הקיא ושלשול הארוך וגרידת המעים וחליקות המעים והתפתח פיות העורקים ממטה. → NM 3:229.

• שלשול (ה)מעיים · I. **abrasion of the intestines:** Arab. سحج الأمعاء · Maimonides, *Šarḥ fuṣūl Abūqrāṭ* · trans. Zeraḥyah Ḥen (*Pirqei Abuqraṭ*), 6.3 (295): אמר המפרש: שינוי הדם בהיותו עם שלשול המעיים הנק׳ סחג׳ פונט ויאריך יוסיף לחפור בעומק האיברים וישוב נגע בעל עיפוש והכאב באצטומ׳ עם השיתוף ויקח בה ההזק. → NM 3:229.

· II. **tenesmus:** Arab. زحير · Maimonides, *Šarḥ fuṣūl Abūqrāṭ* · trans. Zeraḥyah Ḥen (*Pirqei Abuqraṭ*), 7.27 (379): אמר בקראט: כשיתחדש באשה ההרה שלשול מעיים הנק׳ בערבי זחיר תהיה סבה להיותה מפלת. → NM 3:229.

• שלשול וקיא · cholera: Arab. هيضة / Gr. χολέρα · Al-Zahrāwī, *K. al-taṣrīf li-man ʿağiza ʿan at-taʾlīf* · trans. Shem Tov ben Isaac (*Sefer ha-Shimmush*), bk. 27, fol. 136[a], col. a: ויש פחד מן הפטריות שאינם ממיתים שלא יקרה מהן חניקה וגנוח ועלוף וקרירות הידים והרגלים ועל הרוב ירדוף אותן שלשול וקיא חזקים. → NM 4:206.

[שלשל] • *Part. Piʿel* **מְשַׁלְשֵׁל • הסם המשלשל** → **סַם**.

שְׂמָאלִי • הקנה השמאלי → **קָנֶה**.

שָׁמוּר (*Pass. Part.*) → **שָׁמַר**.

שִׁמּוּשׁ · **observation:** Arab. مباشرة · Maimonides, *Šarḥ fuṣūl Abūqrāṭ* · trans. Anonymous (*Pirqei Abuqraṭ*), 1.1 (17): וכן ידע בקלות לאורך שמושו את האנשים ובצורה ההיא הנרשמת בשכלו איך ישתמש בכלים ההם ר״ל המזונות והסמנים ושאר הכלים. זה צריך אל זמן ארוך. → NM 3:230.

[שמט] • *Inf. Nifʿal* **הִשָּׁמֵט • השמט הבטן** · **to suffer from lientery:** Hippocrates, *Aphorisms* · trans. Doʾeg ha-Edomi (*Sefer Agur*), 4.12 (149) (fol. 61[b]): דרך הבטן להשמט אל תשקהו להקיאו. → NM 3:230.

שֶׁמֶט · **dislocation:** Arab. خلع · Maimonides, *K. al fuṣūl fī al ṭibb* · trans. Nathan ha-Meʾati (*Sefer ha-Peraqim*), 15.46: וכפי זה המשל כשיהיה בפרק מן הפרקים הגדולים שמט עם שחין נרפא השחין עד שיבריא ואע״פ שאי אפשר שהשמט יחבש אחר זה. → NM 2:88.

שְׁמִיטָה · **dislocation:** a) Arab. خَلْع · Al-Zahrāwī, *K. al-taṣrīf li-man ʿağiza ʿan at-taʾlīf* · trans. Shem Tov ben Isaac (*Sefer ha-Shimmush*), bk. 30, 1.40 (fol. 206[b]): שער מ׳ בכוית שמיטת הירך. לפעמים תשתפכנה לחויות עבות אל כף הירך ותהיינה סבה לצאתו ממקומו. ואות השמיטה אורך השוק האחד על חברו כשיוקש אחד אל אחר. → NM 1:118.

b) Arab. فكّ · Al-Zahrāwī, *K. al-taṣrīf li-man ʿağiza ʿan at-taʾlīf* · trans. Shem Tov ben Isaac (*Sefer ha-Shimmush*), bk. 30, 3.23 (fol. 237[a]): השמיטה הוא צאת פרק מן הפרקים ממקומו. → NM 1:118.

שְׁמִיעָה • מקום השמיעה → **מָקוֹם**.

שָׁמִיר · I. **Indian iron:** Arab. الحديد الهندي · Al-Zahrāwī, *K. al-taṣrīf li-man ʿağiza ʿan at-taʾlīf* · trans. Shem Tov ben Isaac (*Sefer ha-Shimmush*), bk. 30, 2.19 (fol. 211[b]): וכשיתגלה ויראה בו הפסד או שחרות ראוי לגרדו בכלי כזה ויקרא העץ הראש ראוי לעשותו משמיר. → NM 1:118.

‣ II. **steel**: Arab. فالوذ · Al-Zahrāwī, *K. al-taṣrīf li-man ʿağiza ʿan at-taʾlīf* · trans. Shem Tov ben Isaac (*Sefer ha-Shimmush*), bk. 27, fol. 146[b], col. a: והצלוי בחלוקי אבנים או בחתיכות השמיר עד שתכלה מימיותו יעזור על עצירת הבטן. → NM 4:206.

שְׁמִירָה ‣ I. **diet**: Arab. حمية · a) Ibn al-Jazzār, *Zād al-musāfir wa-qūt al-ḥādir* · trans. Moses ibn Tibbon (*Sefer Ṣedat ha-Derakhim*), bk. 7, 17.5: והנה תועילהו גם כן הכויה ויתמיד השמירה ויעזוב התערובות במאכלים וכבר שאלו לגאליה מה היא הרפואה היותר גדולה? אמר המעצור. → NM 1:69.

b) Maimonides, *K. al-fuṣūl fī al-ṭibb* · trans. Zeraḥyah Ḥen (*Sefer ha-Peraqim*), 13.38: ראוי שיהיה נזהר כל מה שאפשר בשאר מיני ההרקות במי שעניין גופו יהיה חלק ורך ובעל בשר ואספוגי ומהר ניתך. וכן מי שנתרבה בו השומן והרזון ויהיה הרקת אילו בשמירה הממוצעת והחפיפה והקרישטירי המחליקים והנטילות והתחבושות ובעשיית השיאף ובמרחץ ותקיז מי שעניינו כן לפי מה שיורוך בו ענייני החולה. → NM 1:192.

‣ II. **a precautionary (prophylactic) measure**: Arab. احتياط · Maimonides, *Šarḥ fuṣūl Abūqrāṭ* · trans. Moses ibn Tibbon (*Pirqei Abuqraṭ*), 6.47 (339): זה מבואר למי שיצטרך אליו על צד השמירה כמו שיעשו הבריאים תמיד. → NM 3:230.

• **הנהגת השמירה** → הַנְהָגָה.

• **שמירה והנהגה** ‣ **diet**: Arab. حمية · Maimonides, *K. al-fuṣūl fī al-ṭibb* · trans. Nathan ha-Meʾati (*Sefer ha-Peraqim*), 13.38: ויהיה הרקת אלו בשמירה ובהנהגה השוה ובחפיפה וחוקן הרך ויציקת הדברים המבושלים והתחבושות והנחת הפתילות למטה ובמרחץ. → NM 2:88.

• **מעברי השמירה** → מַעֲבָר.

שְׁמָמוֹן ‣ **affliction; distress; grief; sadness**: Arab. كآبة ; كرب · Ibn Zuhr, *Regimen of Health* · trans. Jacob ibn Tibbon (*Hanhagat ha-Beriʾut le-Abu ʿAli ben Zuhr*), ch. 12: ואולם הטחול הוא כלי השחוק כמו שאמ׳ פיתגורש לפי שהוא ינקה הדם השחור וכאשר לא ינוקה ממנו יזון הלב בדם שחור עכור ויחודש ממנו השממון. → NM 4:207.

שָׁמֵן ‣ **thick**: Lat. pinguis · Hippocrates, *Aphorisms* · trans. Hillel ben Samuel, 4.76 (214) (fol. 29[b]): א״א: אותם ששתנם שמן ויש בו כסובין יש להם גרב בשלפוחית. → NM 3:230.

שֶׁמֶן • **שמן טוב** ‣ **oil from unripe olives**: Arab. الزيت الأنفاق / Gr. το ὀμφάκινον [ἔλαιον] · Ibn al-Jazzār, *Zād al-musāfir wa-qūt al-ḥādir* · trans. Moses ibn Tibbon (*Sefer Ṣedat ha-Derakhim*), fol. 29[b]: ויהיה מזונו צלי קדר וצלי אש וכרוב מבושל בבשר צאן או כרוב שלוק מתוקן במוריס ושמן טוב. → NM 4:207.

שָׁמַע • *Part.* **שׁוֹמֵעַ** • **העצב השומע** → עָצָב.

שֶׁמַע • **העצב אשר בו ילך השמע** → עָצָב.

שָׁמַר ‣ **to investigate**: Arab. حدّد · Maimonides, *Šarḥ fuṣūl Abūqrāṭ* · trans. Moses ibn Tibbon (*Pirqei Abuqraṭ*), 1.23 (50): וכבר נסינו זה פעמים רבות לא ימנו ומצאנו אותו מועיל תועלת חזקה ולא נודע בכאבים החזקים המופלגים רפואה יותר חזקה ויותר מופלגת מן ההרקה עד שיקרה העילוף אחר שישמור וידע אם ראוי שיוקז עורק או יעשה השלשול עד שיקרה העלוף. → NM 3:231.

• *Pass. Part.* **שָׁמוּר** ‣ **trustworthy**: Arab. صحيح / Gr. βεβαίαν καὶ ἀσφαλῆ · Galen, *De diebus decretoriis* · trans. Shimshon ben Shlomo (*Qibbuṣei Maʿamarei Galenus bi-Yemei ha-Buḥran*), 18: והבחראן השמור הוא הבחראן שיובטח עמו שהחולי לא ישוב. → NM 2:173.

[שמש] • *Pi'el* **שִׁמֵּשׁ** ‣ **to attend to**: Arab. باشر · Maimonides, *Šarḥ fuṣūl Abūqrāṭ* · trans. Anonymous (*Pirqei Abuqraṭ*), 1.1 (17): וידוע כי ידיעת זה החלק השביעי כלו ושמירתם מן הספרים המוצעים לכל חלק מהם לא יגיע אליו תכלית פעולת הרופא ולא ישיג לזה החכם השלם במלאכה עד שישמש את האנשים בענין בריאותם וענין חוליהם ויגיע אצלו קנין בהכרת הראיות אשר יורו בהם איך יורה. → NM 3:231.

שִׁמְשִׁי • **הצמוקין השמשיים** → **צִמּוּק**.

שֻׁמְשְׁמָנִי ‣ **sesamoid**: Arab. سمسماني · Ibn Sīnā, *K. al-Qānūn fī al-ṭibb* · trans. Nathan ha-Me'ati (*Sefer ha-Qanun*), bk. 1 (fol. 40[a]): ונמלא הריוח בפרקיהם לתוספת ההדוק בעצמות קטנים נקראים שומשמניים. → NM 4:207.

שֵׁן • *Dual* **שִׁנַּיִם** • **אכול השנים** → **אִכּוּל**.

• **בשר השינים** → **בָּשָׂר**.

• **שני החלומות** ‣ **wisdom teeth**: Arab. أسنان الحلم · Ibn Sīnā, *K. al-Qānūn fī al-ṭibb* · trans. Zeraḥyah Ḥen (*Sefer ha-Qanun*), bk. 1 (fol. 18[a]): וארבעה שנים וברוב הם צומחות באמצע זמן הגדול והוא אחר היותו רואה קרי עד שיגיע אל העמידה כי העמידה קרובה משלשים שנה ועל כן נקראות שני החלומות. → NM 4:207–8.

• **שני החלימה** ‣ **wisdom teeth**: Arab. أسنان الحلم · Ibn Sīnā, *K. al-Qānūn fī al-ṭibb* · trans. Joseph Lorki (*Sefer ha-Qanun*), bk. 1 (fol. 11[a]): והקצויות הנקראות נואגיד צומחות ברוב באמצע זמן הגדול והוא אחר הגיע אל העמידה כי העמידה קרוב משלשים שנה לכן נקראים שני החלימה ובער׳ אסנאן אלחלם. → NM 4:208.

• **שני אלחלם כלומר החלימה** ‣ **wisdom teeth**: Arab. أسنان الحلم · Ibn Sīnā, *K. al-Qānūn fī al-ṭibb* · trans. Nathan ha-Me'ati (*Sefer ha-Qanun*), bk. 1 (fol. 31[b]): והקצויות יצמחו ברוב באמצע זמן הגדול והוא אחר ההמרצה אל ההעמדה וזה כי ההעמדה קרובה מל׳ שנה ולכן נקראים שני אלחלם כלו׳ החלימה. → NM 4:208.

• **השנים הכלביים** ‣ **canine teeth**: Lat. canini dentes · Hippocrates, *Aphorisms* · trans. Hillel ben Samuel, 3.25 (131) (fol. 19[a]): א״א: כשצומחים שיניהם יקרה להם חכוך בשר השינים וקדחות וקווץ ודיאריאה וביחוד כשיצמחו השינים הכלביים ובשמן מן הנערים ואשר בטנם עצור. → NM 3:232.

• **השנים אשר כנגד העינים** ‣ **canine teeth**: Arab. أنياب / Gr. κυνόδοντες · Maimonides, *Šarḥ fuṣūl Abūqrāṭ* · trans. Moses ibn Tibbon (*Pirqei Abuqraṭ*), 3.25 (131): וכאשר קרב הילד שיצמחו לו השנים יקרה לו חיכוך בחניכים וקדחות וקווץ ושלשול כל שכן כאשר יצמחו השנים אשר כנגד העינים ולשמן מן הנערים ולמי שבטנו עצור. → NM 3:231–2.

[שנה] • *Part. Pu'al* **מְשֻׁנֶּה** • **מת מיתה משונה** → **[מות]**.

• *Part. Hitpa'el* **מִשְׁתַּנֶּה** ‣ **pallid**: Arab. حائل / Gr. δύσχροος · Maimonides, *Šarḥ fuṣūl Abūqrāṭ* · trans. Moses ibn Tibbon (*Pirqei Abuqraṭ*), 5.42 (262): כשתהיה האשה הרה מזכר תהיה טובת מראה וכאשר תהיה הרה מנקבה יהיה מראה משתנה. → NM 3:147.

שָׁנָה • *Plur.* **שנים** ‣ **young men**: Arab. أسنان / Gr. ἡλικίαι · Hippocrates, *Aphorisms* · trans. Nathan ha-Me'ati, 1.15 (42) (fol. 13[b]): אמר אבוקרט: הגופים בסתיו ובאביב הם יותר חמים שיהיו בטבע והשינה יותר ארוכה שתהיה ולכן ראוי שיהיה בשני העתים האלו מה שיקח האדם מן המזונות יותר וזה שהחום הטבעי בגופים בשני אלו העתים רב ולכן יצטרכו אל מזון רב והאות על זה השנים והמתאבקים. → NM 3:232.

• **עלה בשנים** → **עָלָה**.

שִׁנּוּי · I. **diarrhea**: Arab. اختلاف · Maimonides, *K. al-fuṣūl fī al-ṭibb* · trans. Zeraḥyah Ḥen (*Sefer ha-Peraqim*), 21.11: החלב היותר מעולה משאר החלבים מלבד חלב האשה הוא חלבי בעלי חיים שהם קרובים מטבע האדם כחזירות והצאן והעזים והסוסים. ואם יתקן כשיתחמם חלוקי אבנים אחרי שקדם ותכבס בחלב אחר חממם לאש והתלבנם עד שיחסר מן החלב מימיותו ויותר לחותו ואחרי כן ירד מהאש וישתנה ישכך התרת הבטן המרובה ויפסיק שינוי הדברים הנמצא בהם שמנות. → NM 1:192.

· II. **cure; removal [of a disease]**: Lat. mutatio / Arab. انتقال · Hippocrates, *Aphorisms* · trans. Hillel ben Samuel, 5.7 (227) (fol. 30[b]): האפילינציאה כשתעשה קודם שיבוא הבחרות יש לה שנוי אבל אותה שתעשה מבן עשרים וחמש שנה ומעלה הרבה פעמים ימותו עמה. → NM 3:232–3.

• **שינוי דם** · **dysentery**: Arab. اختلاف دم · Maimonides, *Šarḥ fuṣūl Abūqrāṭ* · trans. Zeraḥyah Ḥen (*Pirqei Abuqraṭ*), 4.26 (163): אמר בקראט: מי שהיה בו שינוי דם ויצא ממנו דומה לחתיכות הבשר זה סימן מות. → NM 3:233.

שְׁנוּן → סְנוּן.

שְׁנִיּוּת • **יותר שניות** · **more frequent**: Arab. أكثر تكرا · Ibn Sīnā, *K. al-Qānūn fī al-ṭibb* · trans. Zeraḥyah Ḥen (*Sefer ha-Qanun*), bk. 1 (fol. 24[b]): כי תנועות איברי הפנים והשפתים יותר מנין ויותר שניות והתמדה. → NM 4:208.

[שסע] • *Pi'el* **שִׁסַּע** · **to incise**: Arab. شقّ · Maimonides, *K. al-fuṣūl fī al-ṭibb* · trans. Nathan ha-Me'ati (*Sefer ha-Peraqim*), 15.48: אם ראית הרפואות לא יוכלו להתיך המוגלא כלה אבל תנצחם המוגלא ותגבר עליהם אז ראוי שתכרות המורסא הנקרא יציאה ושסעה במקום היותר גבוה שבה והיותר רקיק שבה. → NM 2:88.

שִׁעוּר • **השיעור המכוון** · **a moderate amount (measure)**: Arab. المقدار القصد / Gr. μέτριος · a) Maimonides, *Šarḥ fuṣūl Abūqrāṭ* · trans. Moses ibn Tibbon (*Pirqei Abuqraṭ*), 2.3 (55): אמר אבקראט: השינה והיקיצה כאשר עבר כל אחד מהם השעור המכוון הוא סימן רע. → NM 3:131.

b) Maimonides, *K. al-fuṣūl fī al-ṭibb* · trans. Nathan ha-Me'ati (*Sefer ha-Peraqim*), 17.26: אין טוב לאדם שישתה מן היין יותר מן השיעור המכוון. → NM 2:60.

שִׁעוּר • **מי השעור** → מַיִם.

שְׁעִיעוּת · **softening**: Lat. lenificatio · Bruno Longobucco, *Cyrurgia Magna* · trans. Hillel ben Samuel (*Sefer Keritut*), fol. 86[b]: אמנם צריך שעיעות לניפיקציאון בלע׳ למען ישושע העב. → NM 1:40–1.

שְׂעִיף · **branch (of a nerve)**: Arab. شعبة · Ibn Sīnā, *K. al-Qānūn fī al-ṭibb* · trans. Zeraḥyah Ḥen (*Sefer ha-Qanun*), bk. 1 (fol. 31[b]): והשני זוגות השפלים ישלחו שעיף גדול אל צד השוקים ויתערב עמם שעיף מן הזוג השלישי ושעיף ראשון מעצבי העצם הנק׳ הזקן. → NM 4:209.

שָׂעִיר · **rough**: Lat. asper · Bruno Longobucco, *Cyrurgia Magna* · trans. Hillel ben Samuel (*Sefer Keritut*), fol. 100[b]: ומיני האבן רבים ממנה קטנה וממנה גדולה וממנה חלקה וממנה שעירה וממנה קצרה וממנה ארוכה. → NM 1:40.

שְׂעִירוּת · **roughness**: a) Lat. asperitas · Bruno Longobucco, *Cyrurgia Magna* · trans. Hillel ben Samuel (*Sefer Keritut*), fol. 20[a]: אם מיובש אותותיו הקושי והשעירות ומעט הטרי. → NM 1:40.

b) Arab. خشونة · Ibn al-Jazzār, *Zād al-musāfir wa-qūt al-ḥāḍir* · trans. Moses ibn Tibbon (*Sefer Ṣedat ha-Derakhim*), bk. 1, ch. 18 (fol. 26ᵃ): ויקרה לחולה עם עלות החולי וקרוב חזקתו מקרים מפחידים כמו צמא חזק ונגוב פה ושעירות לשון ושחרותה וסער ודפיקת לב. → NM 4:209.

שִׁעֲמוּם · I. **coma; faint; swoon; unconsciousness:** Arab. إغماء · Galen, attr., *Prohibition of Burial* · trans. Judah al-Ḥarizi (*Sefer Issur ha-Qevurah le-Galienus*), par. 15: והשעמום מינים רבים וכולם עם הנשימה ודפיקת העורקים. → NM 4:209.

· II. **(melancholic) delusion:** Arab. وسواس · Maimonides, *K. al-fuṣūl fī al-ṭibb* · trans. Zeraḥyah Ḥen (*Sefer ha-Peraqim*), 2.16: החליים המתחדשים מהמרה השחורה הם הסרטן והצרעת והגרב והחולי אשר יתקלף בו העור וקדחת רביעית והוסוסא הוא השעמום ועובי הטחול. → NM 1:193.

[שעמם] • *Part. Pu'al* **מְשֻׁעֲמָם** · **someone suffering from delusions:** Arab. موسوس · Maimonides, *K. al-fuṣūl fī al-ṭibb* · trans. Zeraḥyah Ḥen (*Sefer ha-Peraqim*), 20.74: התפוחים להריח אותם יחזקו הלב והמוח וריחו יועיל לבעלי הרישפיצי והמשועממים. → NM 1:169.

שַׁעַר • *Part.* **שׁוֹעֵר** · **(lit., gatekeeper); pylorus:** Arab. بوّاب · Ibn Sīnā, *K. al-Qānūn fī al-ṭibb* · trans. Nathan ha-Me'ati (*Sefer ha-Qanun*), bk. 1 (fol. 63ᵇ): והחלק השני מתפרק בשיפולי האסטומ׳ ואצל השער אשר הוא פי האסטומכא. → NM 4:200.

• *Pi'el* **שִׁעֵר** · **to be able to:** Arab. قدر · Maimonides, *K. al-fuṣūl fī al-ṭibb* · trans. Nathan ha-Me'ati (*Sefer ha-Peraqim*), 8.1: מי שיהיה בגופו ליחות רעות רקיקות יחייב זה לזונו יותר ומי שיהיו ליחותיו בהפך זה יורה על הפך. וההעתק אל החסרון כשיעלם ידיעת השיעור הראוי יותר בטוח מן ההעתק אל התוספת כי אתה תשער שתוסיף כשיהיה הכח חזק ולא תשער לחסר מן המאכל אשר כבר ירד אל האסטומכה. → NM 2:89.

שַׁעַר · **the gate of the liver; the portal vein:** Arab. باب · Ibn Sīnā, *K. al-Qānūn fī al-ṭibb* · trans. Nathan ha-Me'ati (*Sefer ha-Qanun*), bk. 1 (fol. 63ᵃ): ונתחיל הנתוח העורק הנק׳ השער ונאמר השער הנה תחלה מתחלק קצהו השוקע בחלל הכבד לה׳ חלקים. → NM 4:209.

שֵׂעָר • **נשירות שער הראש** → **נְשִׁירוּת**.

• **חשער סביב הערוה** · **pubes:** Arab. عانة · Maimonides, *Šarḥ fuṣūl Abūqrāṭ* · trans. Zeraḥyah Ḥen (*Pirqei Abuqraṭ*), 5.7 (227): אמר אבקראט: מי שמצאו חולי הנופל קודם צמיחת השער סביב הערוה הנה יתחדש לו העתק ואולם מי שקרה לו וכבר עברו עליו מן השנים חמישה ועשרים שנה הנה הוא ימות והוא בו. → NM 3:32–3.

• **עצם מקום שער הרגלים** → **עֶצֶם**.

• **צמוח השיער בבית הערוה** → **צָמַח**.

• **צמח השער בשפל הבטן** → **צָמַח**.

• **צמיחת השער בגב הערוה** → **צְמִיחָה**.

• **צמיחת השער סביב הערוה** → **צְמִיחָה**.

• **צמיחת השער בתחתון** → **צְמִיחָה**.

שְׂעָרָה • *Plur.* **שערות** • **הביא שתי שערות** → **[בוא]**.

[שעשע] • *Pi'el* **שִׁעֲשַׁע** · **to soften:** Lat. lenire · Bruno Longobucco, *Cyrurgia Magna* · trans. Hillel ben Samuel (*Sefer Keritut*), fol. 82ᵇ: אחר כן תשוב אל הרפואה המקומית במה שיתיך וישעשע ביחד. → NM 1:41.

שָׂפָה • *Dual* **שְׂפָתַיִם** • **בקיעת השפתים** → **בְּקִיעָה**.

• **פלחי השפתים** → **פֶּלַח**.

שַׁפּוּדִיי • **shaped liked a spit**: Arab. سفّودي · Ibn Sīnā, *K. al-Qānūn fī al-ṭibb* · trans. Nathan ha-Me'ati (*Sefer ha-Qanun*), bk. 1 (fol. 29ª): ושלב מחלק לאורך הראש ישר יאמר לו לבדו חציי וכשיחקר מצד חבורו עם הכלילי אז יאמר לו שפודיי. → NM 4:210.

שִׁפּוּי • **שפוי כובע** • I. **larynx**: Arab. حنجرة · Ibn Sīnā, *K. al-Qānūn fī al-ṭibb* · trans. Nathan ha-Me'ati (*Sefer ha-Qanun*), bk. 1 (fol. 46ᵇ): השפוי כובע אבר שחוסי נברא כלי לקול. → NM 4:210.

• II. **xiphoid [cartilage]**: Arab. خنجري · Ibn Sīnā, *K. al-Qānūn fī al-ṭibb* · trans. Nathan ha-Me'ati (*Sefer ha-Qanun*), bk. 1 (fol. 64ᵇ): עד שהגיע אל השפוי כובע ומשאיר מדי עברו שריגים מתפרדים בעצלים אשר בין הצלעות. → NM 4:210.

שִׁפּוּל • *Plur.* **שפולים** • **שפולי הבטן** • **groin**: Lat. inguen · Bruno Longobucco, *Cyrurgia Magna* · trans. Hillel ben Samuel (*Sefer Keritut*), fol. 62ᵇ: ואין החולה יכול לכוף ברכו לצד שפולי בטנו ומקום השפול נפוח בנפיחה נגלית. → NM 1:41.

• **שפולי הרגלים** • **the soles of the feet**: Arab. أسفل القدمين · Galen, attr., *Prohibition of Burial* · trans. Judah al-Ḥarizi (*Sefer Issur ha-Qevurah le-Galienus*), cf. 144: ותרופת עלות המאמר הרביעי שילקח חלב האתון באשישות רבות אחר יחממוהו בתנור חם ובהקרבו להקפיא יוציאוהו וישימוהו על כל אשישה ליטר דבש ויערבוהו ויטבלוהו החולי וימרחו שפולי רגליו. → NM 4:210–1.

שִׁפּוּעַ • **pronation**: Arab. كبّ · Ibn Sīnā, *K. al-Qānūn fī al-ṭibb* · trans. Joseph Lorki (*Sefer ha-Qanun*), bk. 1 (fol. 15ᵇ): וכשיתנענעו אלו ביחד ימתחו החוליא מתיחה עם מעט שיפוע. → NM 4:211.

שְׁפוֹת • **(fresh) butter; cream**: Arab. زبد · Al-Zahrāwī, *K. al-taṣrīf li-man ʿağiza ʿan at-taʾlīf* · trans. Shem Tov ben Isaac (*Sefer ha-Shimmush*), bk. 27, fol. 146ᵇ, col. b–147ª, col. a: מיץ החלב אמנם כשתוסר שפותו והתחיל להחמיץ הוא טוב לשלשול המתהוה מן המרה הכרכומית עם כחשות הגוף וחולשתו. → NM 4:211.

• **שפות הבקר** • **(fresh) butter; cream**: Arab. زبد · Al-Zahrāwī, *K. al-taṣrīf li-man ʿağiza ʿan at-taʾlīf* · trans. Shem Tov ben Isaac (*Sefer ha-Shimmush*), bk. 27, fol. 139ᵇ, col. a: ודחית נזקם למי שירגילם בהכרח על דרך מזון ויזיקוהו לשתות אחריהם מן השמנים הלחים או מן החמאה או מן שפות הבקר או מן החלב תכף שנחלב. → NM 4:211.

שְׁפִיכָה • **cholera**: Arab. هيضة / Gr. χολέρα · Maimonides, *Šarḥ fuṣūl Abūqrāṭ* · trans. Moses ibn Tibbon (*Pirqei Abuqraṭ*), 3.30 (136): אמר אבקראט: ואולם מי שעבר אלו השנים הנה יקרה לו הרנפלי וחלי הצד וחלי הריאה והקדחת אשר תהיה עמה היקיצה והקדחת אשר יהיה עמה ערבוב השכל והקדחת השורפת והשפיכה והשלשול הארוך וחמרמרות המעים וקלוח המעים ופתיחת פיות העורקים מלמטה. → NM 3:233–4.

שָׁפָל • **נפח הגידים השפלים** → **נֶפַח**.

• **העצם השפל** → **עֶצֶם**.

שֵׁפֶל • **שפל הבטן** • I. **loins**: Arab. قطن · Maimonides, *Šarḥ fuṣūl Abūqrāṭ* · trans. Moses ibn Tibbon (*Pirqei Abuqraṭ*), 4.11 (148): אמר אבקראט: מי שהיו בו צירים וכאב תחת הטבור וכאב בשפל הבטן תמיד ולא יסורו ברפואה משלשלת ולא בזולתה הנה ענינו יבוא אל השקוי היבש. → NM 3:234–5.

‣ II. **lower abdomen:** Arab. ثُنَّة / Gr. ἦτρον · Maimonides, *Šarḥ fuṣūl Abūqrāṭ* · trans. Moses ibn Tibbon (*Pirqei Abuqraṭ*), 2.35 (87): אמר אבקראט: הנה הטוב בכל חולי שיהיה עובי למה שקרוב מן הטבור ושפל הבטן וכאשר היה דק מאד כחוש הנה זה רע וכאשר היה גם כן בשלשול יש בו סכנה. → NM 3:234.

‣ III. **pubes:** Arab. عانة / Gr. κτείς · Maimonides, *Šarḥ fuṣūl Abūqrāṭ* · trans. Moses ibn Tibbon (*Pirqei Abuqraṭ*), 7.39 (391): אמר אבקראט: מי שהשתין דם נקרש והיה בו הטפת השתן כאב בצדי הטבור ושפל הבטן יורה זה על מה סביב מקותו כואב. → NM 3: 234.

• **צֶמַח** → **צמח השער בשפל הבטן**.

• **שפל השדרה** ‣ **loins:** Arab. قطن / Gr. ὀσφῦς · a) Maimonides, *Šarḥ fuṣūl Abūqrāṭ* · trans. Moses ibn Tibbon (*Pirqei Abuqraṭ*), 3.23 (129) (fol. 53[a]): אמר אבקראט: ואולם בסתו יקרה מדוה הצד ומדוה הריאה והרובמאס והבחוחה והשעול וכאבי הצדדים ושפל השדרה וכאב הראש והסבוב והשתוק. → NM 3:235.

b) Maimonides, *K. al-fuṣūl fī al-ṭibb* · trans. Nathan ha-Me'ati (*Sefer ha-Peraqim*), 17.14: וימשחו שפל השדרה אחר הרחיצה בשמנים מקררים. → NM 2:89.

שִׁפְלוּת • **שפלות הקול** ‣ **hoarseness:** Arab. بحوحة الصوت / Gr. βράγχος · Ibn al-Jazzār, *Zād al-musāfir wa-qūt al-ḥāḍir* · trans. Moses ibn Tibbon (*Sefer Ṣedat ha-Derakhim*), introduction, fol. 3[a]: השער הד' בשפלות הקול הוא בחוח אלצות. → NM 4:211.

[שפע] • *Hif'il* **הִשְׁפִּיעַ** ‣ **to produce pronation:** Arab. أكبّ · Ibn Sīnā, *K. al-Qānūn fī al-ṭibb* · trans. Joseph Lorki (*Sefer ha-Qanun*), bk. 1 (fol. 15[b]): ואמנם המשפיעים אותו זוג מונח מחוץ → NM 4:212.

שָׁקַד ‣ **to last:** Arab. دام · Maimonides, *K. al-fuṣūl fī al-ṭibb* · trans. Nathan ha-Me'ati (*Sefer ha-Peraqim*), 10.65: וכל אחד משני המינים שוקדים ימים רבים והיא עונה אחת מתחלת החולי עד עת אחריתו. → NM 2:89.

• **-שקד ב** ‣ **to stick to:** Arab. لزم ل- · Maimonides, *K. al-fuṣūl fī al-ṭibb* · trans. Nathan ha-Me'ati (*Sefer ha-Peraqim*), 10.26: ולפעמים יחשב שהקדחת בלתי שוקדת בסדר והיא שוקדת בסדר וסבת זה היותה הקפים רבים מורכבים לא יאמוד חרופא בחרכבתם. → NM 2:89.

• *Part.* **שׁוֹקֵד** ‣ **inherent:** Arab. لازم · Al-Zahrāwī, *K. al-taṣrīf li-man ʿağiza ʿan at-ta'līf* · trans. Shem Tov ben Isaac (*Sefer ha-Shimmush*), bk. 27, fol. 135[b], col. b: ומסגולותיו השוקדת אותם שהם מולידים קיטורים מחשיכים וחלומות רעים. → NM 4:212.

[שקה] • *Part. Pu'al* **מְשֻׁקֶּה** • *Plur.* **משוקים** ‣ **suffering from dropsy:** Arab. مستسقين / Gr. ὑδρωπικοί · Maimonides, *Šarḥ fuṣūl Abūqrāṭ* · trans. Moses ibn Tibbon (*Pirqei Abuqraṭ*), 6.27 (319): אמר אבקראט: מי שנכוה או נבקע מן הנפוחים או המשוקים ויגר ממנו מן החומר או מן המים שעור רב פתאום הנה הוא ימות בלא ספק → NM 3:147.

• *Hif'il* **הִשְׁקָה** • **השקה הרפואה** ‣ **to administer purgative drugs:** Arab. سقى الدواء · Hippocrates, *Aphorisms* · trans. Nathan ha-Me'ati, 4.1 (138) (fol. 58[b]): אמר אבקראט: ראוי שתשקה למעוברת הרפואה בהיות הליחות בגופה מתעוררות מעת שיגיע על העובר ארבעה חדשים עד יעברו שבעה חדשים. → NM 3:235.

שִׁקּוּי • **בַּעַל** → **בעלי שקוי**.

• **השקוי הבשריי** ‣ **anasarca:** Arab. الاستسقاء اللحمي · Maimonides, *K. al-fuṣūl fī al-ṭibb*

· trans. Nathan ha-Me'ati (*Sefer ha-Peraqim*), 23.50: השקוי הבשריי נקרא גם כן השקוי הלבניי הלבן ונקרא אלחבאן ואלגבאן. → NM 2:90.

• **השקוי הנאדי** · **ascites:** Arab. الاستسقاء الزقّي · a) Al-Zahrāwī, *K. al-taṣrīf li-man ʿağiza ʿan at-taʾlīf* · trans. Shem Tov ben Isaac (*Sefer ha-Shimmush*), bk. 30, 1:32 (fol. 206a): הכויה ראויה בשקוי הנאדי בלבד. → NM 1:118–9.

b) Maimonides, *Šarḥ fuṣūl Abūqrāṭ* · trans. Moses ibn Tibbon (*Pirqei Abuqraṭ*), 4.11 (148): אמר המפרש: כאשר לא יותך זה ברפואה הנה הוא ראיה על הפסד מזג שגבר על האיברים ההם ונשתקע בהם ויחדש השקוי התופי והוא אשר קראו היבש כנגד השקוי הנאדי אשר בו המים והנודי יתחדש מקור נוסף. → NM 3:235–6.

c) Maimonides, *K. al-fuṣūl fī al-ṭibb* · trans. Nathan ha-Me'ati (*Sefer ha-Peraqim*), 4.41: השקוי הנאדי מפני מה שיתקבץ בבטן מן הלחויות יתמתחו העורקים ויתפזרו. → NM 2:90.

• **השקוי התופי(י)** · **tympanites:** Arab. الاستسقاء الطبلي · a) Maimonides, *Šarḥ fuṣūl Abūqrāṭ* · trans. Moses ibn Tibbon (*Pirqei Abuqraṭ*), 4.11 (148): אמר המפרש: כאשר לא יותך זה ברפואה הנה הוא ראיה על הפסד מזג שגבר על האיברים ההם ונשתקע בהם ויחדש השקוי התופי והוא אשר קראו היבש כנגד השקוי הנאדי אשר בו המים והנודי יתחדש מקור נוסף. → NM 3:236.

b) Maimonides, *K. al-fuṣūl fī al-ṭibb* · trans. Nathan ha-Me'ati (*Sefer ha-Peraqim*), 23.50: ואמר בפרושו לרביעי בפרקים שהשקוי התופיי הוא אשר יקראהו אבקרט השקוי היבש. → NM 2:90.

[שקט] • *Piʿel* **שִׁקֵּט** · **to put an end to:** Gr. παύω · Hippocrates, *Aphorisms* · trans. Joseph Delmedigo, 2.2 (54): כשהשינה משקטת ערבוב השכל טוב. → NM 3:236.

• *Hifʿil* **הִשְׁקִיט** · **to put an end to:** Arab. سكّن · Hippocrates, *Aphorisms* · trans. Nathan ha-Me'ati, 2.2 (54) (fol. 20a): כשתשקיט השינה ערבוב השכל הנה זה אות טוב. → NM 3:236.

שְׁקִיעָה · I. **pressing:** a) Arab. غَمْز · Al-Zahrāwī, *K. al-taṣrīf li-man ʿağiza ʿan at-taʾlīf* · trans. Shem Tov ben Isaac (*Sefer ha-Shimmush*), bk. 30, 2:95 (fol. 230a): ויתחדש הרבה צבות ובליטה בעת הקזת הבאסליק וראוי אז לתת עליו היד ואם ימצא מתפשט בעת שקיעת היד עליו בידוע שהבליטה ההיא רעה. → NM 1:119.

b) Arab. كَبْس · Al-Zahrawi, *K. al-taṣrif li-man ʿağiza ʿan at-taʾlīf* · trans. Shem Tov ben Isaac (*Sefer ha-Shimmush*), bk. 30, 2:63 (fol. 219b): אמנם אשר יהיה מצבות הגידים הנחים לא יתפזר ממנו מאומה בעת שקיעת האצבע עליו. → NM 1:119.

· II. **squeezing:** Arab. عَصْر · Al-Zahrāwī, *K. al-taṣrīf li-man ʿağiza ʿan at-taʾlīf* · trans. Shem Tov ben Isaac (*Sefer ha-Shimmush*), bk. 30, 2:59 (fol. 218b): ולעשות בה כמו שנעשה בכיס מקוה המים משקיעת היד עד שיגיע הלחות אל הכיס → NM 1:119.

· III. **torpor:** Arab. استغراق · Maimonides, *K. al-fuṣūl fī al-ṭibb* · trans. Nathan ha-Me'ati (*Sefer ha-Peraqim*), 23.64: בטול הדמיונות יאמר לו השקיעה והקפיאה. → NM 2:90.

• **השקיע שקיעה** → **שָׁקַע**.

שְׁקִיקָה · **migraine:** Arab. شقيقة · Maimonides, *K. al-fuṣūl fī al-ṭibb* · trans. Zeraḥyah Ḥen (*Sefer ha-Peraqim*), 6.35: בעלי השקיקה והוא חולי הנק׳ מיגרניאה קצתם ימצא מישוש הכאב יוצא מהגלגלת וקצתם ימצאנו יגיע אל עומק הראש והכאב יכלה במגרניאה אל הגבול המגיע בין שני צלעות הראש. → NM 1:193.

שָׁקַע · **to form a sediment:** Arab. رسب · Maimonides, *Šarḥ fuṣūl Abūqrāṭ* · trans. Zeraḥyah Ḥen (*Pirqei Abuqraṭ*), 4.79 (216): אמר בקראט: מי שישקע בשתנו כמו החצץ החול נולד בשלפוחיתו. → NM 3:236.

• *Hifʿil* **הִשְׁקִיעַ** · **to press:** a) Arab. أمعن · Al-Zahrāwī, *K. al-taṣrīf li-man ʿağiza ʿan at-taʾlīf* · trans. Shem Tov ben Isaac (*Sefer ha-Shimmush*), bk. 30, 2:45 (fol. 216[a]): ואחר להשקיע היד על הצמח כפי גדלו. → NM 1:119.

b) Arab. غمز · Al-Zahrāwī, *K. al-taṣrīf li-man ʿağiza ʿan at-taʾlīf* · trans. Shem Tov ben Isaac (*Sefer ha-Shimmush*), bk. 30, 2:95 (fol. 230[b]): ואין ראוי כשיש רצון להתיר הקזת הזרוע להוציא מן הדם פעם שנית וכבר נסתם פי הגיד ותקשה יציאת הדם להשקיע עליו בחזקה ביד ולפתול אותו בכח. → NM 1:119.

• **השקיע שקיעה** · **to apply pressure:** Arab. شدّ · Al-Zahrāwī, *K. al-taṣrīf li-man ʿağiza ʿan at-taʾlīf* · trans. Shem Tov ben Isaac (*Sefer ha-Shimmush*), bk. 30, 2:59 (fol. 218[b]): ולהשקיע הכיס ביד על הלחות שקיעה בחכמה עד שירגיש החולה שהלחות ההוא כבר הגיע אל הכיס. → NM 1:119.

• *Hofʿal* **הָשְׁקַע** · **pressure to be applied:** Arab. كبس · Al-Zahrāwī, *K. al-taṣrīf li-man ʿağiza ʿan at-taʾlīf* · trans. Shem Tov ben Isaac (*Sefer ha-Shimmush*), bk. 30, 2:52 (fol. 217[a]): וכשיושקע עליו באצבע יתעלם. → NM 1:119.

שָׁרָה • *Pass. Part.* **שָׁרוּי** • **הלחם השרוי במים עד שיחמיץ** → **לֶחֶם**.

שָׁרוּי (*Pass. Part.*) → **שָׁרָה**.

שֵׁרוּי · **macerating:** Arab. نقيع · Maimonides, *K. al-fuṣūl fī al-ṭibb* · trans. Zeraḥyah Ḥen (*Sefer ha-Peraqim*), 20.64: ראוי שתתנהג בכלל המזונות בכל כי מה שיהיה מהם חריף ומחודד או מר יהיה מזונו מעט. ומה שיהיה מהם אין טעם לו מה שהגיע ממזונו אל הגוף מרובה וברוב מה שיהיה מתוק וכל שכן אם יהיה גרם קשה בין שיהיה אילו הטעמים והמאכלים בטבע או נקנים במלאכה כלומר בבישול ובצלי אש ובקלוי ובשרוי במים ודומה לאילו. → NM 1:193.

• **יין הדבש השרוי** → **יַיִן**.

שָׂרִי · **major:** Arab. رئيس · Maimonides, *K. al-fuṣūl fī al-ṭibb* · trans. Zeraḥyah Ḥen (*Sefer ha-Peraqim*), 25.70: ואמנם הקדמתי לך זאת ההקדמה להעירך מעניין גליאנוס זה החכם המשובח שידעת דעתו באברים השריים שהם שלשה והם הלב והמוח והכבד. → NM 1:193.

שריין → **שרין**.

שרייני · **arterial:** Lat. arterialis · Arnau de Vilanova, *Medicationis Parabole* · trans. Abraham Avigdor (*Pirqei Arnauṭ de Vilanova*), 4.21 (54): אם הדם השרייני יכאיב ויעקוץ אבר מן האיברים כמו העין, לא יספיק בהרקתו הקזת השריין אך יצטרך לחתכו ⟨יועיל⟩, ביחוד אל הנזלים הנושנים. → NM 4:212.

• **הוריד השרייני** → **וָרִיד**.

שרין • **השריין הורידי** · **pulmonary vein; venous artery:** Arab. الشريان الوريدي · Ibn Sīnā, *K. al-Qānūn fī al-ṭibb* · trans. Nathan ha-Meʾati (*Sefer ha-Qanun*), bk. 1 (fol. 60[b]): ולכן נקרא השריין הורידי. → NM 4:212.

• *Plur.* **שריינים** • **השריינים הנרדמים** · **the [two] carotid arteries:** Arab. الشرايين السباتيين · Ibn Sīnā, *K. al-Qānūn fī al-ṭibb* · trans. Nathan ha-Meʾati (*Sefer ha-Qanun*), bk. 1 (fol. 61[b]): וכל אחד משני השריינים הנרדמים מתחלקים אצל כלותו אל המפרקת לשנע חלקים. → NM 4:212.

שריפה → שְׂרֵפָה.

שָׂרַף • *Part.* **שׂוֹרֵף** • **המים השורפים** → מַיִם.

• **הסם השורף** → סַם.

• *Nif'al* **נִשְׂרַף** · **to be cauterized:** Gr. καίομαι · Hippocrates, *Aphorisms* · trans. Joseph Delmedigo, 6.60 (352): המצוערים זמן ארוך מכאב גיד הנשה וינקע ראש הירך ממקומו ר"ל מעצם גב הערוה יעבש להם הכיח ויהיו פסחים אם לא ישרפו. → NM 3:236–7.

• *Hof'al* **הָשְׂרַף** · **to be treated by cautery:** Hippocrates, *Aphorisms* · trans. Judah Shalom, 7.44 (396) (fol. 122[b]): מי שהוא אמפימו ויושרף או יחותך אם יצא מוגלא נקיה ולבנה ירופאו ואם עכורה ומריח רע ימותו. → NM 3:237.

שְׂרָף · **broth:** Arab. حسو · Al-Zahrāwī, *K. al-taṣrīf li-man ʿağiza ʿan at-taʾlīf* · trans. Shem Tov ben Isaac (*Sefer ha-Shimmush*), bk. 27, fol. 124[a], col. b: שרף קמח החטה הוא ממין שרף הגריסין בהולידו הסתומים והלחה הלבנה → NM 4:213.

שְׂרֵפָה · **burn:** Arab. احتراق / Gr. καῦμα · Maimonides, *Šarḥ fuṣūl Abūqrāṭ* · trans. Moses ibn Tibbon (*Pirqei Abuqraṭ*), 7.13 (365): אמר אבקראט: ומהשריפה החזקה הקווץ והמשיכה. → NM 3:236.

שָׂרַץ • *Part.* **שׂוֹרֵץ** • **המורסא השורצת** → מֻרְסָא.

שֹׁרֶשׁ • **שרש האזנים** · **parotid gland:** Arab. أصل الأذن · Al-Zahrāwī, *K. al-taṣrīf li-man ʿağiza ʿan at-taʾlīf* · trans. Shem Tov ben Isaac (*Sefer ha-Shimmush*), bk. 27, fol. 126[b], col. a: והמערב קמח הפול עם קמח התלתן ומחבש בהם יתיכו הנפח אשר יקרה בשרשי האזנים ומה שיקרה מן הכהות מתחת העין. → NM 4:213.

• **שרש הלשון** · **uvula:** Arab. لهاة · Ibn Zuhr, *Regimen of Health* · trans. Jacob ibn Tibbon (*Hanhagat ha-Beri'ut le-Abu 'Ali ben Zuhr*), ch. 8 (variant reading): והרחקת אכילת העצמים הדקים כמו עצם העוף והפרדיך והצפרים והתרנגולים ואכילת הדגים הקוציים, זולת עצמי השיות והתישים הסריסים כאשר יותך מהם לעיסותם ממה שירכך הקנה והלהאה הוא שרש הלשון וירכך הושט וישלשל המעברות ויעזור לירידת המאכל בקערורית האצטומכא → NM 4:213–4. (corr.)

שִׁתּוּף · **affinity; interrelationship; sympathetic affection:** Arab. مشاركة · Maimonides, *Šarḥ fuṣūl Abūqrāṭ* · trans. Moses ibn Tibbon (*Pirqei Abuqraṭ*), 6.29 (257): אמר המפרש: כבר נודע שתוף השדים עם הרחם וכאשר יצמקו יורה על מיעוט המזון המגיע אליהם וכאשר ימעט גם כן המזון המגיע לרחם יפול העובר. → NM 3:237.

שָׁתוּק (*Pass. Part.*) → שָׁתַק.

שִׁתּוּק · **apoplexy; stroke:** Arab. سكتة · a) Ibn al-Jazzār, *Zād al-musāfir wa-qūt al-ḥāḍir* · trans. Moses ibn Tibbon (*Sefer Ṣedat ha-Derakhim*), bk. 1, ch. 22: והכפיה קרוב מן השתוק כי מקום החולי בשניהם אחד והליחה המולידה אותם קרה לחה אבל כי השתוק יהיה בהעדר הכח אשר ילך אל העצבים כלם והכפיה תהיה בתנועה מצטערת. → NM 4:214.

b) Maimonides, *K. al-fuṣūl fī al-ṭibb* · trans. Zeraḥyah Ḥen (*Sefer ha-Peraqim*), 6.1: יורה על השיתוק אם הוא חזק וימית על כל פנים או חלוש ואפשר שיתרפא וזה קשה מענין הניפוש כי העדר תנועת הניפוש בכלל עד שלא יושג ויהיה זה יותר חזק ממה שיהיה מן השיתוק. → NM 1:193.

c) Maimonides, *K. al-fuṣūl fī al-ṭibb* · trans. Nathan ha-Me'ati (*Sefer ha-Peraqim*),

תנועת הלשון הוא מן הזוג השביעי מזוגות עצבי המוח וכשיקבל עלה החלק הימני 6.36: והחלק השמאלי במקום צמיחת זה הזוג השביעי אז בעל העלה הזאת בסכנה מן השתוק. → NM 2:91.

שְׁתִיָּה · **wine**: Lat. potus · Hippocrates, *Aphorisms* · trans. Hillel ben Samuel, 2.21 (73) (fol. 10[b]): השתייה מתירה הרעב. → NM 3:237.

• **שתיית הרפואה** · **taking a purgative drug**: Arab. شرب الدواء / Gr. φαρμακοποσία · Hippocrates, *Aphorisms* · trans. Nathan ha-Me'ati, 6.31 (323) (fol. 115[a]): אמר אבוקרט: כאיבי העינים יתיכם שתיית היין החי או המרחץ או הנחות החמות או הקזת העורק או שתיית הרפואה. → NM 3:237–8.

שתייה → שְׁתִיָּה.

שְׁתִיקָה · **apoplexy; stroke**: Arab. سكتة · Maimonides, *K. al-fuṣūl fī al-ṭibb* · trans. Zeraḥyah Ḥen (*Sefer ha-Peraqim*), 9.12: אפשר שיזדמן שיהיה האדם שוכב על ערפו בלילה כלה ואז התקדם אליו חולי השתיקה וויציאו בהתמלא בטני המוח מאותם המותרות. → NM 1:194.

[שתן] • *Hif'il* הִשְׁתִּין • **השתין במטה** · **to wet the bed (enuresis)**: Arab. بال في الفراش · Ibn al-Jazzār, *Zād al-musāfir wa-qūt al-ḥāḍir* · trans. Moses ibn Tibbon (*Sefer Ṣedat ha-Derakhim*), introduction (fol. 3[b]): השער הי״ט ברפואת מי שישתין במטה. → NM 4:214.

שֶׁתֶן • **דרך השתן** → דֶּרֶךְ.
• **הגרת השתן** → הַגָּרָה.
• **הזלת השתן** → הַזָּלָה.
• **הטפת השתן** → הַטָּפָה.
• **התרת השתן** → הַתָּרָה.
• **טיפות השתן** → טִפָּה.
• **טפטוף השתן** → טִפְטוּף.
• **יציאת השתן במכאוב** → יְצִיאָה.
• **כובד הזלת השתן** → כֹּבֶד.
• **מעבר השתן** → מַעֲבָר.
• **מקום השתן** → מָקוֹם.
• **הסם המגיר השתן** → סַם.
• **הסם המתיר השתן** → סַם.
• **עוצר השתן** → עֹצֶר.
• **עכוב השתן** → עִכּוּב.
• **עיצור השתן** → עִצּוּר.
• **עצירת השתן** → עֲצִירָה.
• **קשי יציאת השתן** → קֹשִׁי.
• **קושי השתן** → קֹשִׁי.
• **שביל השתן** → שְׁבִיל.

שֻׁתָּפוּת · **affinity; interrelationship; sympathetic affection**: Arab. مشاركة · Maimonides, *Šarḥ fuṣūl Abūqrāṭ* · trans. Moses ibn Tibbon (*Pirqei Abuqraṭ*), 6.3 (295): אמר המפרש: שלשול הדם כאשר היה עם חמרמרות המעיים וארך עמידתו יתוספו החפירות בעומק האיברים וישובו נגעים בהם עפוש ותכאב האצטו׳ בשותפות וישיג בשולה הנזק. → NM 3:238.

שָׁתַק • *Pass. Part.* **שָׁתוּק** · **suffering from a stroke:** Arab. مسكوت · Maimonides, *K. al-fuṣūl fī al-ṭibb* · trans. Zeraḥyah Ḥen (*Sefer ha-Peraqim*), 1.38: ולא יקשה עליך היות השכור והשתוק כשלא יעורו בשום דבר מאלו כי אלו הם חולים לא בריאים. → NM 1:194.

• *Part. Pu'al* **מְשֻׁתָּק** · **suffering from an apoplexy:** Arab. مسكوت · Maimonides, *K. al-fuṣūl fī al-ṭibb* · trans. Nathan ha-Me'ati (*Sefer ha-Peraqim*), 24.45: ואחר זכר בזה מינים זרים מרפואות המשותקים. → NM 2:64.

שָׁתַת • *Part.* **שׁוֹתֵת** • **דם שותת** → דָּם.

ת

תַּאֲוָה • התאוה הכלבית › **canine appetite**: Arab. الشّهوة الكلبيّة · Maimonides, *Šarḥ fuṣūl Abūqrāṭ* · trans. Moses ibn Tibbon (*Pirqei Abuqraṭ*), 2.21 (73): אמר המפרש: רצה במשקה היין וזה הרעב רוצה בו התאוה הכלבית כי שתיית היין אשר לו חמום חזק ירפא זה הרעב. → NM 3:238.

• נפילת התאוה → נְפִילָה.

[תאם] • *Part. Hif'il* **מַתְאִים • רפואה מתאימה** → רְפוּאָה.

[תבל] • *Part. Pu'al* **מְתֻבָּל • הבשר המליח המתובל** → בָּשָׂר.

תַּבְשִׁיל • תבשיל האספרגוס › **the asparagus dish**: Arab. الهليونية · Al-Zahrāwī, *K. al-taṣrīf li-man 'ağiza 'an at-ta'līf* · trans. Shem Tov ben Isaac (*Sefer ha-Shimmush*), bk. 27, fol. 145[b], col. b–146[a], col. a: ותבשיל הלפת טוב לכליות וכיס מקוה ⟨המים⟩ ואינו מזיק לבעל ההדרקון כנזק תבשיל הנפוס והוא טוב לבעל הקרירות ובלתי טוב לבעלי החמימות ולא בעתים החמים ותבשיל האספרגוס כמוהו. → NM 4:214

• תבשיל בסר הכרם › **a stew soured with juice of unripe grapes**: Arab. الحسرمية · Al-Zahrāwī, *K. al-taṣrīf li-man 'ağiza 'an at-ta'līf* · trans. Shem Tov ben Isaac (*Sefer ha-Shimmush*), bk. 27, fol. 146[a], col. a: תבשיל בסר הכרם והרמונים והתפוחים והדומה להם ואשר יכנס בהם חומץ כלם ראוים לבעלי החמימות ולבעלי הקרבים החמים ובארצות החמות. → NM 4:214–5.

• התבשיל החמוץ › **the sour dish**: Arab. المخلّل · Al-Zahrāwī, *K. al-taṣrīf li-man 'ağiza 'an at-ta'līf* · trans. Shem Tov ben Isaac (*Sefer ha-Shimmush*), bk. 27, fol. 145[a], col. b: התבשיל החמוץ הנקרא סכבאג' אצל אנשי המזרח והוא בשר וחומץ ותבלין ומי בצל והוא קר. → NM 4:215.

• תבשיל הכרוב › **the cabbage dish**: Arab. الكرنبية · Al-Zahrāwī, *K. al-taṣrīf li-man 'ağiza 'an at-ta'līf* · trans. Shem Tov ben Isaac (*Sefer ha-Shimmush*), bk. 27, fol. 146[a], col. a: תבשיל הכרוב ותבשיל התרובתור מטעמים ערבים מדרכם להוליד תחלאי המרה השחורה וכל שכן תבשיל התרובתור ומסגולת תבשיל הכרוב לשלשל הבטן ולהקל צאת הרוחות ולעזור על רוב שתית היין ולמעט השכרות. → NM 4:215.

• תבשיל הלפת › **the turnip dish**: Arab. اللفتية · Al-Zahrāwī, *K. al-taṣrīf li-man 'ağiza 'an at-ta'līf* · trans. Shem Tov ben Isaac (*Sefer ha-Shimmush*), bk. 27, fol. 145[b], col. b–146[a], col. a: תבשיל הלפת הוא מטעם מנפח רב המזון מוסיף בתאות המשגל. → NM 4:215–6.

• תבשיל הנפוס › **the carrot dish**: Arab. الجزرية · Al-Zahrāwī, *K. al-taṣrīf li-man 'ağiza 'an at-ta'līf* · trans. Shem Tov ben Isaac (*Sefer ha-Shimmush*), bk. 27, fol. 145[b], col. b–146[a], col. a: ותבשיל הלפת טוב לכליות וכיס מקוה ⟨המים⟩ ואינו מזיק לבעל ההדרקון כנזק תבשיל הנפוס. → NM 4:216.

• תבשיל הרמונים › **pomegranate stew cooked mostly with chicken**: Arab. الرمانية · Al-Zahrāwī, *K. al-taṣrīf li-man 'ağiza 'an at-ta'līf* · trans. Shem Tov ben Isaac (*Sefer ha-Shimmush*), bk. 27, fol. 146[a], col. a: תבשיל בסר הכרם והרמונים והתפוחים והדומה להם ואשר יכנס בהם חומץ כלם ראוים לבעלי החמימות ולבעלי הקרבים החמים ובארצות החמות. → NM 4:216.

• **תבשיל התפוחים** › **apple stew:** Arab. التفاحية · Al-Zahrāwī, *K. al-taṣrīf li-man ʿağiza ʿan at-taʾlīf* · trans. Shem Tov ben Isaac (*Sefer ha-Shimmush*), bk. 27, fol. 146^{a}, col. a: תבשיל בסר הכרם והרמונים והתפוחים והדומה להם ואשר יכנס בהם חומץ כלם ראוים לבעלי החמימות ולבעלי הקרבים החמים ובארצות החמות. → NM 4:216.

תָּוֶךְ › **cavity:** Arab. جوف · Maimonides, *Šarḥ fuṣūl Abūqrāṭ* · trans. Zeraḥyah Ḥen (*Pirqei Abuqraṭ*), 7.38 (390): אמר בקראט: הנזילות היורדות אל התוך העליון יבואו לידי מגל בעשרים יום. → NM 3:239.

תּוֹלָדָה • *Plur.* **תולדות** • **הוליד תולדות** → [ילד].

תּוֹלַעַת • *Plur.* **תולעים** • **התולעים הגדולים** › **round worms:** a) Arab. دود · Al-Zahrāwī, *K. al-taṣrīf li-man ʿağiza ʿan at-taʾlīf* · trans. Shem Tov ben Isaac (*Sefer ha-Shimmush*), bk. 27, fol. 140^{b}, col. b: וכשיבושל ביין וישתה ממנו תשע אונקי׳ והוא חם יועיל מן הכאב אשר יקרה מן המותרות העבות ויוציא התולעים הגדולים והקטנים מן הבטן. → NM 4:216–7.

b) Arab. حيّات / Gr. ἕλμινθες στρογγύλαι · Maimonides, *Šarḥ fuṣūl Abūqrāṭ* · trans. Moses ibn Tibbon (*Pirqei Abuqraṭ*), 3.26 (132): אמר אבקראט: וכאשר עבר הילד אלו השנים יקרה לו מורסת הגרון והכנסת חוליות הצואר והרנפלי והאבן והתולעים הגדולים והקטנים והיבלת הנתלית והחזירים ושאר הנגעים. → NM 3:239.

• **התולעים הדלועיים** › **tapeworms:** Arab. حبّ القرع · Maimonides, *K. al-fuṣūl fī al-ṭibb* · trans. Nathan ha-Meʾati (*Sefer ha-Peraqim*), 22.9: אלארביאן מריק התולעים הדלועיים. → NM 2:91.

• **התולעים הדקים** › **intestinal worms (h.l., flat worms):** Gr. ἀσκαρίδες · Hippocrates, *Aphorisms* · trans. Joseph Delmedigo, 3.26 (132): וליותר גדולים יקרו מורסות הגרון ודחיית חוליות הצואר לפנים ורוע הנשימה והולדת האבן במקוה והתולעים העגולים והדקים והיבלת התלויה וצמחים קשים באחורי האזנים וטפטוף השתן והחזירים ושאר צמחים אבל ביותר אלו הנזכרים. → NM 3:239–40.

• **תולעים עגולים** › **round worms:** Hippocrates, *Aphorisms* · trans. Judah Shalom, 3.26 (132) (fol. 77^{b}): ובהיותם יותר גדולים יקרה להם מורסת הגרון ודחית חוליות הצואר לפנים ואשמא ואבן ותולעים עגולים והדלועיים והיבלות וזקיפת האמה וחזירים וצמחים אחרים ויותר נזכרים. → NM 3:240.

• **התולעים הקטנים** › I. **intestinal worms (h.l., flat worms):** Arab. دود / Gr. ἀσκαρίδες · Maimonides, *Šarḥ fuṣūl Abūqrāṭ* · trans. Moses ibn Tibbon (*Pirqei Abuqraṭ*), 3.26 (132): אמר אבקראט: וכאשר עבר הילד אלו השנים יקרה לו מורסת הגרון והכנסת חוליות הצואר והרנפלי והאבן והתולעים הגדולים והקטנים והיבלת הנתלית והחזירים ושאר הנגעים. → NM 3:240.

› II. **tapeworms:** Arab. حبّ القرع · Al-Zahrāwī, *K. al-taṣrīf li-man ʿağiza ʿan at-taʾlīf* · trans. Shem Tov ben Isaac (*Sefer ha-Shimmush*), bk. 27, fol. 140^{b}, col. b: וכשיבושל ביין וישתה ממנו תשע אונקי׳ והוא חם יועיל מן הכאב אשר יקרה מן המותרות העבות ויוציא התולעים הגדולים והקטנים מן הבטן. → NM 4:217.

תּוּנְבָּא (*Aram.*) › **numbness:** Arab. خدر · Al-Zahrāwī, *K. al-taṣrīf li-man ʿağiza ʿan at-taʾlīf* · trans. Shem Tov Ben Isaac (*Sefer ha-Shimmush*), bk. 30, 1.48 (fol. 208^{a}): שער מ״ח בכוית התונבא והיא סור חוש אבר או איברין מן הגוף. → NM 1:120.

תּוֹסֶפֶת · **prominence [of the head]**: Arab. نتوء · Ibn Sīnā, *K. al-Qānūn fī al-ṭibb* · trans. Zeraḥyah Ḥen (*Sefer ha-Qanun*), bk. 1 (fol. 17[a]): ואמנם צורות הראש שאינם טבעיים הם שלשה האחד מהם שיחסר מהם התוספת המקדים. → NM 4:217.

• *Plur.* **תוספות** · I. **excrescences**: Arab. زوائد · Maimonides, *K. al-fuṣūl fī al-ṭibb* · trans. Nathan ha-Me'ati (*Sefer ha-Peraqim*), 15.21: הבשר הנוסף בקצוות העין הנקרא מאק והתוספות אשר בטבעת והם הטחורים יצטרכו שיחותכו. → NM 2:91.

· II. **the lobes [of the liver]**: Arab. زوائد · Maimonides, *K. al-fuṣūl fī al-ṭibb* · trans. Zeraḥyah Ḥen (*Sefer ha-Peraqim*), 24.54: החבלה השוקעת אשר תהיה בתוספות הכבד אפשר שתתרפא. → NM 1:194.

· III. **processes (apophyses) of a bone**: Arab. زائدة, *Plur.* زوائد / Gr. ἀπόφυσις, *Plur.* ἀποφυσέις · Ibn Sīnā, *K. al-Qānūn fī al-ṭibb* · trans. Nathan ha-Me'ati (*Sefer ha-Qanun*), bk. 1 (fol. 32[a]): החוליא הוא עצם באמצעיתו יש נקב יעבור בו החוט ויש לחוליא ארבעה תוספות ימין ושמאל. → NM 4:217.

• **התוספות החיציות** · **the arrow-like processes (i.e., the styloid processes)**: Arab. الزوائد السهمية · Ibn Sīnā, *K. al-Qānūn fī al-ṭibb* · trans. Nathan ha-Me'ati (*Sefer ha-Qanun*), bk. 1 (fol. 47[b]): העצלים המניעים הלשון הם תשעה שנים רחבים באים מהתוספות החיציות ומתחברים בצדדיו. → NM 4:219.

• **התוספות שהם כמו החץ** · **the arrow-like processes (i.e., the styloid processes)**: Arab. الزوائد السهمية · Ibn Sīnā, *K. al-Qānūn fī al-ṭibb* · trans. Joseph Lorki (*Sefer ha-Qanun*), bk. 1 (fol. 15[a]): ואמנם העצלים המניעים הלשון הם תשעה עצלים שנים מתרחבים יבואו מהתוספות שהם כמו החץ ונדבקים בשני צדדיו. → NM 4:219.

• **התוספות הדומות לחצים** · **the arrow-like processes (i.e., the styloid processes)**: Arab. الزوائد السهمية · Ibn Sīnā, *K. al-Qānūn fī al-ṭibb* · trans. Zeraḥyah Ḥen (*Sefer ha-Qanun*), bk. 1 (fol. 25[b]): ואמנם מושקלי המניעים הלשון הם תשעה מושקלי שנים ברחב באים מן התוספות הדומות לחצים ויתדבקו בשני צדדים. → NM 4:217–8.

• **התוספות הדומות למחטים** · **the needle-like processes (i.e., the styloid processes)**: Arab. الزوائد الابرية · Ibn Sīnā, *K. al-Qānūn fī al-ṭibb* · trans. Zeraḥyah Ḥen (*Sefer ha-Qanun*), bk. 1 (fol. 24[b]): אמנם מושקולי של הפעירה וירידת הלחי יצמחו חוטיה מן התוספות הדומות למחטים. → NM 4:218.

• **התוספות המחטייות** · **the needle-like processes (i.e., the styloid processes)**: Arab. الزوائد الابرية · Ibn Sīnā, *K. al-Qānūn fī al-ṭibb* · trans. Nathan ha-Me'ati (*Sefer ha-Qanun*), bk. 1 (fol. 45[a]): ואמנם עצלי הפעירה וירידת הלחי יצמחו פתיליהם מן התוספות המחטייות. → NM 4:219.

• **התוספות הדומות לשתי פטומות** · **nipple-like processes**: Arab. الزوائد الشبيهة بحلمتي الثدي · Ibn Sīnā, *K. al-Qānūn fī al-ṭibb* · trans. Nathan ha-Me'ati (*Sefer ha-Qanun*), bk. 1 (fol. 56[a]): הנה יצמח מן המוח מן העצביים ⟨שבעה⟩ זוגות הזוג הראשון התחלתו מעומק שני החדרים המוקדמים מן המוח אצל שכונת שתי התוספות הדומות לשתי פטומות אשר בהם הריח. → NM 4:218.

• **התוספות הדומות לפיות השדים** · **nipple-like processes**: Arab. الزوائد الشبيهة بحلمتي الثدي · Ibn Sīnā, *K. al-Qānūn fī al-ṭibb* · trans. Zeraḥyah Ḥen (*Sefer ha-Qanun*), bk. 1 (fol. 30[a]):

מן המוח צומחים שבעה זוגות מעצבים הזוג הראשון התחלתו מעומק הבתים שבמקדים של מוח אצל מקום שעוברים שתי התוספות הדומות לפיות השדים אשר בהם יריח האדם. → NM 4:218.

• **התוספות הדומים בשני ראשי השדים** · **nipple-like processes**: Arab. الزوائد الشبيهة بحلمتي الثدى · Ibn Sīnā, *K. al-Qānūn fī al-ṭibb* · trans. Joseph Lorki (*Sefer ha-Qanun*), bk. 1 (fol. 17^{a}): כבר יצמחו מהמוח ז' זוגות מה עצלים הזוג הראשון התחלתם מבפנים החדרים המוקדמים מהמוח אצל השתי תוספות הדומים בשני ראשי)ם(השדים ובהם יהיה הרוח. → NM 4:218–9.

תופי • **ההדרקון התופיי** → הִידְרוֹקָן.

• **השקוי התופי(י)** → שִׁקּוּי.

תּוֹצָאָה • *Plur.* **תוצאות** · I. **emptying; excretion; voiding**: Lat. egestio · Bruno Longobucco, *Cyrurgia Magna* · trans. Hillel ben Samuel (*Sefer Keritut*), fol. 100^{a}: ולי נראה שיבוא זה מהטרדת התוצאות ומן הליחות המשוקעות בשולי הנגע. → NM 1:41.

· II. **evacuations; excrements; stool**: Hippocrates, *Aphorisms* · trans. Do'eg ha-Edomi (*Sefer Agur*), 4.83 (220) (fol. 79^{a}): מי שישתין שתן רב בלילה תדין כי תוצאותיו יהיו מעטים. → NM 3:240–1.

תוקף → תֹּקֶף.

תּוֹשֶׁבֶת · **anus**: Ibn Zuhr, *Regimen of Health* · trans. Jacob ibn Tibbon (*Hanhagat ha-Beri'ut le-Abu 'Ali ben Zuhr*), ch. 15: והאורז מבושל עם החלב החלוב יזון אותם ויחזקם גם כן עד שהוא יועיל מרפיון הרחם ויפתח פיות העורקים אשר בבטן התושבת. → NM 4:219–20.

תחבושת → תַּחְבֹּשֶׁת.

תַּחְבֹּשֶׁת · I. **fomentation; fomenting**: Arab. تكميد · Maimonides, *Šarḥ fuṣūl Abūqrāṭ* · trans. Anonymous (*Pirqei Abuqraṭ*), 5.28 (248): אמר אבוקרט: התחבושת בבושם הנקרא בערבי אפאיה מושך הדם הבא מן הנשים. וכבר היה ראוי שיועיל במקומות אחרים הרבה לולי שיתחדש כובד בראש. → NM 3:241.

· II. **plaster; poultice**: Lat. emplastrum · Bruno Longobucco, *Cyrurgia Magna* · trans. Hillel ben Samuel (*Sefer Keritut*), fol. 61^{b}: ואם לאו תוסיף לעשות התחבושת והקשירות עד שיתחזק. → NM 1:42.

תַּחֲלוּא • **תחלוא השחורה** · **melancholic delusion**: Hippocrates, *Aphorisms* · trans. Do'eg ha-Edomi (*Sefer Agur*), 3.20 (126) (fol. 54^{b}): ספור המדוים אשר יחולו בזמן האביב והם תחלואי הקדחת והדם והאדומה והשחורה גם אפיסת הדעת סתימת הגידים והחולי הנופל וזיבת הדם ונזלת האף שעול ואפיסת הקול. → NM 3:241.

תַּחַת • **תחת הארכובה** · **the back (hollow) of the knee (popliteal fossa)**: Arab. مأبض الركبة · Maimonides, *Šarḥ fuṣūl Abūqrāṭ* · trans. Zeraḥyah Ḥen (*Pirqei Abuqraṭ*), 6.36 (328): תיקן גאלנוס זה הפרק כשאמר יתיר עוצר השתן וזה בהיות סבתו מורסא מדם וריבוי דם. והנשאר מהפרק אמר שהוא נכנס במאמר בקראט והראוי שתהיה ההקזה אז בתחת הארכובה. → NM 3:241–2.

• **תחת החלציים** · **hypochondrium**: Arab. تحت الشراسيف · Al-Zahrāwī, *K. al-taṣrīf li-man 'ağiza 'an at-ta'līf* · trans. Shem Tov ben Isaac (*Sefer ha-Shimmush*), bk. 30, 2.76 (fol. 221^{b}). → NM 1:93; corr. 4:229.

• **מתחת החלצים** · **hypochondrium**: Arab. ما دون الشراسيف · Maimonides, *K. al-fuṣūl* *fī al-ṭibb* · trans. Zeraḥyah Ḥen (*Sefer ha-Peraqim*), 6.52: סימני המראקיא שיהיה לו אחר אכלו רוטו חמוץ ורקיקה לחה בשיעור ושריפה מתחת החלצים. → NM 1:149.

• **תחת הטבור** · **hypochondrium**: Hippocrates, *Aphorisms* · trans. Do'eg ha-Edomi (*Sefer Agur*), 6.40 (332) (fol. 105[b]): לאשר יקרה כאב תחת הטבור בלא צמח אם אחזו קדחת יעבור הכאב מעליו. → NM 3:242.

• **כאב תחת הצלעות** → **כְּאֵב**.

• **תחת הכסלים** · **hypochondrium**: Gr. ὑποχόνδριον · Hippocrates, *Aphorisms* · trans. Joseph Delmedigo, 4.64 (201): בקדחת שיקדם הירקון ביום שביעי או בתשיעי או הי״א או הי״ד הנה זה משובח אם לא יהיה קושי בצד ימין תחת הכסלים ואם לאו אינו משובח. → NM 3:242.

• **תחת הצלעים** · **hypochondrium**: Hippocrates, *Aphorisms* · trans. Do'eg ha-Edomi (*Sefer Agur*), 4.64 (201) (fol. 74[b]): קם בצד ימינו ותחת צלעיו קושי אין זה טוב. → NM 3:242–3.

• **מה שתחת הצלעות** · **hypochondrium**: Arab. ما دون الشراسيف · Maimonides, *K. al-fuṣūl fī al-ṭibb* · trans. Zeraḥyah Ḥen (*Sefer ha-Peraqim*), 6.55: סימני המורסות החדות בכבד שמונה סימנים והם הקדחת השורפת והצמא הגדולה וביטול התאוה בכליות ואודם הלשון תחלה ואחר כך ישתחר ויקיא מרות דומות לאודם הביצה ובסוף הענין יהיה זנגארי הוא וירדידט וכאב בצד הימין עד הקטיולא ילך וכל שכן כשתמשוך מה שתחת הצלעות למעלה. → NM 1:181–2.

• **תחת השחי** · **[the] armpits**: a) Lat. subascellas · Bruno Longobucco, *Cyrurgia Magna* · trans. Hillel ben Samuel (*Sefer Keritut*), fol. 15[b]: ולכן צריך שנקיז בחולה מבלתי שנשגיח על כוחו והעורף והחוט השדרה ותחת השחי תמשח תמיד בשמן חם. → NM 1:42.

b) Arab. الإبطان · Maimonides, *K. al-fuṣūl fī al-ṭibb* · trans. Zeraḥyah Ḥen (*Sefer ha-Peraqim*), 7.71: אמנם השחוק אשר יהיה במישוש הנראה שלתחת השחי ותחת כפות הרגלים וכן השחוק אשר אנו עושים בראותינו הדברים שאדם שוחק עליהם או שישמע אותם אין לי בידיעת הסבה בזה דרך כלל. → NM 1:195.

תַּחְתּוֹן • **הזנאד התחתון** → **זנאד**.

• **הזקן התחתון** → **זָקָן**.

• **המעי התחתון** → **מְעִי**.

• **הנקב התחתון** → **נֶקֶב**.

• **העמוד התחתון** → **עַמּוּד**.

• **צמיחת השער בתחתון** → **צְמִיחָה**.

תַּחְתּוֹנִית • *Plur.* **תחתוניות** · **hemorrhoids**: Hippocrates, *Aphorisms* · trans. Do'eg ha-Edomi (*Sefer Agur*), 6.21 (313) (fol. 100[b]): זה אשר נפל למשכב ונטרפה דעתו בסבת השחורה או נפתח לו המקור הנק׳ דואילי נבקעו לו תחתוניות יעבור מעליו מדויהו. → NM 3:243; cf. *Sefer ha-Yosher* (Ms. Oxford, Bodleian Library, Opp. 180 (cat. Neubauer 2134), fol. 38[a]): שער לתחלואי הטחורי׳ הנקראי׳ תחתוניות והם אמרואידש.

תַּחְתִּית • **תחתית העין** · **eyeball**: Arab. مقلة · Ibn Sīnā, *K. al-Qānūn fī al-ṭibb* · trans. Nathan ha-Me'ati (*Sefer ha-Qanun*), bk. 1 (fol. 56[b]): והזוג השני מזוגות העצבים המוחיים צמיחתו אחורי צמיחת הזוג הראשון ונוטה ממנו אל הצד החיצוני ויצא מן הנקב אשר בנקרה הכולל על אלמקלה הוא תחתית העין. → NM 4:220.

• **תחתית הרחם** ‣ **the fundus of the uterus**: Arab. تقعير الرحم · Maimonides, *Šarḥ fuṣūl Abūqrāṭ* · trans. Zeraḥyah Ḥen (*Pirqei Abuqraṭ*), 5.45 (265): אמר בקראט: בהיות האשה וגופה ממוצע ותפיל בחודש השיני והשלישי מבלתי סבה מבוארת תחתית רחמה מלא ליחות כמו מותרי האף ולא יוכל להחזיק על הוולד אבל יהיה נכאה מהן. → NM 3:243.

• **תחתית השדרה** ‣ **loins**: Hippocrates, *Aphorisms* · trans. Do'eg ha-Edomi (*Sefer Agur*), 4.11 (148) (fol. 61): גזור על אשר רעמו מעיו וכאב רב על טבורו ועל תחתית שדרתו ולא יעבור בכבוס ולא ברפואה אחרת כי נכון הוא לסבול היבש מארבעת מיני המים הרעים. → NM 3:243–4.

תִּיק ‣ I. **an arm or armour with which one protects oneself; a thing with which a person is concealed, covered, hidden, protected, or veiled**: Arab. جُنّة · Ibn Sīnā, *K. al-Qānūn fī al-ṭibb* · trans. Nathan ha-Me'ati (*Sefer ha-Qanun*), bk. 1 (fol. 28[b]): כלל עצמות קדרת המוח הנה הם תיקי המוח למחסה ולמסתור מן הפגעים. → NM 4:220.

‣ II. **cast**: Arab. قالب · Maimonides, *K. al-fuṣūl fī al-ṭibb* · trans. Zeraḥyah Ḥen (*Sefer ha-Peraqim*), 15.68: שברי הרגל צריך אל תיק כדי שלא יסתער האבר בזמן התנועה וראוי שתעיין היטב בחולי המגיע ללב כי אם יהיה ההזק המתחדש מהלב יותר מתועלתו לא תעשנו. → NM 1:194.

• **תיק הרחם** ‣ **fundus of the uterus**: Arab. تقعير الرحم / Gr. κοτυληδόνες · Maimonides, *Šarḥ fuṣūl Abūqrāṭ* · trans. Moses ibn Tibbon (*Pirqei Abuqraṭ*), 5.45 (265): כשתהיה האשה ממוצעת הגוף מפלת בחדש השני והשלישי מבלתי סבה מבוארת תיק הרחם מלא ליחה הדומה לליחה היוצאת מן הנחירים ולא תוכל להחזיק העובר לכבדותו אבל ימעד ממנו. → NM 3:244.

תִּירוֹשׁ • (ה)תירוש (ה)מבושל ‣ I. **inspissated must**: Arab. عقيد العنب · Al-Zahrāwī, *K. al-taṣrīf li-man ʿağiza ʿan at-taʾlīf* · trans. Shem Tov ben Isaac (*Sefer ha-Shimmush*), bk. 27, fol. 142[a], col. a: ושתייתם בתירוש מבושל לוטשת החלט החלוק מן הכליות. → NM 4:220–1.

‣ II. **wine of grape juice cooked down to one third of its original amount, prepared this way, it is a kind of rubb 'concentrated juice,' used dilated with water**: Arab. طلاء · Al-Zahrāwī, *K. al-taṣrīf li-man ʿağiza ʿan at-taʾlīf* · trans. Shem Tov ben Isaac (*Sefer ha-Shimmush*), bk. 27, fol. 131[a], col. b: התירוש המבושל הנקרא בלשונם אל טלא ושאר מיני המבושלים הוא יותר חם ויותר יבש ויותר עב מן היין שהוא בלתי מבושל. → NM 4:220.

• **תירוש ענבים קרוש בבשול** ‣ **concentrated grape juice**: Arab. عقيد العنب · Maimonides, *K. al-fuṣūl fī al-ṭibb* · trans. Nathan ha-Me'ati (*Sefer ha-Peraqim*), 8.35: ראוי לך שיספיק לך בהשקט חוזק הכאב במורסות חיצוני הגוף החדות במה שילקח מתירוש ענבים קרוש בבשול ושמן וורדים ומעט דונג נמס בהם ותטבול צמר דשן ויהיה בסתו פושר ובקיץ קר. → NM 2:91–2.

תַּיִשׁ • זקן התיש → זָקָן.

תְּכוּנָה ‣ I. **consistency**: Arab. قوام · Ibn al-Jazzār, *Zād al-musāfir wa-qūt al-ḥāḍir* · trans. Moses ibn Tibbon (*Sefer Ṣedat ha-Derakhim*), bk. 7, 15.7: תואר אספלנית למורסא אשר אין לה ראש והיה צורך לפתחה והוא מנוסה: יקח זרע פשתן וזבל יונים ופניגריג מזרחי מ״א חמשה שקלים שישמאן שרוף עשרים שקלים יודק השישמאן עד שיהיו כמוח וילושו בו הסמים בעלי עד שישתוה תכונתו. → NM 1:69–70

‣ II. **external appearance:** Arab. سحنة · Ibn al-Jazzār, *Zād al-musāfir wa-qūt al-ḥādir* · trans. Moses ibn Tibbon (*Sefer Ṣedat ha-Derakhim*), bk. 7, 17.3: ואות המותר כאשר הוא חוץ מן העורקים שתפסד תכונת החולה ויפתחו ידיו ויקרה לו נגעים בעלי מוגלא ומורסות. → NM 1:69–70.

תָּכוּף ‣ **spasmodic:** Arab. متواتر · Maimonides, *K. al-fuṣūl fī al-ṭibb* · trans. Nathan ha-Me'ati (*Sefer ha-Peraqim*), 4.17: כשיתך הכח ישים הדפק קטן וחלוש ותכוף מאד. → NM 2:92.

תַּכְלִית ‣ I. **climax; culmination; peak:** a) Arab. منتهى · i. Ibn al-Jazzār, *Zād al-musāfir wa-qūt al-ḥādir* · trans. Moses ibn Tibbon (*Sefer Ṣedat ha-Derakhim*), bk. 1, ch. 18 (fol. 26[b]): ואולם הערבוב המתחדש בתכלית הקדחות החמות יהיה כשיעלה אל המוח עשן נושך חם וכאשר סרה הקדחת ינוח אותו הערבוב והשגעון. → NM 4:221.

· ii. Ibn al-Jazzār, *Zād al-musāfir wa-qūt al-ḥādir* · trans. Moses ibn Tibbon (*Sefer Ṣedat ha-Derakhim*), bk. 7, 15.3: ובתכלית המורסא ישתמש באלו הרפואות אשר זכרנו ממה שיתיך. → NM 1:70.

· iii. Maimonides, *K. al-fuṣūl fī al-ṭibb* · trans. Nathan ha-Me'ati (*Sefer ha-Peraqim*), 9.81: רפואות בעלת הצד בהקזה וההנחות החמות ורכוך הבטן. והזהר מלתת כשך השעורים בעת תכלית בעלת הצד כדי שלא יעכב הגבול הנקרא בחראן. → NM 2:92.

b) Arab. انتهاء · Maimonides, *K. al-fuṣūl fī al-ṭibb* · trans. Nathan ha-Me'ati (*Sefer ha-Peraqim*), 3.103: אותם שימותו בלי בחראן הנה ביום העונה תהיה המות וימותו קצת מהם בתחלת העונות לקדחות ולפעמים ימותו בתכלית העונה. → NM 2:92.

‣ II. **extent:** Arab. مبلغ · Maimonides, *K. al-fuṣūl fī al-ṭibb* · trans. Zeraḥyah Ḥen (*Sefer ha-Peraqim*), 8.8: והמזון לפי תכלית תוספתו בכח החולי ואיחורו בבישול יהיה תכלית חיזוקו ותטה לעולם לצד היותר צריך לעזור. → NM 1:194–5.

• **העמדת התכלית** → הַעֲמָדָה.

• **תכלית ההעמדה** ‣ **culmination:** Arab. منتهى · Maimonides, *K. al-fuṣūl fī al-ṭibb* · trans. Nathan ha-Me'ati (*Sefer ha-Peraqim*), 11.25: וכפי חדות החולי יהיה קורבת תכלית העמדתם. → NM 2:92.

תַּכְלִיתִיּוּת • **תכליתיות בעין** ‣ **cataract:** Arab. زرقة / Gr. γλαύκωσις · Hippocrates, *Aphorisms* · trans. Nathan ha-Me'ati, 3.3 (137) (fol. 57[b]): אמר אבוקרט: ואמנם הישישים יקרה להם רוע הנשימה הנקרא רבו והנזל אשר יקרה עמו השעול וטפטוף השתן וקושי יציאתו וכאבי הפרקים וכאבי הכליות וסבוב הראש והשתוק ושחינים רעים וחכוך הגוף והתעורה ורכות בטן ולחות בעינים והנחירים ומחשך הראות וכובד השמע ותכליתיות בעין. → NM 2:240–1.

[תלה] • *Nif'al* **נִתְלָה** ‣ **to cleave:** Arab. علق · Maimonides, *K. al-fuṣūl fī al-ṭibb* · trans. Nathan ha-Me'ati (*Sefer ha-Peraqim*), 9.124: הנהגת החולה ההוה בהנהגה מדקדקת בתכלית. ורבים יצטרכו לשלשול הבטן ברפואה בהתחלה. ואמנם בעת שיולד הדשבד אז תזונהו במזון טוב הכימוס רב המזון דבק והרפואות אשר מחוץ מה שיסתבך ויתדבק ונתלה ומהדק בעצמיותו ומחמם מעט ומנגב בשווי. → NM 2:92–3.

• *Part. Nif'al* **נִתְלָה** • **החוטים הנתלים** → חוּט.

תְּלוּלִית • *Plur.* **תלוליות** • **תלוליות של בשר** ‣ **cysts:** Arab. سلع · Al-Zahrāwī, *K. al-taṣrīf li-man ʿağiza ʿan at-taʾlīf* · trans. Shem Tov Ben Isaac (*Sefer ha-Shimmush*), bk. 30,

2.42 (fol. 215[b]): ויהיה אשר יקרה מהם בצואר אחד או רבים ויתילדו קצתם מקצתם וכל חזיר מהם יהיה בתוך קרום מיוחד לו כמו שיהיה בתלוליות של בשר וצמחי הראש כמו שזכרתי. → NM 1:120.

[תמד] • *Hif'il* **הִתְמִיד** · **to apply**: Arab. ألزم · Ibn al-Jazzār, *Zād al-musāfir wa-qūt al-ḥādir* · trans. Moses ibn Tibbon (*Sefer Ṣedat ha-Derakhim*), bk. 7, 12.1: או יקח קישואים ותבושל ותכתוש אותה ויתמידה על המקום. → NM 1:70.

תִּמָּהוֹן · I. **confusion**: Gr. ἔκστασις · Hippocrates, *Aphorisms* · trans. Joseph Delmedigo, 7.5 (357): מהשגעון שלשול דם או שקוי או תמהון טוב. → NM 3:247.

· II. **stupor**: Gr. ἔκπληξης · Hippocrates, *Aphorisms* · trans. Joseph Delmedigo, 7.14 (336): מקבלת פצע בראש תמהון או בלבול דעת רע. → NM 3:244–5.

תְּמוּנָה · **volume**: Arab. حجم · Maimonides, *Šarḥ fuṣūl Abūqrāṭ* · trans. Anonymous (*Pirqei Abuqraṭ*), introduction (9): ויש מי שכונתו ההארכה והרבוי ולהגדיל תמונת הספר ולהרבות מספר חלקיו ואף אם יקבץ זה כלו ענינים מעטים. → NM 3:245.

• **תמונת הפנים** · **complexion**: Arab. سحنة · Ibn al-Jazzār, *Zād al-musāfir wa-qūt al-ḥādir* · trans. Moses ibn Tibbon (*Sefer Ṣedat ha-Derakhim*), ch. 18 (fol. 26[a]): ויקרה לחולה עם עלות החולי וקרוב חזקתו מקרים מפחידים כמו צמא חזק ונגוב פה ושעירות לשון ושחרותה וסער ודפיקת לב ושלא יראה ועלוף ושינוי תמונת הפנים מן הענין הטבעי אל ענין יוצא מהטבע. → NM 4:221.

תמרי · **date-**: Arab. تمري · Al-Zahrāwī, *K. al-taṣrīf li-man ʿağiza ʿan at-taʾlīf* · trans. Shem Tov ben Isaac (*Sefer ha-Shimmush*), bk. 27, fol. 141[b], col. b: והמרבה מאכילת השקדים הרטובים החדשים ראוי לקחת עליהם ממרקחת התמרי או ממרקחת החבושים המשלשל. → NM 4:221.

• **מרקחת התמרי** → **מִרְקַחַת**.

תְּנוּךְ · **cartilage**: Lat. cartilago · Hippocrates, *Aphorisms* · trans. Hillel ben Samuel, 6.19 (311): אם יכרת העצם או התנוך או הדק מהלחיים או האמה לא ידבקו ולא יצמחו. → NM 3:245.

תְּנוּמָה • *Plur.* **תנומות** · **lethargus**: Gr. λήθαργος, *Plur.* λήθαργοι · Hippocrates, *Aphorisms* · trans. Joseph Delmedigo, 3.30 (136): וליוצאים מאלו השנים יקרם קוצר הנשימה וחולי הצד ומורסת הריאה ותנומות ומורסות קרומי המוח וקדחות בוערות ושלשולי הבטן ארוכים והרקת הירוקה מלמעלה ומלמטה ושלשול הדם וחלקות הבטן והטחורים. → NM 3:245.

תְּנוּעָה · **stimulant; stimulation**: Arab. تهييج / Gr. ἐρέθισμα · Maimonides, *Šarḥ fuṣūl Abūqrāṭ* · trans. Moses ibn Tibbon (*Pirqei Abuqraṭ*), 1.20 (47): אמר אבקראט: הגופות אשר יבא אליהם או שכבר בא להם הנקיון על השלמות אין ראוי שיונעו ולא שיחודש בהם חדוש לא ברפואה משלשלת ולא בזולתה מן התנועות אבל יונחו. → NM 3:245–6.

• **תנועה מצטערת** · **convulsion**: Arab. حركة مضطربة · Ibn al-Jazzār, *Zād al-musāfir wa-qūt al-ḥādir* · trans. Moses ibn Tibbon (*Sefer Ṣedat ha-Derakhim*), bk. 22, ch. 1: והכפיה קרוב מן השתוק כי מקום החולי בשניהם אחד והליחה המולידה אותם קרה לחה אבל כי השתוק יהיה בהעדר הכח אשר ילך אל העצבים כלם והכפיה תהיה בתנועה מצטערת. → NM 4:221–2.

תנועי • **העצבים התנועיים** → **עָצָב**.

תעב · **to force**: Arab. استكره · Maimonides, *Šarḥ fuṣūl Abūqrāṭ* · trans. Anonymous (*Pirqei Abuqraṭ*), 2.37 (89): אמר המפרש: הבריאים כשיעשו הקיא או השלשול יקרה להם סבוב והמיה

ויקשה צאת מה שיצא מהם וימהר להם עם זה העלוף כי הסם תשתדל להמשכת הכימוס הניאות המחובר לו וכשלוא מצאהו ימשוך הבשר ⟨והדם⟩ ויתעבום להסיר מהם מה שבם ממה שיאות לו.
→ NM 3:246.

תְּעָלָה • *Plur.* **תעלות** • **תעלות העורקים** · **intestinal canal; mesentery**: Arab. جدول العروق, *Plur.* جداول العروق · Ibn Sīnā, *K. al-Qānūn fī al-ṭibb* · trans. Nathan ha-Me'ati (*Sefer ha-Qanun*), bk. 1 (fol. 62[b]): ואחר יתפרק מן השריין הזה הגדול שני שריינים מתפרדים בתעלות העורקים אשר סביב המעי הישר. → NM 4:222.

תַּעַר · **a sharp knife**: Lat. novacula · Bruno Longobucco, *Cyrurgia Magna* · trans. Hillel ben Samuel (*Sefer Keritut*), fol. 40[a]: ואם החולה לא יסבול חתוך הבשר המעופש בתער אז תעשה זולתי החתוך של הפתוח עד העומק. → NM 1:42.

• **תער הגלבים** · **razor**: Arab. موسى · Al-Zahrāwī, *K. al-taṣrīf li-man ʿağiza ʿan at-taʾlīf* · trans. Shem Tov Ben Isaac (*Sefer ha-Shimmush*), bk. 30, 1.1 (fol. 203[b]): וצורת הכויה להריק החולה בתחלה בסם משלשל מנקה הראש שלש לילות או ארבע כפי חיוב כחו ושניו ומנהגו ואחר להעביר שער ראשו בתער הגלבים. → NM 1:120; corr. 4:229.

תַּעֲרֹבֶת • *Plur.* **תערובות** · **humors**: Arab. أخلاط · Maimonides, *Šarḥ fuṣūl Abūqrāṭ* · trans. Anonymous (*Pirqei Abuqraṭ*), 1.8 (35): וזה כי אינו צריך שיתעסק הטבע בבשול המזון שירד עליו וימנענו מלבשל החולי ר״ל התערובות המולידים לחולי כאשר הטבע בעת ההיא מתעורר עליהם בכחותיו כלם ואמנם נשאר לו מעט כח עד שישלם להתגבר עליהם. → NM 3:246.

תערובת → **תַּעֲרֹבֶת**.

תְּפוּחַ · **soft**: Arab. رخو · Al-Rāzī, *K. al-Manṣūrī* · trans. Shem Tov ben Isaac (*Sefer Almansur*), Ḥet 10 (38): חצץ ובלע׳ ליסיאום: בינוני בחום ובקור יועיל למורסות החמות בעין כשיוטח בו עליהם ולמורסות התפוחות. → NM 2:19–20.

תַּפּוּחַ • *Plur.* **תפוחים** • **תבשיל התפוחים** → **תַּבְשִׁיל**.

תְּפִיחָה · **swelling**: Arab. تربل · Al-Zahrāwī, *K. al-taṣrīf li-man ʿağiza ʿan at-taʾlīf* · trans. Shem Tov ben Isaac (*Sefer ha-Shimmush*), bk. 27, fol. 129[b], col. b: המים הקובצים מועילים משלשול המעים ומתפיחת הגוף. → NM 4:222.

תְּפִירָה · **suture**: Lat. ligatura · Bruno Longobucco, *Cyrurgia Magna* · trans. Hillel ben Samuel (*Sefer Keritut*), fol. 10[b]: אבל אם המכה תהיה כל כך גדולה שלא תוכל לאסוף החלקים הנפרדים אז צריך לך התפירה. → NM 1:42.

• *Plur.* **תפירות** · **sutures**: Arab. خياطات · Al-Zahrāwī, *K. al-taṣrīf li-man ʿağiza ʿan at-taʾlīf* · trans. Shem Tov Ben Isaac (*Sefer ha-Shimmush*), bk. 30, 2.1 (fol. 209[a]): ואם יהיה הלחות מתחת העצם ואותותיו הראות תפירות הראש פתוחות מכל צד והמים נשפכים לתוך הראש כשיוסחטו ביד וזה דבר בלתי נעלם מן הרופא צריך לבקע באמצע הראש שלש בקיעות על זאת הצורה. → NM 1:120.

תְּפִישָׂה · **objection**: Arab. اعتراض · Maimonides, *K. al-fuṣūl fī al-ṭibb* · trans. Nathan ha-Me'ati (*Sefer ha-Peraqim*), Introduction: אז נשיבהו לתפישה הזאת. → NM 2:93.

תָּפֵל · **crude; raw**: Arab. خام · Al-Rāzī, *K. al-Manṣūrī* · trans. Shem Tov ben Isaac (*Sefer Almansur*), Qof 3 (68): קנטוריון ובלעז סינטוריא: ישלשל הליחה התפלה טוב למכאובי העצבים וההדרקון. → NM 2:20.

[תקן] • *Part. Pu'al* **מְתֻקָּן** · **seasoned**: Arab. مطيّب · Maimonides, *K. al-fuṣūl fī al-ṭibb* ·

trans. Nathan ha-Me'ati (*Sefer ha-Peraqim*), 20.61: וכשיהיה אדם מעונג בהנהגתו משתדל אז איפשר לו שיקרר וירטיב מה שיתחדש מן היגיעה במין אחר מההנהגה בהכנסת המרחץ ויזון אחריו במזונות טובי הכימוס מתוקנים בחומץ וכיוצא בזה. → NM 2:64–5.

תֹּקֶף ‣ **culmination**: Gr. ἀκμή · Hippocrates, *Aphorisms* · trans. Joseph Delmedigo, 2.30 (82) בהתחלת החולאים ובסופם כל המקרים חלושים וכשהם בתוקפם המקרים חזקים. → NM 3:247.

תרדי → נרדי.

תרדימה → תַּרְדֵּמָה.

תרדימיי → תרדמיי.

תַּרְדֵּמָה ‣ I. **apoplexy**: Arab. سكات / Gr. ἀπόπληκτοι · Maimonides, *Šarḥ fuṣūl Abūqrāṭ* · trans. Zeraḥyah Ḥen (*Pirqei Abuqraṭ*), 3.16 (122): אמר בקראט: אמנם החליים המתחדשים בהתרבות מטר ברוב העניינים הם קדחות ארוכים והתרת הבטן ועיפושים וויציאו ותרדימה ואישקוינכציאה. → NM 3:247.

‣ II. **lethargy; torpor**: Arab. سبات / Gr. καταφορά · a) Ibn al-Jazzār, *Zād al-musāfir wa-qūt al-ḥādir* · trans. Moses ibn Tibbon (*Sefer Ṣedat ha-Derakhim*), bk. 1, ch. 16 (fol. 23[a]): התרדמה היא הנטיה אל השינה עם סתימת העינים ויהיה זה על אחד משני פנים אם שנשקע החולה בשינה עד שיקשה להקיצו ואם שתהיה שנתו קלה. → NM 4:222–3.

b) Maimonides, *K. al-fuṣūl fī al-ṭibb* · trans. Nathan ha-Me'ati (*Sefer ha-Peraqim*), 23.58: כשיגבר בראש לחות הנקרא מררות יתחדש מזה התעורה וערבוב שכל. וכשיגבר בו ליחות עבות לבניות יתחדש מזה עם תרדמה הבהלה והבהלה הוא ערבוב שכל מועט. → NM 2:93–4.

‣ III. **numbness**: Arab. خدر / Gr. νάρκη · a) Ibn al-Jazzār, *Zād al-musāfir wa-qūt al-ḥādir* · trans. Moses ibn Tibbon (*Sefer Ṣedat ha-Derakhim*), bk. 7, 8.2: וכאשר יקרה ממשוש מזון או משקה שרפה או תרדמה או קווץ בצפרנים או נפח לאצבע. → NM 1:70.

b) Maimonides, *Šarḥ fuṣūl Abūqrāṭ* · trans. Moses ibn Tibbon (*Pirqei Abuqraṭ*), 5.25 (245): אמר אבקראט: המורסות אשר יהיו בפרקים והכאבים אשר יהיו מבלתי נגע וכאבי בעלי הנקרס ובעלי הקווץ המתחדש במקומות שיש בהם עצבים ורוב מה שדומה לאלו הנה אם נשפך עליהם מים קרים הרבה ישקיטום ויכמישום ויניחו הכאב בחדשם תרדמה והתרדמה גם כן המעט ממנה משקיטה הכאב. → NM 3:247.

• **תרדמת האברים** ‣ **numbness [of the limbs]**: a) Arab. تخدير · Ibn al-Jazzār, *Zād al-musāfir wa-qūt al-ḥādir* · trans. Moses ibn Tibbon (*Sefer Ṣedat ha-Derakhim*), bk. 7, 17.1: ומסגולת הליחה הלבנה תרדמת האברים. → NM 1:70.

b) Arab. خدر / Gr. νάρκη · i. Ibn al-Jazzār, *Zād al-musāfir wa-qūt al-ḥādir* · trans. Moses ibn Tibbon (*Sefer Ṣedat ha-Derakhim*), bk. 7, 17.2: ואם התילד החולי הזה מפני עפוש ליחה לבנה ושריפתה הנה אותותיו לחות הגוף וריבוי הגרנדולש ורפיון ורבוי הגרת העינים ולובן המראה ותרדמת האיברים. → NM 1:70–1.

· ii. Ibn al-Jazzār, *Zād al-musāfir wa-qūt al-ḥādir* · trans. Moses ibn Tibbon (*Sefer Ṣedat ha-Derakhim*), bk. 1, ch. 25 (fol. 39[b]): ואולם תרדמת איברים הנה היא מקרה גם כן מתערב במה שבין הטבע ובין החולי. → NM 4:223.

· iii. Maimonides, *K. al-fuṣūl fī al-ṭibb* · trans. Nathan ha-Me'ati (*Sefer ha-Peraqim*), 22.43: הזכרים שביוני שובך מבריא מן הרפיון ותרדמת האברים והשתוק והרעש. → NM 2:94.

• **תרדמת הגוף** · **apoplexy**: Hippocrates, *Aphorisms* · trans. Do'eg ha-Edomi (*Sefer Agur*), 3.23 (129) (fol. 55[b]): צרות יום הקור הם כאב הצדדים ותחת הצלעות והריאה וזוב הנחירים והשזרה סתימת המקורות ותרדמת הגוף. → NM 3:248.

• **תרדמת החוש** · **numbness**: Arab. خدر · Maimonides, *K. al-fuṣūl fī al-ṭibb* · trans. Nathan ha-Me'ati (*Sefer ha-Peraqim*), 7.66: הכאב עם תרדמת החוש ברגלים בחליי הכליות יהיה מפני השתוף אשר בין הכליות והרגלים בשני עורקים יורדים על השדרה. → NM 2:94.

תרדמיי · **lethargic**: Arab. سباتي · Maimonides, *K. al-fuṣūl fī al-ṭibb* · trans. Nathan ha-Me'ati (*Sefer ha-Peraqim*), 9.38: לפעמים תערב ברפואות רקיקת הדם רפואות מרדימות לישנם שינה תרדימיית. → NM 2:93.

• **העורק התרדמיי** → **עוֹרֶק**.

תְּרוּבְתוּר · **cauliflower**: Arab. قنّبيط · Al-Zahrāwī, *K. al-taṣrīf li-man ʿağiza ʿan at-ta'līf* · trans. Shem Tov ben Isaac (*Sefer ha-Shimmush*), bk. 27, fol. 134[b], col. b–135[a], col. a: התרובתור יותר עב ויותר מתאחר להתעכל באסטומ׳ מן הכרוב. → NM 4:223.

תְּרִיסִי • **ציניי ותריסי** → **צְנִי**.

תַּרְנְגוֹל • *Plur.* **מרק תרנגולים קטנים** • **תרנגולים** → **מָרָק**.

תַּרְעֵלָה · **vertigo**: Arab. سدر / Gr. ἴλιγγος, σκοτοδινία · Al-Zahrāwī, *K. al-taṣrīf li-man ʿağiza ʿan at-ta'līf* · trans. Shem Tov ben Isaac (*Sefer ha-Shimmush*), bk. 27, fol. 135[b], col. b: ואמר הכנדי כשישתה מסחיטת הכוסבר משקל ארבע אונקיאו׳ יורגש ריחו בגוף כלו ויחדש נחרת הגרון ותרעלה או שבוש הדעת עד שוב שותהו כשכור מנבל פיו. → NM 4:224.

תרקוה · **collarbone**: Arab. ترقوة · Ibn Sīnā, *K. al-Qānūn fī al-ṭibb* · trans. Nathan ha-Me'ati (*Sefer ha-Qanun*), bk. 1 (fol. 36[b]): פרק ששה עשר בנתוח התרקוה. התרקוה העצם המונח על כל אחד משני צדי עליוני החזה. → NM 4:224.

תשיה • **תשית הבשר** · **softening of the flesh**: Gr. σαρκῶν ἐκθήλυνσις · Hippocrates, *Aphorisms* · trans. Joseph Delmedigo, 5.16 (236): החום יגרום אלו ההזקים לנוהגים בו לרוב תשית הבשר רפיון העצבים תרדמת הדעת שפיכות דמים עילופים ואלה דברים מביאים לידי מיתה. → NM 3:248.

www.ingramcontent.com/pod-product-compliance
Lightning Source LLC
LaVergne TN
LVHW091039021026
849161LV00002BA/163